REVIEW FOR

S U R G E R Y

SCIENTIFIC PRINCIPLES AND PRACTICE

THIRD EDITION

REVIEW FOR

SURGERY

SCIENTIFIC PRINCIPLES AND PRACTICE

THIRD EDITION

EDITED BY

Lazar J. Greenfield, MD
Frederick A. Coller Distinguished
Professor of Surgery
Chairman, Department of Surgery
University of Michigan Medical School

Surgeon-in-Chief
University of Michigan Hospitals
Ann Arbor, Michigan

Keith D. Lillemoe, MD
Professor and Vice-Chairman
Department of Surgery
Johns Hopkins University School of Medicine
Johns Hopkins Hospital
Baltimore, Maryland

Michael W. Mulholland, MD, PhD
Section Head, General Surgery
Department of Surgery
University of Michigan Medical School
University of Michigan Hospitals
Ann Arbor, Michigan

Keith T. Oldham, MD
Surgeon-in-Chief and
Marie Z. Uihlein Chair
Department of Pediatric Surgery
Medical College of Wisconsin
Milwaukee, Wisconsin

Gerald B. Zelenock, MD
Chairman, Department of Surgery
Chief, Surgical Services
William Beaumont Hospital
Royal Oak, Michigan

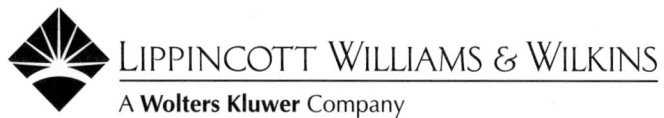

LIPPINCOTT WILLIAMS & WILKINS
A **Wolters Kluwer** Company
Philadelphia • Baltimore • New York • London
Buenos Aires • Hong Kong • Sydney • Tokyo

Acquisitions Editor: Lisa McAllister
Developmental Editor: Delois Patterson
Production Editor: Thomas Boyce
Manufacturing Manager: Timothy Reynolds
Cover Designer: Christine Jenny
Compositor: Lippincott Williams & Wilkins Desktop Division
Printer: Courier Westford

© 2002 by LIPPINCOTT WILLIAMS & WILKINS
530 Walnut Street
Philadelphia, PA 19106 USA
LWW.com

Printed in the USA

Library of Congress Cataloging-in-Publication Data
Review for Surgery : scientific principles and practice / edited by Lazar J. Greenfield ... [et al.].— 3rd ed.
    p. ;   cm.
    ISBN 0-7817-3189-5
    1. Surgery.   2. Medicine.   3. Surgery—Examinations, questions, etc.   I. Greenfield, Lazar J.,
1934-   II. Surgery.
    [DNLM: 1. Surgical Procedures, Operative—Examination Questions.   WO 100 S9617 2001 Suppl.]
    RD31 .S922 2001 Suppl.
    617—dc21
                                                                                          2001038037

Care has been taken to confirm the accuracy of the information presented and to describe generally accepted practices. However, the authors, editors, and publisher are not responsible for errors or omissions or for any consequences from application of the information in this book and make no warranty, expressed or implied, with respect to the currency, completeness, or accuracy of the contents of the publication. Application of this information in a particular situation remains the professional responsibility of the practitioner.

The authors, editors, and publisher have exerted every effort to ensure that drug selection and dosage set forth in this text are in accordance with current recommendations and practice at the time of publication. However, in view of ongoing research, changes in government regulations, and the constant flow of information relating to drug therapy and drug reactions, the reader is urged to check the package insert for each drug for any change in indications and dosage and for added warnings and precautions. This is particularly important when the recommended agent is a new or infrequently employed drug.

Some drugs and medical devices presented in this publication have Food and Drug Administration (FDA) clearance for limited use in restricted research settings. It is the responsibility of the health care provider to ascertain the FDA status of each drug or device planned for use in their clinical practice.

10 9 8 7 6 5 4 3 2 1

PREFACE

If the optimal educational process is an interactive exchange between teacher and student, then the closest we can come to this approach with written material is for authors to pose questions to their readers. We have attempted to extend the effectiveness of the third edition of *Surgery: Scientific Principles and Practice* by providing a revised edition of this review book. The inclusion of new authors and extensive revisions by previous authors ensures that the material presented will be fresh and comprehensive. Although it is not possible to cover all of the information in the text, the most important concepts are reviewed in a challenging and comprehensive manner.

Positive feedback from the inclusion of computer software in the previous edition of the *Review* has encouraged us to extend this approach and allow the reader to use the disc for rapid and effective guidance to specific topics and procedures. Concise discussions, appropriate referencing to the text, and immediate feedback on correct responses remain the focus of our efforts. Combining questions of authors and editors assures that the material presented will satisfy the needs of surgeons at all levels of training or practice.

We hope that this review will stimulate the next as well as the current generation of surgeons to continue to question established concepts and promote further progress in the expanding field of surgery.

For the editors and authors,

Lazar J. Greenfield, MD
Editor-in-Chief

ACKNOWLEDGMENTS

Most importantly, we thank all of the contributors to *Surgery: Scientific Principles and Practice,* for their excellent material from which these questions and answers were taken. This review book could not have been done without their efforts.

CONTENTS

PART I. SCIENTIFIC PRINCIPLES

PART II. SURGICAL PRACTICE

A. HEAD AND NECK

B. ESOPHAGUS

C. STOMACH AND DUODENUM

D. SMALL INTESTINE

ONE

SCIENTIFIC PRINCIPLES

CHAPTER 1

CELL STRUCTURE AND FUNCTION

1. Which of the following statements is/are true concerning the cell plasma membrane?
   a. The plasma membrane is composed of amphipathic molecules
   b. The hydrophobic core of the lipid bilayer of the cell membrane contains specialized transport proteins that maintain the intracellular ionic milieu separately from the extracellular fluid
   c. Plasma membrane proteins extend externally and bear phospholipid moieties that contribute to the cell coat
   d. The membrane proteins of nerve cells are highly voltage dependent

COMMENT: The plasma membrane defines the boundary of the cell and contains and concentrates enzymes and other macromolecule constituents. The plasma membrane is composed of amphipathic molecules, mainly phospholipids and proteins that contain distinct regions that are either insoluble in water (hydrophobic) or soluble in water (hydrophilic). The plasma membrane forms a continuous barrier between the aqueous extracellular and intracellular fluids. Transport proteins in the membrane act as regulated channels or transporters to maintain the intracellular ionic milieu, which is clearly different from the extracellular milieu. In some cells, membrane proteins are diversified, as in nerve cells, where the ion channels are highly voltage dependent, and provide the basis for information transmission in the form of electrical impulses. Most plasma membrane proteins extend externally and bear carbohydrate moieties primarily as oligosaccharide chains that contribute to the cell coat or glycocalyx.

ANSWER: a, b, d

REFERENCE: *Chapter 1—Cell Structure and Function: Cell Structure*

2. Intracellular organelles involved with protein synthesis include:
   a. Mitochondria
   b. Endoplasmic reticulum
   c. Golgi complex
   d. Lysosomes

COMMENT: Mitochondria are the main source of energy production in eukaryotic cells. The endoplasmic reticulum is the network of interconnected membranes that form closed vesicles, tubules, and saccules. The endoplasmic reticulum has a number of functions and is primarily involved in the synthesis of proteins and lipids. Adjacent to the rough endoplasmic reticulum and functionally involved in the sorting and package of secreted protein is the Golgi complex. Lysosomes are membrane-limited organelles that contain acid hydrolytic enzymes that degrade polymers such as proteins, carbohydrates, and nucleic acids.

ANSWER: b, c

REFERENCE: *Chapter 1—Cell Structure and Function: Cell Structure*

3. The activities of the cytoskeleton depend on which of the following types of filaments?
   a. Microtubules
   b. Intermediate filaments
   c. Actin filaments
   d. None of the above

COMMENT: The cytoskeleton is a collection of filamentous protein structures that allow cells to assume and maintain a variety of shapes, to produce directed movement of organelles within the cell, and to effect movement of the entire cell relative to other cells. These activities depend on three main types of filaments: actin filaments, intermediate filaments, and microtubules.

ANSWER: a, b, c

REFERENCE: *Chapter 1—Cell Structure and Function: Cell Structure*

4. Which of the following statements is/are correct concerning cell junctions?

   a. The main occluding junction is the tight junction or zonula occludens

   b. Tight junctions usually are located near the basal pole of the cell

   c. Desmosomes are button-like points of attachment that weld together adjacent cells

   d. Gap junctions are a type of cell junction specialized for cell communication

COMMENT: Cell junctions are classified as occluding, anchoring, and communicating. The main occluding junction is the tight junction or zonula occludens, which connects cells in epithelia and thereby allows epithelia to serve as selective permeability barriers. Tight junctions are normally located near the apical pool of the cell and form a belt that completely encircles the cell. Anchoring junctions connect the cytoskeleton of the cell to the extracellular matrix or neighboring cells. Morphologically these are adherens junctions, or desmosomes. Desmosomes are button-like points of attachment with a prominent intracellular plaque that welds together adjacent cells by serving as anchoring sites for intermediate filaments within the cell. The third functional type of cell junction is a gap junction, which is specialized for communication. This junction mediates both electrical and chemical coupling.

ANSWER: a, c, d

REFERENCE: *Chapter 1—Cell Structure and Function: Cell-Cell Interaction*

5. A striking feature of living cells is a marked difference between the composition of the cytosol and the extracellular milieu. Which of the following statements is/are true concerning the mechanisms of maintenance of these differences?

   a. The cell membrane is able to maintain a 10,000-fold gradient between the extracellular concentration of ionized calcium and the intracellular concentration

   b. The key to these differences is the fact that the plasma membrane is normally impermeable to sodium, potassium, and calcium

   c. The selectivity of biologic membranes is highly consistent and seldom changes

   d. The selectivity of cell membranes relates only to ions and not to organic compounds

COMMENT: The survival of the cell requires that cytosolic composition be maintained within narrow limits despite the constant influx of nutrients and the simultaneous outflow of waste. A familiar example of the distribution of ions across the cell membrane is that of sodium and potassium. Cells are typically rich in potassium and contain very little sodium, although they are constantly bathed by fluid that is precisely the opposite composition. Even more impressive is the distribution of ionized calcium. The extracellular concentration of this ion is typically on the order of 10^{-3} mol/L, whereas that of cytosol is typically 10^{-7} M, a 10,000-fold gradient. Such nonequilibrium ion distributions are even more remarkable in light of the fact that the plasma membrane is, to varying degrees, leaky to ions such as sodium, potassium, and calcium. The plasma membrane is leaky to a variety of substances, but it exhibits an astonishing ability to discriminate or select one substance over another. This selectivity relates not only to ions but also to organic compounds, such as glucose. Finally, the selectivity of biologic membranes can be altered drastically as a result of regulatory or signaling processes that occur within the cell.

ANSWER: a

REFERENCE: *Chapter 1—Cell Structure and Function: Membrane Transport*

6. There are two properties of the cell necessary to maintain nonequilibrium cellular composition; the first is selectivity and the second is energy conversion. Which of the following statements is/are true concerning energy-converting transport?

   a. The site of energy conversion and transport in the plasma membrane involves the phospholipid component

   b. Na^+-K^+-ATPase derives energy from hydrolysis of extracellular adenosine triphosphate (ATP)

   c. In some systems, energy inherent in the transmembrane ion gradient can be used to drive transport of a second species

   d. Examples of species transported by means of secondary active transport include hydrogen ions, calcium, amino acids, and glucose

COMMENT: The selectivity of the plasma membrane, although impressive, cannot account for the non-equilibrium composition of living cells. A cell can be maintained in a nonequilibrium state only through continual expenditure of energy. Maintenance of steady-state, nonequilibrium cellular composition is possible because the plasma membrane is the site of energy converters, membrane proteins that function as biologic transport machines using energy derived from metabolic processes to perform transport work. The archetype of the biologic transport machine is Na^+-K^+-ATPase, a membrane protein that hydrolyses cytosolic ATP and couples the resulting free energy to transport of Na^+ and K^+. A second equally important type of energy-converting transporter is one in which the energy inherent in a transmembrane ion gradient, usually that of Na^+, can be used to drive the transport of a second species, such as protons, calcium, amino acids, or glucose.

ANSWER: c, d

REFERENCE: *Chapter 1—Cell Structure and Function: Membrane Transport*

7. Which of the following statements is/are true concerning water movement across cell membranes?

   a. Water moves only actively through cell membrane transport proteins

   b. For most cells of the body, the transmembrane hydrostatic pressure is 0

   c. Water distribution is determined entirely by solute distribution

   d. Specialized cells such as the glomeruli of the kidney actively transport water to maintain hydrostatic pressure

COMMENT: The energetics of water transport across cell membranes is simplified by the fact that water moves only passively owing to gradients of hydrostatic pressure or water concentration. Hydrostatic pressure is an important driving force only for certain specialized cells—the capillary endothelium and the glomeruli of the kidney. For most cells of the body, transmembrane hydrostatic pressure is 0, and water moves only in response to water concentration gradients. Because the concentration of water is determined by the amount of dissolved solute, the difference in water concentration is typically expressed as a function of the difference in solute concentration or osmotic pressure difference. Because there are no specialized, energy-converting transport mechanisms for water, water is distributed at equilibrium. Water distribution is determined entirely by solute to solute distribution.

ANSWER: b, c

REFERENCE: *Chapter 1—Cell Structure and Function: Membrane Transport*

8. Which of the following statements is/are true concerning cellular ion channels?
   a. Ion channels are transmembrane proteins that form pores that can conduct ions across the plasma membrane
   b. Ion channels are formed by membrane-spanning peptides arranged so that polar moieties line a central core
   c. Ion channel proteins undergo conformational changes between open states and closed states
   d. Ion channels can be blocked

COMMENT: Ion channels are transmembrane proteins that form pores that can conduct ions across the plasma membrane. Ion channels are formed by membrane-spanning peptides arranged so that polar moieties line a central pore. These polar groups take the place of the water of hydration, which stabilizes an ion in an aqueous solution. The polar groups in essence produce a water-like environment into which the ion can partition and move in the presence of the appropriate driving force. Ion channels are permissive transport elements. Ions flow through a channel only because of the presence of an appropriate driving force. Ion channels do not conduct all the time; rather the channel protein undergoes conformational changes between a conducting (open) state and nonconducting (closed) state. These conformational changes are collectively called *gating*. The conduction process also can be blocked by ions or organic compounds that enter the channel, bind there, and occlude the pore.

ANSWER: a, b, c, d

REFERENCE: *Chapter 1—Cell Structure and Function: Membrane Transport*

9. Examples of ion channel blockers include:
   a. Tetrodotoxin
   b. Amiloride
   c. Lidocaine
   d. None of the above

COMMENT: Channel blockade is an important mechanism of action of toxins and some therapeutic agents. The deadly toxin of the puffer fish, tetrodotoxin, acts by blocking the Na^+ channels responsible for conduction of nerve impulses. The diuretic amiloride blocks the Na^+ channels that inhabit the apical membrane of the epithelial cells of the distal nephron. Local anesthetics such as lidocaine also block ion channels.

ANSWER: a, b, c

REFERENCE: *Chapter 1—Cell Structure and Function: Membrane Transport*

10. Which of the following statements is/are true concerning carrier proteins?
   a. Carrier proteins are distinguished by three types of mechanisms: carrier type, channel type, and conduction type
   b. Conformational changes in the membrane protein occur between the conducting and the nonconducting states
   c. A channel-type carrier protein has two states—closed and open
   d. Carrier-type transport proteins are equally accessible from either side of the membrane

COMMENT: Most transport proteins appear to function as carriers rather than channels. Important distinctions can be made between types of carrier proteins on the basis of transport kinetics. Two primary types can be distinctly identified on the basis of carrier-type and channel-type mechanisms. The most important difference between the channel mechanism and the carrier mechanism is the role in the transport event played by conformational changes in the membrane protein. The channel is depicted as having two states, closed and open, so that it operates as a switch. In contrast, carrier transport is envisioned as requiring a cycle of conformational changes. The transport of one molecule of substrate requires one complete cycle of the protein. In a channel mechanism, binding sites within the open pore are equally accessible from either side of the membrane, whereas in a carrier mechanism, the binding site is available on only one side of the membrane at any instant.

ANSWER: b, c

REFERENCE: *Chapter 1—Cell Structure and Function: Membrane Transport*

11. Which of the following statements is/are true concerning DNA?
    a. DNA is contained only in the nucleus of the cell
    b. DNA strands are encoded by the sequence of four bases—adenine, guanine, cytosine, and uridine
    c. The basic unit of information of DNA is the intron, a sequence of three bases
    d. There are an infinite number of possible codons

COMMENT: The genetic blueprint of an organism is carried in the nucleus of every cell, encoded by the sequence of four bases—adenine, guanine, cytosine, and thymine. Together these bases make up two long chains bound together by hydrogen bonds to form a DNA double helix. A gene is a segment of DNA that is transcribed into a corresponding RNA molecule that either codes for a protein or forms a structural RNA molecule. Genes are commonly between 10,000 and 100,000 base pairs long and include, in addition to the coding sequence, flanking regions and intervening sequences, called *introns.* Introns are removed from the primary RNA transcript by means of a process called *splicing.* The basic unit of information is the codon, a sequence of a triplet of bases. The four nucleotide bases arranged as triplets lead to 64 possible codons. Sixty-one of these code for amino acids, and three are termination signals called *stop codons.*

ANSWER: a

REFERENCE: *Chapter 1—Cell Structure and Function: Intracellular Synthesis, Transport, and Organization of Macromolecules*

12. An important step in protein synthesis is transcription. Which of the following statements is/are true concerning this process?
    a. The first step in gene transcription involves separating the double helix of DNA with an enzyme known as DNA polymerase
    b. The initial product of DNA transcription is called *heterogeneous nuclear RNA,* which codes directly for proteins
    c. After processing is complete, the messenger RNA (mRNA) is exported from the nucleus to the cytoplasm
    d. Only one protein can be produced from an initial mRNA strand

COMMENT: Transcription of a gene begins at an initiation site associated with a specific DNA sequence, called a *promoter region.* After binding to DNA, RNA polymerase opens a short region of the double helix to expose the nucleotides. Once the two strands of DNA are separated, the strand containing the promoter acts as a template to which ribonucleoside triphosphates form base pairs by means of hydrogen bonds. The initial products of transcription are known as *heterogeneous nuclear RNA* because of their large size variation. These primary transcripts are then processed to form mRNA. Because of RNA splicing, mature RNA is much shorter than nuclear RNA. Alternative splicing can lead to production of different mRNA molecules and in some cases different proteins from the same gene. Messenger RNA is exported from the nucleus only after processing is complete.

ANSWER: c

REFERENCE: *Chapter 1—Cell Structure and Function: Intracellular Synthesis, Transport, and Organization of Macromolecules*

13. Which of the following statements is/are true concerning translation of the mRNA message to protein synthesis?

    a. An adaptor molecule, transfer RNA (tRNA), recognizes specific nucleic acid bases and unites them with specific amino acids
    b. Covalent attachment of tRNA to amino acids is energy dependent
    c. The formation of a peptide bond between the growing peptide chain and the free amino acid occurs in the free cytoplasm
    d. Complete protein synthesis takes hours

COMMENT: Synthesis of protein involves conversion from a four-letter nucleotide language to one of 20 chemically distinct amino acids. This process is called *translation*. There is no mechanism for direct chemical recognition between specific nucleic acid bases and specific amino acids. Instead, an adaptor molecule, tRNA, is used. Each tRNA carries only one amino acid and must be recognized by a distinct enzyme that catalyzes the covalent attachment of the carboxyl end of the amino acid to the end of the tRNA in a process in which ATP is used. Protein synthesis occurs by means of formation of a peptide bond between the carboxyl terminal of the growing peptide chain and the free amino acid of deactivated amino acid tRNA. This event occurs not in free solution but within ribosomes. Ribosomes are protein-synthesizing machines that bring all of the necessary components together in the correct sequence and spacial orientation. Protein synthesis consumes a great deal of energy because four high-energy phosphate bonds must be split to make each peptide bond. Complete synthesis of a single protein takes 30 seconds to a few minutes, but multiple ribosomes can initiate translation and be moving down the mRNA molecules simultaneously to increase the rate of protein synthesis.

ANSWER: a, b

REFERENCE: *Chapter 1—Cell Structure and Function: Intracellular Synthesis, Transport, and Organization of Macromolecules*

14. Proteins destined to be secreted from the cells must pass through a series of organelles. These organelles include:

    a. Endoplasmic reticulum
    b. Golgi apparatus
    c. Mitochondria
    d. Lysosomes

COMMENT: Protein targeted for the secretory pathway most commonly begin with translocation from the cytoplasm across the lipid bilayer into the lumen of the endoplasmic reticulum. It must then pass through a number of compartments, including the Golgi apparatus, where it is further processed and sorted to end up in a secretory vesicle or lysosome.

ANSWER: a, b, d

REFERENCE: *Chapter 1—Cell Structure and Function: Intracellular Synthesis, Transport, and Organization of Macromolecules*

15. The transport of proteins out of the cell is called *exocytosis.* Which of the following statements is/are true concerning this process?

    a. Secretory vesicles fuse with the plasma membrane
    b. The process can be either constitutive or regulated
    c. Regulated secretion is triggered by a stimulus, most likely a hormone or a neurotransmitter
    d. A decrease in cytoplasmic calcium occurs as part of secretion

COMMENT: Transport vesicles that bud off the Golgi network carry both material to be secreted from the cell and protein destined to become components of the plasma membrane. These vesicles can fuse with the plasma membrane in a process called *exocytosis.* Vesicular transport to the cell surface can be divided into two components—constitutive and regulated secretion. Regulated secretion occurs in cells secreting digestive enzymes, hormones and other regulatory molecules, and neurotransmitters. In regulated secretion, the material to be secreted is sorted in a storage vesicle or granule; fusion with the plasma membrane in exocytosis occurs in response to external stimulation. Regulated secretion is triggered in most instances by a hormone or neurotransmitter. The ensuing process is called *stimulus-secretion coupling.* In most instances, coupling involves an increase in cytoplasmic concentration of Ca^{2+}, but it also can involve generation of diacylglycerol or production of cyclic adenosine monophosphate (cAMP), which activate kinases or phosphatases.

ANSWER: a, b, c

REFERENCE: *Chapter 1—Cell Structure and Function: Intracellular Synthesis, Transport, and Organization of Macromolecules; Transport to the Cell Surface—Exocytosis*

16. Which of the following statements is/are true concerning the cell function of phagocytosis?

    a. Phagocytosis is a mechanistically distinct process of endocytosis performed by special cells to take up larger particles such as bacteria or erythrocytes
    b. Lymphocytes are the primary blood cell involved with this process
    c. The process involves a coating of the cytoplasmic surface known as *clathrin*
    d. Phagocytosis is performed only by white blood cells and tissue macrophages

COMMENT: Phagocytosis is a specialized form of endocytosis by which large particles are internalized by specialized cells, primarily macrophages and neutrophils. To undergo phagocytosis, particles must bind to the surface of the phagocytic cell, usually because specific antibodies coat the particle. The phagocytic cell then extends pseudopods that engulf the particle. This event is followed by membrane fusion and pinching off. Unlike endocytosis, this process does not involve the membrane protein clathrin but involves actin. A physiologically relevant site of phagocytosis is the thyroid gland, where thyroid follicular cells phagocytose and digest thyroglobulin from the lumen of the thyroid follicle and release the thyroid hormones thyroxine and tri-iodothyronine.

ANSWER: a

REFERENCE: *Chapter 1—Cell Structure and Function: Intracellular Synthesis, Transport, and Organization of Macromolecules—Endocytosis*

17. Cell regulation can be thought of as the effector side of cell communication. Cell regulation most commonly occurs by means of extracellular chemical messengers. Which of the following statements is/are true concerning these messengers?

   a. Paracrine regulation involves a messenger that is produced and acts systemically
   b. The extracellular signal or stimulus is received by a receptor on or in the target cell
   c. Neurocrine regulation depends on a physical connection between the neuron and the target cell
   d. Most hormones, local mediators, and neurotransmitters readily cross the cell plasma membrane

COMMENT: Depending on how the extracellular messenger arrives, cell regulation can be classified as paracrine, endocrine, or neurocrine. In paracrine regulation, a chemical messenger or mediator is produced and acts locally. In endocrine regulation, the extracellular messengers (hormones) are released into the blood and act on target cells anywhere in the body that has appropriate receptors. In neurocrine regulation, neurons secrete transmitters into highly localized regions, the synaptic cleft, so that the regulation depends on a physical connection between the neuron and the target cell as well as the presence of a specific receptor. In almost all cases of cell regulation, the extracellular signal or stimulus is restricted to being an informational molecule. This information is received by receptors on or in the target cell, which generally has an affinity for the signal molecule. Most hormones, local mediators, and neurotransmitters are water soluble and cannot readily cross the plasma membrane.

ANSWER: b, c

REFERENCE: *Chapter 1—Cell Structure and Function: Regulation of Cell Function*

18. Most hormone receptors are localized on the cell membrane and transduce hormone binding into altered levels of intracellular messengers. A limited number of intracellular receptors do exist. Which of the following statements is/are true concerning intracellular receptors?

   a. The messengers or hormones must be lipophilic
   b. These intracellular receptors generally regulate protein synthesis
   c. The intracellular receptors are located entirely in the nucleus of the cell
   d. A heat shock protein serves as an inhibitor protein that blocks the DNA-binding domain of the steroid receptor

COMMENT: Although most hormone and other messenger receptors are extracellular, intracellular receptors have been identified. The hormone messengers involved for these receptors are primarily steroid and thyroid hormones and are lipophilic. Because of their hydrophobic nature, these molecules readily penetrate the lipid portion of the cell membrane. Receptors for these hormones exist intracellularly in the cytoplasm or in the nucleus and generally act as regulators of gene expression. These hydrophobic signaling molecules exist in plasma bound to protein, so the concentration of this class of regulators does not fluctuate rapidly in plasma and the actions are generally slower in onset and more prolonged than are those of the water-soluble class. Some types of steroid receptors, particularly for glucocorticoids, are located in the cytosol in the inactive state. Once the ligand binds, the receptor undergoes conformational change, called *activation*. This allows cytoplasmic receptors to move into the nucleus and bind to DNA. Receptors already in the nucleus increase their affinity for DNA. In the case of glucocorticoid receptors and probably others of this class, the inactive receptor is associated with another protein, heat shock protein. These proteins block the DNA-binding domain of the receptor. Activation involves dissociation of the inhibitor protein.

ANSWER: a, d

REFERENCE: *Chapter 1—Cell Structure and Function: Regulation of Cell Function*

19. Which of the following statements is/are true concerning cell membrane receptors?

    a. The largest family of cell surface receptors are the G protein–linked receptors

    b. Activity of G protein involves binding and hydrolysis of ATP

    c. The G-protein receptor generates an intracellular messenger commonly through the use of adenylate cyclase

    d. Tyrosine kinase receptors are considered G protein–linked receptors

COMMENT: All water-soluble regulatory molecules bind to the cell surface receptor proteins. Binding of the appropriate ligand evokes an intracellular signal that usually regulates enzyme activity, membrane transport, or in some cases gene expression. Most cell surface receptors belong to one of three functional classes—ion channel receptors, catalytic receptors, and G protein–linked receptors. Ion channel receptors are multisubunit assemblies that with each subunit have a multiple-membrane spanning segment. Together these subunits form an ion-selected pore that can be gated by a change in transmembrane electrical potential or binding of a ligand to one of the subunits. Catalytic receptors are membrane proteins that have enzymatic activity. The best understood receptors of this class are the tyrosine kinases. The largest family of cell surface receptors are the G protein–linked receptors. G proteins are a family of proteins that bind and hydrolyze guanosine triphosphate (GTP). The final component of single transduction by G protein–linked cell surface receptors is the effector that generates the intracellular messenger. The two best understood effectors are adenylate cyclase, which converts ATP to cAMP, and polyphosphoinositide-specific phospholipase C.

ANSWER: a, c

REFERENCE: *Chapter 1—Cell Structure and Function: Regulation of Cell Function*

20. The best understood intracellular messenger is cyclic adenosine monophosphate. Which of the following statements is/are correct concerning this intracellular messenger?

    a. Intracellular cAMP is constantly degraded by a specific enzyme, cAMP phosphodiesterase

    b. Most of the actions of cAMP are mediated by activation of protein kinase A

    c. Intracellular levels of cAMP are relatively stable and change solely in response to activation of adenylate cyclase

    d. cAMP is the only cyclic nucleotide active as an intracellular messenger

COMMENT: The prototypic intracellular messenger is cAMP. To function as a mediator, the concentration of cAMP must change rapidly. In resting cells, cAMP is continuously being degraded by a specific enzyme, cAMP phosphodiesterase. Levels of cAMP can increase 10-fold or more within seconds of receptor binding through activation of adenylate cyclase. Cyclic AMP acts as an allosteric regulator, and most, if not all, of its actions are mediated by activation of cAMP-dependent protein kinase A. Cyclic AMP is not the only cyclic nucleotide active as an intracellular messenger. Most animal cells produce cyclic guanosine monophosphate. Intracellular calcium ions also serve as second messengers in a large number of cells.

ANSWER: a, b

REFERENCE: *Chapter 1—Cell Structure and Function: Regulation of Cell Function; Intracellular Messengers*

CHAPTER 2

NUTRITION AND METABOLISM

1. Total body mass is composed of an aqueous component and a nonaqueous component. The nonaqueous component is made up of which of the following?
   a. Liver
   b. Tendons
   c. Skeletal muscle
   d. Extracellular fluid
   e. Adipose tissue

COMMENT: The nonaqueous portion of total body mass is made up of bones, tendons, and mineral mass as well as adipose tissue. The aqueous component contains the body cell mass, which is made up of skeletal muscle, intraabdominal and intrathoracic organs, skin, and circulating blood cells. Also contributing to the aqueous portion is the interstitial fluid and intravascular volume.

ANSWER: b, e

REFERENCE: *Chapter 2—Nutrition and Metabolism: Basic Nutritional Biochemistry*

2. Which of the following statements is/are true concerning body fuel reserves?
   a. The largest fuel reserve in the body is skeletal muscle
   b. Fat provides about 9 calories per gram
   c. Free glucose and glycogen stores are a trivial fuel reserve
   d. Body protein is a valuable storage form of energy

COMMENT: The body contains fuel reserves that it can mobilize and utilize during times of starvation or stress. By far the greatest energy component is fat, which is calorically dense because it provides about 9 calories per gram. Body protein composes the next largest mass of useable energy, but amino acids yield only about 4 kcal/g. Unlike fat reserves, body protein is not a storage form of energy but serves as a structural functional component of the body; loss of body protein, if severe, is associated with functional consequences. Glycogen stored in muscle and liver and free glucose have a trivial caloric value of less than 1,000 kcal for a 70-kg man.

ANSWER: b, c

REFERENCE: *Chapter 2—Nutrition and Metabolism: Basic Nutritional Biochemistry*

3. Fatty acids are an important energy source for the body. Which of the following statements is/are true concerning the use of fatty acids as an energy source?
   a. Fatty acids are stored in adipocytes as triglycerides
   b. Hormone-sensitive lipase is present only in adipose tissue
   c. Fatty acids are released into the circulation to travel freely in plasma
   d. Approximately 25% of total nonprotein caloric needs supplied by means of total parenteral nutrition should be in the form of fat

COMMENT: In most tissues, fatty acids are readily oxidized for energy. They are especially important energy sources for the heart, liver, and skeletal muscle. In adipose tissue, fatty acids can be re-esterified with glycerol and stored as triglycerides in adipocytes. Stored fat is mobilized during starvation and stress. Hormone-sensitive lipase, present only in adipose tissue, catalyzes the breakdown of stored triglycerides into glycerol and fatty acids. The fatty acids produced are released in the circulation. The major lipids in plasma do not circulate in a free form, thus free fatty acids must be bound to albumin. During stress, the activity of hormone-sensitive lipase is increased, and the increased activity leads to mobilization of fat stores. However, fat remains an important fuel source for critically ill patients. As a rule, the amount of fat administered to patients receiving total parenteral nutrition (TPN) should compose 5% to 30% of total nonprotein caloric needs.

ANSWER: a, b, d

REFERENCE: *Chapter 2—Nutrition and Metabolism: Energy Metabolism*

4. Which of the following statements is/are true concerning human energy requirements?

    a. Among healthy persons, less than 5% of basal energy requirement is spent on cardiac output and the work of breathing
    b. Mechanical ventilation can decrease the energy expenditure for normal respiration
    c. For a 70-kg man, average resting energy consumption is almost 1,500 kcal/d
    d. Similar increases in energy expenditures are associated with elective surgery and trauma or thermal injury

COMMENT: Basal energy requirements are measured with the person at rest when no external work is being done. The energy is used mainly for transport and synthetic work within cells. A surprisingly small percentage (<5%) of this energy is spent on cardiac output, and the work of breathing of healthy persons. In contrast, the work of breathing performed by persons with chronic obstructive lung disease or patients using a ventilator can account for 15% to 20% of caloric expenditure. The average resting postabsorptive 70-kg man consumes about 1,500 kcal/d. Energy needs increase as severity of illness increases. The expenditure of calories is only minimally increased after elective surgery. The largest increase in energy expenditure occurs among patients with severe multiple trauma or severe thermal injury. An average-sized adult who sustains a severe burn rarely needs more than 3,500 kcal/d for maintenance.

ANSWER: a, c

REFERENCE: *Chapter 2—Nutrition and Metabolism: Energy Metabolism*

5. Which of the following statements is/are true concerning protein and amino acid metabolism for humans?

    a. The main source of amino acids is breakdown of circulating proteins
    b. The recommended daily allowance for protein may triple for critically ill patients
    c. Urinary nitrogen losses approach 0 in the face of protein starvation
    d. Negative nitrogen balance refers to a decrease in nitrogen taken into the body versus the amount of nitrogen lost

COMMENT: Approximately 15% of the total body weight is made up of proteins, about one half of which are intracellular and one half extracellular. In humans and other animals, dietary protein is the source of most amino acids. Intestinal absorption is the only physiologic pathway by which the body obtains exogenous amino acids. Digestion of ingested protein provides free amino acids that are absorbed by the small intestine and transported to the liver, where they can be incorporated into new proteins or other biosynthetic products. Excess amino acids are degraded, and their carbon skeleton is oxidized to produce energy or it is incorporated into glycogen or into free fatty acids. In addition to the metabolism of dietary amino acids, the existing proteins in the cell are continuously recycled, such that total protein turnover in the body is about 300 g/d. Vertebrates cannot reuse nitrogen with 100% efficiency; therefore obligatory nitrogen losses occur, mainly in the urine. Urinary nitrogen losses diminish when persons are fed a protein-free diet, but the losses never become 0 because of the inability of the body to completely reuse nitrogen. Among stressed patients, this ability to adapt to starvation is compromised such that proteolysis of body proteins continues at a high rate. This increases the amount of obligatory nitrogen losses, which are accentuated by the catabolic disease state. This results in negative nitrogen balance, in which the amount of nitrogen taken in by the patient is exceeded by the amount of nitrogen lost in the urine, stool, skin wounds, and fistula drainage.

ANSWER: b, d

REFERENCE: *Chapter 2—Nutrition and Metabolism: Protein and Amino Acid Metabolism*

6. Which of the following hormones can be expected to be released as part of the stress response?

    a. Antidiuretic hormone (ADH)

    b. Aldosterone

    c. Insulin

    d. Epinephrine

COMMENT: Several important responses occur in response to stress. The body immediately attempts to compensate for a reduction in circulating blood volume to maintain adequate organ perfusion. Afferent nerve signals are initiated that stimulate the release of both ADH and aldosterone. The pain and fear associated with the stress response lead to excessive production to catecholamines, which increase metabolic rate and stimulate lipolysis, hepatic glycolysis, and gluconeogenesis. Glucagon, which has a potent glycogenolytic and gluconeogenic effect in the liver, is released. This hormone has the opposite effect of insulin, which promotes glucose storage and uptake by the cells.

ANSWER: a, b, d

REFERENCE: *Chapter 2—Nutrition and Metabolism: Specific Components of the Stress Response*

7. Which of the following determine(s) the host response to surgical stress?

    a. Sex

    b. Age

    c. Nutritional status

    d. Body composition

COMMENT: The pattern of physiologic changes elicited in response to surgical stress results from the specific interaction of an individual patient with a stressful stimulus. Several factors specific to the patient determine the nature of the host response to stress. Body composition is an important determinant of metabolic responses during surgical illness. Posttraumatic nitrogen excretion is directly related to the size of the body protein mass. A strong relation between protein depletion and postoperative complications has been found among nonseptic, nonimmunosuppressed patients undergoing elective gastrointestinal operations. Protein-depleted patients have diminished preoperative respiratory muscle strength and vital capacity, a high incidence of postoperative pneumonia, and long postoperative hospital stays. Impaired wound healing and respiratory, hepatic, and muscle function of protein-depleted patients awaiting surgery also has been reported. Many of the changes in the metabolic responses to surgical illnesses that occur with aging can be attributed to alterations in body composition and to long-standing patterns of physical activity. Fat mass tends to increase with age, and muscle mass tends to decrease. Loss of strength that accompanies immobility, starvation, and acute surgical illness can have marked functional consequences. The prevalence of cardiovascular and pulmonary diseases increases with age. Thus delivery of oxygen to tissues can be impaired among elderly persons. Observed differences in metabolic responses of men and women generally reflect differences in body composition. Women have less lean body mass than do men. This difference is thought to account for the lower net loss of nitrogen after elective abdominal procedures among women than among men.

ANSWER: a, b, c, d

REFERENCE: *Chapter 2—Nutrition and Metabolism: Determinants of Host Responses to Surgical Stress*

8. The neurohormonal component of the stress response is well defined. Less is known about the inflammatory component mediated primarily by cytokines. Which of the following statements is/are true concerning this component of the surgical stress response?

a. Cytokines primarily work locally through direct cell-to-cell communication
b. Cytokines are never detectable in the systemic bloodstream
c. Cytokines are produced only by immune cells attracted to the site of injury
d. Cytokine release can stimulate the release of other cytokines and initiate an important cascade of events

COMMENT: Cytokines, which are produced at the site of injury by endothelial cells and by diverse immune cells throughout the body, occupy a pivotal position in the stress response. Cytokines differ from classic endocrine hormones in that they are produced by a variety of cell types and they can exert their tissue effects locally through direct cell-to-cell communication in a paracrine or autocrine manner. Cytokines can stimulate production of other cytokines and initiate important cascades that both amplify and diversify the effects of the proximal cytokine. When in excess, cytokines occasionally act as hormones and spill over into the systemic circulation and become detectable in the bloodstream.

ANSWER: a, d

REFERENCE: *Chapter 2—Nutrition and Metabolism: Mediators of the Stress Response*

9. Cytokines that have an important role in the metabolic response to injury include:

a. Tumor necrosis factor α (TNF)
b. Interleukin-1 (IL-1)
c. Interleukin-6 (IL-6)
d. Interferon-γ

COMMENT: Tumor necrosis factor α, or cachectin, is considered the primary mediator of the systemic effects of endotoxin. It produces anorexia, fever, tachypnea, and tachycardia at low doses and hypotension, organ failure, and death at higher doses. Tumor necrosis factor α is produced primarily by macrophages, but lymphocytes, Kupffer cells, and a number of other cell types have been identified as sources. Interleukin-1, like TNF, has a variety of proinflammatory activities. Interleukin-6 is a primary mediator of the altered hepatic protein synthesis known as the *acute-phase protein synthetic response*. Glucocorticoid hormones augment the cytokine effects on acute-phase protein synthesis. Interferons are a family of proteins readily identified for their ability to inhibit viral replication in infected sells. Interferon-γ can up-regulate the number of TNF receptors on various cell types.

ANSWER: a, b, c, d

REFERENCE: *Chapter 2—Nutrition and Metabolism: Mediators of the Stress Response*

10. Interleukin-6 is recognized as the cytokine primarily responsible for the alteration in hepatic protein synthesis recognized as the acute-phase response. Which of the following statements is/are true concerning acute-phase protein response to surgical stress?

    a. Glucocorticoid hormones inhibit this response

    b. Levels of proteins such as albumin and transferrin that serve in serum transport are generally increased in this response

    c. Examples of acute-phase proteins include fibrinogen and C-reactive protein

    d. In general, the physiologic role of acute-phase proteins is to reduce the systemic effects of tissue damage

COMMENT: Interleukin-6 is recognized as the cytokine primarily responsible for the alteration in hepatic synthesis recognized as the acute-phase response. Glucocorticoid hormones augment this response. The primary metabolic component of the acute-phase response is qualitative alteration in hepatic protein synthesis that alters in plasma protein composition. The quantity of proteins that act as serum transport in binding molecules (albumin, transferrin) characteristically decreases, and that of acute-phase proteins (fibrinogen, C-reactive proteins) increases. Acute-phase proteins are elaborated for the purpose of reducing the systemic effects of tissue damage. Many act as antiproteases, opsonins, or coagulation and wound healing factors that inhibit the tissue destruction associated with the local initiation of inflammation.

ANSWER: c, d

REFERENCE: *Chapter 2—Nutrition and Metabolism: Mediators of the Stress Response*

11. Under certain circumstances, the intestine can become a source of sepsis and serve as the motor of systemic inflammatory response syndrome. Microbial translocation is the process by which microorganisms migrate across the mucosal barrier to invade the host. Which of the following mechanisms can promote bacterial translocation?

    a. An increased number of intestinal bacteria

    b. Altered intestinal mucosal permeability

    c. Decreased host defense mechanisms

    d. Lack of enteral feeding

COMMENT: Translocation is promoted in three general ways: (a) altered permeability of the intestinal mucosa as caused by shock, sepsis, distant injury, or cell toxins, (b) decreased host defense caused by administration of glucocorticoids, immunosuppression, or protein depletion, and (c) an increase in the number of bacteria in the intestine. Because many factors that facilitate bacterial translocation occur simultaneously in surgical patients, these effects can be either additive or cumulative. In addition, many patients in surgical intensive care units do not receive enteral feedings, and current parenteral therapy causes intestinal atrophy that further promotes translocation.

ANSWER: a, b, c, d

REFERENCE: *Chapter 2—Nutrition and Metabolism: Gut Mucosal Barrier Dysfunction as a Mediator of the Stress Response*

12. A 55-year-old man undergoes total abdominal colectomy. Which of the following statements is/are true concerning the hormonal response to the surgical procedure?
    a. Corticotropin is secreted from the anterior pituitary gland
    b. Corticotropin stimulation results in elevation of serum cortisol levels for as long as 1 week after the operation
    c. Increased secretion of aldosterone and ADH contributes to postoperative fluid retention
    d. An increase in serum level of insulin and a decrease in glucagon level accelerate production of hepatic glucose and maintain gluconeogenesis

COMMENT: One of the earliest consequences of a surgical procedure is an increase in levels of circulating cortisol in response to a sudden outpouring of corticotropin from the anterior pituitary gland. The increase in corticotropin secretion stimulates the adrenal cortex to elaborate cortisol, the level of which remains elevated for 24 to 48 hours after an operation. The neuroendocrine responses to the operation also modify the mechanisms that regulate salt and water excretion. Alterations in serum osmolarity and tonicity of body fluids caused by anesthesia and operative stress stimulate secretion of aldosterone and ADH. Thus the ability to excrete a water load after elective surgical procedures is restricted, and weight gain due to salt and water retention is usual after an operation. Alterations occur in response to function of the endocrine pancreas after elective operations. Insulin elaboration is diminished and glucagon concentrations increase. The increase in glucagon concentration and the corresponding decrease in insulin level are important signals to accelerate hepatic glucose production, and with other hormones (epinephrine and glucocorticoids), gluconeogenesis is maintained.

ANSWER: a, c

REFERENCE: *Chapter 2—Nutrition and Metabolism: Elective Operations; Physiologic Responses to Surgery*

13. Which of the following statements about perioperative nutrition is true concerning the patient described in question 12?
    a. Because the patient's weight had been stable with no preoperative nutritional deficit, 5% dextrose intravenous solution is adequate for the initial postoperative source of nutrition
    b. Preoperative immunologic status should be determined, including total peripheral lymphocyte count and delayed hypersensitivity reaction to determine skin-test response to common antigens
    c. Routine postoperative fluid administration with intravenous 5% glucose solutions can provide the calories to meet basal energy requirements
    d. A jejunal feeding catheter should be placed at the time of surgery for postoperative enteral feeding

COMMENT: Most patients undergoing elective operations are adequately nourished. Unless the patient has suffered severe preoperative malnutrition, characterized by weight loss greater than 10% to 15%, or has serious intraoperative or postoperative complications, solutions containing 5% dextrose can be administered for 5 to 7 days before initiation of enteral nutrition with no detrimental effect on outcome. The usual postoperative surgical patient given intravenous glucose at 125 mL/h receives approximately 500 kcal/d, far less than the amount needed to meet energy requirements. The increased cost of feeding and the potential complications associated with intravenous nutrition cannot be justified. Although the use of jejunal feedings in the postoperative period may be useful in the care of some patients, especially those undergoing extensive gastrointestinal surgery, this technique does not appear indicated for this patient.

ANSWER: a

REFERENCE: *Chapter 2—Nutrition and Metabolism: Nutritional Support for Elective Surgical Patients*

14. Which of the following statements is/are true concerning a patient who has sustained multiple trauma as opposed to undergoing an elective operation?

    a. Basal metabolic rates are similar

    b. The patient is highly sensitive to insulin

    c. Utilization of the amino acids glutamine and alanine is similar to their composition in skeletal muscle

    d. Fat and protein stores are rapidly depleted

COMMENT: The degree of hypermetabolism is generally related to the severity of injury. Patients with fractures of long bones have a 15% to 25% increase in metabolic rate, whereas those with multiple injuries have a 50% increase. These metabolic rates among trauma patients contrast with those among postoperative patients, who rarely have more than a 10% to 15% increase in basal metabolic rate after an operation. Studies have shown that uninjured volunteers dispose of exogenous glucose loads much more readily than do injured patients. Other studies have shown a failure to suppress hepatic glucose production among trauma patients during glucose loading or insulin infusion. Thus profound insulin resistance occurs among injured patients. Skeletal muscle is the main source of nitrogen lost in the urine after extensive injury. Although it is recognized that amino acids are released by muscle in increased quantities after injuries, it has only been recently appreciated that the composition of amino acid reflux does not reflect the composition of muscle protein. The release is skewed toward glutamine and alanine, each of which constitutes about one third of the total amino acids released by skeletal muscle. To support hypermetabolism, stored triglyceride is mobilized at an accelerated rate. Although mobilization and use of free fatty acids are accelerated among injured patients, unfed severely injured patients rapidly deplete their fat and protein stores.

ANSWER: b, d

REFERENCE: *Chapter 2—Nutrition and Metabolism: Trauma*

15. Which of the following statements is/are true concerning nutritional support of an injured patient?

    a. The goal of nutritional support is maintenance of body cell mass and limitation of weight loss to less than 25% of preinjury weight

    b. Undernutrition may compromise the available defense mechanisms

    c. Nutritional support is an immediate priority for the trauma patient

    d. Fifty percent of non-nitrogen caloric requirements should be provided in the form of fat

COMMENT: Metabolic response to injury results in increased energy expenditure. If energy intake is less than expenditure, oxidation of body fat stores and erosion of lean body mass occurs with resultant loss of weight. When weight loss exceeds 10% to 15% of body weight, the complications of malnutrition interact with disease processes, and morbidity and mortality rates increase. The goal of nutritional support is maintenance of body cell mass and limitation of weight loss to less than 10% of preinjury weight. The most important effect of nutritional support of trauma patients is to aid host defense. Undernutrition can compromise the available host defense mechanism and thus increase the likelihood of invasive sepsis, multiple organ system failure, and death. Resuscitation, oxygenation, and arrest of hemorrhage are immediate priorities for survival. Nutritional support is an essential part of the metabolic care of critically ill patients and should be instituted after resuscitation before considerable weight loss occurs. The nutritional requirements of a trauma patient can be determined by determining basal metabolic rate; appropriate increases are based on extent of injury and hospital activity. After initial determination of nitrogen requirements, caloric requirements are distributed at a ratio of 70% as glucose and 30% as fat.

ANSWER: b

REFERENCE: *Chapter 2—Nutrition and Metabolism: Trauma*

16. Sepsis causes a marked metabolic response. Which of the following statements is/are true concerning the metabolic response to sepsis?

    a. Oxygen consumption increases in the face of infection
    b. For a patient with a maximal metabolic rate due to trauma, the presence of infection increases the rate further
    c. Metabolic rate increases approximately 10% for each increase of 1°C in central temperature
    d. The extent of increase in oxygen consumption relates to the severity of infection

COMMENT: The oxygen consumption of patients with infection usually is elevated. The extent of this increase is related to the severity of infection, peak elevations reaching 50% to 60% greater than normal. If the metabolic rate is already elevated to a maximal extent because of severe injury, no further increase occurs. For patients with only a slightly accelerated rate of oxygen consumption, the presence of infection causes an increase in metabolic rate added to the preexisting state. A portion of the increase in metabolism can be ascribed to an increase in reaction rate associated with fever. Calculations suggest that the metabolic rate increases 10% to 13% for each elevation of 1°C in central temperature.

ANSWER: a, c, d

REFERENCE: *Chapter 2—Nutrition and Metabolism: Sepsis*

17. Which of the following metabolic effects can be observed among patients with sepsis?

    a. Increased gluconeogenesis
    b. Accelerated proteolysis
    c. Increased lipolysis
    d. Impaired intestinal metabolism of glutamine

COMMENT: A number of metabolic responses to sepsis have been defined. Glucose production increases in patients with infection, and the increase appears to be additive to the augmented gluconeogenesis that occurs after injury. Accelerated proteolysis, increased nitrogen excretion, and prolonged negative nitrogen balance also occur after infection with a response pattern similar to that described for injury. Severe infection often is associated with a hypercatabolic state that initiates marked changes in interorgan glutamine metabolism. This process results in accelerated muscle proteolysis and net skeletal muscle glutamine release. The bulk of glutamine is taken up by the liver at the expense of the intestine. It appears that sepsis can impair intestinal metabolism of glutamine. Fat is a major fuel oxidized in patients with infection, and increased metabolism of lipids from peripheral fat stores is especially prominent during a period of inadequate nutritional support.

ANSWER: a, b, c, d

REFERENCE: *Chapter 2—Nutrition and Metabolism: Sepsis*

18. A number of changes in trace mineral metabolism occur during sepsis. Which of the following changes can be observed in a patient with sepsis or trauma?

    a. Plasma iron levels decrease
    b. Plasma copper levels decrease
    c. Plasma serum zinc levels may decrease
    d. Administration of iron is appropriate

COMMENT: Changes in the balance of magnesium, inorganic phosphate, zinc, and potassium generally follow alterations in nitrogen balance. Although the iron-binding capacity of transferrin usually is unchanged in early infection, iron disappears from the plasma, especially during severe pyogenic infection; similar alterations in serum zinc levels are observed. The administration of iron to an infected host, especially early in the disease, is contraindicated, however, because increased serum iron concentration can impair resistance. Unlike levels of iron and zinc, copper levels generally increase, and the increased plasma concentrations can be ascribed almost entirely to the levels of the ceruloplasmin produced by the liver.

ANSWER: a, c

REFERENCE: *Chapter 2—Nutrition and Metabolism: Sepsis*

19. A 59-year-old trauma patient has multiple septic complications, including severe pneumonia, intraabdominal abscess, and major wound infection. He has signs of multiple system organ failure. Which of the following statements is/are true concerning necessary changes in nutritional management?

    a. Carbohydrate load should be reduced in the face of respiratory failure
    b. For patients with renal failure, protein intake should be diminished
    c. During hemodialysis protein intake should be limited to the same extent
    d. For patients with hepatic failure, carbohydrate load should be increased

COMMENT: The most severe complication of sepsis is multiple system organ dysfunction syndrome, which may result in death. The development of organ failure necessitates changes in nutritional requirements and causes special feeding problems. A problem associated with systemic infection is oxygenation and elimination of carbon dioxide. Most enteral and parenteral formulas used to provide nutritional support for critically ill patients contain large amounts of carbohydrate, which generates large amounts of carbon dioxide after oxygenation. Such a large carbon dioxide load can worsen pulmonary function or delay weaning from the respirator. If this factor becomes a problem, the carbohydrate load should be decreased to 50% of metabolic requirements, and fat emulsion should be administered to provide additional calories. When renal failure becomes progressive, use of hemodialysis minimizes the effect of uremia superimposed on the metabolism of sepsis. Metabolic studies involving patients with acute and chronic renal failure have limited the intake of nonessential amino acids in an attempt to lower urea production. Proteins of high biologic value, but in much smaller quantities than usually given, are administered along with adequate calories, usually in the form of glucose. When enteral feeding is not feasible, central venous infusion of an essential amino acid solution and hypertonic dextrose provides calories and a small quantity of nitrogen to reduce protein catabolism while simultaneously controlling the increase in blood urea nitrogen level. During dialysis, protein intake is liberalized, but the blood urea nitrogen level should be maintained at less than 100 mg/dL. Hepatic dysfunction is a common manifestation of septicemia. The carbohydrate load usually is decreased to consist of no more than 50% of metabolic requirements. The additional calories should be provided as fat emulsion. If encephalopathy develops, protein load should be reduced.

ANSWER: a, b

REFERENCE: *Chapter 2—Nutrition and Metabolism: Nutritional Requirements and Special Feeding Problems*

20. Which of the following statements is/are true concerning the indications and administration of nutritional support to cancer patients?

    a. Preoperative nutritional support should be provided to all patients with cancer

    b. To be effective, preoperative nutrition must be given for at least 2 weeks preoperatively

    c. Parenteral nutrition is the preferred route of feeding for all cancer patients

    d. Standard TPN solutions maintain integrity of the small bowel

    e. None of the above

COMMENT: The role of nutritional support of cancer patients remains an important component of overall therapy. Preoperative nutritional support should be given only to patients who do not need an emergency operation and who have severe weight loss (>15% of pre-illness body weight) and a serum albumin level <2.9 mg/dL. Preoperative nutrition (enteral or parenteral) should not be given for longer than 7 to 10 days. Enteral nutrition is always the preferred route of feeding cancer patients if the gastrointestinal tract is functional. There are several benefits of using the bowel lumen for nutrient delivery. The trophic effects of enteral feeding on the small-bowel mucosa have been well described. The integrity of the mucosal lining is maintained, and it may provide an effective barrier to intraluminal enteric organisms, which might otherwise translocate into the systemic circulation. Atrophic changes can be seen in the intestinal epithelium after several days of bowel rest; this atrophy is not reversed with currently available TPN solutions.

ANSWER: e

REFERENCE: *Chapter 2—Nutrition and Metabolism: Nutrition and Metabolism in the Cancer Patient*

21. A number of prospective clinical trials have addressed the role of TPN in the care of cancer patients. The results have been somewhat conflicting. Which of the following statements has/have been proved correct in prospective trials?

    a. Preoperative TPN is beneficial to surgical patients with severe preoperative nutrition

    b. Postoperative TPN is of value after pancreatic resection

    c. Routine use of perioperative (before and after an operation) TPN is of benefit in the care of patients undergoing hepatectomy for hepatoma

    d. Total parenteral nutrition is of no benefit to patients undergoing bone marrow transplantation

COMMENT: Numerous clinical trials have failed to yield a consensus with regard to the efficacy of TPN in the care of cancer patients. In 1991, a multicenter Veterans Affairs cooperative trial showed that preoperative TPN was of benefit to surgical patients (many of whom had cancer) with severe preoperative malnutrition. Another study examined the use of routine postoperative TPN after major pancreatic resection. Patients randomized to receive TPN starting on postoperative day 1 were found to have an increased incidence of intraabdominal abscess and a tendency toward an increased incidence in peritonitis and bowel obstruction. These investigators concluded that routine use of postoperative TPN is not indicated and may be harmful after pancreatic resection. Another study, however, showed that patients undergoing hepatectomy for hepatocellular carcinoma and receiving a regimen of perioperative (starting 7 days before the planned procedure) TPN had a statistically lower incidence of infectious complications than did patients who did not receive TPN. This was one of the few studies that showed routine TPN (without the requirement of severe preoperative malnutrition) was of benefit. The use of TPN in the care of patients receiving bone marrow transplants has also been shown to be a valuable component of overall care.

ANSWER: a, c

REFERENCE: *Chapter 2—Nutrition and Metabolism: Total Parenteral Nutrition in the Cancer Patient*

22. Appropriate guidelines for the use of TPN in the care of cancer patients include:
    a. Long-term TPN for patients with rapid progressive tumor growth unresponsive to other therapy
    b. Mildly malnourished patients undergoing surgery for a curable cancer
    c. Preoperatively administered TPN before surgery or other therapy in the care of patients with severe malnutrition
    d. Patients for whom treatment toxicity precludes the use of enteral nutrition

COMMENT: As a rule, the most important factor to consider when making decisions about the use of TPN in the care of patients with cancer is the response of the tumor to antineoplastic therapy. Appropriate guidelines include the following: Short-term TPN is indicated for severely malnourished patients or in those in whom gastrointestinal or other toxicities preclude adequate enteral intake for 7 days or longer. Total parenteral nutrition is not indicated in the care of well-nourished or mildly malnourished patients undergoing therapy or surgery who would be expected to be able to resume adequate nutrition in approximately 7 days. Long-term TPN is indicated in the care of patients with treatment-associated toxicities that preclude use of enteral nutrition and represent the primary impediment to the restoration of performance status. These patients are expected to respond to antitumor therapy. Long-term TPN is not indicated when there is rapidly progressive tumor growth, which is unresponsive to such therapy.

ANSWER: c, d

REFERENCE: *Chapter 2—Nutrition and Metabolism: Total Parenteral Nutrition in the Cancer Patient*

23. A 47-year-old patient undergoing complicated laparotomy for bowel obstruction has a postoperative enterocutaneous fistula. Which of the following statements is/are true concerning parenteral nutritional support in the postoperative period?
    a. Oral intake can cause severe dehydration, electrolyte abnormalities, and perifistular skin injury
    b. Total parenteral nutrition increases the spontaneous closure rate of intestinal fistulas
    c. Total parenteral nutrition decreases the mortality rate among patients with intestinal fistulas
    d. The use of TPN better prepares the patient for surgery if surgical intervention proves necessary

COMMENT: Patients with gastrointestinal-cutaneous fistulas have the classic indication for TPN. In the care of such patients, oral intake almost invariably increases fistula output with associated metabolic disturbances, dehydration, skin breakdown, and death. Authors of several comprehensive reviews concluded that TPN clearly affects the course of treatment of patients with gastrointestinal fistulas. The following conclusions can be drawn from studies evaluating the use of TPN in the care of patients with enterocutaneous fistula. First, TPN increases the rate of spontaneous closure of enterocutaneous fistulas but does not markedly decrease the mortality rate among patients with fistulas. Second, if spontaneous closure of the fistula does not occur, patients are better prepared for operative intervention because of the nutritional support they have received. Third, certain fistulas are associated with a lower rate of spontaneous closure than are others, and aggressive surgical management should be provided after a defined period of nutritional support, unless closure occurs.

ANSWER: a, b, d

REFERENCE: *Chapter 2—Nutrition and Metabolism: Choice of Nutrition in Surgical Patients; Enteral vs. Parenteral*

24. A 16-year-old boy has midgut volvulus with massive loss of small intestine. Which of the following statements is/are true concerning his nutritional requirements and treatment?

    a. If at least 18 inches (45 cm) of residual small intestine survives, the patient may tolerate some form of enteral nutrition

    b. A nutritional regimen consisting of supplemental glutamine, growth hormone, and a modified high-carbohydrate, low-fat diet may be beneficial to this patient

    c. The regimen described in *b.* may decrease the cost of care

    d. The need for TPN will increase after discontinuation of growth hormone

COMMENT: Before TPN became available, most patients with short-bowel syndrome from either surgery or a catastrophic event died. Some patients with residual small intestine (at least 18 inches [45 cm]), however, have postresection hyperplasia that eventually allows enteral feeding. Studies have shown the requirement for TPN can be decreased or even eliminated in the care of patients with short-bowel syndrome if they are given a nutritional regimen of supplemental glutamine, growth hormone, and a modified high-carbohydrate, low-fat diet. The studies showed marked improvement in absorption of nutrients with this combination of therapy and a decrease in stool output. In addition, TPN requirements were decreased 50%, as were costs associated with the care of these patients. Discontinuation of growth hormone did not increase TPN needs once the patient had undergone successful intestinal rehabilitation.

ANSWER: a, b, c

REFERENCE: *Chapter 2—Nutrition and Metabolism: Choice of Nutrition in Surgical Patients; Enteral vs. Parenteral*

25. Altering the amino acid profile in TPN solutions can be of benefit in certain conditions. Which of the following conditions is/are associated with benefit from supplementation with the amino acid type listed?

    a. Acute renal failure and essential amino acids

    b. Hepatic failure and aromatic amino acids

    c. Short-bowel syndrome and glutamine

    d. Chronic renal failure and essential amino acids

COMMENT: In a number of conditions, altering the amino acid profile of the TPN solution can be of benefit. Total parenteral nutrition with amino acids of high biologic value can decrease mortality among patients with acute renal failure. These solutions, which contain high-quality amino acids, can improve nitrogen balance and diminish urea nitrogen level. Provision of essential amino acids only allows the body to maximally utilize nitrogen for synthesis of nonessential amino acids and thereby helps prevent rapid increases in blood urea nitrogen level. There appear to be no advantages to using essential amino acids if the patient is already undergoing dialysis every other day; therefore a balanced standard amino acid solution is recommended. Because of liver damage and portosystemic shunting, patients with hepatic failure have derangements in circulating levels of amino acids. The plasma aromatic to branched-chain amino acid ratio is increased in favor of the transport of aromatic amino acids across the blood-brain barrier. These amino acids are precursors of false transmitters that contribute to lethargy and encephalopathy. Treatment of patients with liver failure with solutions enriched in branched-chain amino acids and deficient in aromatic amino acids improves tolerance to administration of protein and results in clinical relief of encephalopathic states. Glutamine-enriched TPN partially attenuates villous atrophy and may be useful in the management of short-bowel syndrome.

ANSWER: a, c

REFERENCE: *Chapter 2—Nutrition and Metabolism: Choice of Nutrition in Surgical Patients; Enteral vs. Parenteral*

26. Which of the following complications of TPN is/are appropriately managed with the listed treatment?

    a. Air embolism—place patient in reverse Trendelenburg and left lateral decubitus position and aspirate venous air
    b. Hyperchloremic metabolic acidosis—give sodium and potassium as acetate salts
    c. Carbon dioxide retention—decrease glucose calories and replace with fat
    d. Line sepsis—administer intravenous antibiotics

COMMENT: A number of complications of TPN can occur that can be divided into three types: mechanical, metabolic, and infectious.

ANSWER: b, c

REFERENCE: *Chapter 2—Nutrition and Metabolism: Choice of Nutrition in Surgical Patients; Enteral vs. Parenteral*

27. Although it has beneficial effects on patients and specific organ systems, TPN has a limitation related to disuse of the intestine. Which of the following statements is/are true concerning the effects of TPN on the gastrointestinal tract?

    a. Patients receiving TPN have an accentuated systemic response to endotoxin challenge compared with enterally fed volunteers
    b. Total parenteral nutrition can disrupt the intestinal microflora
    c. In experimental models, bacterial translocation from the intestine increases
    d. The effects of TPN on the intestine can lead to multiple organ failure

COMMENT: A number of studies have examined the effects of TPN on intestinal function and immunity. Although most of these studies have been performed with animal models, TPN has consistently been shown to have some detrimental effects. In experiments with rats, TPN markedly disrupted the intestinal microflora and caused bacterial translocation of the intestine to the mesenteric lymph nodes. In addition, when stress such as a burn injury, chemotherapy, or irradiation is introduced into these models, animals receiving TPN have a much higher mortality. Most results reported in the literature suggest that TPN under certain circumstances predisposes patients to an increase in intestine-derived infectious complications. In a study with human volunteers, persons receiving TPN had an accentuated systemic response to endotoxin challenge compared with enterally fed volunteers. The results of this study suggested impairment of intestinal barrier function during parenteral feeding may promote the release of bacteria or cytokines and cause pronounced systemic responses and possibly multiple organ failure.

ANSWER: a, b, c, d

REFERENCE: *Chapter 2—Nutrition and Metabolism: Choice of Nutrition in Surgical Patients; Enteral vs. Parenteral*

28. Which of the following statements is/are true concerning the role of glutamine in TPN?

    a. Glutamine is an essential amino acid
    b. Glutamine appears to be of primary benefit in critical illness
    c. Glutamine is included in most standard TPN solutions
    d. Glutamine is the primary energy source for intestinal mucosal cells of the small bowel and colon

COMMENT: Glutamine is the most studied intestine-specific nutrient. Glutamine has been classified as a nonessential or nutritionally dispensable amino acid because glutamine can be synthesized in adequate quantities from other amino acids and precursors. Glutamine is not included in most nutritional formulas and has been eliminated from TPN solutions because of its relative instability and short half-life compared with other amino acids. With few exceptions, glutamine is present in oral enteral diets but only at relatively low levels characteristic of the concentration in most animal and plant stores (approximately 7% of total amino acids). Several studies, however, have shown that glutamine may be an essential amino acid during critical illness, particularly in supporting the metabolic requirements of the intestinal mucosa. The results of these studies show that dietary glutamine is not required during health but appears to be beneficial when glutamine depletion is severe or when the intestinal mucosa is damaged by insults such as chemotherapy or radiation therapy. The addition of glutamine to an enteral diet decreases the incidence of intestinal translocation, but these improvements depend on the amount of supplemental glutamine and the type of insult studied. Glutamine-enriched TPN partially attenuates villous atrophy that develops during parenteral nutrition. The use of intravenous glutamine to treat patients appears to be safe and effective in ability to maintain muscle glutamine stores and improve nitrogen balance. Unlike glutamine, short-chain fatty acids are a primary energy source for colonocytes.

ANSWER: b

REFERENCE: *Chapter 2—Nutrition and Metabolism: Choice of Nutrition in Surgical Patients; Enteral vs. Parenteral*

29. A 17-year-old patient involved in an automobile accident is paralyzed with multiple peripheral extremity injuries. Nutritional support is instituted with a transnasal feeding catheter. Which of the following statements is/are true concerning the patient's treatment?

    a. Feeding into the stomach results in stimulation of the biliary-pancreatic axis, which is probably trophic for the small bowel
    b. Gastric secretions dilute the feedings and increase the risk of diarrhea
    c. The most serious risk for this patient is tracheobronchial aspiration
    d. Placement of the feeding catheter through the pylorus into the first portion of the duodenum decreases the risk of regurgitation and aspiration

COMMENT: The use of transnasal feeding catheters for intragastric feeding or for duodenal intubation is a popular adjunct for providing nutritional support by the enteral route. The stomach is easily accessed by means of passage of a soft, flexible feeding tube. Intragastric feeding provides several advantages to the patient. The stomach has the capacity and reservoir for bolus feedings. Feeding into the stomach stimulates the biliary-pancreatic axis, which is probably trophic for the small bowel. Gastric secretions have a dilutional effect on the osmolarity of the feedings, and this effect decreases the risk of diarrhea. The most important risk of intragastric feeding is regurgitation of gastric contents, which causes aspiration into the tracheobronchial tree. This risk is highest among patients who have an altered sensorium or who are paralyzed. Placement of the feeding tube through the pylorus into the fourth portion of the duodenum decreases the risk of regurgitation and aspiration of feeding formulas.

ANSWER: a, c, d

REFERENCE: *Chapter 2—Nutrition and Metabolism: Techniques of Nutritional Support*

30. Which of the following statements is/are true concerning intravenous nutritional support?

    a. Concentrations of glucose no higher than 5% should be used to avoid peripheral venous sclerosis

    b. An important disadvantage of the peripheral technique is limited caloric delivery

    c. If TPN is needed, access to the superior vena cava through the external jugular vein is the most suitable site

    d. Venous thrombosis is an uncommon complication for long-term central venous catheterization

COMMENT: Although peripheral access can be used for intravenous nutrition, the main disadvantage of this technique is limited caloric delivery to meet catabolic demands within tolerated fluid limits. Infusion of glucose (up to 10%), amino acid solutions, and fat emulsions can be administered peripherally, but these solutions must be nearly isotonic to avoid peripheral venous sclerosis. The preferred method of access for TPN is into the superior vena cava by means of cutaneous cannulation of the subclavian vein. Alternative sites include the internal and external jugular veins, but the catheter exiting from the neck region makes it more difficult to secure and maintain a sterile dressing. Complications of long-term central venous catheterization include venous thrombosis and infection related to the venous catheter. Thrombosis of central vessels is a complication that often is overlooked. Clinical suspicion of subclavian venous thrombosis is only approximately 3%, whereas studies with phlebography or radionucleotide venography indicate the incidence is as high as 35%.

ANSWER: b

REFERENCE: *Chapter 2—Nutrition and Metabolism: Techniques of Nutritional Support*

CHAPTER 3

WOUND HEALING

1. Scar formation is part of the normal healing process after injury. Which of the following tissues has/have the ability to heal without scar formation?

    a. Liver
    b. Skin
    c. Bone
    d. Muscle

COMMENT: Every tissue in the body undergoes reparative processes after injury. Bone has the unique ability to heal without scarring, and the liver can regenerate parenchyma, the only organ that has maintained that ability in adult humans. Although liver does regenerate, it often heals with scarring (cirrhosis). With these exceptions, all other mature human tissues heal with scars.

ANSWER: c

REFERENCE: *Chapter 3—Wound Healing: Normal Wound Healing*

2. Products of platelet degranulation include:

    a. Tumor necrosis factor
    b. Interleukin-1
    c. Transforming growth factor β
    d. Platelet-derived growth factor

COMMENT: The initial response to injury and disruption of a blood vessel is bleeding. The hemostatic response to this is clot formation to stop hemorrhage. Platelet plug formation initiates the hemostatic process along with clotting factors activated by collagen and the basement membrane proteins exposed by the injury. Platelets then degranulate and release the contents of their α granules and dense granules, most notably platelet-derived growth factor and transforming growth factor β. These substances initiate chemotaxis and proliferation of inflammatory cells, beginning the inflammatory response that ultimately heals the wound. Tumor necrosis factor and interleukin-1 also stimulate fibroblast proliferation; however, they are produced by macrophages.

ANSWER: c, d

REFERENCE: *Chapter 3—Wound Healing: Inflammatory Phase*

3. Which of the following statements is/are true concerning the vascular response to injury?

    a. Vasoconstriction is an early event in the response to injury

    b. Vasodilation is a detrimental response to injury, and normal body processes work to avoid this process

    c. Vascular permeability is maintained to prevent further cellular injury

    d. Histamine, prostaglandin E_2 (PGE_2), and prostacyclin (PGI_2) are important mediators of local vasoconstriction

COMMENT: After wounding, transient vasoconstriction is mediated by catecholamines, thromboxane, and prostaglandin F_2 (PGF_2). This period of vasoconstriction lasts for only 5 to 10 minutes. Once a clot has been formed and active bleeding has stopped, vasodilation occurs in and around the wound. Vasodilatation increases local blood flow to the wounded area and supplies the cells and substrate necessary for further wound repair. The vascular endothelial cells also deform, and the deformity increases vascular permeability. Vasodilation and increased endothelial permeability are mediated by histamine, PGE_2, prostacyclin, and vascular endothelial cell growth factor (VEGF). These vasodilatory substances are released by injured endothelial cells and mast cells and enhance the egress of cells and substrate into the wound and tissue.

ANSWER: a

REFERENCE: *Chapter 3—Wound Healing: Inflammatory Phase*

4. Which of the following cells or blood elements play(s) a role in the initial phases of wound healing?

    a. Polymorphonuclear leukocytes (PMNs)

    b. Platelets

    c. Monocytes

    d. Lymphocytes

COMMENT: Soon after the initial injury, the wound is full of debris, which is cleared over the next several days by recruited and activated phagocytic cells. Polymorphonuclear leukocytes begin to arrive immediately, reaching large numbers within 24 hours. The PMNs are followed by macrophages, which appear in wounds in significant numbers within 2 to 3 days. Macrophages are mononuclear phagocytic cells derived from circulating monocytes or resident tissue macrophages. They complete the process of removing all material not necessary for the ensuing steps of wound healing. Lymphocytes also appear in wounds in small numbers during the inflammatory response. The role of lymphocytes in the wound healing process remains to be clarified, but these cells are thought to be more related to the chronic inflammatory processes than to the initial response to wounding. Platelets are anuclear discoid blood elements derived from bone marrow megakaryocytes. They have a role in the initial hemostatic process and release chemotactic factors and factors that lead to fibroblast proliferation.

ANSWER: a, b, c, d

REFERENCE: *Chapter 3—Wound Healing: Inflammatory Response*

5. Which of the following statements is/are true about the role of macrophages in wound healing?

   a. Macrophages are the dominant cell type during the inflammatory phase of wound healing

   b. Macrophages are not essential for wound healing

   c. The macrophage role in wound healing is limited to phagocytosis

   d. Macrophages are a source of a number of humoral factors essential for wound healing

COMMENT: Within 3 or 4 days after injury, macrophages become the dominant cell type in the inflammatory phase of wound healing. The role of macrophages is not limited to phagocytosis. Macrophages also are the source of more than 30 different growth factors and cytokines. These growth factors induce fibroblast proliferation, endothelial cell proliferation (angiogenesis), extracellular matrix production, and recruit and activate additional macrophages. The result is induction of a wound healing amplification cycle as growth factors recruit macrophages and elicit additional growth factor release. Experimental studies in which antibodies, which either destroy PMNs or block aspects of their function, have shown that wounds heal normally but that healing is impaired without functional macrophages. The results of these studies confirm the dominant role of the macrophage in the inflammatory phase of wound healing.

ANSWER: a, d

REFERENCE: *Chapter 3—Wound Healing: Inflammatory Phase*

6. Which of the following statements is/are true concerning the proliferative phase of wound healing?

   a. The macrophage is the predominant cell type

   b. The pink or purplish-red appearance of a wound is caused by ingrowth and proliferation of endothelial cells

   c. Collagen, the dominant structural molecule of the wound matrix, contains two unique amino acids—hydroxyproline and hydroxylysine

   d. The predominant collagen type in a scar is type III

COMMENT: The proliferative phase of wound healing begins with formation of a provisional matrix of fibrin and fibronectin as part of the initial clot formation. The provisional matrix initially is populated by macrophages; however, by day 3 fibroblasts appear in the fibronectin-fibrin framework and initiate collagen synthesis. Fibroblasts that proliferate in response to growth factors become the dominant cell type during this phase. Growth factors produced by macrophages simultaneously induce angiogenesis, which results in ingrowth and proliferation of endothelial cells, and new capillaries form. This neovascularity is visible through the epithelium and gives the wound a pink or purplish-red appearance.

Collagen is the dominant structural molecule in the wound matrix and in the final scar. Collagen is synthesized into an organized cable-like network in a multistep process with both intra- and intercellular components. The collagen molecule has quantities of two unique amino acids—hydroxyproline and hydroxylysine. The hydroxylation that forms these amino acids requires ascorbic acid (vitamin C) and is necessary for the subsequent stabilization and cross-linkage of collagen. The principal collagen type in scars is type I; lesser amounts of type III collagen also are present.

ANSWER: b, c

REFERENCE: *Chapter 3—Wound Healing: Proliferative Phase*

7. Which of the following statements is/are true concerning the remodeling phase of wound healing?
   a. Total collagen content increases steadily through this phase
   b. The normal adult ratio of collagen is approximately 4:1 of type I to type III collagen
   c. Eventually a scar achieves the strength of unwounded skin
   d. The proteoglycans are responsible for the ground substance of the extracellular matrix

COMMENT: The transition from the proliferative phase to the remodeling phase of wound healing is defined by reaching collagen equilibrium. Collagen accumulation within the wound becomes maximal by 2 to 3 weeks after wounding. Although supramaximal rates of synthesis and degradation continue throughout remodeling, there is no further change in total collagen content. During the initial phase of wound healing, there is a relative abundance of type III collagen in the wound. With remodeling, the normal adult ratio of 4:1 (type I to type III) collagen is restored. The other important component of the extracellular matrix is the ground substance or proteoglycans. These substances are composed of a protein background with long hydrophilic carbohydrate side chains. The hydrophilic nature of these molecules accounts for much of the water content of scars.

Scars never achieve the degree of order advanced by collagen in normal skin or tendons, but they do increase in strength for 6 months or more, eventually reaching 70% of the strength of unwounded skin.

ANSWER: b, d

REFERENCE: *Chapter 3—Wound Healing: Remodeling Phase*

8. Reconstitution of the epithelial barrier (epithelialization) begins within hours of the initial injury. Which of the following statements is/are true concerning the process of epithelialization?
   a. Bacteria, protein exudate, and necrotic tissue all compromise this process
   b. Epithelial cells exhibit contact proliferation
   c. Epithelialization occurs only from the margins of the wound
   d. Visible scarring can occur only when the injury extends deeper than the superficial dermis

COMMENT: The initial step of epithelialization involves epithelial cells from the basal layer of the wound edge that flatten and migrate across the wound to complete wound coverage within 24 to 48 hours in a co-opted surgical wound. Epithelial cells exhibit contact inhibition. That is, they continue to migrate across an appropriate bed until a single continuous layer is formed. Epithelial cell migration occurs by means of a process in which the epithelial cells send out pseudopods that attach to the underlying extracellular matrix by integrin receptors. Bacteria, large amounts of protein exudate from leaky capillaries, and necrotic tissue compromise this process and delay epithelialization. In the case of open wounds, epithelialization results from migration of epithelial cells from remaining dermal appendages, sweat glands, and hair follicles, if the dermis is not completely destroyed. In a full-thickness injury, the entire dermis is destroyed or removed. Epithelialization occurs only at the margins of a wound, at a dermal rate of 1 to 2 mm/d.

Visible scarring occurs only when the injury extends deeper than the superficial dermis. Superficial abrasions and burns usually heal without scarring, whereas deeper abrasions and burns can scar considerably. Whenever the dermis is incised, a scar forms.

ANSWER: a, d

REFERENCE: *Chapter 3—Wound Healing: Epithelialization*

9. Which of the following surgical techniques lead(s) to improved wound healing?
   a. Atraumatic handling of tissue
   b. Approximation of underlying fatty tissue to obliterate dead space
   c. Protecting the wound from water for at least 1 week
   d. Meticulous hemostasis

COMMENT: There are numerous practical implications for the care of wounds and surgical incisions. Meticulous hemostasis reduces the inflammation of phagocytosis necessary to clear the wound of blood. Atraumatic handling of tissue decreases the load of necrotic or nonviable cells at the wound margin. Deep sutures are best placed only into collagen-laden structures that will hold tension, that is, fascia and dermis. These tissues have a tensile strength to hold sutures under tension. Fat does not contain collagen and does not hold tension. Therefore fatty tissue should not be sutured as a separate layer. Given that epithelialization of an incision is normally complete within 24 to 48 hours, there is no reason to protect the incision from water beyond this time. Allowing the patient to wash or shower 1 or 2 days after surgery has a useful purpose in débridement of the wound.

ANSWER: a, d

REFERENCE: *Chapter 3—Wound Healing: Clinical Implications*

10. A patient with gross fecal contamination and peritonitis from a ruptured sigmoid diverticulum has a midline wound left open to heal by secondary intention. Which of the following statements describe(s) this healing process?
    a. Wounds that heal in this manner have an altered sequence of healing compared with primarily closed wounds
    b. A bed of granulation tissue forms over exposed subcutaneous tissue
    c. Epithelialization is enhanced in the face of bacterial colonization
    d. The ability of a wound to form granulation tissue depends on the blood supply of the tissue

COMMENT: Open wounds, whether they be ulcers or open surgical incisions closing by secondary intention, heal with the same sequence of inflammation, matrix deposition, epithelialization, and scar maturation as do all wounds. The main difference is that in healing incisional wounds, the healing progresses in an orderly, temporal sequence. In an open wound, the healing events are spatially separated. In a healing wound, a bed of granulation tissue forms over the exposed subcutaneous tissue. Granulation tissue is composed of new capillaries, proliferating fibroblasts, an immature matrix of collagen, proteoglycans, substrate adhesion molecules, and acute and chronic inflammatory cells. Granulation tissue is the cobblestone pink surface of the healthy new tissue in an open wound. The ability of an open wound to form granulation tissue is governed by the blood supply to the tissue and the relative absence of devitalized tissue and bacteria. Epithelialization is therefore enhanced by limitation of bacterial growth, which is presumed to interfere through the action of bacterial and phagocytic cell products such as proteases, collagenases, elastases, and other enzymes.

ANSWER: b, d

REFERENCE: *Chapter 3—Wound Healing: Open Wounds (Acute)*

11. Which of the following statements is/are true concerning wound contraction?
    a. Wound contraction accounts for similar rates of reduction of wound size regardless of location
    b. The fibroblast, at the cellular level, is the primary force driving wound contraction
    c. Excessive wound contraction over a joint can lead to disability
    d. Actin microfilaments are present in fibroblasts and may have a role in wound contracture

COMMENT: Wound contraction is an important event that contrasts healing open wounds and closed incisions. When open wounds contract, the surrounding skin is pulled over the open wound to reduce its size. This can occur much faster than does epithelialization. Unlike that of other animals, the skin of humans does not have a substantial degree of mobility in most sites. Specifically on the lower leg, the skin is tightly adherent and less elastic than skin in other areas. Although contraction may account for 90% of reduction of wound size on the perineum, it accounts for, at most, 30% to 40% of healing of a lower leg ulcer. All healing wounds generate a strong contractile force. When this force is exerted across a joint, it can cause scar contracture, which can limit the functional range of motion. At the cellular level, the force that drives wound contraction comes from fibroblasts. Fibroblasts, like muscle cells, contain actin microfilaments. When these filaments increase in number, the cells take a morphologic appearance of myofibroblasts. Myofibroblasts are present in increased number in contracting wounds and are believed to have an active role in the process of wound contraction.

ANSWER: b, c, d

REFERENCE: *Chapter 3—Wound Healing: Wound Contraction*

12. Which of the following statements is/are true concerning the clinical management of an open wound?
    a. A wet-to-dry dressing is the most optimal form of wound management
    b. A moist occlusive dressing promotes epithelialization and reduces pain
    c. The protein-rich plasma exudate covering the open wound facilitates healing
    d. Irrigation of the wound disrupts epithelialization and inhibits healing

COMMENT: Epithelialization is more rapid under moist conditions than under dry conditions. Without dressings, a superficial wound or one with minimal devitalized tissue forms a scab or crust, meaning that the blood and serum coagulate, dry, and form a protective moisture barrier over the open wound. If a wound is kept moist with an occlusive dressing, epithelial migration is optimized. The pain of an open wound is dramatically reduced under an occlusive dressing. The traditional wet-to-dry dressing if truly left to dry simply produces desiccation and necrosis of the surface layer of the wound, and epithelialization is delayed. Although wet-to-dry dressings can be effective for débridement of wound exudate, they are generally less desirable than a moist healing environment combined with effective cleaning of the wound (water irrigation). Any open wound leaks plasma. With more inflammation, plasma capillary permeability increases further. This exudate of serum proteins and inflammatory cells serves as a rich culture medium. This continues to cycle bacterial proliferation and leads to further exudate formation. The result of this cycle is delayed or no wound healing. The edema that results from capillary dysfunction increases the distance for diffusion from sources of oxygen and nutrients to their metabolic targets.

ANSWER: b

REFERENCE: *Chapter 3—Wound Healing: Open Wounds (Acute); Clinical Features*

13. Which of the following tissues contain(s) significant collagen useful for placing sutures to allow the prolonged tension necessary to maintain tissue approximation?
    a. Dermis
    b. Intestinal submucosa
    c. Muscular fascia
    d. Blood vessel wall

COMMENT: It takes at least 3 weeks for collagen to undergo sufficient remodeling and cross-linking to attain moderate strength. Because most skin sutures are removed 1 to 2 weeks after they are placed, the wound has only a small fraction of its eventual strength and can disrupt with even modest stress. Therefore deep sutures are placed in collagen-containing structures to maintain the prolonged tension needed. Dermis, intestinal submucosa, muscular fascia, tendon, ligament, Scarpa's fascia, and blood vessel wall represent a partial list of tissues with high collagen content.

ANSWER: a, b, c, d

REFERENCE: *Chapter 3—Wound Healing: Wound Management*

14. Which of the following statements is/are correct concerning the management of an open wound?
    a. Frequent surgical débridement usually is necessary
    b. Water irrigation is effective for débridement of most wounds
    c. Hydrogen peroxide is particularly useful in the management of open wounds
    d. A number of the newer dressing products have been shown to be clearly better than simple moist occlusive dressing in promoting wound healing

COMMENT: Although numerous dressing products are commercially available, no treatment has been demonstrated to improve healing beyond that of standard treatment that adheres to basic principles. In the absence of large amounts of necrotic tissue, wound débridement does not have to be surgical. Simple water irrigation with a whirlpool or a hand-held shower can generate enough power for effective débridement of most wounds. Frequent changes of moist dressings can accomplish this as well. In some cases, occlusive absorptive dressings can generate enough tissue proteases to effectively degrade proteins, which the absorptive dressings remove. Deeper portions of a wound can accumulate exudate and bacteria. In such cases, water irrigation can be particularly useful. Commonly used agents such as hydrogen peroxide actually may be harmful to normal tissue, are weak oxidants, and do a poor job of débridement. Enzymatic débriding agents can be effective when used properly. Most of the newer dressing products have been designed to be more absorptive and to achieve moist healing without infection from excess exudate. However, as long as moist healing is achieved, there has been no evidence that one product is better than another.

ANSWER: b

REFERENCE: *Chapter 3—Wound Healing: Wound Management*

15. Which of the following factors has/have been demonstrated to promote wound healing among healthy persons?
    a. Vitamin A supplementation
    b. Vitamin C supplementation
    c. Application of vitamin E to the wound
    d. Zinc supplementation
    e. None of the above

COMMENT: Several important systemic factors or conditions influence wound healing. No known systemic condition enhances or accelerates wound healing. Overall nutrition and adequate vitamin levels play an important role in wound healing. Vitamin A is involved in stimulation of fibroplasia, collagen cross-linking, and epithelialization. Although there is no conclusive evidence among humans, vitamin A may be useful clinically for steroid-dependent patients who have difficult wounds or who are undergoing extensive surgical procedures. Vitamin C is a necessary cofactor in hydroxylation of lysine and proline in collagen synthesis and cross-linkage. The benefit of vitamin C supplementation to patients who otherwise eat a normal diet has not been established. Vitamin E is applied to wounds and incisions empirically by many patients. The evidence to support this practice is entirely anecdotal. In fact, large doses of vitamin E have been found to inhibit wound healing. Zinc and copper are important cofactors for many enzyme systems that are important to wound healing. Deficiency states occur with parenteral nutrition, but they are rare and readily recognized and controlled with supplements. Overall, vitamin and mineral deficiencies are extremely rare in the absence of parenteral nutrition or other extreme dietary restrictions. There is no evidence to support the concept that supranormal provision of these factors enhances wound healing among normal patients.

ANSWER: e

REFERENCE: *Chapter 3—Wound Healing: Systemic Factors Affecting Wound Healing*

16. Which of the following statements describe(s) the effects of aging on wound healing?
    a. A finer, more cosmetic scar can be expected
    b. Results of in vitro studies show decreased proliferative potential of fibroblasts and epithelial cells
    c. Skin sutures should be left in for a longer period of time
    d. Wound infection occurs more frequently among elderly patients because of diminished ability to fight infection

COMMENT: There are important age-dependent aspects of wound healing. The elderly heal more slowly and with less scarring. There is a gradual attenuation of the inflammatory response with age, and decreased wound healing is one of the consequences. In vitro studies have shown an age-dependent decrease in proliferative potential of fibroblasts and epithelial cells. Clinically this accounts for formation of finer scars and better appearance among the elderly. Sutures should be left in place longer to allow for the slow regain of tensile strength among the aged. This can also be done without concern for formation of suture marks because slower epithelialization occurs along the sutures. There is no evidence to suggest that wound infections occur more commonly among elderly patients.

ANSWER: a, b, c

REFERENCE: *Chapter 3—Wound Healing: Systemic Factors Affecting Wound Healing*

17. Which of the following factors can be associated with impaired wound healing?
    a. Chemotherapy
    b. Long-term use of steroids
    c. Peripheral vascular disease
    d. Radiation therapy
    e. Diabetes mellitus

COMMENT: Bone marrow suppression, a common consequence of chemotherapy, is detrimental to wound healing. Quantitative and qualitative lymphocyte and monocyte deficiency impairs cellular proliferation in the inflammatory phase of wound healing. Any chemotherapeutic agent that suppresses the bone marrow impairs healing. Glucocorticoids inhibit wound healing because of their antiinflammatory and immunosuppressive effects. The antiinflammatory effect of steroids is in part the result of inhibition of arachidonic acid metabolism through impairment of macrophage migration and alteration of neutrophil function. Glucocorticoids also inhibit the synthesis of procollagen by fibroblasts; the result is delayed wound contraction. Radiation injury leads to arteriolar fibrosis and impairment of oxygen delivery. In addition, there is progressive obliteration of blood vessels in the radiated area. Radiation also causes intranuclear and cytoplasmic damage to fibroblasts, and this appears to limit their proliferative potential. Diabetes mellitus often is associated with decreased healing of open wounds and increased susceptibility to infection. Many factors contribute to poor healing among patients with diabetes; most of these factors reflect local wound ischemia. However, healing is not impaired in a normally perfused area when diabetes is well controlled. Peripheral arterial occlusive disease due to atherosclerosis can be a primary cause of impaired healing and can be a cofactor with other conditions.

ANSWER: a, b, c, d, e

REFERENCE: *Chapter 3—Wound Healing: Systemic Factors Affecting Healing*

18. A multitude of dressings are available. Which of the following statements is/are true concerning options for surgical dressings?
    a. Hydrocolloids, such as karaya compounds, offer the primary advantage of increased absorptive ability
    b. Films, such as OpSite, provide a water impermeable environment to achieve a dry wound
    c. Impregnates are fine gauze impregnated with a variety of substances such as antibiotics or moisturizing agents that adhere tightly to the wound and do not require a secondary dressing
    d. Absorptive powders and paste are highly useful in débridement of necrotic and fibrous material from wounds and in absorption of wound serum

COMMENT: Although the simplest dressing of gauze and tape combined with the use of antibacterial ointment can achieve moist wound healing for most patients, a multitude of other products are available. These can be classified into films, foams, hydrocolloids, hydrogels, and absorptive powders. Films are semipermeable to water, generally made of polyurethane, and are nonabsorptive. They are useful to achieve a moist wound-healing environment over a minimally exudative wound such as split-thickness skin graft donor sites. The hydrocolloids deserve special mention because they have achieved widespread use. These agents contain hydrophilic materials such as karaya or carboxymethyl cellulose with an adhesive material and are covered by a semipermeable polyurethane film. The material adheres to the skin surrounding the wound, is highly absorptive, and achieves a moist healing environment. Impregnates are generally fine-mesh gauze impregnated with either moisturizing, antibacterial, or bactericidal compounds. They are generally not adherent and require a secondary dressing. They promote reepithelialization and have an antiinfective effect when combined with antibacterial or bactericidal agents. The variety of absorptive powders and pastes consist of starch copolymers or colloidal hydrophilic particles. These agents have high absorbency for tissue wound fluid and débride necrotic and fibrous material from a wound.

ANSWER: a, d

REFERENCE: *Chapter 3—Wound Healing: Agents to Optimize Wound Healing*

19. Which of the following statements is/are true concerning the role of antibiotics in wound care?
   a. Systemic antibiotics are indicated for all open wounds
   b. Bacterial resistance can occur with systemic but not topical antibiotics
   c. An indication for systemic administration of antibiotics is a granulation tissue bacterial count in excess of 105 organisms per gram of tissue on quantitative analysis
   d. Silver sulfadiazine is useful only for the management of burns

COMMENT: The role of antibiotics in wound care is controversial. All open wounds are colonized with bacteria. Only when surrounding tissue is invaded (cellulitis) are systemic antibiotics clearly indicated. Antibiotics can be useful in other situations, such as when granulation tissue has a high bacterial count (more than 105 organisms per gram tissue), or in the case of reduced resistance to bacteria, such as in a diabetic foot ulcer. The routine use of systemic antibiotics to manage chronic wounds should be avoided to reduce the development of resistant bacterial strains within the wound. Topical ointments can be useful. The topical vehicle can help keep the wound moist, and the bacterial count in the wound may decrease as the result. As with most antibiotics, however, resistant organisms quickly emerge. Silver sulfadiazine, frequently used for burn care, also is useful in the management of chronic wounds. Its broad spectrum of activity, lack of relevant drug-resistant plasmids in bacteria, and its low cost make it a good choice.

ANSWER: c

REFERENCE: *Chapter 3—Wound Healing: Agents to Optimize Wound Healing*

20. Which of the following statements is/are true concerning pharmacologic agents used to accelerate wound healing?
   a. A number of these agents are now currently approved for use in the United States
   b. Platelet-derived growth factor (PDGF) promotes fibroblast proliferation, chemotaxis, and collagenase synthesis
   c. Platelet-derived growth factor has been found in a number of clinical trials to promote healing of chronic wounds
   d. Growth hormone functions by promoting fibroblast proliferation and collagen synthesis

COMMENT: No approved clinical agent accelerates normal healing. Although a number of clinical trials are in progress, no agents are currently approved. Platelet-derived growth factor accelerates wound healing by promoting fibroblast proliferation and chemotaxis and collagenase synthesis. Clinical trials have shown that PDGF accelerates healing in the treatment of patients with chronic wounds, such as pressure sores and diabetic ulcers. Growth hormone has been used successfully in some situations to reverse the catabolic effect of severe injuries. Wound healing is fundamentally an anabolic event, and in the setting of a severe burn, administration of growth hormone accelerates donor site healing, presumably because of its effects in minimizing catabolism.

ANSWER: b, c

REFERENCE: *Chapter 3—Wound Healing: Agents to Optimize Wound Healing*

21. Which of the following statements is/are true concerning excessive scarring?
    a. Keloids occur randomly regardless of sex or race
    b. Hypertrophic scars and keloids are histologically different
    c. Keloids tend to develop early and hypertrophic scars late after the surgical injury
    d. Simple reexcision and closure of a hypertrophic scar can be useful in certain situations, such as a wound that closes by secondary intention

COMMENT: True keloids are uncommon and occur predominantly among dark-skinned persons with a genetic predisposition to keloid formation. In most cases, the gene appears to be transmitted in an autosomal dominant pattern. The primary difference between a keloid and a hypertrophic scar is that a keloid extends beyond the boundary of the original tissue injury. It behaves as a tumor and extends into or invades the normal surrounding tissue to produce a scar larger than the original wound. Keloids and hypertrophic scars are histologically similar. Both contain an overabundance of collagen. Although the absolute number of fibroblasts do not increase, production of collagen continually outpaces the activity of collagenase. The result is a scar of ever-increasing dimensions. Hypertrophic scars respect the boundaries of the original injury and do not extend into normal unwounded tissue. There is less of a genetic predisposition, but hypertrophic scars also occur more frequently among Asian and black populations. Hypertrophic scars often occur on the upper part of the torso and across flexor surfaces. Some improvement in a keloid can be obtained with excision followed by intralesional steroid injection. However, the resulting scar is unpredictable and potentially worse. Reexcision and closure should be considered, however, for hypertrophic scars, if the condition of closure can be improved. This is especially pertinent for wounds that originally healed by secondary intention or are complicated by infection. Keloids typically develop several months after an injury and rarely, if ever, subside. Hypertrophic scars usually develop within the first month after wounding and often subside gradually.

ANSWER: d

REFERENCE: *Chapter 3—Wound Healing: Excessive Scarring*

CHAPTER 4

HEMOSTASIS

1. Which of the following substances, not normally present in the circulation, trigger(s) the initiating events in the hemostatic process?
    a. Thrombin
    b. Platelet factor 3
    c. Tissue factor
    d. Collagen

COMMENT: The initiating agents for hemostasis involve two substances not normally present in the circulation—collagen and tissue factor. Tissue factor is released from injured cells, and this release begins activation of the extrinsic pathway of coagulation. Disruption of the protective endothelial barrier of blood vessels exposes the underlying collagen to the activation of platelets. In the bloodstream, tissue factor forms a complex with factor VII, which activates factor X to factor Xa. At the same time, activated platelets change from their discoid shape with procoagulant phospholipid (platelet factor 3) buried on the inner side of the surface membrane to a spreading shape to allow for externalization of activity of platelet factor 3. Activated factor X, activated factor V, ionized calcium, and factor II (prothrombin) assemble on the platelet phospholipid surface to form the so-called prothrombinase complex, which catalyzes formation of thrombin.

ANSWER: c, d

REFERENCE: *Chapter 4—Hemostasis: Basic Considerations*

2. As thrombin generation proceeds, the body has natural anticoagulant systems that oppose further thrombus formation. Natural anticoagulants include:

a. Tissue plasminogen activator (TPA)
b. Antithrombin III
c. Activated protein C
d. Heparin cofactor II

COMMENT: As thrombin generation is the key to coagulation, antithrombin III is the most central anticoagulant protein. This glycoprotein binds to thrombin and prevents its removal of fibrinoprotein A and B from fibrinogen and prevents activation of factor V and VIII and activation and aggregation of platelets. The second line of defense is activated protein C, which inactivates factors Va and VIIIa. This inactivation decreases the ability of the prothrombinase complex to accelerate the rate of thrombin formation. A third natural anticoagulant is heparin cofactor II. Its concentration in plasma is estimated to be approximately fourfold lower than that of antithrombin III. The action of heparin cofactor II is primarily implicated in the regulation of thrombin formation in extravascular tissues. Tissue plasminogen activator is a natural catalyst for activation of plasminogen to plasmin, the main fibrinolytic enzyme in the body. Therefore TPA is part of the fibrinolytic system rather than a natural anticoagulant.

ANSWER: b, c, d

REFERENCE: *Chapter 4—Hemostasis: Natural Anticoagulant Mechanisms*

3. Which of the following statements is/are true concerning heparin-associated thrombocytopenia?

a. Heparin-associated thrombocytopenia occurs only with excessive anticoagulation with heparin
b. Severe thrombocytopenia (platelet count less than 100,000/μL) occurs among fewer than 10% of patients treated with heparin
c. Heparin-associated thrombocytopenia is caused by aggregation of platelets and can result in thrombosis or embolic episodes
d. Heparin-associated thrombocytopenia can occur within hours of initiation of heparin therapy

COMMENT: Heparin-associated thrombocytopenia occurs among 0.6% to 30% of patients who receive heparin, although severe thrombocytopenia (platelet counts less than 100,000/μL) occurs among fewer than 10% of patients treated with heparin. It is caused by a plasma factor, most likely a heparin-dependent platelet antibody, that causes aggregation of platelets when exposed to heparin. Activation of platelets in this setting results in thrombocytopenia, thrombosis, and embolic episodes, which can lead to death. Both bovine and porcine heparin have been associated with this syndrome, which usually begins 5 to 15 days after initiation of heparin therapy. Even trivial exposure with heparin, such as coating on pulmonary arterial catheters or low-rate infusion into arterial catheters, can cause this syndrome.

ANSWER: b, c

REFERENCE: *Chapter 4—Hemostasis: Procoagulant States*

4. A number of hypercoagulable states can be associated with arterial or venous thrombosis and embolic phenomena. These include:

    a. Heparin-associated thrombocytopenia
    b. Antithrombin III deficiency
    c. Von Willebrand disease
    d. Vitamin C deficiency

COMMENT: A number of hypercoagulable states exist. These include heparin-associated thrombocytopenia, in which heparin-dependent platelet antibodies cause aggregation of platelets when the patient is exposed to heparin. Activation of platelets in this setting results in thrombocytopenia, thrombosis, and embolic episodes. Antithrombin III deficiency accounts for about 2% of venous thrombotic events and has been described in association with pulmonary embolism, mesenteric venous thrombosis, lower extremity venous thrombosis, arterial thrombosis, and dialysis fistula failure. Von Willebrand disease is a hereditary complex coagulation factor deficiency manifested by a reduction of factor VIII activity. Von Willebrand factor is an adhesive protein that mediates platelet adhesion to collagen. Severe vitamin C deficiency results in a disorder in soft tissue that increases vascular permeability and fragility; the result is risk of bleeding disorders.

ANSWER: a, b

REFERENCE: *Chapter 4—Hemostasis: Procoagulant States*

5. Antithrombin III deficiency is a commonly observed hypercoagulable state. Which of the following statements is/are true concerning this condition?

    a. A patient with this deficiency usually has thrombosis while taking heparin or has an inability to achieve adequate anticoagulation with heparin
    b. This deficiency can be either congenital or acquired
    c. Thrombotic episodes are related to predisposing events such as operations, childbirth, and infection
    d. Immediate treatment involves administration of fresh frozen plasma followed by long-term treatment with warfarin

COMMENT: Antithrombin III deficiency accounts for approximately 2% of venous thrombotic events. This deficiency has been described among patients with pulmonary embolism, mesenteric venous thrombosis, lower extremity venous thrombosis, arterial thrombosis, and dialysis fistula failure. Antithrombin III is a serine protease inhibitor of thrombin and factors Xa, IXa, and XIa. Because one of the main actions of heparin is to potentiate the anticoagulant effects of antithrombin III, a patient with this deficiency usually has thrombosis while taking heparin or has an inability to achieve adequate anticoagulation with heparin. This deficiency can be either congenital (1 in 2,000 to 5,000 births) or acquired. Acquired defects occur with inadequate production, as in liver disease, malignant disease, nephrotic syndrome, disseminated intervascular coagulation, malnutrition, or increased protein catabolism. Thrombotic episodes are related to predisposing events such as operations, childbirth, and infections. Once the diagnosis of antithrombin III deficiency is established, fresh frozen plasma is administered and is followed by long-term treatment with warfarin.

ANSWER: a, b, c, d

REFERENCE: *Chapter 4—Hemostasis: Procoagulant States*

6. A 67-year-old man with advanced cholangiocarcinoma has gram-negative sepsis. Excessive bleeding is detected around vascular catheters and from needle puncture sites. The diagnosis of disseminated intervascular coagulation (DIC) is considered. Which of the following laboratory tests is/are indicative of DIC?

a. Decreased platelet count
b. Decreased fibrinogen level
c. Normal prothrombin time
d. Elevated fibrin split products

COMMENT: Disseminated intravascular coagulation is the primary form of acute thrombosis. Causes of this syndrome include abruptio placentae, gram-positive and gram-negative sepsis, endotoxemia, malignant tumors, pelvic operations, certain snake bites, hematologic malignant diseases, and hepatic failure. Blood coagulation is activated by the release of tissue factor into the circulation, which activates factor VII of the extrinsic pathway to VIIa and causes massive thrombin production and fibrin generation. This activates the fibrinolytic system and leads to bleeding in the later stages of the syndrome as the result of consumption of coagulation factors, depletion of fibrinogen, and unchecked plasma activities. Laboratory values for DIC usually include a decline in platelet count and fibrinogen level along with an elevation of fibrin split products.

ANSWER: a, b, d

REFERENCE: *Chapter 4—Hemostasis: Procoagulant States*

7. Which of the following statements is/are true concerning hemophilia A?

a. Hemophilia A is inherited as a sex-linked recessive deficiency of factor VIII
b. All patients have a family history of bleeding disorders
c. Laboratory tests reveal a prolongation of activated partial thromboplastin time (aPTT), prothrombin time (PT), thrombin clotting time (TCT), and platelet aggregation
d. Spontaneous bleeding is unusual with factor VIII levels greater than 10% of normal

COMMENT: Hemophilia A is inherited as a sex-linked recessive deficiency of factor VIII, although no cases are caused by spontaneous mutation. The incidence of this abnormality is approximately 1/10,000 births. Laboratory screening tests usually reveal prolongation of aPTT but normal PT, TCT, and platelet aggregation. The minimum level of VIII required for hemostasis is 30% for minor bleeding; spontaneous bleeding is unusual with factor levels greater than 5% to 10% of normal. In severe genetic deficiency states, however, factor levels as low as 1% have been found, and patients are at risk of spontaneous bleeding.

ANSWER: a, d

REFERENCE: *Chapter 4—Hemostasis: Bleeding Disorders*

8. Which of the following statements is/are true concerning treatment of a patient with hemophilia A undergoing an elective surgical procedure?

    a. Concentrates of factor VIII should be given several days before elective surgical procedures
    b. The half-life of factor VIII concentrates is less than 24 hours
    c. A dose of 40 to 50 IU/kg of factor VIII concentrate should be given before the planned surgical procedure
    d. Factor VIII concentration should be given for the first 24 hours after surgery but can be stopped if no abnormal bleeding has been observed
    e. A new recombinant preparation of factor VIII offers the advantage of being virus free

COMMENT: Although the half-life of factor VIII is 2.9 days in healthy persons, the half-life of factor VIII concentrates is 9 to 18 hours. Levels 80% to 100% of normal should be obtained for surgical bleeding or life-threatening hemorrhage. A dose of 40 to 50 IU/kg factor VIII should be given; one half of this dose is then administered every 12 hours. After surgery, transfusion of factor VIII concentrates should be continued for at least 10 days. Unfortunately, past use of concentrates of factor VIII obtained from donors led to a high incidence of human immunodeficiency virus (HIV) infection among persons with hemophilia. A new recombinant preparation of factor VIII offers the advantage of being virus free.

ANSWER: b, c, e

REFERENCE: *Chapter 4—Hemostasis: Bleeding Disorders*

9. Von Willebrand disease is a common, congenital bleeding disorder. Which of the following statements is/are true concerning von Willebrand disease?

    a. As is hemophilia, it is much more common among men
    b. A history of spontaneous bleeding is common
    c. Screening laboratory test results include a prolonged aPTT with a normal PT
    d. Pretreatment for elective surgery requires administration of cryoprecipitate to achieve levels of 23% to 50% normal

COMMENT: Von Willebrand factor is an adhesive protein that mediates platelet adhesion to collagen. In addition, it protects and prevents rapid removal of factor VIII from blood. The classic deficiency state, von Willebrand disease, is caused by a reduction of factor VIII activity (although not as great as in hemophilia A) and von Willebrand factor. Clinical manifestations include epistaxis, gingival bleeding, menorrhagia, rare joint or muscle bleeding, and subcutaneous bleeding. Spontaneous bleeding is not as common as in classic hemophilia A. The syndrome is transmitted as both an autosomal dominant (heterozygous) and an autosomal recessive (homozygous) trait. Therefore there is no sex predilection. Screening laboratory test results include a prolonged aPTT with a normal PT. Because of the importance of this factor in platelet adhesion, patients have a prolonged bleeding time, and decreased level of factor VIII activity, decreased immunoreactive levels of von Willebrand antigen, and abnormal platelet aggregation responses to ristocetin. The most reliable source of von Willebrand factor is cryoprecipitate.

ANSWER: c, d

REFERENCE: *Chapter 4—Hemostasis: Bleeding Disorders*

10. Which of the following statements is/are correct concerning laboratory studies used in monitoring during intravenous heparinization?

 a. The platelet count should be followed because of the risk of heparin-associated thrombocytopenia
 b. The PT should be followed if prolonged treatment is necessary
 c. The aPTT should be maintained at approximately 1.5 times normal
 d. The serum concentration of creatinine should be measured daily to allow adjustments in dose based on renal function

COMMENT: In monitoring the effect of heparin, an aPTT 1.5 times control or a TCT 2 times control reflects adequate anticoagulation. The PT remains normal. Heparin-associated thrombocytopenia from an immune mechanism is a potential complication of use of this anticoagulant. Any patient undergoing heparin therapy should have a platelet count measured every other day after the fourth day of therapy or earlier if he or she is known to have been exposed to heparin in the past. Heparin is not excreted through the kidneys or the liver but is cleared through the reticuloendothelial system. Therefore the dose of heparin need not be adjusted in cases of liver or renal dysfunction.

ANSWER: a, c

REFERENCE: *Chapter 4—Hemostasis: Pharmacologic and Nonpharmacologic Interventions*

11. Minidose heparin has been shown to be useful in the prophylaxis of postoperative venous thrombosis. Mechanism(s) by which low-dose heparin is/are thought to protect against venous thrombosis include:

 a. Enhancement of antithrombin III activity
 b. A decrease in thrombin availability
 c. Inhibition of platelet aggregation and subsequent platelet release action
 d. Mild prolongation of aPTT

COMMENT: Low-dose heparin is thought to protect against venous thrombosis through three different mechanisms. First, antithrombin III activity with its inhibition of activated factor X is enhanced by only trace amounts of heparin. Second, a decrease in thrombin availability prevents activation and thus its fibrin-stabilizing effect. Third, small doses of heparin can inhibit the second wave of platelet aggregation and subsequent platelet release reaction. The standard dosage of heparin (5,000 units twice a day) does not affect aPTT.

ANSWER: a, b, c

REFERENCE: *Chapter 4—Hemostasis: Pharmacologic and Nonpharmacologic Interventions*

12. Which of the following statements is/are true concerning the results of a National Institutes of Health consensus conference on venous thrombosis and low-dose heparin prophylaxis?

   a. The odds of development of deep venous thrombosis with low-dose heparin prophylaxis decrease 67%
   b. The risk of pulmonary embolism decreases almost 50%
   c. There is no increase in mortality from other causes among patients treated with low-dose heparin
   d. There is no difference in the incidence of bleeding complications

COMMENT: In a metaanalysis of 70 randomized trials involving 16,000 patients and comparing low-dose heparin prophylaxis with standard therapy, the odds of development of deep venous thrombosis with low-dose heparin prophylaxis decreased 67%. For pulmonary embolism (both fatal and nonfatal), the odds decreased 47%. For fatal pulmonary embolism, the odds reduction was even greater (64%). No increase in mortality from other causes was found among patients treated with low-dose heparin. Bleeding complications were more frequent among the heparin-treated patients; there was no difference between 5,000 units twice a day and 5,000 units three times a day. Whether dosage was two or three times a day did not influence the effectiveness of prophylaxis.

ANSWER: a, b, c

REFERENCE: *Chapter 4—Hemostasis: Pharmacologic and Nonpharmacologic Interventions*

13. Standard oral anticoagulant therapy for long-term management of venous thromboembolism is with the drug warfarin. Which of the following statements is/are true concerning the administration of warfarin?

   a. An important complication of warfarin therapy is skin necrosis among patients with protein C deficiency
   b. Warfarin interferes with vitamin K–dependent clotting factors II, VII, IX, and X
   c. For effective anticoagulation, PT should be kept at 2 times control value
   d. It is recommended that warfarin be continued for at least 1 year after the initial episode of deep venous thrombosis

COMMENT: Warfarin interferes with the vitamin K–dependent clotting factors II, VII, IX and X, protein C, and protein S. An important complication of warfarin is skin necrosis among patients with and those without protein C deficiency. This syndrome usually involves full-thickness skin slough over fatty areas such as the breasts and buttocks. Warfarin therapy should be monitored with the one-stage PT. The PT should be kept at 1.3 to 1.4 times control value for effective anticoagulation. At higher levels, there is a fivefold increase in the frequency of bleeding complications. Two important complications of warfarin therapy are recurrent thrombosis and bleeding. It is recommended that warfarin be continued 4 months after an initial episode of deep venous thrombosis. Between 10 weeks and 4 to 6 months after deep venous thrombosis, the rate of recurrent thrombosis is 8.3 episodes per 1,000 patient-months. Between 4 months and 3 years, the recurrence rate decreases to 4 episodes per 1,000 patient-months. At 4 months, the risk of bleeding complications matches and exceeds the benefit from anticoagulant therapy and thus is the basis for discontinuation of administration of warfarin at this time.

ANSWER: a, b

REFERENCE: *Chapter 4—Hemostasis: Pharmacologic and Nonpharmacologic Interventions*

14. Fibrinolytic therapy is based on activation of plasminogen, the inactive proteolytic enzyme of plasma that binds to fibrin during the formation of thrombi. Activation of plasminogen to plasmin results in selective thrombolysis at the fibrin clot surface. Which of the following statements is/are true concerning agents used in thrombolytic therapy?

    a. Streptokinase is a bacterial protein that is antigenic in humans, causing allergic reactions in as many as 15% of cases

    b. Tissue plasminogen activator acts directly on plasmin without an intermediate drug-plasmin complex

    c. The half-life of urokinase, streptokinase, and TPA all exceed 30 minutes

    d. Streptokinase is considerably less expensive than urokinase or TPA

COMMENT: Streptokinase is a bacterial protein produced by group C β-hemolytic streptococci. It is therefore antigenic in humans and can be associated with allergic reactions in 2% to 18% of cases. An unusual form of serum sickness also has been associated with administration of streptokinase. Neither urokinase nor TPA, which is manufactured with recombinant DNA technology, is associated with allergic side effects or antigenicity. Streptokinase acts through a streptokinase plasmin complex, whereas urokinase and TPA act directly on plasmin without an intermediate drug plasmin complex. The level of the lytic state is greatest with streptokinase, intermediate with urokinase, and least with TPA. All half-lives are less than 30 minutes. Although the relative efficacy of the three agents has been compared in a number of studies, there appears to be no appreciable benefit of one agent over another. Streptokinase, however, is markedly less expensive than either urokinase or TPA.

ANSWER: a, b, d

REFERENCE: *Chapter 4—Hemostasis: Pharmacologic and Nonpharmacologic Interventions*

15. Bleeding complications are frequently associated with fibrinolytic therapy. Which of the following statements is/are true concerning the complications of fibrinolytic therapy?

    a. Careful monitoring of PT and aPTT are necessary to avoid bleeding complications

    b. A level of serum fibrinogen less than 100 mg/dL is associated with an increased risk of bleeding

    c. Recent (less than 10 days) major surgery is a contraindication to systemic but not regional fibrinolytic therapy

    d. A patient who has had a cerebrovascular event less than 2 months previously can be treated with fibrinolytic therapy if the results of computed tomography of the head are normal

COMMENT: Fibrinolytic therapy induces a hemostatic defect through a combination of factors. Hypofibrinogenemia and fibrin degradation products inhibit fibrin polymerization. In combination with a decrease in the clotting factors V and VIII, they prolong the ability of blood to clot. However, results of coagulation tests in general do not correlate well with the occurrence of bleeding complications. A level of fibrinogen less than 100 mg/dL is associated with increased risk of bleeding. Absolute contraindications to thrombolytic therapy include active internal bleeding, recent (less than 2 months previously) cerebral vascular accident, and documented left-heart thrombosis. Recent (less than 10 days previously) major surgery, obstetric delivery, organ biopsy, or major trauma is considered a relative contraindication to either regional or systemic thrombolytic therapy.

ANSWER: b

REFERENCE: *Chapter 4—Hemostasis: Pharmacologic and Nonpharmacologic Interventions; Fibrinolytic Agents*

16. Thrombolytic therapy has become a useful adjunct in the management of peripheral arterial occlusion. In this setting, direct intraarterial rather than intravenous administration has been advocated to decrease the risk of systemic bleeding. Which of the following statements is/are true concerning the use of thrombolytic agents for arterial occlusion?

   a. A standard technique involves infusing high-dose urokinase, 4,000 units per minute for 1 to 2 hours, directly into the clot through a catheter embedded in the thrombus
   b. If progress is made, additional fibrinolytic therapy is given at 1,000 to 2,000 units per minute until clot lysis has occurred
   c. The usual infusion time in *c.* usually exceeds 24 hours
   d. Successful clot lysis occurs more frequently in arterial graft occlusions than in native arterial occlusions
   e. The use of intraoperative thrombolytic therapy may be indicated for situations in which complete clot evacuation cannot be accomplished surgically

COMMENT: The most popular method of intraarterial thrombolytic therapy for arterial occlusion involves passing a guidewire through the thrombus with arteriographic guidance and then infusing high-dose urokinase, 4,000 units per minute for 1 to 2 hours, directly into the clot. If progress is made, further fibrinolytic therapy is given at 1,000 to 2,000 units per minute for 6 to 12 hours or until clot lysis has occurred. With this technique, the mean infusion time has been found to be 18 hours, and the incidence of bleeding complications has been markedly decreased. Selective intraarterial infusion of urokinase was associated with complete clot resolution in 77% of native arterial occlusions versus only 41% with arterial graft occlusion. After thrombolytic therapy has reopened an occluded vessel or graft, radiologic or surgical correction of the lesion that caused thrombosis must be addressed for any hope of long-term success. The use of intraoperative thrombolytic therapy is advocated in situations in which complete clot resolution cannot be accomplished, such as after balloon embolectomy for acute arterial occlusion, or when occlusion of distal blood vessels precludes appropriate inflow patency.

ANSWER: a, b, e

REFERENCE: *Chapter 4—Hemostasis: Pharmacologic and Nonpharmacologic Interventions*

17. External pneumatic compression has been advocated for the prevention of deep venous thrombosis during operative procedures. Which of the following statements is/are true concerning the use of external pneumatic compression devices?

   a. Intermittent pneumatic compression is as effective as low-dose heparin in prevention of venous thrombosis
   b. These devices function by compressing the lower extremities and augmenting venous return
   c. Pneumatic compression devices can exert their antithrombotic effect through stimulation of local and systemic fibrinolysis
   d. The duration of intermittent pneumatic compression includes the entire operation and at least several days in the postoperative period

COMMENT: In many well-controlled studies of venous prophylaxis, intermittent pneumatic compression has been found to be as effective as low-dose heparin therapy. In addition to augmentation of venous return with these devices, local and systemic fibrinolysis appears to be stimulated. Fibrinolytic activity usually decreases for 7 to 10 days after an operation. Studies have shown that the pneumatic compression devices exert their antithrombotic effect through prevention of this fibrinolytic shutdown, even when the devices are applied to the upper extremity. The duration of intermittent pneumatic compression has not been adequately determined. Most data suggest that devices should be used through the operation and for at least 5 days in the face of prolonged immobilization.

ANSWER: b, c, d

REFERENCE: *Chapter 4—Hemostasis: Pharmacologic and Nonpharmacologic Interventions*

18. Laboratory monitoring of coagulation and anti-coagulation includes testing of platelet function. Which of the following statements is/are true concerning tests of platelet function?

    a. A platelet count of 50,000/µL or more usually ensures hemostasis
    b. Bleeding time assays are used to assess the ability of platelets to form hemostatic plugs and is determined from a sample of blood drawn in an EDTA-coated test tube
    c. Aspirin therapy can be associated with a bleeding time in the range of 8 to 15 minutes
    d. Tests of platelet aggregation should be part of the standard preoperative evaluation of patients using aspirin

COMMENT: Tests of platelet function include peripheral platelet count, bleeding times, and platelet aggregation. A platelet count of 50,000/µL or more usually ensures adequate hemostasis, whereas counts less than 10,000/µL are dangerous and can lead to spontaneous bleeding. Bleeding time, measured by means of observing the clotting of blood induced with a small needle stick, is used to assess the ability of platelets to form hemostatic plugs and usually is shorter than 8 minutes. A bleeding time between 8 and 15 minutes most often reflects a low plasma level of von Willebrand factor or use of antiplatelet drugs. A bleeding time greater than 15 minutes is clearly prolonged and indicates severe impairment of platelet function. Platelet aggregation studies involve the use of a number of different agonists. Although a relatively straightforward technique, platelet aggregation is not available in most laboratories, probably because of the observer-dependent nature of the test.

ANSWER: a, c

REFERENCE: *Chapter 4—Hemostasis: Laboratory Monitoring of Coagulation and Anticoagulation*

19. Tests of coagulation are used to monitor anticoagulation treatment and detect intrinsic abnormalities in coagulation. Which of the following statements is/are true concerning coagulation tests?

    a. Prothrombin time is a measurement of both the intrinsic and extrinsic clotting pathways and fibrinogen
    b. Activated partial thromboplastin time can be used to monitor both oral anticoagulation with warfarin and intravenous anticoagulation with heparin
    c. Thrombin clotting time is a measurement of the time it takes for exogenously administered thrombin to turn plasma fibrinogen into fibrin clot
    d. Whole-blood activated clotting time (ACT) is a measurement of the ability of whole blood to clot and is used for intraoperative monitoring of heparin levels during cardiovascular and peripheral vascular operations

COMMENT: Coagulation tests include PT, which is a measurement of the intrinsic and extrinsic pathways of fibrinogen production and is the most common method for measuring a level of oral anticoagulant therapy. The aPTT is used to identify abnormalities of the contact and intrinsic phases of coagulation. Values of aPTT have variably been shown to correlate with heparin doses and serum heparin levels and are therefore most commonly used in monitoring heparin therapy. Activated partial thromboplastin time is of no value in long-term care of patients undergoing oral warfarin therapy. Thrombin clotting time is the time it takes for exogenously administered thrombin to turn plasma fibrinogen into fibrin clot. It is extremely sensitive to levels of heparin and is an excellent measurement of the level of heparin-induced anticoagulation. The beauty of TCT is that it is not specific for any disease or condition; it can be used to differentiate factor deficiencies from the presence of heparin or to separate lupus anticoagulant from abnormalities in fibrinogen levels. Whole-blood ACT is a measurement of the ability of whole blood to clot. As such it can be used for intraoperative monitoring of heparin levels. The ACT responds in a linear manner to increasing heparin doses and correlates well with observed clinical anticoagulation. Adequate anticoagulation for extracorporeal circulation is defined as an ACT of 480 seconds or more. For peripheral vascular applications, values of 250 seconds or greater are considered appropriate.

ANSWER: a, c, d

REFERENCE: *Chapter 4—Hemostasis: Laboratory Monitoring of Coagulation and Anticoagulation*

20. Transfusions of blood products can be associated with a number of complications, including immediate and delayed hemolytic reactions, nonhemolytic reactions, infectious disease transmission, and complications of massive transfusions. Which of the following statements is/are true concerning complications of blood transfusion?

a. Immediate hemolytic transfusion reactions are caused by major ABO blood group incompatibility
b. Nonhemolytic transfusion reactions usually are caused by Rh factor incompatibility and are therefore more common among women of childbearing age
c. The most common complication of massive blood transfusion is dilutional thrombocytopenia
d. Routine empiric calcium supplementation is necessary during most massive transfusion episodes

COMMENT: Immediate hemolytic reactions usually are caused by blood group ABO incompatibility, although they can be caused by antigens of other blood group systems on the transfused red blood cells. The clinical manifestations revolve around the antigen on the red blood cell stroma and the antibody in the patient's serum. The manifestations include production of bradykinin, complement activation, release of vasoactive agents from platelets, and initiation of systemic clotting. Chills and fever, chest and lumbar pain, tachycardia, and hypotension if the patient is conscious and diffuse bleeding if the patient is anesthetized or unconscious constitute this syndrome. Although the reaction occurs immediately, death related to the syndrome is uncommon, unless more than 100 mL of blood has been transfused. Death usually occurs from acute renal failure or hemorrhage due to DIC. Nonhemolytic reactions occur with a frequency of 1% to 2% of all transfusions and consist primarily of chills and fevers during the transfusion or in the first 2 to 3 hours after the transfusion is complete. The mechanism of these reactions includes the presence of antibodies to white blood cell antigens in the transfused blood, especially if the patient has had numerous transfusions or is multiparous. Complications of massive transfusion are related to the rate and volume of blood transfused. The most common complication is dilutional thrombocytopenia. Factor deficiency of the labile factors V and VIII rarely is of sufficient magnitude to cause problems with hemostasis. For hypocalcemia to occur with massive transfusion, citrated blood must be administered 1 unit every 5 minutes. Routine empiric calcium supplementation is unnecessary during most massive transfusion episodes. Hypothermia is a problem, especially when associated with massive transfusion during complex operative procedures such as resection of a thoracoabdominal aneurysm.

ANSWER: a, c

REFERENCE: *Chapter 4—Hemostasis: Risks of Blood Transfusions*

21. Transmission of infectious diseases during blood transfusions is of clinical significance to surgeons and of importance to patients considering undergoing operations associated with the possible need for blood administration. Which of the following statements is/are true concerning the transmission of infectious disease during blood transfusions?

a. Posttransfusion hepatitis usually is caused by hepatitis B virus
b. Transmission of hepatitis virus and HIV is greatest with administration of pooled plasma products such as serum albumin
c. The most important cause of posttransfusion disease among immunosuppressed patients is cytomegalovirus (CMV) infection
d. The risk of transmission of HIV in blood transfusions is considerably less than the risk of hepatitis transmission

COMMENT: The most common infectious diseases transmitted during blood transfusions are viral hepatitis, CMV, and HIV infection. In 90% of cases posttransfusion hepatitis consists of non-A, non-B hepatitis, known as *hepatitis C.* All blood products except for immune serum globulin and albumin can carry and transmit this form of hepatitis. Because heat treatment eliminates the risk of virus transmission, heat-treated products from pooled plasma, such as albumin, are not at risk of transmission of HIV or hepatitis virus. Transmission of CMV exists in three forms—primary, reinfection, and reactivation. Primary exposure results in an IgM response to the virus. Reactivation is most commonly related to pregnancy, transplantation, and immunosuppression. It is the most important cause of posttransfusion disease accompanying immunosuppression. Although the degree of the public concern for transmission of HIV disease associated with blood transfusions has outweighed that of transmission of other infectious diseases, the risk of HIV transmission is markedly less than that of hepatitis.

ANSWER: c, d

REFERENCE: *Chapter 4—Hemostasis: Risks of Blood Transfusions*

CHAPTER 5

CYTOKINES

1. Cytokines with clearly defined actions in acute inflammation and early tissue injury include which of the following?

a. Cysteine-X-cysteine (C-X-C) chemokines
b. Tumor necrosis factor α (TNF-α)
c. Transforming growth factor β (TGF-β)
d. Interleukin-6 (IL-6)
e. Platelet-derived growth factor (PDGF)

COMMENT: Polypeptide mediators, such as TNF-α and IL-1, are considered "early response" cytokines and are actively involved in the initiation of the cascade of events that precipitate acute inflammation. In addition to being important triggers for the induction of other cytokines important in the inflammatory network, TNF-α and IL-1 appear to be key mediators in promoting the adherence of inflammatory cells to the endothelium. Interleukin-1 is a complex, multifunctional molecule that shares many overlapping biologic properties with TNF-α. Interleukin-1 and TNF-α potentiate the effects of one another. The most important function of IL-6 appears to be regulation of the hepatic acute-phase response. After injury, a number of physiologic changes occur within several hours. Interleukin-6 is one of the primary stimuli for the production of acute-phase proteins from the liver. Endotoxin, IL-1, TNF-α, and PDGF can induce IL-6 synthesis.

At least 12 C-X-C chemokines have been identified. These include IL-8, one of the most potent mediators of chemotaxis. Tumor necrosis factor-α and IL-1 are key molecules for the induction of IL-8, which is important for induction of neutrophil recruitment and activation. Similar properties are apparent for other members of this chemokine family.

Platelet activation and degranulation occur during coagulation after injury and lead to deposition of a number of cytokines into the provisional matrix. These cytokines include TGF-α, TGF-β, PDGF, and neutrophil-activating peptide 2 (NAP-2). These cytokines are either important growth factors or chemotaxis for leukocytes, endothelial cells, fibroblasts, and keratinocytes, which are key components in the process of tissue repair. Thus coagulation and platelet activation provide the initial foundation for subsequent cellular recruitment.

ANSWER: a, b, c, d, e

REFERENCE: *Chapter 5—Cytokines*

2. Which of the following statements is/are true regarding TNF-α?

    a. Tumor necrosis factor-α has a marked procoagulant effect

    b. Passive immunization of patients with neutralizing antibodies to TNF-α improves survival from multiple organ system failure

    c. Tumor necrosis factor-α up-regulates expression of E-selectin

    d. The most potent known stimulus for production and release of TNF-α is IL-1

COMMENT: Tumor necrosis factor-α has a marked procoagulant effect on endothelial cells and precipitates intravascular thrombosis. Tumor necrosis factor-α causes endothelial cells to release procoagulant activity (tissue factor), platelet activating factor, and von Willebrand factor, all of which favor thrombosis. Tumor necrosis factor-α also down-regulates the expression of thrombomodulin, which can block the assembly of protein C and protein S complexes and further decrease the anticoagulant properties of the endothelial cell surfaces.

Administration of recombinant TNF-α to experimental animals produces a clinical syndrome similar to septic shock and multiple organ system failure among humans. Passive immunization of animals with neutralizing antibodies against TNF-α before infusion of TNF-α or endotoxin has been shown to prevent development of this syndrome. No such evidence exists for human patients. Tumor necrosis factor-α up-regulates a variety of leukocytic adhesion molecules, including ICAM-1, PECAM-1, VCAM-1, E-selectin, and P-selectin. A variety of exogenous and endogenous factors, including IL-1, are capable of inducing cells to produce TNF-α; however, the most potent stimulus for production and release of TNF-α is endotoxin.

ANSWER: a, c

REFERENCE: *Chapter 5—Cytokines: Inflammation; Table 5.1*

3. Which of the following statements is/are correct regarding IL-1?

    a. Although IL-1 and TNF-α share many biologic effects, IL-1 appears to be more potent

    b. Interleukin-1 expression is autoregulated in part

    c. Interleukin-1 inhibits prostaglandin production

    d. The ability of IL-1 to up-regulate endothelial cell neutrophil adhesion molecules is relatively limited

COMMENT: Interleukin-1 and TNF-α share many biologic properties. In addition, each potentiates the effects of the other when given concurrently. Overall, IL-1 alone probably has weaker effects than does TNF-α with respect to the induction of shock. The role of IL-1 is likely to be important with respect to its marked potentiating abilities as it relates to TNF-α. Expression of IL-1 is regulated by a host of factors, including IL-2, granulocyte-macrophage colony-stimulating factor (GM-CSF), TGF-β, TNF-α, all of the interferons, and IL-1 itself. Other endogenous stimuli of IL-1 production include antigen-antibody complex, the Fc region of IgG, and C5a. Other nonspecific exogenous stimuli include silica particles and ultraviolet radiation.

One of the key proinflammatory features of IL-1–induced inflammation is stimulation of arachidonic acid metabolism. Interleukin-1 stimulates the release of pituitary stress hormones and increases the synthesis of collagenases. The result is destruction of cartilage, bone, and other collagen-rich structures. Interleukin-1 stimulates prostaglandin production.

One of the most important properties of IL-1 involves its interaction with the vascular endothelium. This includes the adherence of neutrophils, basophils, eosinophils, monocytes, and lymphocytes to the vascular endothelium through interaction between adhesion molecules on leukocytes and adhesion-receptor complexes on the endothelial cells. By inducing expression of ICAM-1, E-selectin, and VCAM-1 on endothelial cells, IL-1 provides a key step in the extravasation of leukocytes to sites of local inflammation and injury.

ANSWER: b

REFERENCE: *Chapter 5—Cytokines: Inflammation*

4. A 65-year-old patient has carcinoma of the colon metastatic to the liver and lungs. He has had a weight loss of 10 kg. Cytokine-dependent tumor cachexia is attributable to which of the following?

a. Increased glucose uptake and increased glycogen breakdown occur in this circumstance.
b. Suppressed activity of lipoprotein lipase results from presence of TNF-α
c. Tumor necrosis factor-α stimulates lipolysis
d. The differentiation process of preadipocytes is impaired
e. Partial reversal of differentiated adipocytes to preadipocyte morphologic features and gene expression occurs

COMMENT: Tumor cachexia appears to be mediated by TNF-α. Lipopolysaccharide and other cytokines activate a variety of inflammatory cells, most importantly macrophages, to produce TNF-α. Both long-term administration of TNF-α to rats and implantation of tumors secreting TNF-α in mice induce a syndrome of cachexia. In vitro, higher TNF-α concentrations alter glucose metabolism in cultured myotubules by increasing glucose uptake and glycogen breakdown. It has also been demonstrated that purified TNF-α suppresses lipoprotein lipase activity and stimulates lipolysis in cultured adipocytes. Further, TNF-α not only inhibits differentiation of preadipocytes but also partially reverses differentiated adipocytes to a preadipocyte structure and pattern of gene expression. All of these metabolic effects at least partially explain the chronic syndromes of anorexia, weight loss, and cachexia associated with both chronic infection and malignant disease.

ANSWER: a, b, c, d, e

REFERENCE: *Chapter 5—Cytokines: Inflammation; Table 5.2*

5. Leukocyte activation and adhesion to vascular endothelial cells is a critical step in the inflammatory process. This process is regulated by which of the following molecules?

a. The selectins
b. The β_5 integrins
c. The immunoglobulin supergene family
d. Nitric oxide
e. Interleukin-8

COMMENT: The temporal events that initiate and propagate neutrophil recruitment and inflammation include endothelial cell activation and expression of endothelium-derived neutrophil adhesion molecules, neutrophil-endothelial cell adherence, and neutrophil transendothelial migration through established neutrophil chemotactic gradients. Three major families of adhesion molecules are expressed on the surface of leukocytes and endothelial cells and are important for leukocyte-endothelial cell interactions. These include the immunoglobulin supergene family (ICAM-1, VCAM-1, and PECAM-1), the selectins (E-selectin, P-selectin, and L-selectin), and the integrins. The leukocyte β_2 integrin adhesion molecule family consists of three members with heterodimeric glycoproteins displayed as a variable α and a constant β chain. Nitric oxide regulates adhesion by means of both direct influence on leukocyte binding and regulation of regional blood flow. Interleukin-8 is one of the most potent mediators of chemotaxis in the C-X-C chemokine family. It serves an important role in neutrophil recruitment and activation and continued propagation of the inflammatory response.

ANSWER: a, c, d, e

REFERENCE: *Chapter 5—Cytokines: Inflammation*

6. Neutrophil chemotaxis is a fundamental aspect of inflammatory injury in conditions such as adult respiratory distress syndrome. Neutrophil chemotaxis is directly attributable to which of the following molecules?

   a. C5a
   b. Tumor necrosis factor-α
   c. Lipopolysaccharide
   d. Interleukin-1
   e. Epithelial neutrophil-activating protein

COMMENT: A large collection of peptide, polypeptide, and lipid mediators have chemotactic properties. Although TNF-α, IL-1, and lipopolysaccharide were initially reported to have direct neutrophil chemotactic activity, studies have shown that these molecules are not directly chemotactic for neutrophils. This finding suggests that cytokine networks may be operative in vivo and depend on the initial expression of early response cytokines. This initial interaction is followed by the generation of more distal inflammatory mediators that directly influence neutrophil chemotaxis and activation. A particularly important group of novel chemotactic cytokines share homologic features with the presence of four conserved cysteine amino acid residues. These cytokines in their monomeric forms are all less than 10 kd, are characteristically basic heparin-binding proteins, have specific neutrophil chemotactic activity, and display four highly conserved cysteine amino acid residues, the first two cysteines separated by one nonconserved amino acid residue. Because of their chemotactic properties and the presence of C-X-C cysteine motif, these have been designated the *C-X-C chemokine family*. Twelve different chemokines have been identified in the last decade. These include IL-8, epithelial neutrophil activating protein, and others. Among the other endogenous chemoattractants are several complement-derived peptides. Perhaps the most potent of these is the short-lived C5a peptide.

ANSWER: a, e

REFERENCE: *Chapter 5—Cytokines: Inflammation*

7. Which of the following statements is/are true regarding angiogenesis?

   a. Angiogenesis is a seminal biologic event with clinical relevance limited to its effect on tumor growth
   b. C-X-C chemokines regulate angiogenesis
   c. Platelet factor 4 has angiogenic properties
   d. Sites of atherosclerosis demonstrate chronic angiogenic activity

COMMENT: An important component of tissue repair and wound healing is angiogenesis. This normal, physiologic process is a local, transient event that is regulated strictly. A biologic imbalance in the production of angiogenic and angiostatic factors contributes to the pathogenesis of several angiogenesis-dependent disorders. These include both malignant and nonmalignant disorders, such as rheumatoid arthritis, scleroderma, psoriasis, atherosclerosis, and idiopathic pulmonary fibrosis. Persistent neovascularization in these benign disorders is a prerequisite for the perpetuation of fibroproliferation. Interleukin-8 and possibly other C-X-C chemokines are involved in angiogenesis. Interleukin-8 is a potent angiogenic factor. In contrast, another member of the C-X-C chemokine family, platelet factor 4, has angiostatic properties. This suggests that the C-X-C chemokines may function as either angiostatic or angiogenic factors and that the biologic balance between these factors may govern overall angiogenic potential in a variety of physiologic and pathophysiologic states.

ANSWER: b, d

REFERENCE: *Chapter 5—Cytokines: Wound Healing*

8. Which of the following statements is/are true regarding fibroblasts and their function in wound healing?
   a. Interleukin-1 has both inhibitory and promotional effects on fibroblast growth
   b. Tumor necrosis factor-α stimulates fibroblast collagen synthesis
   c. Interleukin-1 and TNF-α have opposite effects on the healing of bone
   d. In clinical trials, epithelial growth factor (EGF) has been found to accelerate epidermal regeneration in cutaneous wounds

COMMENT: Interleukin-1 appears to be important in the process of normal wound repair. Interleukin-1 has been shown to stimulate skin fibroblast and keratinocyte growth, fibroblast collagen synthesis, and keratinocyte chemotaxis. Interleukin-1 also promotes increased transcription of the matrix degradative enzymes collagenase and stromelysin. These are important and potent tissue-degrading proteinases. Other studies have shown that IL-1 inhibits fibroblast growth and matrix synthesis and stimulates collagenase production. These actions are at least partly caused by the ability of IL-1 to up-regulate production of prostaglandin E_2, which results in down-regulation of matrix synthesis. Interleukin-1 has both promoting and inhibiting effects on fibroblast collagen synthesis; therefore the overall activity in this area is somewhat unclear in comparison with other well-defined fibroblast growth-promoting cytokines. Tumor necrosis factor α inhibits fibroblast collagen synthesis, but it also has potent mitogenic effects. The mitogenic response correlates well with increased stimulation of tyrosine phosphorylation. Interleukin-1 and TNF-α have similar effects on bone. Both stimulate cartilage resorption and release of proteoglycans from cartilage by limited proteolytic degradation, and both inhibit proteoglycan synthesis. Studies also have shown that TNF-α inhibits fracture healing in experimental animals. This is the result of inhibition of cartilage formation and new bone synthesis and inhibition of mesenchymal cell differentiation into chondroblasts. The family of EGF-like molecules induces mitogenesis and has a role in wound healing. In clinical trials, EGF has been found to accelerate epidermal regeneration in cutaneous wounds. In vitro data show that recombinant EGF enhances keratinocyte migration. Epithelial growth factor also is a potent chemoattractant for granulation tissue fibroblasts.

ANSWER: a, d

REFERENCE: *Chapter 5—Cytokines: Wound Healing*

9. Which of the following statements is/are true regarding TGF-β?
   a. Expression of TGF-β is autoregulated
   b. Transforming growth factor β enhances collagen synthesis
   c. Transforming growth factor β inhibits extracellular matrix production
   d. Transforming growth factor β can inhibit or promote cellular proliferation

COMMENT: Transforming growth factor β appears to be one of the key cytokines in control of tissue repair. It is strongly chemotactic for neutrophils, T cells, monocytes, and fibroblasts. Transforming growth factor b activates inflammatory cells to elaborate fibroblast growth factor, TNF-α, and IL-1 and to increase synthesis of extracellular matrix proteins. Transforming growth factor β also induces both infiltrating cells and resident cells to produce more TGF-β. This autoinduction amplifies the biologic effects of TGF-β at the site of injury and may play an important role in the development of chronic fibrosis in a variety of pathologic states. Transforming growth factor b also enhances collagen synthesis. It also may function as a mitogen or growth inhibitor for a variety of cell types, including selected cell types of mesenchymal origin. Whether TGF-β stimulates or inhibits proliferation depends on the presence of other growth factors, the concentration of TGF-β, and cell density. At low doses, TGF-β stimulates the proliferation of densely plated human marrow fibroblasts but is inhibitory at high concentrations.

ANSWER: a, b, d

REFERENCE: *Chapter 5—Cytokines: Wound Healing; Table 5.6*

10. Which of the following belong(s) to the family of C-X-C chemokines?

    a. Interleukin-8
    b. Interleukin-10
    c. Growth related oncogene-α
    d. Leukotriene B_4
    e. β-Thromboglobulin

COMMENT: A particularly important group of novel chemotactic cytokines has been elucidated. The following 12 are known:

C-X-C chemokines
Connective tissue activating protein III
β-Thromboglobulin
Growth-regulated oncogene α
Growth-regulated oncogene β
Growth-regulated oncogene γ
Interleukin-8
Epithelial neutrophil activating protein
Granulocyte chemotactic protein-2
Platelet factor 4
γ-Interferon-inducible protein
Monokine induced by interferon-γ

Each has unique biologic functions. Important in vivo cytokine networks appear to involve these molecules and regulate chemotaxis and other fundamental aspects of inflammation.

ANSWER: a, c, e

REFERENCE: *Chapter 5—Cytokines: Inflammation; Table 5.7*

CHAPTER 6

INFLAMMATION

1. Which of the following acute-phase protein levels is/are increased in human plasma after acute inflammation?

    a. C-reactive protein
    b. HSP Fo
    c. Chaperonics
    d. Fibrinogen
    e. Albumin

COMMENT: The acute-phase response is a series of homeostatic responses of the organism to tissue injury infection and inflammation. After an inflammatory stimulus, a number of events occur within hours. These reflect altered set points for various physiologic mechanisms, including thermoregulation (fever), nitrogen balance (negative), and changes in levels of various plasma proteins (increases or decreases). Erythrocyte sedimentation rate, which increases with inflammatory states, is an example of this phenomenon. The increase in sedimentation rate is caused by increases in levels of fibrinogen and some of the other acute-phase reactants in plasma. The heat shock proteins are important participants in this stress response, particularly HSP Fo and the HSP Fo family (chaperonins). Some proteins have a large increase (approximately 1,000-fold), some a twofold to fivefold increase, and others an approximately 50% increase over resting, nonstressed levels. These are summarized in Table 6.1. Albumin is an acute-phase reactant. Levels of albumin decrease after an inflammatory stimulation, usually 30% to 50% of the level before injury. The reason for the decrease in production is poorly understood.

ANSWER: a, b, c , d

REFERENCE: *Chapter 6—Inflammation: Integration of the Inflammatoy Components; Acute-phase Response*

Table 6.1. RESPONSES OF SOME HUMAN ACUTE-PHASE PROTEINS

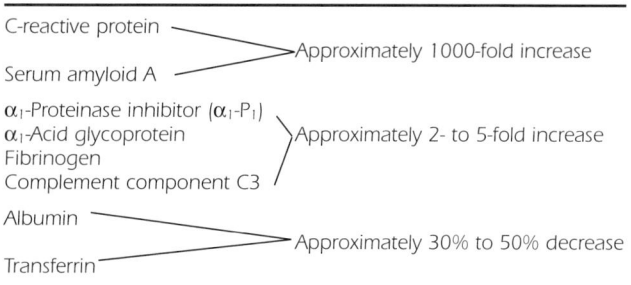

C-reactive protein
Serum amyloid A
— Approximately 1000-fold increase

α_1-Proteinase inhibitor (α_1-P$_1$)
α_1-Acid glycoprotein
Fibrinogen
Complement component C3
— Approximately 2- to 5-fold increase

Albumin
Transferrin
— Approximately 30% to 50% decrease

2. Which of the following statements regarding the complement system is/are true?

a. Complement activation yields products that are directly cytotoxic as well as products that act indirectly through activated leukocytes

b. Complement products called *anaphylatoxins* include C1, C3a, C4a, and C5a

c. The principal role of C5a is bacterial opsonization

d. The alternative and classic pathways converge proximal to the site of generation of the membrane attack complex (C5b-9)

COMMENT: The complement system is composed of two different but linked sequences—the classic and alternative pathways. The pathways involve serum proteins that amplify the inflammatory-immune response and directly mediate tissue injury. Complement activation along either pathway has been associated with a cascade of events, some of which are mediated directly at a physiologic level by complement products and some of which occur indirectly through activated leukocytes. The direct physiologic effects mediated by C3a and C5a, and to a lesser extent C4a, include increased vascular permeability and contraction of smooth muscle. These are key elements of anaphylaxis. C1 is not an anaphylatoxin because it is the initial complement component that binds to antigen-antibody complex to initiate activation of the classic pathway. C5a acts principally to alter the behavioral characteristics of leukocytes. Effects include enhanced adherence, enhanced chemotactic activity, release of proteinases, and production of toxic metabolites of oxygen. C3, on the other hand, plays a key role in bacterial opsonization; the result is enhanced phagocytosis of invading microorganisms. The alternative and classic complement pathways converge at the C5 level proximal to the site of generation of the membrane attack complex (C5b-9) (Fig. 6.3).

ANSWER: a, d

REFERENCE: *Chapter 6—Inflammation: Humoral Components of Inflammation; The Complement System*

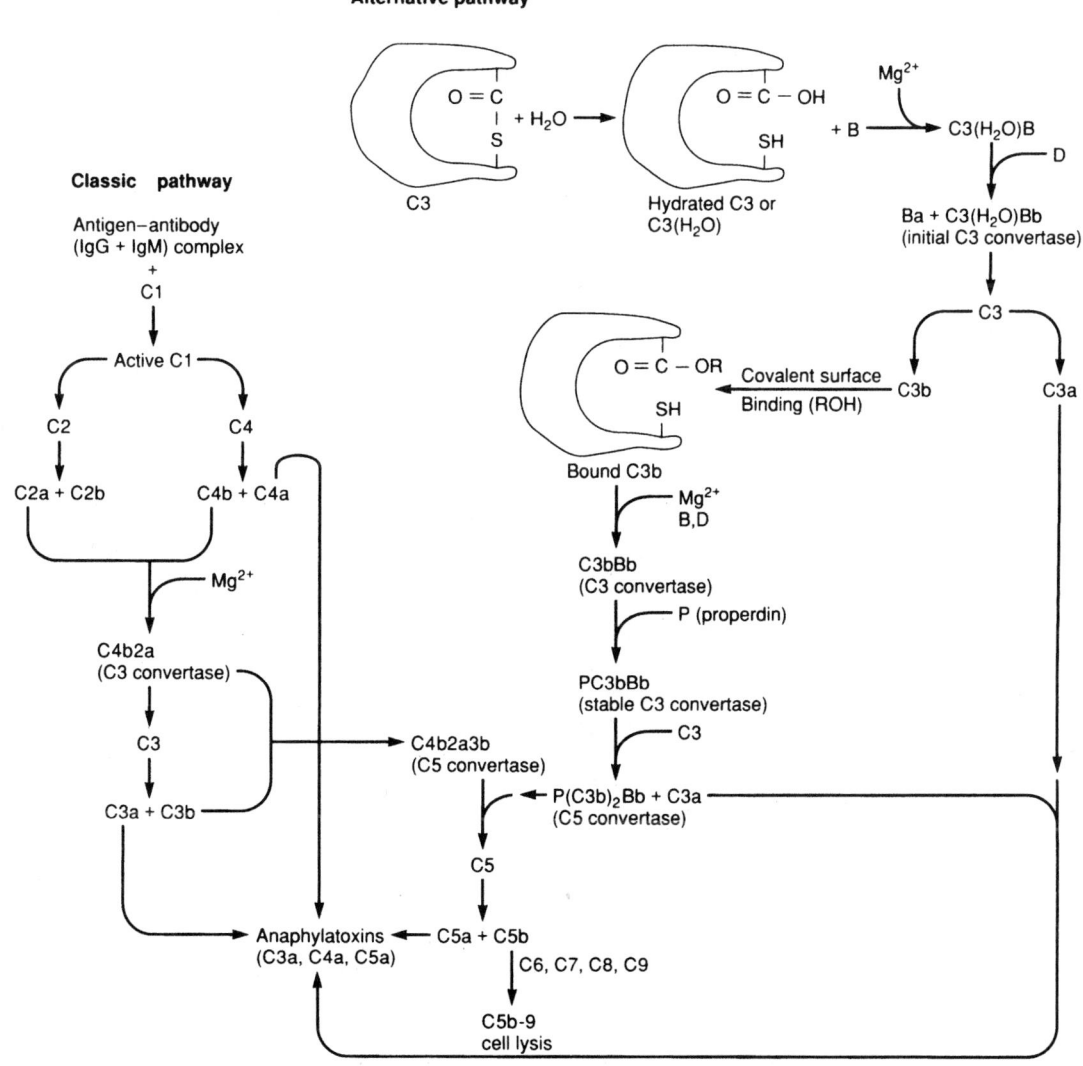

Figure 6.3

3. Which of the following statements regarding the alternative complement pathway is/are true?

   a. C1, C4, and C2 are involved
   b. Ammonia NH_3 apparently activates complement along this pathway
   c. Factors B and D are involved
   d. Endotoxin activates complement along the alternative pathway

COMMENT: The alternative pathway differs from the classic pathway in that the first steps involving C1, C4, and C2 are bypassed. (See Fig. 6.14 previously reproduced.) This pathway can be directly activated by agents other than antigen-antibody complex (e.g., complex polysaccharides such as endotoxin and zymosan). Other serum protein factors (e.g., factors B and D) are involved in the activation sequence. Ammonia can attack the thiol ester, produce amidated C3, and activate the alternative pathway. This leads to formation of the membrane attack complex (C5b-9) and activation of a number of phagocytic cell functions, including production of toxic oxidants. This phenomenon may have relevance to several in vivo disease states. In animal models of renal failure, elevated levels of renal vein ammonia have correlated with impaired renal function and the presence of complement components at the sites of renal injury.

ANSWER: b, c, d

REFERENCE: *Chapter 6—Inflammation: Humoral Components of Inflammation; The Complement System*

4. Eicosanoids mediate inflammation in a variety of ways. Of the following statements, which is/are true with regard to this?

   a. Eicosanoids are stored in cytoplasmic granules for release after receptor-mediated signaling
   b. Eicosanoids include prostaglandins, thromboxanes, leukotrienes, and lipoxins
   c. Eicosanoids generally have a plasma half-life measured in hours
   d. Physiologic responses to eicosanoids include vasodilation, vasoconstriction, increased vascular permeability, and both chemotaxis and chemoattractant inhibition

COMMENT: The eicosanoids are derived from arachidonic acid (eicosatetraenoic acid) and consist of prostaglandins, thromboxanes, leukotrienes, and lipoxins. The eicosanoids are not stored in cells but are rapidly synthesized by cells in response to a variety of stimuli. They have potent effects on vascular and bronchial smooth muscle, including vasodilation, vasoconstriction, bronchodilation, and bronchoconstriction. They also directly regulate vascular permeability. Leukotriene B_4 is a potent neutrophil chemoattractant, whereas lipoxin A_4 inhibits other chemoattractants. It appears that eicosanoids are important regulators of the endogenous inflammatory response. The rapid destruction of eicosanoids in the circulation limits their role primarily to that of mediators of local inflammatory changes. The local effects can be substantial. In general, the eicosanoids are rapidly metabolized or are so chemically unstable that they primarily exert their effects near the site of synthesis. Arachidonic acid does not exist in cells but is esterified to membrane phospholipids. Thus the first step in production of eicosanoids is phospholipase action, which liberates arachidonic acid (Fig. 6.15).

ANSWER: b, d

REFERENCE: *Chapter 6—Inflammation: Humoral Components of Inflammation; Lipid Mediators*

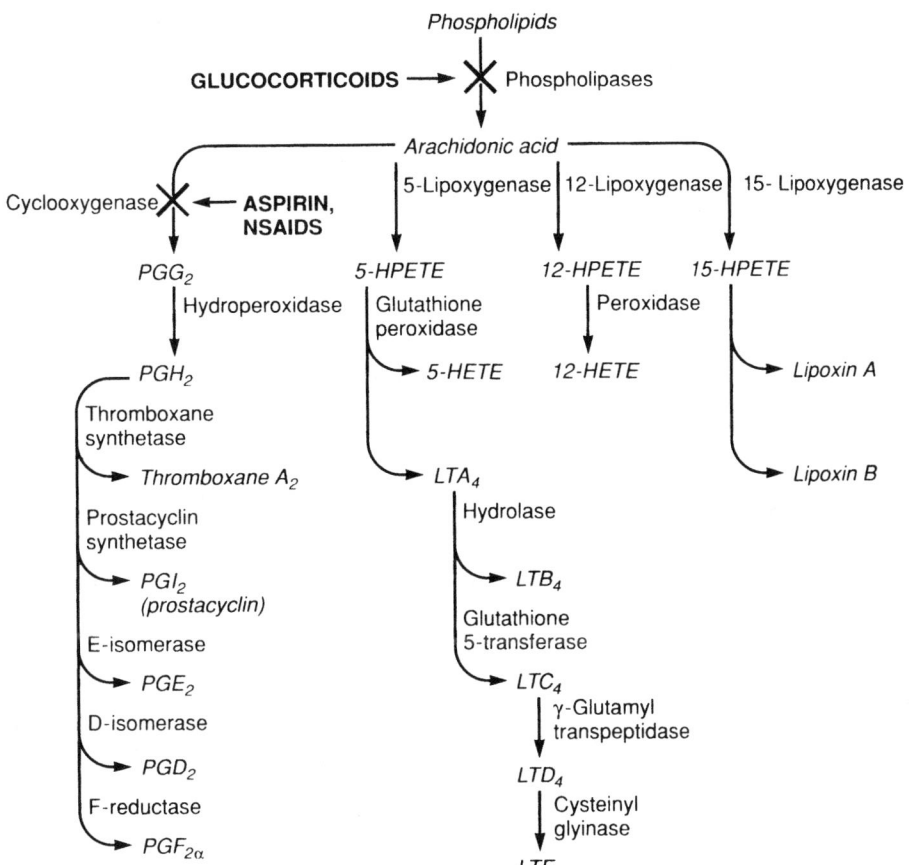

Figure 6.15A

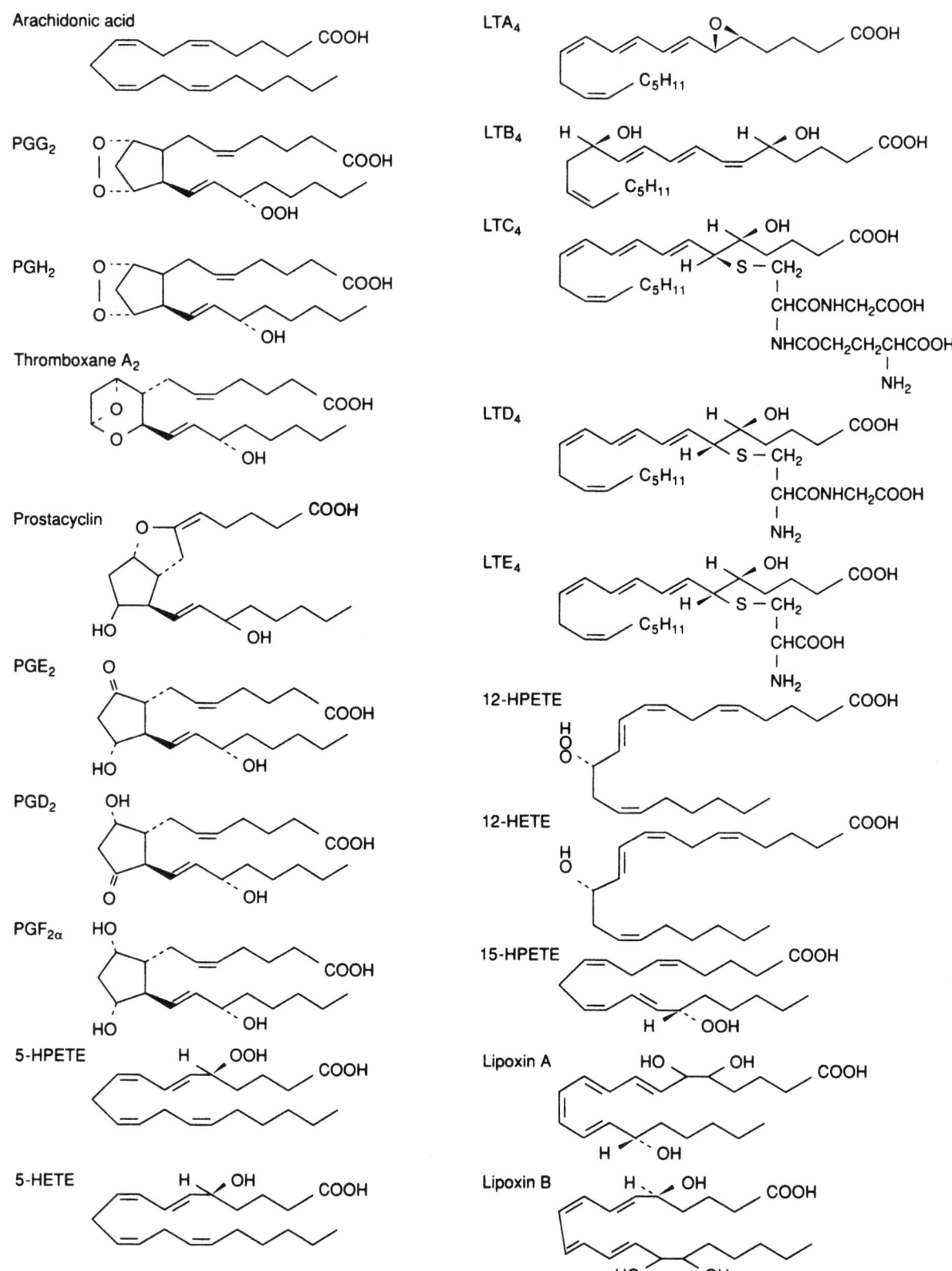

Figure 6.15B

5. Platelet-activating factor (PAF):

   a. Is generated by the action of phospholipase A$_2$ on membrane phospholipids
   b. Is antiinflammatory in most of its actions
   c. Is synthesized by endothelial and other cells
   d. Exerts a variety of platelet-independent biologic effects

COMMENT: Like the eicosanoids, PAF is not stored in cells but is rapidly produced during inflammation. Platelet-activating factor exerts a variety of platelet-independent biologic effects. Synthesis of PAF is initiated by activation of phospholipase A$_2$. Activation of phospholipase A$_2$ releases arachidonic acid in addition to lyso-PAF. Hence, PAF synthesis and eicosanoid production are coordinately regulated. Platelet-activating factor is synthesized on activation of a variety of inflammatory cells, including platelets, neutrophils, basophils, mast cells, mononuclear phagocytes, eosinophils, and vascular endothelium. Platelet-activating factor is a stimulatory agonist for many inflammatory cells and for smooth muscle cells, vascular endothelium, and others. Platelet-activating factor enhances the ability of neutrophils to respond to challenge with *N*-formyl peptides and leukotriene B$_4$. There is considerable overlap and redundancy in the effects produced by PAF and eicosanoids.

ANSWER: a, c, d

REFERENCE: *Chapter 6—Inflammation: Humoral Components of Inflammation; Lipid Mediators*

6. Which of the following statements regarding neutrophils is/are true?

   a. The neutrophil undergoes final maturation after release into the circulation
   b. Patients with chronic granulomatous disease have a defective neutrophil NADPH oxidase system
   c. Neutrophil killing of bacteria is achieved by oxidants, proteinases, and cationic proteins
   d. A normal human neutrophil circulates in the blood for 7 to 10 days

COMMENT: The neutrophil is a migratory phagocytic cell that defends the host against bacteria and eliminates necrotic tissue. The neutrophil matures in the bone marrow and is released into the circulation as a fully differentiated cell. It is loaded with granules containing a variety of proteinases, hydrolases, antimicrobial agents, and cationic proteins. The material undergoes phagocytosis by the cell, and the granules fuse with the phagocytic vacuoles to degrade the foreign material. When the cells are challenged with a large amount of material, the granule contents can be released into the extracellular space, where damage to surrounding tissue occurs. The neutrophil normally circulates in the human bloodstream for 7 to 10 hours. Neutrophils are thought to exist 1 to 2 days thereafter in the tissues before being cleared from the system. Granule constituents are formed during differentiation, and replenishment of spent granules does not occur once the cells are in the circulation.

The neutrophil is a fully differentiated end-cell poised to respond rapidly to stimuli, but it is rapidly spent in the process. Neutrophils have a NADPH oxidase enzyme system on the plasma membrane that can be activated to produce toxic oxygen species, including the superoxide anion (O$_2^{-}$). Patients with chronic granulomatous disease have a defective NADPH oxidase system in their neutrophils and are thus unable to generate oxygen. Although neutrophils from patients with chronic granulomatous disease are able to phagocytose bacteria, they are unable to kill the intracellular microbes, and chronic, unresolved infections result.

ANSWER: b, c

REFERENCE: *Chapter 6—Inflammation: Neutrophils*

7. Which of the following statements is/are true?

   a. Eosinophils are the main, if not sole, source of histamine in the blood
   b. Basophils are effector cells in allergic reactions because of IgE receptors
   c. Mast cells are the main source of tissue histamine except in the stomach and central nervous system
   d. Mononuclear phagocytes release a variety of proinflammatory cytokines and growth factors

COMMENT: Eosinophils constitute 1% to 3% of the leukocyte population of the bloodstream. They also reside in tissues and have phagocytic capabilities. They are less effective as bactericidal cells than are neutrophils, but they play an important role in defense against parasites. Eosinophils are primary effectors in allergic reactions because of IgE receptors, which are not present on neutrophils.

Basophils are fully differentiated cells released into the circulation from bone marrow. Basophils are the main, if not sole, source of histamine in the blood. Histamine is a vasoactive amine and the main mediator of the IgE-mediated immediate hypersensitivity response. Histamine release from basophils is induced by complement products and IgE receptors.

Mast cells are formed from bone marrow precursors that differentiate and proliferate in connective tissue. Mast cell granules contain histamine and proteoglycans. They represent the main source of histamine in most tissues except the stomach and central nervous system.

The monocyte-macrophage system consists of phagocytic cells scattered throughout the body. During acute inflammation, monocytes respond to chemoattractants released and are recruited to the site of inflammation. Mononuclear phagocytes respond to inflammatory stimuli by releasing macrophage colony-stimulating factor (M-CSF), granulocyte-macrophage colony-stimulating factor (GM-CSF), interleukin-1 (IL-1), and tumor necrosis factor (TNF), in addition to a variety of growth factors. These factors increase production of mononuclear phagocytes, and several of these factors enhance the ability of effector cells to respond to chemotactic stimuli released at the site of injury. Thus the mononuclear phagocytes are important in initiating and augmenting the cycle of events that results in recruitment and activation of inflammatory cells at sites of inflammation.

ANSWER: b, c, d

REFERENCE: *Chapter 6—Inflammation: Cell Development*

8. Platelets have a wide array of functions in inflammation. Which of the following is/are among these?

   a. Synthesis and release of vasoactive eicosanoids
   b. Release of chemotactic factors
   c. Adherence to and coating of bacterial and tumor cells
   d. Increase of vascular permeability
   e. Phagocytosis of bacteria

COMMENT: Platelets are anucleated cells derived from megakaryocytes in the bone marrow. Their central role in hemostasis is well known. Platelets have a wide array of functions in inflammation, including the following:

- Synthesis and release of vasoactive eicosanoids
- Release of chemotactic factors
- Interaction with other inflammatory cells
- Interaction with endothelial cells
- Adherence to and coating of bacterial and tumor cells

Platelets are not capable of phagocytosis. Few of the factors released or the functions carried by platelets during inflammation are unique to this cell type. Other inflammatory cells often have the same or similar capabilities. Some platelet functions may reflect vestigial functions inherited from a primitive precursor inflammatory cell. Platelets serve primarily as an amplifier or modulator of the inflammatory response (see Table 6.4).

ANSWER: a, b, c, d

REFERENCE: *Chapter 6—Inflammation: Platelets*

9. Which of the following statements regarding endothelial cells in acute inflammation is/are true?
   a. Endothelial cells are characterized by phenotypic homogeneity
   b. Specific patterns of receptor expression regulate leukocyte adherence
   c. Endothelial cell nitric oxide generation regulates regional blood flow and leukocyte adhesion
   d. Endothelial cells may be capable of phagocytosis

COMMENT: Endothelial cells are increasingly recognized as being phenotypically heterogeneous. Specific receptor molecules are expressed at various sites, where they help to direct lymphocytes and other leukocytes to their appropriate target organ. In the high endothelial venules, these receptor molecules are known as *vascular addressins.* Endothelial cells play a major role in regulating vascular tone. This is the result of the presence of angiotensin-converting enzyme on the cell surface and the production of both endothelin (a potent vasoconstrictor) and nitric oxide (a potent vasodilator). Both play important physiologic roles in determining the distribution of blood flow. In addition, evidence suggests that nitric oxide may have direct effects on expression of a variety of leukocyte adhesion molecules. Under unusual circumstances, endothelial cells can have macrophage-like properties in that they can act as antigen-presenting cells and consume particles through phagocytosis. Endothelial cells also may be an important source of oxidants in inflammatory reactions after ischemic injury. Endothelial cells are not passive participants in inflammatory processes; they possess the ability to direct and focus many aspects of an inflammatory event.

ANSWER: b, c, d

REFERENCE: *Chapter 6—Inflammation: Cellular Effector Mechanisms in Inflammation*

10. Cellular injury from oxidants may be manifested by which of the following?
    a. Cell membrane lipid peroxidation
    b. DNA strand breaks
    c. Cytoskeletal disassembly
    d. Depletion of adenosine triphosphate

COMMENT: Free oxygen radicals are chemical species that are intermediates in the normal process of cellular respiration. Oxidants that are free radicals have been implicated as initiators of reactions that lead to a variety of cellular injuries. Oxidants are derived from several sources, notably phagocytes. Among the effects of oxygen free radicals are membrane lipid peroxidation, DNA strand breaks, cytoskeletal disassembly, and inhibition of glucose metabolism, which lead to decreased cellular concentrations of adenosine triphosphate.

ANSWER: a, b, c, d

REFERENCE: *Chapter 6—Inflammation: Reactive Oxygen Species*

CHAPTER 7

DIAGNOSIS, PREVENTION, AND TREATMENT OF INFECTION IN SURGICAL PATIENTS

1. The first line of host defense is the barrier presented to the external environment. Which of the following statements is/are true concerning host barriers?

   a. Sebaceous glands secrete chemical compounds that maintain a relatively high pH and provide effective bacterial stasis
   b. Within the respiratory tract, ciliary function extrudes microorganisms trapped within the mucous secretion layer
   c. The low pH within the stomach markedly decreases the bacterial content of the upper gastrointestinal tract
   d. Intestinal peristalsis prevents microbial adherence and invasion

COMMENT: The skin, mucous membranes, and epithelial layers of various organs of the body constitute effective physical barriers against microbial invasion. In certain portions of the body, these barriers have developed ancillary adaptations to increase the effectiveness of the barrier functions. Skin structures such as sebaceous glands secrete chemical compounds that maintain a relatively low pH and provide effective bacterial stasis. Mucous secretion by specialized glands within the bronchi and gastrointestinal tract provides a mucous layer that represents a physical and chemical barrier to microbial invasion. Within the respiratory tract, ciliary function extrudes microorganisms trapped within this mucous layer. In the alimentary tract, the low pH within the stomach and intestinal peristalsis both prevent microbial adherence and invasion.

ANSWER: b, c, d

REFERENCE: *Chapter 7—Diagnosis, Prevention, and Treatment of Infection in Surgical Patients: Host Defenses*

2. Which of the following statements is/are correct concerning the gastrointestinal microflora?

   a. The gastrointestinal microflora evolves constantly throughout development
   b. The gastrointestinal microflora can contribute to the physical and chemical barriers at the mucous membrane level
   c. Most of the microorganisms in the oropharynx eventually pass into the intestine
   d. In the colon, anaerobic organisms outnumber aerobic organisms in a ratio greater than 100:1

COMMENT: The composition of the gastrointestinal microflora is established in neonates after ingestion of microbes acquired during contamination from the birth canal and during initial feeding. It stays relatively constant thereafter. Although this flora promotes development of the immune system, the specific interactions that produce this effect have not been fully elucidated. The microflora also contributes to physical and chemical barriers at the mucous membrane level in that many autochthonous microbes have adhesion proteins by which they can bind to certain areas of the mucosal cell or to specific types of bacteria, occupy potential binding sites of pathogenic organisms, and produce a substantial physical mucobacterial layer. The oropharynx contains a number of aerobic and anaerobic microorganisms; however, these microbial inhabitants do not usually pass into the intestine, because the stomach itself is a barrier to invading microorganisms because of its low pH, which kills most microbes. The upper part of the small intestine contains few organisms, mainly gram-positive aerobes and lactobacilli. The lower part of the small intestine contains a large number of aerobes and anaerobic forms, especially if the ileocecal valve allows free backwash of cecal contents into the terminal ileum. Within the colon, a wide diversity and a large number of facultative and strict anaerobic isolates are present. Only a small number of aerobes are present and are outnumbered 100:1 to 300:1 by anaerobes.

ANSWER: b, d

REFERENCE: *Chapter 7—Diagnosis, Prevention, and Treatment of Infection in Surgical Patients: Host Defenses*

3. Initiation of a humoral immune response involves a complex interaction of antigen, cells, and intercellular messengers. Which of the following statements is/are correct concerning the initiation of the humoral immune response?

   a. Helper T lymphocytes stimulate B lymphocytes through secretion of cytokines such as interleukin-4 (IL-4) and IL-6
   b. A number of cells can aid in presenting the antigen to the helper T cell, including B lymphocytes and macrophages
   c. All antigens require coordinated efforts of the various cellular components of the immune system
   d. An antigen must be a living microorganism

COMMENT: Stimulation of the immune system occurs after a variety of antigen-presenting cells (B lymphocytes, macrophages, dendritic cells, and Langerhans cells) engulf, process, and present antigen to T lymphocytes of the helper lineage. These T lymphocytes stimulate B lymphocytes to become mature plasmacytes, through secretion of cytokines such as IL-4 and IL-6, dedicated to the production of antibody directed against the specific antigen. An antigen can be defined as any substance that stimulates the host immune response; that is, that the host immune system recognizes as foreign. Thus an antigen can be an invading microorganism, an inert particle, or any type of chemical compound that triggers the host immune system. Although some antigens directly stimulate B lymphocytes in and of themselves to produce antibody (many polysaccharides), most antigens require coordinated efforts of the various cellular components of the immune system.

ANSWER: a, b

REFERENCE: *Chapter 7—Diagnosis, Prevention, and Treatment of Infection in Surgical Patients: Host Defenses*

4. Which of the following statements is/are true concerning the antibody response to an invading antigen?

   a. All antibodies are composed of one type of heavy and one type of light protein chain
   b. The carboxyl terminus of the heavy chain is the antigen binding site
   c. Antibody of the IgG class is the initial antibody produced in response to an antigenic stimulus
   d. Immunoglobulins A, D, and E play an active role in the circulating humoral response

COMMENT: Humoral defenses consist of antibody (immunoglobulin) and complement. All immunoglobulin classes (IgM, IgG, IgA, IgE, and IgD) and IgG subclasses are composed of one type (M, G, A, E, D) of heavy and one type (K and γ) of light protein chains that consist of several domains both structurally and functionally. Each immunoglobulin molecule contains one or more units that consist of two heavy and two light chains linked by disulfide bonds. The amino terminus of both heavy and light chains contains several hypervariable regions that fold in three dimensions to produce the antigen-binding site. The carboxyl terminus of the heavy chains contain regions that activate complement and bind Fc receptors, by which direct adherence to polymorphonuclear leukocytes (PMNs) and macrophages takes place after antigen binding occurs.

Antibody of the IgM class initially is produced in response to an antigenic stimulus. A second exposure to the same antigen, or a cross-reactive antigen, leads to the so-called second set response, in which antibody of the IgG class with two binding sites is produced more rapidly and in larger quantity than is the initial IgM primary response. Immunoglobulin of the IgA class is secreted by gastrointestinal tract–associated lymphoid tissue and is combined with secretory components of protein to form a dimer termed *secretory IgA*. This antibody acts at a variety of epithelial sites to prevent microbial adherence and invasion. Immunoglobulin D and IgE exist in smaller amounts in the circulation and do not appear to play a major role as host defense components.

ANSWER: a

REFERENCE: *Chapter 7—Diagnosis, Prevention, and Treatment of Infection in Surgical Patients: Host Defenses*

5. The complement system consists of a series of serum proteins that exist in a quiescent or very low-level state of activation in the uninfected host. Which of the following statements is/are true concerning complement activation?

a. The alternative (properdin) pathway of complement activation can occur directly through contact with fungal or bacterial cell wall compounds

b. Complement component fragments can decrease vascular permeability

c. Excessive complement activation can produce deleterious effects

d. Fragments of certain complement components serve as chemoattractants to additional cellular components of the host defense mechanism

COMMENT: Complement activation can occur through the classic or the alternative (properdin) pathway, both of which end in deposition of terminal complement pathway components on the antigenic cell surface. The classic pathway of complement activation usually begins with IgG binding, which also binds the antigen. Activation of the alternative pathway occurs in response to activation of direct binding of the antigen or directly through contact with fungal and bacterial cell wall compounds such as zymosan and gram-negative bacterial lipopolysaccharide (LPS endotoxin). Several complement components represent important host defenses that recruit or augment cellular host defenses or directly inactivate invading microbes through lytic activity. The production of complement component fractions C3a and C5a during activation of this cascade primarily markedly increases vascular permeability. C5a functions as a PMN and macrophage chemoattractant. This process leads to the recruitment of additional humoral and cellular defenses to the specific area of infection. Excessive complement activation can produce deleterious effects in some instances. Complement activation causes enhanced PMN adhesion, margination, and release of lysosomal enzymes that can directly damage certain target tissues, such as the lung.

ANSWER: a, c, d

REFERENCE: *Chapter 7—Diagnosis, Prevention, and Treatment of Infection in Surgical Patients: Host Defenses*

6. Which of the following statements is/are true concerning cellular defense mechanisms?

a. Macrophages function solely as antigen processing cells in the initial reaction to exposure to an antigen

b. Macrophages can become activated and secrete cytokines

c. Macrophages serve as phagocytic cells in the tissues but not within the bloodstream

d. Polymorphonuclear leukocytes are normally present in only small numbers within the tissue and enter an area of infection through diapedesis

COMMENT: A variety of cell types provide host defense at several levels. Macrophages act as the initial antigen processing cell that presents antigen to helper T cells, thus initiating the immune response. Macrophages, however, are pluripotent cells that, in the process of engulfing and processing antigen, can become activated. Activated macrophages secrete a variety of cytokines. Macrophages also act as phagocytic cells in the tissues and within the bloodstream. Because of their resident nature in many tissues, macrophages also represent the first line of host defenses in many areas of the body, even before activation. Polymorphonuclear leukocytes are present within the bloodstream but only in small numbers within the tissue. They enter an area of infection through diapedesis after chemotactic stimuli are excluded by macrophages, bacterial breakdown products, and complement activation.

ANSWER: b, d

REFERENCE: *Chapter 7—Diagnosis, Prevention, and Treatment of Infection in Surgical Patients: Host Defenses*

7. Cytokines are low-molecular-weight polypeptides that exert a variety of biologic effects at both local and systemic levels. Which of the following statements is/are true concerning the production and actions of cytokines?

    a. Cytokines are produced solely by macrophages
    b. Cytokines act only on other cells within the local environment
    c. Cytokines can have both protective and deleterious effects on the host
    d. Each specific cytokine is produced by a single cell type

COMMENT: Macrophages, endothelial cells, lymphocytes, and other cells secrete a large number of compounds called *cytokines,* which most probably evolved for the purpose of local intercellular and intracellular signaling. Cytokines frequently are secreted after initial lymphocyte or macrophage activation and can act on the secreting cell itself (autocrine activation) or on other cells within the local environment (paracrine activation) to cause increased secretion of the same cytokine or other cytokines, respectively. Some cytokines are produced by several cell types, and most produce a wide array of effects. The duality of the effects of the cytokine component of host defenses, exerting both salutatory and deleterious effects on the host, has become increasingly evident.

ANSWER: c

REFERENCE: *Chapter 7—Diagnosis, Prevention, and Treatment of Infection in Surgical Patients: Host Defenses*

8. Which of the following statements is/are true concerning initial microbiologic diagnostic techniques?

    a. Appropriate expeditious transport of specimens to the microbiology laboratory is essential for obtaining accurate clinical information
    b. The use of potassium hydroxide in preparing a specimen slide for light microscopic examination is useful in identification of anaerobic bacteria
    c. Antibiotic sensitivity is determined by means of exposing the specific microorganism to varying amounts of antibiotic. The concentration of the antibiotic inhibiting growth is called the minimum inhibitory concentration (MIC)
    d. Serum levels of antimicrobial agents should achieve more than a fourfold to eightfold increase over MIC to be considered clinically efficacious.

COMMENT: Because most surgical infections are polymicrobial, specimens are cultured for aerobic and anaerobic bacteria as well as fungi. Although aerobic and aerotolerant microorganisms often do not require special transport media, a delay in specimen processing can markedly reduce the yield. Anaerobic transport media have been found to increase markedly the cultural yield of this type of organism. The initial piece of information gained concerning possible infection may come from simple staining of a specimen. Gram staining, which helps identify the staining characteristics and number of the organisms, is performed on all specimens. Potassium hydroxide is useful in that it causes lysis of bacteria and other cellular elements within a preparation and allows observation of yeast and mycelial elements.

Initial culture results may indicate solely that microorganisms are growing; full characterization can take 2 or 3 days. Once a specific microorganism is identified, a sample is inoculated during the log phase into broth containing varying amounts of an antibiotic. After an 18- to 24-hour period, the tube or well that exhibits no visible growth is documented, and the reciprocal of this dilution is the MIC. This value can be compared with either measured or known achievable serum levels for a particular antibiotic. In general, antimicrobial agents that achieve more than a fourfold to eightfold increase over MIC during the peak serum level have been found to be clinically efficacious.

ANSWER: a, c, d

REFERENCE: *Chapter 7—Diagnosis, Prevention, and Treatment of Infection in Surgical Patients: Microbiologic Diagnostic Techniques*

9. Which of the following statements is/are true concerning newer detection methods of systemic infection?
    a. Enzyme-linked immunosorbent assay (ELISA) is a rapid immunologic assay used to detect both antigen and antibody
    b. Southern, Northern, and Western immunoblot techniques are used to detect DNA, RNA, and proteins, respectively
    c. Polymerase chain reaction (PCR) is a sensitive assay used to detect small amounts of microbial DNA and thus infection in the early stages
    d. Infectious agents detected with advanced molecular techniques include cytomegalovirus (CMV) and human immunodeficiency virus (HIV)

COMMENT: Although the classic detection of infection based on clinical signs of infection and bacterial culture are the most common clinical tools, increasing reliance has been placed on assays in which cultural data are not used. Antibody and cytokine host responses are being intensely examined. Extremely sensitive amplified assays that rely on antigen, antibody, or microbial DNA detection are used in the clinical setting. Enzyme-linked immunosorbent assay is a rapid, antigen-based, immunologic assay that can be used for antigen and antibody detection, determination of antibody titer, and screening for production of monoclonal antibodies. Transblot techniques are being used increasingly in the clinical setting. These include Southern, Northern, and Western immunotransblot techniques used to detect DNA, RNA, or proteins, respectively. The PCR is being used in some centers as a sensitive assay to detect small amounts of microbial DNA. This technique involves extraction of the DNA from the test sample by means of in vitro amplification through repeated nucleic acid denaturing and polymerization so that the gene copy number increases exponentially. This marked amplification of the gene copy number results in extremely sensitive tests for detecting infection in the early stages. These detection methods are being used clinically to detect a wide variety of infectious agents, including CMV and HIV. Preliminary investigations into detection of fungal pathogens are underway.

ANSWER: a, b, c, d

REFERENCE: *Chapter 7—Diagnosis, Prevention, and Treatment of Infection in Surgical Patients: Microbiologic Diagnostic Techniques*

10. Antibacterial agents can be classified with regard to structure, mechanism of action, and activity pattern against various types of bacterial pathogens. Which of the following statements is/are true concerning antimicrobial classes?
    a. Penicillins and cephalosporins share the compound structure of a β-lactam ring, which binds to bacterial division plate proteins
    b. Tetracyclines and macrolides such as erythromycin inhibit bacterial ribosomal activity and therefore protein synthesis
    c. Aminoglycosides act in a manner similar to that of tetracyclines and therefore are bacteriostatic
    d. Sulfonamides and trimethoprim act synergistically to inhibit purine synthesis

COMMENT: Penicillins, cephalosporins, and monobactams have a β-lactam ring of some type. They bind bacterial division plate proteins, thus inhibiting cell wall peptidoglycan synthesis and either causing or inducing autolytic bacteriolysis. Because gram-positive and gram-negative bacteria have different types of division plate proteins, many of these agents have differential activity between these two types of microorganisms. Tetracyclines, chloramphenicol, and macrolides inhibit bacterial ribosomal activity and thus overall protein synthesis by a variety of different mechanisms. Aminoglycosides inhibit protein synthesis and presumably act on a different target site, a supposition based on the fact that aminoglycosides are bacteriolytic and the other agents are bacteriostatic. Vancomycin inhibits assembly of peptidoglycan polymers, whereas quinolones bind to DNA helicase proteins and inhibit bacterial DNA synthesis. Sulfonamides and trimethoprim act in different mechanisms to inhibit protein synthesis; therefore two agents in combination act synergistically.

ANSWER: a, b, d

REFERENCE: *Chapter 7—Diagnosis, Prevention, and Treatment of Infection in Surgical Patients: Antimicrobial Agents*

11. The use of prophylactic antibiotics has become commonplace. Which of the following statements is/are true concerning the prophylactic use of antibiotics?

    a. The appropriate use of prophylactic antibiotics must include the initiation of administration of the agent before the surgical procedure

    b. Continuing the antibiotic into the postoperative period has led to improved results in antibiotic prophylaxis

    c. Prophylactic administration of broad-spectrum agents (third-generation cephalosporins) has been shown to be particularly advantageous

    d. The topical use of antimicrobial agents is of no advantage in the prophylactic setting

COMMENT: Intravenous administration of an antibiotic is clearly indicated for patients undergoing clean-contaminated operations. These antibiotics should be administered before surgery to obtain adequate tissue levels at the time of potential contamination. However, no added benefit has been found for postoperative use of antibiotics with regard to prophylaxis. The choice of antibiotic is a complex issue that remains unresolved largely because both superficial and deep wound infections can occur as a result of either or both skin (superficial wound) flora (e.g., *Staphylococcus aureus*), and body site (deep wound) infection. For this reason, administration of agents with activity directed against these expected agents is reasonable. Although administration of a first-generation cephalosporin is acceptable, second-generation cephalosporins or extended-spectrum penicillins with gram-positive and gram-negative activity and biliary tract excretion may be more suitable for patients undergoing gastrointestinal or biliary tract procedures. The use of agents with additional anaerobic activity for patients undergoing gastrointestinal procedures involving the small intestine or colon should be considered. Administration of broad-spectrum agents such as third-generation cephalosporins for prophylaxis does not seem to provide additional benefit in comparison with the aforementioned types of antibiotics and may foster development of resistant organisms within a given institution or superinfection within a given patient. There is evidence that in some cases topical use of antimicrobial agents is equivalent to administration of intravenous antimicrobial agents.

ANSWER: a

REFERENCE: *Chapter 7—Diagnosis, Prevention, and Treatment of Infection in Surgical Patients: Antimicrobial Agents*

12. The use of antibiotics can be either based on clinical course without the benefit of well-defined microbiologic data (empiric therapy) or targeted at specific identified pathogens once sensitivity reports are available (directed therapy). Which of the following statements is/are true concerning these therapies?

    a. The issue of toxic side effects of antibiotics is important only in dealing with empiric therapy

    b. Single-agent therapy is generally inferior to specific multidrug therapy (aminoglycoside plus an antianaerobic agent) for the management of secondary bacterial peritonitis due to appendicitis, diverticulitis, penetrating gastrointestinal injury, or anastomotic leak

    c. With the empiric use of antibiotics, a diligent search for the septic source should be undertaken and continued until identified

    d. In clinical situations in which polymicrobial infection is identified, specifically directed therapy for the predominant organism is satisfactory

COMMENT: The use of empiric therapy without the benefit of well-defined microbiologic data is appropriate when there is sufficient clinical evidence to support the diagnosis such that it would be imprudent to withhold antimicrobial therapy. In this setting, however, a diligent search for the septic focus source, as with cultures and radiographic procedures, should be undertaken and continued. Initial limits should be placed in the course of empiric therapy, and continued reevaluation should be based on the clinical course. The choice of antibiotic agents should be based on the clinical situation and known activity patterns within the institution. Single broad-spectrum agents, although they have a lack of individual pathogen specificity, are useful in this setting because they provide broad coverage against several groups of pathogens and may avoid some of the toxic effects of specific combined-modality regimens. For directed therapy, single-agent therapy has been found to be equivalent to combined therapy and should be chosen in an attempt to select agents with appropriate sensitivities that retain suitable clinical efficacy but have minimal toxicity. After review of culture reports, many patients have been found to have polymicrobial infection. Because experimental clinical evidence supports the concept of aerobic-anaerobic synergy, therapy should be directed against all possible components of the infection if the body site is such that these microorganisms may be present.

ANSWER: c

REFERENCE: *Chapter 7—Diagnosis, Prevention, and Treatment of Infection in Surgical Patients: Antimicrobial Agents*

13. Wounds are classified according to the likelihood of bacterial contamination. Which of the following statements is/are true concerning wound classifications?

    a. A clean-contaminated wound is associated with elective colon resection with adequate mechanical and antibiotic bowel preparation

    b. A contaminated wound includes resection of obstructed bowel with gross spillage of intestinal contents

    c. In a clean wound, no viscus is entered

    d. Antibiotic prophylaxis is administered for all clean-contaminated and contaminated wounds and selectively to patients with clean wounds

COMMENT: Wounds are classified according to the likelihood of bacterial contamination, as follows: (1) clean (no viscus is entered; e.g., herniorrhaphy), (2) clean-contaminated (minimal contamination; e.g., elective colon resection with adequate mechanical and antibiotic bowel preparation), and (3) contaminated (heavily contaminated operation; e.g., resection of unprepared, obstructed bowel with gross spillage of intestinal contents or stool, drainage of abscesses, débridement of traumatic neglected wounds). Antibiotic prophylaxis generally should be administered for class 2 and 3 wounds, but patients undergoing clean operations do not always need antimicrobial prophylaxis. An exception to this tenet involves operations in which a prosthetic material may be used (e.g., artificial joint, heart valve, tissue patch).

ANSWER: a, b, c, d

REFERENCE: *Chapter 7—Diagnosis, Prevention, and Treatment of Infection in Surgical Patients: Approaches to Diagnosis of Infection in the Surgical Patient*

14. Which of the following statements is/are true concerning host defense mechanisms to intraabdominal infection?

    a. Bacterial clearance can occur by means of translymphatic absorption

    b. Phagocytic activity and bacterial killing are caused by resident phagocytic cells and an influx of PMNs

    c. A fibrinogen-rich inflammatory exudate is released into the peritoneal cavity and traps large numbers of bacteria and other particulate matter

    d. Perforation of the bowel can be walled off but seldom sealed by the omentum and other mobile viscera

COMMENT: Introduction of microorganisms into the normally sterile peritoneal environment invokes several potent specialized host antimicrobial defense mechanisms. Bacterial clearance, also called *translymphatic absorption,* occurs through specialized structures present only on the peritoneal mesothelium on the underside of the diaphragm that act as conduits for both fluid and particulate matter. Lymphatic channels eventually form that drain into the venous circulation through the thoracic duct. Bacteria not cleared by means of translymphatic absorption are rapidly engulfed by resident and recruited phagocytic cells, including resident macrophages on the peritoneal surface and omentum and attracted PMNs. The final primitive host defense mechanism is sequestration by which a fibrinogen-rich exudate containing plasma opsonins appears during peritoneal infection and fibrin polymerization occurs. Fibrin can trap large numbers of bacteria and other particulate matter. With omentum and other mobile viscera, perforations are sealed and the contaminated enteric contents walled off to prevent continued soilage of the peritoneal cavity.

ANSWER: a, b, c

REFERENCE: *Chapter 7—Diagnosis, Prevention, and Treatment of Infection in Surgical Patients: Approaches to Diagnosis of Infection in the Surgical Patient*

15. A 67-year-old man has an intraabdominal abscess caused by perforated sigmoid diverticulitis. Which of the following statements is/are true concerning the intraabdominal abscess?

a. Culture will likely reveal a solitary organism
b. Both aerobic and anaerobic islets are encountered in 50% of specimens
c. The most common aerobic islets likely are *Escherichia coli* and other gram-negative enteric bacilli
d. The most common anaerobic islet is a *Bacteroides* organism

COMMENT: Intraabdominal infection typically results in perforation of a hollow viscus and contamination of a normally sterile peritoneal cavity. The normal bacterial flora and the particular location of the alimentary tract thus determines the initial inoculum. In parallel with the overall quantity of microorganisms—aerobes but predominantly anaerobes—perforation of the lower small bowel and colon produces a high frequency of infections with anaerobic microorganisms. Certain predictable patterns of bacterial islets are found, but on average four or five islets are present in patients with established intraabdominal infection, more than half of which are anaerobes. Both aerobes and anaerobes are encountered in 80% to 90% of specimens. Commonly encountered aerobes isolated are *E. coli* and other gram-negative enteric bacilli, such as *Enterobacter* and *Klebsiella* organisms. Among the anaerobes, *Bacteroides* organisms, especially *B. fragilis,* Clostridium organisms, and anaerobic cocci are most consistently isolated.

ANSWER: b, c, d

REFERENCE: *Chapter 7—Diagnosis, Prevention, and Treatment of Infection in Surgical Patients: Approaches to Diagnosis of Infection in the Surgical Patient*

16. Treatment of the patient in *15.* should include:

a. Initial empiric therapy directed against both aerobes and anaerobes
b. The addition of antifungal therapy because the patient is elderly
c. A minimum of 2 weeks of antibiotic therapy
d. The addition of appropriate antibiotic therapy has made surgical therapy unnecessary in such cases
e. Either a single agent or combination therapy if the agents selected have activity against both aerobic and anaerobic bacteria

COMMENT: Primary management of a perforated viscus is surgical; however, antimicrobial therapy is an extremely important adjunct. Empiric antibiotic therapy for secondary bacterial peritonitis and intraabdominal abscess is directed against both aerobes and anaerobes. Administration of an agent directed against only one component of the infection is inferior to combined therapy. Results of several studies indicate that the results of using several agents in combination are equivalent to use of single-agent therapy as long as the agents selected have activity against both components of the infection. The addition of antientercoccal or antifungal agents as initial therapy has not been substantiated. The most beneficial duration of antibiotic therapy must be based on the setting for the specific patient. Minimal peritoneal contamination with adequate surgical treatment can be managed with a 3- to 5-day course of antibiotics. Longer periods are indicated for immunosuppressed patients and patients with extensive contamination.

ANSWER: a, e

REFERENCE: *Chapter 7—Diagnosis, Prevention, and Treatment of Infection in Surgical Patients: Approaches to Diagnosis of Infection in the Surgical Patient*

17. Which of the following statements is/are true concerning necrotizing fascitis?

    a. Mortality rates as high as 40% can be expected

    b. The infection involves only the superficial fascia and spares the deep muscular fascia

    c. An impaired immune system is a common factor predisposing to this condition

    d. The infection usually is polymicrobial

    e. Necrotizing fascitis is most likely to develop in the face of impairment of the fascial blood supply

COMMENT: Necrotizing fascitis is an uncommon infection of the deep and superficial fascia that is associated with mortality as high as 40%. Although many underlying diseases predispose patients to necrotizing fascitis, the following three common factors are almost invariably present: (1) impairment of the immune system; (2) compromise of fascial blood supply, and (3) microorganisms that are able to proliferate within this environment. Infections of this type are usually polymicrobial, gram-positive organisms such as staphylococci and streptococci, gram-negative enteric bacteria, and gram-negative anaerobic organisms being frequently identified. These polymicrobial cultural results are assuredly indicative of the occurrence of a synergistic process, perhaps in large part accounting for the severity of these infections. Some microorganisms have virulence factors that, in conjunction with an underlying host predisposition, allow this disease to occur without dependence on other bacteria. Examples of such bacteria include *Clostridium, Pseudomonas,* and *Aeromonas* organisms. In these patients, the process is often fulminant and is frequently associated with cellulitis, myositis, fascitis, and bacteremia with attendant high mortality.

ANSWER: a, c, d, e

REFERENCE: *Chapter 7—Diagnosis, Prevention, and Treatment of Infection in Surgical Patients: Approaches to Diagnosis of Infection in the Surgical Patient*

18. If a necrotizing soft-tissue infection is likely, therapy mandates:

    a. Empiric administration of antibiotics active against gram-positive, gram-negative, and anaerobic bacteria

    b. Because of resistant species, penicillin is not indicated

    c. Immediate operative intervention and aggressive resection of all involved tissues are mandatory

    d. The use of hyperbaric oxygen has been demonstrated to be clearly advantageous

COMMENT: Identification of a necrotizing soft-tissue infection mandates immediate operative intervention with aggressive resection of all involved tissues and empiric administration of antibiotics active against gram-positive, gram-negative, and anaerobic bacteria. In most cases, this involves the use of several antimicrobial antibiotics in combination. Because of concern in all cases about the presence of *Clostridium* infection, high doses of aqueous penicillin G are administered. Gram-positive organisms are controlled with vancomycin or a semisynthetic penicillin. Gram-negative organisms are controlled with an aminoglycoside or a monobactam agent. Anaerobic coverage typically is achieved by use of metronidazole or clindamycin. The use of hyperbaric oxygen therapy is controversial, and because of the rarity of the disease, data from prospective, randomized studies are not available. The literature remains without results of controlled trials that show additional benefits of hyperbaric oxygen therapy.

ANSWER: a, c

REFERENCE: *Chapter 7—Diagnosis, Prevention, and Treatment of Infection in Surgical Patients: Approaches to Diagnosis of Infection in the Surgical Patient*

19. A patient with diabetes has a severe perineal infection with skin necrosis, subcutaneous crepitance, and drainage of a thin, watery, grayish, and foul-smelling fluid. Management should consist of:

a. Gram stain of the fluid, which will likely show multiple bacteria, including predominantly gram-positive rods
b. Computed tomography is indicated in the evaluation of a patient in stable condition to define the extent of the disease
c. Therapy with broad-spectrum antibiotics followed by prompt, extensive débridement is indicated
d. A safe guideline is to resect infected necrotic tissue so that a several-centimeter margin of grossly normal, healthy tissue can be achieved
e. Colostomy is of little benefit in this situation

COMMENT: The presence of severe perineal infection (called *Fournier gangrene* when this process involves the perineum and scrotum) is associated with a high mortality despite aggressive and appropriate therapy. The clinical description provided suggests underlying soft-tissue necrosis. If the patient is in stable condition, radiologic studies, including CT, to define the extent of the disease and the presence of pelvic infection are indicated. Gram stain will likely show evidence of polymicrobial organisms, but the presence of *Clostridium* organisms marked by gram-positive rods suggests involvement of this organism. Prompt, aggressive, and extensive débridement to remove all devitalized and affected tissue and administration of broad-spectrum antibiotics, fluid resuscitation, hemodynamic monitoring, and nutritional support appear to afford the patient the best chance of survival. The clearest guidelines to determine the limits of resection involve removal of clearly infected, necrotic tissue so that margins several centimeters into grossly normal, healthy tissue are achieved. Because the entire perineal region and buttocks are frequently involved, fecal stream diversion by means of colostomy often improves wound care, although the outcome is not invariably positive.

ANSWER: a, b, c, d

REFERENCE: *Chapter 7—Diagnosis, Prevention, and Treatment of Infection in Surgical Patients: Approaches to Diagnosis of Infection in the Surgical Patient*

20. Which of the following statements is/are true concerning gram-negative bacterial sepsis?

a. Mortality due to this condition has almost been eliminated through therapeutic intervention with antibiotics, aggressive hemodynamic monitoring, and fluid resuscitation
b. The incidence of this condition is decreasing
c. Predisposing factors include old age, malnutrition, and immunosuppression
d. Pseudomonal bacteremia is the most common cause of gram-negative sepsis
e. Polymicrobial sepsis is generally considered a more serious problem than sepsis caused by a single organism

COMMENT: Gram-negative bacterial sepsis is a serious disease that produces substantial morbidity and mortality among both healthy (10% to 20% lethality) and immunosuppressed patients (30% lethality) despite therapeutic intervention with antimicrobial agents, aggressive hemodynamic monitoring, fluid resuscitation, and metabolic support. Nosocomial infections due to gram-negative pathogens have increased in frequency with a resultant increase in the incidence of gram-negative bacteremia to between 3 and 13 cases per 1,000 hospital admissions. Factors that predispose to these infections include underlying host disease processes such as malignant tumors and diabetes, old age and disability, malnutrition, previous or concurrent antimicrobial antibiotic therapy, major operations, respiratory or urinary manipulation or intubation, and immunosuppression.

Although many organisms cause this form of sepsis, *E. coli* predominates in overall frequency. Also common are isolates of *Klebsiella, Enterobacter,* and *Serratia; Pseudomonas* bacteremia is less common. Results of some studies, however, have suggested that *Pseudomonas* sepsis is associated with the highest lethality. In several series, 10% to 20% of patients have had polymicrobial sepsis. Most investigators agree that polymicrobial sepsis is more lethal than infection with a single organism.

ANSWER: c, e

REFERENCE: *Chapter 7—Diagnosis, Prevention, and Treatment of Infection in Surgical Patients: Approaches to Diagnosis of Infection in the Surgical Patient*

21. Increasing evidence has implicated gram-negative bacterial LPS endotoxin as the portion of the gram-negative bacterial cell membrane responsible for many if not all the toxic effects that occur during gram-negative bacterial sepsis. Which of the following statements is/are true concerning LPS and the host response?

a. The LPS molecule itself can in cause physiologic responses similar to that during gram-negative bacterial sepsis
b. Lipopolysaccharide triggers host macrophages to release a variety of cytokines, including tumor necrosis factor α (TNF-α), IL-1α, IL-1β, IL-6, and interferon-α (IFN-α)
c. Excessive cytokine production is not associated with detrimental consequences
d. Tumor necrosis factor-α and IL-1β appear to be the primary mediators within the host and exert deleterious effects on the host when excessive amounts reach the systemic circulation

COMMENT: The LPS molecule exerts diverse effects on the mammalian host. Immunologic responses to LPS include nonspecific polyclonal B-cell proliferation, macrophage activation and cytokine secretion, tolerance of subsequent LPS or bacterial challenge, and production of antibody directed against various portions of the LPS molecule after repeated challenge. Physiologic responses similar to those during gram-negative bacterial sepsis occur during LPS administration alone. They include hypotension, hypoxemia, acidosis, bacterial translocation across the gastrointestinal barrier, activation of the complement and coagulation cascade, white blood cell and platelet margination, and death. Indirect effects result from LPS triggering of host macrophages. Activated macrophages secrete a wide array of cytokines, including TNF-α, IL-1α, IL-1β, IL-6, and IFN-α. Excessive secretion of cytokines produces substantial systemic effects in the mammalian host. Tumor necrosis factor α and IL-1β appear to be the primary mediators within the local host milieu. They exert deleterious effects on the host only after large amounts are secreted and reach the systemic circulation.

ANSWER: a, b, d

REFERENCE: *Chapter 7—Diagnosis, Prevention, and Treatment of Infection in Surgical Patients: Approaches to Diagnosis of Infection in the Surgical Patient*

22. Which of the following statements is/are true concerning hospital-acquired infections?

a. Vascular catheter infections are most frequently associated with high-virulence organisms such as *E. coli* and *Klebsiella*
b. The most common cause of gram-negative bacterial sepsis among patients in the hospital is urinary tract infection
c. The most common organisms associated with parotitis in an elderly postoperative patient are *Streptococcus* species
d. Catheter removal is mandatory for any patient with infection involving long-term use of indwelling vascular catheters

COMMENT: As the complexities of medical care have advanced, so have the associated infectious complications related to these treatments. Prosthetic device and catheter infections frequently are caused by low-virulence organisms such as *Staphylococcus epidermidis,* although *Staphylococcus aureus* also is a frequent pathogen, and infection due to gram-negative bacteria can occur. Treatment generally consists of device removal and administration of antimicrobial agents directed against the infecting organism. Although this is a simple proposition with regard to percutaneously inserted catheters, many types of long-term indwelling catheters and devices must be removed surgically. A prolonged course of antibiotic therapy eradicates infection in some cases but not when overt bacteremia or fungemia is present. This approach may be indicated in the care of patients with relatively few systemic manifestations due to infection and who would be adversely affected by removal of the device. Removal never should be delayed, nor should antimicrobial agents be withheld from a patient who has obvious purulence in the region of the catheter or evidence of systemic sepsis.

Urinary tract infections are of concern, particularly among patients in the hospital, because they represent the most common cause of gram-negative bacterial sepsis. An indwelling urinary catheter, even for a short period of time, predisposes patients for such infection. Gram-negative bacilli are frequent pathogens in these infections, but gram-positive organisms such as enterococci and staphylococci are not uncommonly identified. Parotitis can also occur among surgical patients, particularly elderly, dehydrated patients. Therapy should be directed at rehydration, enhancing salivation, ensuring that no mechanical obstruction to the duct of Stensen is present, and administration of antibiotics against *S. aureus,* which is the most common offending organism.

ANSWER: b

REFERENCE: *Chapter 7—Diagnosis, Prevention, and Treatment of Infection in Surgical Patients: Approaches to Diagnosis of Infection in the Surgical Patient*

23. A 55-year-old recipient of a renal transplant has been hospitalized in a surgical intensive care unit receiving a prolonged course of antibiotics after an attack of acute cholecystitis. Which of the following statements is/are true concerning his treatment?

    a. Because of the risk of *Candida* infection, prophylaxis with oral nystatin should be instituted early
    b. A *Candida* urinary tract infection should be managed with systemic amphotericin B
    c. The changes of *Candida* retinitis are of little importance
    d. The presence of a virulent *Candida* bacteremia suggests the need for a reduction in dosage of immunosuppressive agents until the infection can be adequately controlled

COMMENT: Infections caused by fungal pathogens have become increasingly common. They occur frequently among patients undergoing prolonged hospitalization in surgical intensive care units and among immunosuppressed persons. Prophylaxis with an oral antifungal agent (nystatin) is warranted, especially during periods of maximal immunosuppression for transplant recipients, for patients with uncontrolled diabetes, or during some cases of prolonged antibacterial microbial therapy. In general, local, apparently noninvasive *Candida* infections involving the integument and mucous membranes are managed with oral decontamination and topical antifungal therapy with topical agents such as nystatin. *Candida* urinary tract infections can be managed with either an oral antifungal agent or with topical amphotericin B as continuous bladder irrigation. Several studies have shown that patients with three positive sites of *Candida* infection or with peritoneal or blood cultures positive for *Candida* have higher survival rates when amphotericin B therapy is instituted early in the course of infection. The presence of retinal changes compatible with *Candida* retinitis or of *Candida* organisms in the peritoneal cavity is considered an indication for a limited course of amphotericin B therapy (300 to 500 mg). Patients receiving exogenous immunosuppressive agents should undergo a marked dosage reduction, and some agents should be discontinued until evidence of infection is absolutely controlled or eradicated.

ANSWER: a, d

REFERENCE: *Chapter 7—Diagnosis, Prevention, and Treatment of Infection in Surgical Patients: Fungal Infections*

24. Which of the following statements is/are true concerning viral infections?

    a. The most common posttransplantation viral infections are caused by herpes viruses, including CMV and herpes simplex virus
    b. Viral infections occur at equal frequency anytime during the posttransplantation period
    c. Cytomegalovirus infection in a patient who has undergone transplantation is most likely a pulmonary process
    d. Herpes simplex virus infection primarily manifests as a mononucleosis-type syndrome with fever, lethargy, and cough

COMMENT: Patients who undergo solid-organ transplantation are prone to the development of viral infection because of exogenous immunosuppression. The most common posttransplantation viral infections are caused by herpes viruses (CMV, herpes simplex virus, Epstein-Barr virus, and varicella-zoster virus). All are most common during periods of maximal host immunosuppression immediately after transplantation and during periods of allograft rejection. Cytomegalovirus is a common cause of fever after solid-organ transplantation, and evidence of CMV infection is present among approximately 30% of patients. The most common presentation of CMV infection is fever, leukopenia, a cough, diffuse interstitial infiltrates on a chest radiograph, and hypoxia.

Herpes simplex virus infection causes primarily oral pharyngeal ulcerations in most cases, although sporadic cases of disseminated disease have been reported. Epstein-Barr virus causes an occasional case of mononucleosis-type syndrome but has also been clearly indicated in the pathogenesis of posttransplantation lymphoma. Varicella-zoster virus infection can manifest as disseminated and occasionally life-threatening infection among nonimmune transplant recipients or as painful herpes zoster among patients who have had chicken pox.

ANSWER: a, c,

REFERENCE: *Chapter 7—Diagnosis, Prevention, and Treatment of Infection in Surgical Patients: Viral Infections*

25. Which of the following statements is/are true concerning HIV infection?

a. Initial screening with ELISA is highly sensitive but can be associated with a false-positive rate of 25%
b. Treatment with zidovudine (AZT) appears to prolong survival when administered early in the disease
c. Predisposition to infection associated with HIV infection is primarily caused by a reduction in the number of helper T cells
d. Common infections among patients with AIDS are *Pneumocystis carinii* pneumonia, CMV pneumonitis, *Cryptococcus* meningitis, and disseminated infection due to atypical mycobacteria

COMMENT: Acquired immunodeficiency syndrome (AIDS) is caused by the human retrovirus (HIV-1) that infects T lymphocytes and causes severe immunosuppression. Persons who become infected with HIV are prone to a variety of infections and different types of malignant tumors. A spectrum exists in which patients regress from asymptomatic infection to development of the AIDS-related complex (ARC) of diseases to AIDS itself. Common infections among patients with AIDS are *Pneumocystis carinii* pneumonia, CMV pneumonitis, gastritis, hepatitis and meningitis due to *Cryptococcus neoformans* infection, and pneumonia and disseminated infection caused by atypical mycobacteria. Predisposition to these infections is due in part to the lymphotrophic nature of HIV, which markedly reduces the number of helper T cells and the absolute number of T cells. Detection of HIV typically consists of initial ELISA screening, but this test has about a 1% to 3% false-positive rate, thus mandating that all positive test results be confirmed by means of Western immunoblot analysis. Management of ARC and AIDS consists of aggressive antiinfective therapy once a specific infection occurs and the use of AZT. Treatment with AZT has been shown to prolong survival when administered early in the course of disease and is considered routine therapy.

ANSWER: b, c, d

REFERENCE: *Chapter 7—Diagnosis, Prevention, and Treatment of Infection in Surgical Patients: Viral Infections*

26. Treatment modalities designed to modulate host defense mechanisms that have been found conclusively to be of benefit include:

a. Gastrointestinal decontamination
b. Anti-LPS antibody
c. Anti-TNF antibody
d. Thymopentin
e. None of the above

COMMENT: Selective intestinal decontamination involves the use of orally administered antibiotics that achieve a high intraluminal level directed against gram-negative aerobes and yeast, leaving the host anaerobic intestinal microflora relatively undisrupted. Although reduction and alteration of the microorganisms responsible for infectious episodes have been found in certain groups of patients, a clear effect on host mortality has not been found. Because LPS may be responsible for toxicity both directly and through host mediator systems, the availability of agents to bind against this portion of gram-negative bacteria to reduce mortality has been intensively examined. Large multicenter randomized trials have provided no evidence of benefit for this treatment. Because many of the systemic manifestations of gram-negative bacteremia are mediated by cytokines, the effect of an anti-TNF antibody preparation is in clinical trial. No proven benefits have been identified. The use of immunostimulants to enhance the state of activation of host defenses has been proposed. Thymopentin is a peptide that contains active thymopoietin, a thymic molecule that stimulates T-lymphocyte activity. Results of preliminary trials indicate that this agent ameliorates host septic response after major operations and trauma, but conclusive evidence that concurrent reduction of infection-related mortality occurs is not available.

ANSWER: e

REFERENCE: *Chapter 7—Diagnosis, Prevention, and Treatment of Infection in Surgical Patients: New Treatment Modalities*

CHAPTER 8

SHOCK

1. Which of the following statements is/are true concerning the consequences of inadequate or untimely resuscitation of shock?

a. Cells switch from oxidative phosphorylation to more anaerobic metabolic pathways
b. The lack of sufficient high-energy phosphates leads to a failure to maintain important cellular electrochemical gradients
c. The accumulation of end products of anaerobic metabolism—lactic acid—is the most important event in cell death
d. Improvements in oxygen extraction at the cellular level can sufficiently support oxidative phosphorylation and maintain cell function indefinitely

COMMENT: If resuscitation of shock is untimely or incomplete the consequences are predictable and often lethal. Cells initially switch from oxidative phosphorylation to the more anaerobic metabolic pathways. End products of metabolic metabolism, notably lactic acid, accumulate. More importantly, the electrochemical gradients across cytoplasmic and subcellular membranes, normally maintained by a constant supply of high-energy phosphates, start failing. As gradients fail, water and salt on either side equilibrate, disrupting the 3-dimensional organization of proteins. Disrupted proteins can not be repaired because the repair mechanisms also require high-energy phosphates. Disrupted proteins can not be recycled because the recycling mechanisms also require high-energy phosphates. Beyond a salvage threshold of failed gradients and disrupted proteins, the affected cell becomes necrotic. Unfortunately, clean-up of necrotic tissue also requires energy. The result is a collective, accelerating spiral of deteriorating function of cells, tissues, and organs. Normally approximately ¼ of available oxygen is removed from circulation during each circuit through vital organs and tissues. Even if every oxygen molecule could be unloaded from hemoglobin to cells, unreplenished oxygen delivery would be exhausted in approximately 4 minutes. This is important for three reasons. It points to oxygen as a critical nutrient; it points to the importance of efficient resuscitation; and it points to the restoration of oxygen delivery as imperative in resuscitation from shock.

ANSWER: a, b

REFERENCE: *Chapter 8—Shock: Introduction*

2. The catecholamine response results in many of the clinically apparent manifestations of shock. Catecholamines, in this setting, are known to:

a. Accelerate heart rate
b. Divert blood from peripheral arterial beds and splanchnic beds into the systemic circulation
c. Shift potassium into the extracellular fluid
d. Markedly increase diastolic blood pressure

COMMENT: Several classes of hormones are released during the initial response to shock. The catecholamines, epinephrine and norepinephrine, are agonists for both α-adrenergic and β-adrenergic receptors. The catecholamines cause three early events. First, the heart rate accelerates, second peripheral arterial beds and splanchnic beds empty into the systemic circulation, and third, potassium is shifted to intracellular compartments. These events are appreciated as tachycardia; as delayed capillary refill and a slight rise in diastolic blood pressure; and as mild hypokalemia. Catecholamine secretion is prominent in all forms of shock and the effects of catecholamines are nearly always the first physical signs of shock.

ANSWER: a, b

REFERENCE: *Chapter 8—Shock: Introduction*

3. The renin-angiotensin-aldosterone axis is also activated in shock. Which of the following statements is/are true concerning this neuroendocrine response?

   a. Renin is released from the kidneys in response to hypovolemia.
   b. The release of renin is inhibited by epinephrine.
   c. The increase in circulating angiotensin causes splanchnic vasoconstriction, mobilizing up to 30% of total blood volume.
   d. The entire hormonal response causes the kidneys to retain water and sodium

COMMENT: Renin is released from the kidneys in response to hypovolemia, and the release is potentiated by epinephrine. The release catalyzes the conversion of angiotensinogen to the angiotensins. The sudden rise in circulating angiotensins contributes substantially to overall splanchnic vasoconstriction. Such constriction can mobilize up to 30% of the total blood volume compensating for, but also masking the loss of blood from the systemic circulation. The combination of catecholamines, renin, and antidiuretic hormone released early in response to shock causes the kidneys to retain water and sodium and decreases splanchnic perfusion. Urine output is therefore modulated relatively early in the response to shock.

ANSWER: a, c, d

REFERENCE: *Chapter 8—Shock: Introduction*

4. Later in the course of shock, other hormones play an important role including:

   a. Glucagon
   b. Cortisol
   c. Insulin
   d. Growth hormone

COMMENT: Other hormones secreted later in response to shock include glucagon, cortisol, and growth hormone. Collectively, they alter physiology to create a state similar to diabetes, including mild hyperglycemia and insulin resistance. Both muscle protein and fat stores are mobilized during recovery from shock to augment plasma glucose through gluconeogenesis.

ANSWER: a, b, d

REFERENCE: *Chapter 8—Shock: Introduction*

5. Shock due to fluid or blood loss is the most common form encountered by the surgeon. Which of the following statements is/are true concerning hypovolemic shock?

   a. Acute volume loss of approximately 10%, such as seen with voluntary blood donation, is well tolerated often with no clinically apparent affect
   b. Neuroendocrine response to shock becomes apparent with blood loss greater than 20%
   c. Compensatory redistribution fails at approximately 30% volume loss
   d. Neuroendocrine compensatory mechanisms will maintain viability up to 50% of volume loss

COMMENT: The surgeon most commonly encounters shock through the perfusate pathway. The associated clinical symptoms are hypovolemic shock due to dehydration and hemorrhagic shock due to acute loss of blood volume. Mild perfusate loss is common and does not cause clinical symptoms. For example, voluntary blood loss corresponds to acute loss of approximately 10% of the circulating volume. The skin and skeletal muscle vasculature experience a slight decease in perfusion, however, such an acute loss is well tolerated because intravascular volume can be quickly recruited from the interstitial and intracellular reserves. Beyond 10% loss, however, the neuroendocrine response to shock becomes clinically apparent. This results in compensatory increase in heart rate and redistribution of blood from the splanchnic bed. This compensatory redistribution fails at approximately 30% volume loss; a failure clinically manifested as the onset of systolic and diastolic hypotension. Once hypotension occurs, further blood flow distribution occurs in favor of the brain, but at the expense of the heart and kidneys. A 40%–50% volume loss exhausts all compensatory mechanisms.

ANSWER: a, c

REFERENCE: *Chapter 8—Shock: The Pathways to Shock*

6. Cardiogenic shock or pump failure can be caused by:
   a. Myocardial failure such as with infarction or cardiomyopathy
   b. Valvular failure such as with a ruptured papillary muscle
   c. Obstruction to flow by tension pneumothorax or pericardial tamponade
   d. Airlock due to a large air embolus

COMMENT: The pump pathway to shock has two important entrances: primary pump failure and inability of the pump to accept the perfusate. The latter is commonly termed obstructive shock. The causes of pump failure, or cardiogenic shock, are familiar: acute failure of the cardiac muscle or a cardiac valve, and acute dysrhythmias. The specific diagnoses include myocardial infarction, rupture of a papillary muscle, and fracture of the chordae tendineae. The obstructive pathway to shock, the inability of the pump to accept the perfusate, is frequently traversed by injured patients. The specific diagnoses causing obstruction in the acutely injured are tension pneumothorax and pericardial tamponade. Acute embolism of a blood clot from the systemic veins into the heart (pulmonary embolism) is also a common cause of obstructive shock among surgical patients. A less common, but deadly cause of obstructive shock is air embolism consequent to under filled systemic veins brought into contact with the atmosphere either during surgery or by a central venous catheter. A large air embolus obstructs the right ventricular outflow track, whereas slow entrapment of air causes distal pulmonary arteries to become obstructed with acute right ventricular dysfunction.

ANSWER: a, b, c, d

REFERENCE: *Chapter 8—Shock: The Pathways to Shock*

7. Various types of shock result in distinct clinical parameters and measured cardiovascular correlates. Which of the following observations is/are true?
   a. A patient with hypovolemic shock will have cool pale skin, decreased cardiac output, and increased myocardial oxygen consumption
   b. Cardiogenic shock will manifest cool pale skin, decreased cardiac output, increased right heart filling pressure, and decreased myocardial oxygen consumption
   c. Early septic shock will manifest warm pink skin, increased cardiac output, decreased vascular resistance, and increased myocardial oxygen consumption
   d. Spinal shock will manifest warm pink skin below the level of injury, decreased cardiac output, increased vascular resistance, and decreased right heart filling pressure

COMMENT: Table 8.2.

ANSWER: b, c

REFERENCE: *Chapter 8—Shock: The Pathways to Shock*

Table 8.2. CLINICAL PARAMETERS AND MEASURED CORRELATES IN SHOCK

Class	Skin	Right heart filling pressure	Cardiac output	Left heart pressure	Vascular resistance	Myocardial oxygen consumption
Hypovolemic	Cool, pale	↓	↓	↓	↑	↓
Cardiogenic	Cool, pale	↑	↓	↑	↑	↓
Septic (early)	Warm, pink	↔	↑	↓	↓	↑
Septic (late)	Cool, pale	↓	↓	↓	↑	↓
Spinal	Warm, pink below lesion	↓	↓	↓	↓	↔
Obstructive	Cool, pale	↑	↓	↓	↑	↓

8. Hypovolemic shock is classified based on the percent volume loss and clinical response. Which of the following statements is/are true concerning the classification of hypovolemic shock?

   a. Urine output will be decreased in Class I shock with estimated blood loss of less than 15%
   b. Confusion and anxiety will be seen with Class II shock with estimated blood loss of 15%–30%
   c. Blood replacement is indicated with Class III shock (30%–40% blood loss)
   d. Class IV shock with an estimated blood loss of 40% or more will manifest a narrow, but obtainable pulse pressure

COMMENT: Table 8.3.

ANSWER: c

REFERENCE: *Chapter 8—Shock: Types of Shock*

9. Which of the following statements is/are true concerning the manifestations of septic shock and its resuscitation?

   a. Early sepsis causes marked vessel constriction
   b. Sepsis can result in a beneficial afterload reduction
   c. Hypotension in advanced septic shock is primarily due to hypovolemia because of volume redistribution
   d. Aggressive volume resuscitation will restore systemic blood pressure although venous resistance will remain constant

COMMENT: Septic shock is the most common form of distributive shock encountered by the surgeon. Absent medical intervention, the venodilatation of sepsis will restore systemic blood pressure to normal value, but now with markedly decreased venous resistance. The competing cardiac effects of sepsis are modeled with appropriate shifts in the cardiac function curve. Afterload reduction, occurring during early septic shock, tends to increase cardiac performance while direct myocardial depression overwhelms this advantage in late uncompensated shock.

ANSWER: b

REFERENCE: *Chapter 8—Shock: Types of Shock*

Table 8.3. **CLASSIFICATION OF HYPOVOLEMIC SHOCK (ASSOCIATED WITH ACUTE BLOOD LOSS)**

	Class I	Class II	Class III	Class IV
Estimated blood loss (% blood volume)	≤15%	15%–30%	30%–40%	40%
Typical pulse rate	<100	>100	>120	>140
Typical blood pressure	Normal	Normal mean, with declining systolic and rising systolic pressures	Decreased	Markedly decreased
Pulse pressure	Normal	Narrowed	Narrowed	Unobtainable
Central nervous system/mental status	Normal to slightly anxious	Mildly anxious	Anxious and confused	Confused or lethargic
Urine output	Normal	~0.5 mL/kg/h	<0.5 mL/kg/h	Nil
Volume required	Often none	Crystalloid	Crystalloid and blood	Blood

10. Which of the following statements is/are correct concerning neurogenic shock?

   a. Cardiac function is depressed regardless of the level of injury
   b. If cardiac function is unaffected, limited volume resuscitation and treatment with a β-agonist is appropriate therapy.
   c. Phenylephrine is an appropriate treatment in all settings of neurogenic shock
   d. Neuraxial anesthesia, if extended beyond its intended effect, results in significant neurogenic shock

COMMENT: Surgeons encounter neurogenic shock in two arenas: the trauma resuscitation bay and the operating room. Traumatic spinal injury occurs when the cord is severed at a level within or above the sympathetic chain, where as neurogenic shock encountered in the operating room is the consequence of neuraxial anesthetic that is extended beyond its intended effect. Bearing in mind that the heart also receives sympathetic input, there is an important functional distinction between an injury above T-4 and one below T-4. The former depresses cardiac function in addition to affecting venous return, where the latter leaves cardiac performance unaffected. When cardiac performance is unaffected, limited volume resuscitation and treatment with a pure α-agonist such as phenylephrine is sufficient therapy. However, if cardiac sympathetic intervention is compromised, vagal parasympathetic intervention may predominate and administration of phenylephrine may aggravate reflex bradycardia.

ANSWER: d

REFERENCE: *Chapter 8—Shock: Types of Shock*

11. Resuscitation from shock must begin immediately on recognition. Which of the following statements is/are correct concerning the early stages of resuscitation?

   a. The absence of a carotid pulse indicates a systolic blood pressure less than 60 mm Hg.
   b. A blood sample for type and cross match and hemoglobin determination should be obtained early.
   c. An initial rapid fluid bolus of crystalloid will increase cardiac preload and diminish venous resistance.
   d. Care should be taken to determine the etiology of shock prior to fluid bolus administration

COMMENT: The absence of central pulses (femoral, carotid) mandates cardiac life support including cardiopulmonary resuscitation, determination of rhythm, and cardioversion defibrillation. More commonly, a faint pulse is palpable. The carotid pulse is ordinarily present in adults with systolic blood pressure greater than 60 mm Hg. A short, wide-bore intravenous catheter should be inserted into a peripheral vein and an aliquot of blood taken for analysis. Given the frequency of hypovolemic shock in the surgical population, one of the most important steps is the immediate crossmatching of blood. A hemoglobin determination is also desirable. The venous catheter then serves as a conduit for rapid infusion of a balanced salt solution. Ringer's lactate at 20 mL/kg should be administered as rapidly as practical. The fluid bolus serves to increase preload, diminish venous resistance, and possibly decrease arterial afterload, all of which augment cardiac performance. Stroke volume improves by this mechanism even in patients who have sustained an acute myocardial infarction or have pericardial tamponade. Fluid bolus should therefore only be withheld when there is incontrovertable evidence that the cause is cardiogenic and associated with frothy pink pulmonary adema.

ANSWER: a, b, c

REFERENCE: *Chapter 8—Shock: Shock Recognition and Resuscitation; Practical Aspects*

12. Which of the following are valuable in the assessment of the success of resuscitation and shock reversal?
    a. Urine output
    b. Arterial blood gas
    c. Serum lactate
    d. Anion gap

COMMENT: The best first proxy for the adequacy of organ perfusion appears to be urine output, which should be measured every 30 minutes by indwelling bladder catheter. The best first proxy for the adequacy for shock reversal is the pH of arterial blood gas analysis. During shock, the pH falls into the acid range as a consequence of anaerobic metabolism with obligatory accumulation of lactic acid. Once resuscitation is adequate, the lactic should be metabolized and the anion gap should normalize. Persistent anion gap acidosis suggests inadequate resuscitation or frankly nonviable tissue. A non-anion gap acidosis is less worrisome and may follow resuscitation with normal saline. The most immediately valuable measures of tissue perfusion include arterial blood gas analysis for pH and the by-product of anaerobic metabolism, lactate.

ANSWER: a, b, c, d

REFERENCE: *Chapter 8—Shock: Shock Recognition and Resuscitation; Practical Aspects*

13. Patients with severe shock or with preexisting medical diseases often lack sufficient compensatory mechanisms. Which of the following statements is/are correct concerning adjunctive therapy for shock?
    a. In order to decrease metabolic requirements, the patient's temperature should be cooled
    b. Calcium should be administered early in the resuscitation of all patients
    c. Sodium bicarbonate should be administered to correct serum pH to normal range
    d. Circulation can not be readily restored at temperatures less than 33°C

COMMENT: Because severe hypocalcemia and severe acidosis both can thwart shock resuscitation, the ionized calcium and base deficit should be determined early in the resuscitation. Calcium should be administered to bring the ionized calcium into the normal range, and consideration should be given to giving sufficient bicarbonate to bring the plasma pH up to 7.2. There is no benefit to the administration of calcium or bicarbonate in excess of these targets. Temperature should also be measured, and patients whose temperatures are less then 30–34°C actually should be rewarmed because the circulation can not be readily restored at lower temperatures.

ANSWER: d

REFERENCE: *Chapter 8—Shock: Adjuncts to Resuscitation*

14. Several classes of drugs serve as adjuncts to resuscitation from shock. Sympathetic and sympathomimetic amines are widely used. These drugs can manifest their effects through either α, β^1, or β^2 receptor effects. Which of the following statements is/are true concerning the relative affects of these drugs?

    a. Phenylephrine has a pure α effect

    b. Epinephrine has a comparable affect at all receptor sites

    c. Norepinephrine has its predominant effect on β receptors

    d. Dobutamine offers the advantage of having a selective β^1 effect

COMMENT: Table 8.4.

ANSWER: a, b, d

REFERENCE: *Chapter 8—Shock: Adjuncts to Resuscitation*

Table 8.4. RELATIVE EFFECTS OF VASOACTIVE DRUGS

Drug	α	β_1	β_2
Phenylephrine	++/+++	—	—
Norepinephrine	+++	++	+
Epinephrine	+++	+++	+++
Dopamine	+ to +++	++	++
Dobutamine	+	+++	+
Isoproterenol	—	+++	+++

15. Which of the following statements is/are true concerning vasoactive agents used in the treatment of shock?

    a. Sympathomimetic amines are most effective in a slightly acid milieu (pH 7.2–7.4)

    b. Dopamine has a unique characteristic of accumulating effects with increasing dose allowing titration of desired effect

    c. The affects sympathomimetic amines is primarily through extracellular mechanisms

    d. Dobutamine is effective as a long-term agent in the treatment of cardiogenic shock

COMMENT: Dopamine differs from other pressors by having accumulating effects with increasing doses. In order, the receptors occupied are dopaminergic on the kidney and splanchnic beds that augment regional blood flow; β receptors with vasodilitation dominating as well as an increasing heart rate; and finally, at higher doses, the α receptors become occupied with vasoconstriction. The effects of sympathomimetic amines are modulated by several factors. In addition to being more effective in a slightly acid milieau (pH 7.2–7.4), the hemodynamic effects depend on receptor number and occupancy, and coupling of the receptors to second messengers. All sympathomimetic amines appear to act through one or more internal cell signaling systems. Receptor numbers and second messenger coupling appears to be especially important for dobutamine because tachyphylaxis can render the drug ineffective after just a few days administration.

ANSWER: a, b

REFERENCE: *Chapter 8—Shock: Adjuncts to Resuscitation*

16. Which of the following statements is/are true with respect to the use of pulmonary artery catheters (Swan-Ganz catheters) in patients with shock?
    a. A pulmonary artery catheter may improve the outcome in patients with myocardial infarction and cardiogenic shock
    b. The use of a pulmonary artery catheter has been shown to decrease mortality in critically ill patients.
    c. A pulmonary artery catheter is useful in patients with septic shock who have not responded to initial fluid resuscitation.
    d. Pulmonary artery catheters should be used more frequently for determining the management of patients with hemodynamic instability or shock.

COMMENT: Pulmonary artery catheters (Swan-Ganz catheters) are a non-therapeutic device in which the performance depends heavily on the skill of the operator and expertise of the interpreter. With this in mind, pulmonary artery catheters appear to be over used. A multi-center trial reported in 1996 showed that pulmonary artery catheters increased attributable mortality in patients with critical illness. There likely are specific indications for a pulmonary artery catheter in shock. Grade E evidence suggests that these catheters will lead to an improvement in outcome of patients with myocardial infarction complicated by cardiogenic shock. A pulmonary artery catheter may also be useful in patients with septic shock who have not responded to initial aggressive fluid resuscitation and low-dose isotropic/vasoconstrictor therapy. The paucity of data, however, from randomized prospective trials still leaves questions with respect to the use of this device.

ANSWER: a, c

REFERENCE: *Chapter 8—Shock: Pulmonary Artery Catheter in Shock Management; Whether and When*

17. Recognition of sepsis in the intensive care unit patient can be extremely difficult. Which of the following conditions may suggest underlying sepsis?
    a. Mental status changes
    b. Decreased minute ventilation
    c. Glucose intolerance
    d. Feed intolerance
    e. Rising platelet count

COMMENT: Objective clues contributing to the impression of underlying sepsis in the intensive care unit patient include the following: (1) mental status changes. The brain is exquisitely sensitive to the metabolic derangements of sepsis. Sudden, unexplained deterioration of responsiveness must always suggest either an oxygen delivery problem or sepsis. (2) Increased minute ventilation. Sepsis causes tachypnea. This is difficult to appreciate in the mechanically ventilated patient. Respiratory therapists provide a diagnostic tool in their charting of minute ventilatory volume. Increasing minute ventilatory volume, particularly when oxygen saturations have been adequate, suggest sepsis or pulmonary embolism. (3) Glucose intolerance. Sepsis renders patients resistant to endogenous or administered insulin. New-onset hyperglycemia or glycosuria or an increase in previously stable dose of insulin, suggests sepsis. (4) Feed intolerance. Non-ICU patients who contact infections typically become anorectic: they decline food. ICU patients who are typically fed by tube into the proximal GI tract, become intolerant of those feedings. This intolerance presents as either "residuals," which are evacuated per tube by the nurse, or more dramatically as regurgitation and vomiting. (5) Falling platelet count. Leukocytosis is a poor indicator of sepsis in surgical patients, for two reasons. First, elective surgery, trauma, and drug reactions cause leukocytosis in many patients. Second, leukopenia is common in advanced sepsis. The clue to sepsis in the hemogram in the surgical patient is the platelet count: thrombocytopenia is common owing to the remarkable sensitivity of megacaryocytes to infection. Although thrombocytopenia may be caused by several drugs, sepsis should always be considered. Occult sepsis-induced thrombocytopenia is more common in many ICUs than drug-induced thrombocytopenia.

ANSWER: a, c, d

REFERENCE: *Chapter 8—Shock: Problems of Secondary Sepsis*

18. Which of the following should be considered as a cause of shock for a patient in the operating room?

    a. Inadequate ventilation
    b. Arrhythmia
    c. Tension pneumothorax
    d. Air embolism
    e. Transfusion reaction

COMMENT: Although anesthetics and operations have become progressively safer, most surgeons are eventually confronted with sudden circulatory collapse of a patient in the operating room. Such situations can be salvaged only if the surgeon and anesthesiologist work rapidly to analyze and correct the problem. After recognition that the patient is "in extremis," the most important next step is to determine whether it is ventilation or/and circulation. The presence of carbon dioxide in the end-tidal gas confirms that both are present. Conversely, the absence of end-tidal carbon dioxide means that either ventilatory or circulation or both has failed. Such failure requires immediate confirmation that the endotracheal tube is in the airway, immediate ventilation, and initiation of cardiac compression while the underlying cause of the arrest is sought. The cardiac rhythm should be inspected on the monitor, and the anesthesiologist should be asked about any changes in morphology (suggestive of myocardial ischemia or infarction) before the collapse. If a life-threatening arrhythmia is noted, it should be treated using advanced cardiac life support guidelines. If ventilation and circulation are present, but there is a circulatory collapse in the context of a reasonably normal cardiac rhythm, the next step is to look at the operative field while asking the anesthesiologist about airway pressures. The surgeon must look for excessive bleeding and at the shape of the diaphragms. If significant bleeding is observed, isolation and control becomes the next priority. The reason to inspect the diaphragms while asking about airway pressures is that pneumothoraces are not only common, but quickly become tension pneumothoraces under positive-pressure ventilation. The diaphragm on the affected side blows into the abdomen and remains relatively distended throughout the ventilatory cycle. The airway pressures are higher than previously observed.

While the surgeon's inspecting the diaphragms, the anesthesiologist should be listening for breath sounds and heart sounds. The reason for listening to heart sounds is to exclude the rarer cause of obstructive shock, air embolism, a cause that should be suspected in any patient who has either a central venous catheter or who has had a large vein open in the operative field. Diagnosis is based entirely on suspicion, but the central venous catheters should be inspected and the heart should be auscultated for a continuous murmur. If air embolism is thought likely, an attempt should be made to aspirate air back through the central catheter while the patient is placed in Trendelenburg position. Finally, the possibilities of anaphylaxis to a recently administered drug or of a major transfusion reaction need to be considered.

ANSWER: a, b, c, d, e

REFERENCE: *Chapter 8—Shock: Specific Perioperative Problems with Shock*

19. The following pairs of statements include a cause for shock and a specific time period in the postoperative care when such an event would be *most* likely. Which of the following causes are associated with shock in the specific time period noted?

    a. Bleeding/greater than 24 hours
    b. Myocardial infarction/4–24 hours
    c. Pulmonary embolism/greater than 24 hours
    d. Severe wound infection/greater than 24 hours

COMMENT: Shock in the immediate postoperative period is attributed to bleeding until proven otherwise. More often than not, bleeding is either an obvious cause of the shock state or is suggested by a lower-than-expected hematocrit. Although exploration of the surgical site is mandatory, the cause of bleeding is not always surgical, and appropriate coagulation studies should be ordered along with blood products as soon as immediate postoperative shock is recognized.

As anesthetics and pain medications wear off in the period 4–24 hours after surgery, patients often experience significant pain and respond with a catecholamine surge. The associated increase in heart rate can cause or mask an evolving myocardial infarction in patients with cardiovascular risk. Surgical site pain can extinguish anginal pain, and an EKG and biochemical tests for myocardial damage should be obtained promptly. Also in the 4- to 24-hour period, serious surgical site infections can cause shock. These site infections, typically streptococcal, cause a brawny cellulitis (sometimes associated with brown edema fluid) that mask a necrotizing myofascial infection. For this reason, shock appearing during the immediate postoperative period mandates at least an inspection of the wound. If cellulitis is present, the wound should be promptly explored in the operating room where radical débridement is undertaken. Aggressive antibiotic therapy, an adjunct to surgical débridement (not a substitute) may be life saving. There are four common causes of unexplained shock in the late postoperative period. Sepsis is by far the most common including surgical site infections, blood stream infections, urinary tract infections, and pneumonias. Pulmonary embolism in a setting of occult deep venous thrombosis also tends to occur somewhat later because the operation and consequently immobility are usually the cause of deep venous thrombosis, and pulmonary embolism must follow its formation. Shock and unexplained hypoxemia should suggest pulmonary embolism.

ANSWER: b, c

REFERENCE: *Chapter 8—Shock: Specific Perioperative Problems with Shock*

CHAPTER 9
CRITICAL CARE

1. Which of the following statements is/are true concerning oxygen consumption ($\dot{V}O_2$)?

    a. $\dot{V}O_2$ is normally 100 to 120 mL/m^2 per minute
    b. Resting $\dot{V}O_2$ is controlled by the level of thyroid and catecholamine hormones
    c. Under steady-state conditions, the amount of oxygen consumed exceeds the amount of oxygen taken up by the pulmonary capillaries
    d. $\dot{V}O_2$ depends on the status of pulmonary function

COMMENT: Oxygen consumed in the process of metabolism is expressed as the volume of oxygen per minute ($\dot{V}O_2$). $\dot{V}O_2$ is normally 100 to 120 mL/m^2 per minute, or 200 mL/min for a typical adult. Resting $\dot{V}O_2$ is a function of metabolizing body cell mass. Fine-tuning is provided by the level of thyroid and catecholamine hormones. $\dot{V}O_2$ decreases under conditions of hypothermia, paralysis, and hypothyroidism. $\dot{V}O_2$ increases during exercise or muscular activity, hyperthermia, profound hypothalamic injury, hyperthyroidism, and use of catecholamines or inflammatory mediators, particularly interleukin cytokines. Under steady-state conditions, the amount of oxygen consumed in systemic metabolism equals the amount of oxygen taken up by the pulmonary capillaries through the airway. This is true regardless of the status of pulmonary function or dysfunction, so $\dot{V}O_2$ is measured across the lung, and it is assumed that this amount is consumed in the systemic metabolism.

ANSWER: a, b

REFERENCE: *Chapter 9—Critical Care: Oxygen Kinetics; Integrating Hemodynamics, Respiratory, and Metabolic Physiology*

2. Which of the following statements is/are true concerning oxygen delivery?
   a. The amount of oxygen delivered to peripheral tissues depends on the oxygen content in arterial blood and cardiac output
   b. Oxygen content is commonly measured in arterial blood
   c. The normal arterial-venous difference is 4 mL oxygen per deciliter
   d. Normal systemic oxygen delivery for a typical adult is approximately 1,000 mL/min

COMMENT: The amount of oxygen delivered to peripheral tissues is the product of the oxygen content in arterial blood and cardiac output. The oxygen content of arterial blood normally is approximately 20 mL/dL, and the normal cardiac index is 5 L/min. Therefore, the normal systemic oxygen delivery is approximately 1,000 mL/min. Although oxygen content is the most important measurement of oxygen in the blood, partial pressure of oxygen (P_{O_2}) and oxyhemoglobin saturation are more commonly measured in intensive care units, hence it is necessary to convert between these measurements. The normal oxygen content of venous blood is 16 mL/dL. Hence the normal arterial-venous difference is 4 mL oxygen per deciliter.

ANSWER: a, c, d

REFERENCE: *Chapter 9—Critical Care: Oxygen Kinetics; Integrating Hemodynamics, Respiratory, and Metabolic Physiology*

3. Which of the following statements is/are true concerning the autoregulation necessary to maintain $\dot{V}_{O_2}$ and oxygen delivery?
   a. A change in $\dot{V}_{O_2}$ is followed by a proportionate change in oxygen delivery
   b. A change in oxygen delivery is followed by a change in $\dot{V}_{O_2}$
   c. Increases in oxygen delivery are caused solely by an increase in cardiac output
   d. The normal ratio of oxygen delivery to consumption is 2:1

COMMENT: The relation between $\dot{V}_{O_2}$ and oxygen delivery represents one of the most interesting regulation systems in homeostasis. If one of the three components of oxygen delivery is abnormal, endogenous mechanisms regulate the other two until normal oxygen delivery has been restored. The various combinations of compensatory mechanisms supply adequate oxygen for systemic metabolism through a wide range of variations in oxygen delivery. When there is a change in $\dot{V}_{O_2}$, a proportionate change in oxygen delivery occurs almost immediately and is mediated completely by a change in cardiac output. A primary change in oxygen delivery is not followed by a change in $\dot{V}_{O_2}$. The normal ratio of oxygen delivery to consumption is approximately 5:1.

ANSWER: a

REFERENCE: *Chapter 9—Critical Care: Oxygen Kinetics; Integrating Hemodynamics, Respiratory, and Metabolic Physiology*

4. Which of the following statements is/are true concerning oxygen venous saturation monitoring?

   a. The normal saturation of mixed venous blood is 50%
   b. Mixed venous blood obtained for saturation monitoring can be obtained from any peripheral vein
   c. If arterial blood is fully saturated, the saturation of mixed venous blood is 80%
   d. In less than fully saturated blood, the difference between arterial and venous saturation corresponds to oxygen extraction

COMMENT: The relation between oxygen delivery and $\dot{V}O_2$ is reflected in the amount of oxygen in venous blood. Under normal circumstances, oxygen delivery is 1,000 mL/min, and $\dot{V}O_2$ is 200 mL/min. The amount of oxygen extracted is 20% of that delivered, and 80% of oxygen is still present in venous blood returning to the heart. Arterial blood usually is fully saturated, and under normal circumstances, the saturation of mixed venous blood ($S\dot{V}O_2$) is 80%. This measurement must be made in mixed venous blood because the relative extractions of organs served by the superior and inferior venae cavae and coronary sinus are quite different. As long as arterial blood is fully saturated, this observation holds true regardless of the absolute level of $\dot{V}O_2$ or oxygen delivery. If the arterial blood is less than fully saturated, the difference between arterial and venous saturation corresponds to oxygen extraction, hence the oxygen delivery to consumption ratio.

ANSWER: c, d

REFERENCE: *Chapter 9—Critical Care: Oxygen Kinetics; Integrating Hemodynamics, Respiratory, and Metabolic Physiology*

5. Which of the following statements is/are true concerning oxygen kinetics in a critically ill, febrile patient?

   a. $\dot{V}O_2$ likely is greater than three times normal
   b. The high cardiac output and pulse rate are designed to increase oxygen delivery
   c. The hyperdynamic response can increase oxygen delivery to exceed the increase in $\dot{V}O_2$
   d. The patient can maintain adequate compensation as long as the oxygen delivery to consumption ratio is greater than 2:1

COMMENT: In critically ill patients $\dot{V}O_2$ may be elevated or depressed, but slight to moderate elevation in $\dot{V}O_2$ is the most common abnormality among critically ill patients. $\dot{V}O_2$ is elevated in proportion to the amount of inflammation. Oxygen delivery of a febrile patient with signs of septic toxicity typically is 1.5 to 2 times normal. It is unusual for a critically ill patient to have $\dot{V}O_2$ more than twice normal. This occurs only in situations of severe muscular exercise, such as seizures or tetanus. During hypermetabolism, a change in $\dot{V}O_2$ is followed promptly by a proportionate change in oxygen delivery. Hence, it is "normal" for a hypermetabolic patient to have a high cardiac output and pulse rate. In rare instances the hyperdynamic response exceeds the increase in $\dot{V}O_2$, reflected in a ratio greater than 5:1 and $S\dot{V}O_2$ greater than 80%. Some patients cannot mount increased oxygen delivery in response to increased $\dot{V}O_2$ because of the combination of hypoxemia, anemia, and myocardial failure. If this occurs, the oxygen delivery to consumption ratio is less than 5:1. The patient compensates with increased oxygen extraction, however, and remains in stable condition as long as the ratio is greater than 2:1.

ANSWER: b, d

REFERENCE: *Chapter 9—Critical Care: Oxygen Kinetics; Integrating Hemodynamics, Respiratory, and Metabolic Physiology*

6. Which of the following statements is/are true concerning carbon dioxide kinetics?

   a. The amount of carbon dioxide produced is equivalent to the amount of oxygen consumed
   b. Carbon dioxide levels in blood, present mostly as a bicarbonate ion, can quickly change
   c. Normally the amount of carbon dioxide excreted through the lung equals the amount of carbon dioxide produced in peripheral tissues
   d. The amount of carbon dioxide excreted is a function of ventilation of perfused alveoli

COMMENT: The total amount of carbon dioxide produced by systemic metabolism is roughly equivalent to the amount of oxygen consumed (100 to 120 mL/m^2 per minute, 200 mL/min for a typical adult). Production of carbon dioxide increases or decreases by each of the factors that causes an increase or decrease in $\dot{V}O_2$. Most of the carbon dioxide in blood is present as bicarbonate ion, which cannot be changed quickly. However, metabolically produced carbon dioxide is mostly present as dissolved carbon dioxide, added to the blood in the peripheral tissues and excreted in the lung. In a steady state, the amount of carbon dioxide excreted through the lung equals the amount of carbon dioxide produced in peripheral tissues. The amount of carbon dioxide excreted is a function of ventilation of perfused alveoli (alveolar ventilation per minute).

ANSWER: a, c, d

REFERENCE: *Chapter 9—Critical Care: Respiratory Physiology and Pathophysiology*

7. Which of the following statements is/are true concerning the pathophysiologic mechanism of gas exchange?

   a. Hypoventilation in relation to perfusion can result in an oxygen saturation of less than 100%
   b. Diffusion block and ventilation-perfusion ($\dot{V}O_2/\dot{Q}$) mismatch can almost completely be overcome by breathing 100% oxygen
   c. Transpulmonary shunting does not occur under normal circumstances
   d. Normal arterial oxygen saturation is 100%

COMMENT: Under normal conditions, red blood cells in the pulmonary capillaries become fully saturated, and oxygen dissolves in plasma. The result is a blood Po_2 of 100 mm Hg and oxygen saturation of 100%. This equilibration can be disturbed by means of hypoventilation in relation to the perfusion ($\dot{V}O_2/\dot{Q}$ mismatch), diffusion block caused by interstitial fibrosis, or perfusion of nonventilated alveoli. Diffusion block and $\dot{V}O_2/\dot{Q}$ mismatch can be almost completely overcome by breathing 100% oxygen, hence hypoxemia during exposure to high alveolar Po_2 is caused by total $\dot{V}O_2/\dot{Q}$ mismatch, so-called transpulmonary shunting or venous admixture. Under normal circumstances, approximately 5% of the blood entering the left atrium has been shunted away from the pulmonary capillaries, either as the result of bronchial nutritive blood flow or through thebesian veins that open directly into the left side of the heart. This phenomenon, combined with a normal minor $\dot{V}O_2/\dot{Q}$ mismatch associated with breathing at rest and positional changes in pulmonary blood flow, result in a normal arterial Po_2 of 90 to 100 mm Hg and normal oxygen saturation of 98%.

ANSWER: a, b

REFERENCE: *Chapter 9—Critical Care: Respiratory Physiology and Pathophysiology*

8. Which of the following statements is/are true concerning carbon dioxide transfer in the lung?

   a. Carbon dioxide excretion is a direct function of alveolar ventilation
   b. Normally end-tidal partial pressure of carbon dioxide should be identical to $Paco_2$
   c. The gradient between end-tidal and arterial carbon dioxide can be an indirect measure of nonperfused alveoli
   d. Positive pressure ventilation under normal airway pressure causes a marked gradient between end-tidal and arterial partial pressures of carbon dioxide

COMMENT: The amount of carbon dioxide excreted is directly related to alveolar ventilation. Whereas oxygenation is a function of matching blood flow to alveoli, carbon dioxide excretion is a direct function of ventilation or hyperventilation of alveoli with some blood flow. The normal end-tidal partial pressure of carbon dioxide represents mixed alveolar gas at equilibrium with pulmonary capillary blood and hence with arterial blood. Therefore the end-tidal carbon dioxide value and $Paco_2$ should be identical. End-tidal carbon dioxide measurement is a useful continuous measurement of $Paco_2$ that can be used for monitoring when the lung is normal, as in ventilator weaning. The gradient between end-tidal and arterial carbon dioxide, when it is large, is an indirect measure of nonperfused alveoli and compression volume. For patients using a ventilator with positive pressure ventilation, a marked gradient between the partial pressure of end-tidal and arterial carbon dioxide occurs only when peak airway pressures are greater than 30 cm water, and the compression volume is an important component of each exhaled breath.

ANSWER: a, b, c

REFERENCE: *Chapter 9—Critical Care: The Pathophysiology of Gas Exchange*

9. Which of the following statements is/are true concerning pulmonary mechanics?

   a. The standard compliance or volume pressure curve is measured during lung inflation
   b. The decreased compliance in acute respiratory failure occurs because the lung is smaller, not because it is stiffer
   c. In acute respiratory failure, higher pressures are needed to achieve the same level of inflation
   d. Areas of normal lungs are more vulnerable to overdistension, which can lead to progressive lung dysfunction

COMMENT: The standard compliance or volume pressure curve is drawn by means of measuring volume and pressure at stages of lung deflation after total inflation. The decreased compliance in acute respiratory distress syndrome occurs because the lung is smaller, not stiffer. In acute respiratory failure, the cause of decreased compliance is almost always associated with a decrease in functional residual capacity (FRC). The decreased FRC represents lost alveoli, which are either collapsed or filled with fluid but still perfused with blood. Because the lung is smaller, the compliance curve has shifted to the right, and much higher pressures are needed to achieve the same level of inflation. Lung damage can be caused by high airway pressure, so overdistension is detrimental in addition to being inefficient. Because the areas of lung that are closest to normal have the best compliance, they are most vulnerable to overdistension. This vulnerability contributes to the steady progression of lung dysfunction among patients undergoing ventilation at high peak pressure.

ANSWER: b, c, d

REFERENCE: *Chapter 9—Critical Care: Pulmonary Mechanics*

10. Which of the following result(s) in a decrease in functional residual capacity?

    a. Shallow breathing
    b. Partial airway occlusion
    c. Absorption atelectasis
    d. Hemothorax

COMMENT: A decrease in FRC is caused by incomplete alveolar inflation related to (a) shallow breathing, (b) partial or complete airway occlusion, which can be generalized, as in bronchospasm, or localized, as in gastric aspiration, (c) absorption atelectasis, which occurs when oxygen is substituted for nitrogen in the inspired gas, or (d) conditions in which air or fluid occupies a potential alveolar space in the chest, such as pneumothorax, hemothorax, or pulmonary edema.

ANSWER: a, b, c, d

REFERENCE: *Chapter 9—Critical Care*

11. Which of the following statements is/are true concerning the response to a decrease in FRC?

    a. Supplying supplemental oxygen always improves the situation
    b. Respiratory alkalosis can occur
    c. A decrease in compliance is a common occurrence
    d. Respiratory rate and depth of breathing generally decrease

COMMENT: Pulmonary arterial spasm in response to local hypoxia autoregulates pulmonary blood flow and maintains adequate gas exchange during alveolar collapse—up to a point. However, when the loss in ventilation exceeds the decrease in perfusion, $\dot{V}o_2/\dot{Q}$ mismatch occurs and results in incomplete oxygenation of blood perfusing that area of the lung. The resultant hypoxemia stimulates an increased rate and depth of breathing, which can reexpand the inflated area of lung. If it does not, hypoxemia continues, but increased ventilation in other areas of the lung results in excess carbon dioxide excretion, hypocapnia, and respiratory alkalosis. The blood gas abnormality, hypoxemia with respiratory alkalosis, is the most common abnormality of gas exchange among surgical patients and is a hallmark of $\dot{V}o_2/\dot{Q}$ imbalance.

Oxygenation of blood in poorly ventilated areas of the lung can be improved by means of increasing the concentration of oxygen in the inspired gas. The use of supplemental oxygen, however, addresses the symptom rather than the cause and can worsen the problem by adding to absorption atelectasis, which deprives the poorly ventilated area of nitrogen to hold alveoli open. This can cause total alveolar collapse. In this circumstance, blood perfusing the non-ventilated area mixes with blood from other areas of the lung; the result is hypoxemia that does not improve appreciably in response to administration of oxygen. Aside from the effects on gas exchange, loss of alveolar space results in changes in the volume-pressure relations in the lung. A decrease in functional residual capacity always results in a shift in the volume-pressure relation toward a condition of decreasing compliance.

ANSWER: b, c

REFERENCE: *Chapter 9—Critical Care: Pathophysiology of Respiratory Failure*

12. Which of the following statements is/are true concerning pulmonary edema?

    a. Pulmonary edema effectively narrows bronchi and increases pulmonary vascular resistance

    b. Ventilation and perfusion are decreased equally

    c. Positive pressure ventilation improves gas exchange by decreasing lung edema

    d. The condition is frequently caused by decreased plasma protein levels

COMMENT: The causes of pulmonary edema are (a) increased hydrostatic pressure, (b) increased capillary permeability, and (c) decreased plasma oncotic pressure. The latter, however, is rarely a problem unless the concentration of plasma protein is very low. When it begins to collect in the lung interstitium, fluid migrates to the loose areolar portion of the microanatomic regions of the lung that surround the small bronchioles and pulmonary arteries. The edema in these areas narrows bronchi and increases resistance in the pulmonary vasculature. This decreases both ventilation and perfusion in the edematous area, but ventilation often is affected more than blood flow; the result is a decreased $\dot{V}_{O_2}/\dot{Q}$ ratio, with all of its attendant effects on gas exchange. Ventilator management of pulmonary edema, which increases airway pressure, tends to hold the alveoli open, spread out the space available for water accumulation, and overcome the effect of small bronchial occlusion. Positive pressure ventilation therefore does not affect the amount of edema in the lung; it affects only the manifestations.

ANSWER: a

REFERENCE: *Chapter 9—Critical Care: Pathophysiology of Respiratory Failure*

13. Useful steps to optimize systemic oxygen delivery include:

    a. Maintaining mean arterial blood pressure between 50 and 90 mm Hg

    b. Optimizing positive end-expiratory pressure (PEEP) levels by means of monitoring mixed venous saturation

    c. Turning the patient prone

    d. Sedation or paralysis

COMMENT: Optimizing systemic oxygen delivery in relation to oxygen requirement is the primary goal of management. Improving oxygenation of the blood itself by improving alveolar inflation is only one of the steps in optimizing oxygen delivery. Equally or more important are managing anemia and optimizing cardiac output. Cardiac output should be optimized to maintain delivery of four to five times consumption. In general, this means avoiding factors that decrease cardiac output rather than actively trying to increase cardiac output. Blood pressure should be maintained high enough to provide coronary perfusion (more than 50 mm Hg mean pressure) but not so high as to limit left ventricular function (more than 90 mm Hg mean arterial pressure).

Alveolar collapse is managed by means of cleaning the airways, avoiding 100% oxygen, moving fluid from the lung or chest, and by the use of PEEP to hold open alveoli opened with other measures. The optimal level of PEEP is that which maintains arterial oxygenation but does not decrease venous return or cardiac output. This optimal level is best determined by means of monitoring mixed venous saturation. Another step in optimizing lung function is to take advantage of the gravitational effects on pulmonary blood flow by turning the patient prone or to a full lateral position to direct blood flow to areas of optimal alveolar function. This step often results in opening in the closed posterior alveoli compressed by the weight of the fluid in the lungs. At the same time that oxygen delivery is optimized, $\dot{V}_{O_2}$ should be decreased to normal or even less than normal if necessary. Managing infection, providing adequate sedation, and establishing muscular paralysis decrease $\dot{V}_{O_2}$, and decrease the need for oxygen delivery.

ANSWER: a, b, c, d

REFERENCE: *Chapter 9—Critical Care: Management of Respiratory Failure*

14. Which of the following statements is/are true concerning the use of a ventilator in the management of respiratory failure?

    a. The assist-control mode is appropriate in the care of paralyzed patients
    b. Peak inspiratory pressure should be optimized at a level greater than 40 cm water
    c. A patient receiving excessive carbohydrate for nutritional support may have an elevated minute ventilation and may tire with spontaneous breathing
    d. In general, weaning requires an adequate inspiratory force, vital capacity, and a minute ventilation less than 10 L/min

COMMENT: Most intensive care specialists favor setting the ventilator on the assist-control mode at a low sensitivity. With this setting, the patient breathes at a rate that regulates the $Paco_2$ to normal, but each breath is mechanically assisted to provide maximal inflation. The volume of each breath is set by limiting the maximal pressure or maximal volume of each breath. Whichever method is used, the peak inspiratory pressure should not generally exceed 40 cm water. If the patient is comatose or paralyzed, the assist mode cannot be used, and the rate in addition to the volume is set.

Adequate weaning indices are inspiratory force greater than 20 cm water, vital capacity twice tidal volume, adequate gas exchange with assisted ventilation at Fio_2 of 0.3 and 5 cm water of PEEP, and minute ventilation less than 10 L/min. If the patient is hypermetabolic or is receiving excessive carbohydrate as nutritional support, the minute ventilation will be elevated, even during assisted mechanical ventilation. If this is the case, the patient will tire rapidly with spontaneous breathing.

ANSWER: c, d

REFERENCE: *Chapter 9—Critical Care: Management of Respiratory Failure*

15. Which of the following statements is/are true concerning the management of pulmonary interstitial edema?

    a. Diuresis and blood transfusion are a valuable step
    b. Salt-poor albumin leaks through the capillaries and worsens the condition
    c. Mannitol is contraindicated as a diuretic in this clinical situation
    d. Isoproterenol is a poor choice as an inotropic agent

COMMENT: Management of pulmonary edema has two important goals. The first is to improve oxygenation if it is impaired, and the second is to minimize fibrosis and bacterial infection, which often accompany pulmonary edema caused by capillary injury. The management of interstitial edema is to maintain the hydrostatic pressure as low as compatible with adequate cardiac output and to increase oncotic pressure selectively in the vascular space. These measures, combined with fluid restriction and diuresis, decrease the amount of pulmonary edema. Because it is desirable to maintain filling pressures of the left ventricle as low as possible while maintaining good cardiac output, inotropic drugs to improve left ventricular contractility are helpful. Isoproterenol or dopamine should be used, with serial cardiac output and filling pressure measurements.

The first step in decreasing pulmonary edema is to decrease pulmonary capillary hydrostatic pressure to as low as is compatible with adequate cardiac output. This is done by means of diuresis and fluid restriction. As the patient falls behind in blood volume, signs of hypovolemia may appear. Blood volume is replenished with a fluid that stays in the vascular space. Packed red blood cells are ideal for this application. When the hematocrit is normal, concentrated salt-poor albumin should be used. This hyperoncotic fluid replenishes the blood volume by attracting interstitial fluid from all areas of the body into the vascular space and supplements diuresis. This technique is useful even in the care of septic patients, who may have increased capillary permeability and may lose albumin from the vascular space at a rapid rate. Even if albumin "leaks out," the short-term effects of expanding blood volume and a decrease in edema will appear.

ANSWER: a

REFERENCE: *Chapter 9—Critical Care: Management of Respiratory Failure*

16. Which of the following statements is/are true concerning the relation between cardiac function and effective blood volume?

    a. A pulmonary capillary wedge pressure of 5 to 10 mm Hg rules out fluid overload as a cause of pulmonary edema
    b. A shift to the right in the Frank-Starling curve is associated with compromised cardiac function
    c. Dilutional anemia can contribute to tachycardia even though blood volume and filling pressures are normal
    d. The sole purpose of a pulmonary arterial catheter is to measure pulmonary arterial pressure and cardiac output

COMMENT: Although physical findings often are adequate to establish a diagnosis and institute management of cardiac failure, direct measurement of filling pressures of the right side of the heart (central venous pressure) or the left side of the heart (pulmonary arterial pressure) may be needed. Placement of a pulmonary arterial catheter allows measurement of cardiac output by means of thermodilution. More important, it allows sampling of mixed venous blood for saturation measurements that determine the ratio between systemic oxygen delivery and $\dot{V}o_2$. All these measurements are used to determine whether cardiac output is normal for the level of filling pressure of the left ventricle or contractility is decreased. In the latter case, cardiac output is lower than predicted for a given level of filling pressure. In the Frank-Starling curve, if the patient is to the right of the normal range, cardiac function is compromised because of valvular disease, extrinsic pressure such as pericardial tamponade, or more commonly, a decrease in contractility. If cardiac function and anatomic relations are normal, blood volume, filling pressure, and cardiac function are related to the Starling curve. The intake and output of fluid and salt is autoregulated to maintain the filling pressure of the left ventricle at approximately 10 mm Hg.

Extracellular fluid expansion usually is associated with normal blood volume. Gross expansion of the extracellular space with all the deleterious effects of tissue edema can and does exist with normal blood volume. In other words, a pulmonary capillary wedge pressure of 5 to 10 mm Hg does not rule out fluid overload as a cause of pulmonary or gastrointestinal dysfunction. In the care of critically ill patients, fear of hypotension and the effects of perfusion usually results in infusion of intravenous salt and water in quantities that exceed losses. Consequently, most patients in the intensive care units have anemia, dilutional hypoproteinemia, and a compensatory increase in cardiac output. In response to anemia, these patients have tachycardia, even though blood volume is normal, filling pressures are normal, and total body extracellular fluid is excessive.

ANSWER: b, c

REFERENCE: *Chapter 9—Critical Care: Blood Volume and Hemodynamics*

17. Which of the following statements is/are true concerning estimation and measurement of energy requirements for critically ill patients?
    a. One can only estimate energy expenditure; actual measurement is not technically feasible
    b. The amount of oxygen absorbed through the lungs equals the amount of oxygen consumed by metabolic processes
    c. Metabolic rate, normalized to body surface area, can underestimate metabolism in a fat person
    d. To convert milliliters of oxygen per minute to calories per day, a conversion factor of 10 kcal of energy per liter of oxygen should be used

COMMENT: The actual metabolic rate of any patient can be estimated from the predicted basal rate according to the clinical situation. The amount of energy is most conveniently expressed in calories per day. The metabolic rate is normalized to body surface area; however, the actively metabolizing tissue is the lean body cell mass. Consequently, reporting "per square meter" underestimates the metabolism of a fat person and overestimates that of a very lean person. Although most of the studies on nutrition in critical illness have been based on estimated energy expenditure, actual measurement is much more accurate and has become an important aspect of critical care. The most commonly used method of measurement is indirect calorimetry. In this method, the amount of oxygen absorbed across the lungs into the pulmonary blood is measured over a given time. With the assumption that the patient is at metabolic steady state during this time, the amount of oxygen absorbed across the lungs equals the amount of oxygen consumed in the metabolic process. The metabolic rate, measured in milliliters of oxygen per minute, can be converted to calories per hour or per day if the oxygenated substrates are known. For practical purposes, a conversion factor of 5 kcal of energy per liter of oxygen consumed is a reasonable approximation.

ANSWER: b, c

REFERENCE: *Chapter 9—Critical Care: Metabolism and Nutrition*

18. Which of the following statements is/are true concerning various energy sources?
    a. Carbohydrate is the most efficient source of energy
    b. Endogenous fat is the main source of energy during starvation
    c. The respiratory quotient of carbohydrate is greater than that of either fat or protein
    d. Ketones can be used as a source of energy during starvation

COMMENT: The major sources of energy are carbohydrates and fats. Carbohydrates are a major source of energy during normal, nonstarving existence. The brain, red blood cells, and some other organs are obligate glucose users. The brain and red blood cells can develop the capability to use ketones as an energy source, a process known as *starvation adaptation*. Fat is the most efficient source of energy. Fat produces 9 calories of energy per gram of substrate metabolized, whereas carbohydrate produces only 4 calories. The respiratory quotient represents the number of molecules of carbon dioxide for each molecule of oxygen consumed. For carbohydrates the respiratory quotient is 1.0, whereas for fat it is 0.7. Endogenous fat is the main source of energy during starvation. Glycogen stores are basically depleted after a day of fasting, and fat becomes a major energy source. Protein breakdown supplies glucose through the process of gluconeogenesis.

ANSWER: b, c, d

REFERENCE: *Chapter 9—Critical Care: Metabolism and Nutrition*

19. Which of the following statements is/are true concerning assessment of protein reserve?

 a. Conventional serum proteins such as albumin and globulin are early indicators of malnutrition
 b. The total lymphocyte count reflects immune status, not nutrition
 c. Antigen skin testing reflects patient immunity, not nutrition
 d. Measurement of urea excretion in urine can be used as a measurement of protein breakdown

COMMENT: Because protein is the functional and structural chemical of the body, most nutritional assessment techniques are estimates of protein reserves. Actual nitrogen balance can be measured by means of measuring the amount of nitrogen excreted. This is most conveniently done by means of measuring the amount of urea excreted in the urine, if it is assumed that urea constitutes 85% of the total nitrogen excretion. When nitrogen excretion is known, the amount of protein catabolized can be estimated and compared with the amount of protein ingested by the patient. Indirect assessment of protein reserves is based on single measurements of body substances dependent on rapid protein synthesis for maintenance of normal levels. Conventional serum proteins such as albumin and globulin are not affected by malnutrition until it is severe. Proteins such as prealbumin and transferrin, which turn over rapidly, are better indicators of protein status than are conventional serum proteins.

Lymphocytes are rapidly destroyed, and protein is required for formation of new cells. Consequently, the absolute lymphocyte count is a useful measurement of the status of protein reserves. The lymphocyte count is considered by some the best single "static" measurement characterizing nutritional status. Protein also is required for synthesis of the cells and mediators involved in skin test reactivity. Although skin test reactivity is a manifestation of lymphocyte-mediated immunity, its usefulness in patient assessment is probably assessment of the inflammatory response rather than lymphocyte activity per se. Some patients with chronic or acute malnutrition convert from reactive to anergic, and reactivity can be restored by means of nutritional repletion.

ANSWER: d

REFERENCE: *Chapter 9—Critical Care: Metabolism and Nutrition*

20. Which of the following statements is/are true concerning methods of nutritional support?

 a. Optimal results for enteral feedings are achieved with approximately one half of calories supplied as carbohydrate and one half as fat
 b. Diarrhea is the most common complication of enteral feeding and is caused by the high osmolarity of the carbohydrate components
 c. The hyperosmolar nature of parenteral fat solutions requires central venous administration
 d. Approximately 25% to 50% of calories should be provided as fat emulsion to patients receiving total parenteral nutrition

COMMENT: Most formulas for enteral feeding range from 1.0 to 2 cal/mL and include 3% to 7% protein. Most of the calories are supplied as glucose or sucrose so that the solutions have a high osmolarity. Cramps or diarrhea can occur when these highly osmolar solutions are placed into the stomach or intestine. Diarrhea is the main complication of use of most tube feeding formulas. Diarrhea can be minimized by the use of starch or fat as an energy source in tube feedings. This can be supplied as part of the commercial preparation or added in the form of medium chain triglycerides or other oils. The best results usually are achieved when approximately one half the calories are supplied as carbohydrate and one half as fat. For patients receiving total parenteral nutrition, the energy source is carbohydrate, fat, and amino acid solutions. Parenteral feeding with carbohydrate is limited by the sclerotic effect of hyperosmolar solutions on veins. Fat is a more efficient energy source and can be given through peripheral veins in concentrations of 10% or 20%. Most intensive care specialists favor supplementing standard total parenteral nutrition solution with intravenous fat to provide at least 100 g fat emulsion each week to preclude fatty acid deficiency. Giving up to 25% to 50% of calories each day as fat emulsion may optimize caloric delivery.

ANSWER: a, b, d

REFERENCE: *Chapter 9—Critical Care: Nutritional Supplies*

21. Which of the following statements is/are true concerning various causes of acute renal failure?

   a. Acute tubular necrosis is the most common pathologic finding of acute renal failure
   b. Drug-induced renal failure is compounded in situations of hypovolemia
   c. Myoglobin-induced renal failure can be prevented with diuretics and alkalization of urine
   d. Radiographic contrast medium–induced renal failure occurs independently of preexisting conditions
   e. Myoglobin is a direct nephrotoxin

COMMENT: Acute tubular necrosis results from ischemia to the renal parenchyma and is the most common pathologic finding of acute renal failure. In conditions of diminishing renal blood flow, perfusion to the kidneys is first maintained by vasomotor responses that dilate the afferent arterioles and constrict the efferent arterioles. As hypotension continues, the renin-angiotensin system is activated, and vasoconstriction of the afferent arterioles occurs and exacerbates corticohypoperfusion. Pigment nephropathy is a common cause of acute renal failure after trauma, burns, operations, or hemodynamic catastrophe. With ischemia or blunt injury to large muscles, myoglobin is released into the circulation. In the kidney, it is filtered from blood and reabsorbed by the tubule. Although myoglobin is not a direct nephrotoxin, in the presence of aciduria, myoglobin is converted to ferrihemate, which is toxic to renal cells.

Prevention of myoglobin-induced renal failure may include diuretics and alkalinization of urine. Drug-induced acute renal failure is responsible for approximately 5% of all cases of acute renal failure. Through normal reabsorption and secretion, the kidney is exposed to high concentrations of drugs and solutes, which may be toxic. This problem is compounded by hypovolemia, which increases reabsorption of water and solutes and exposes the lumen to even higher concentrations of toxins. The incidence of radiographic contrast medium–induced nephropathy is 1% to 10%. This reaction can be predicted according to a number of risk factors, including contrast load, age, preexisting renal insufficiency, and diabetes. The incidence among patients with normal renal function is 1% to 2%.

ANSWER: a, b, c

REFERENCE: *Chapter 9—Critical Care: Application of Metabolic Economics to the Critically Ill Patient*

22. A 64-year-old patient with diabetes has acute renal failure after repair of an aortic aneurysm. Which of the following statements is/are true concerning diagnosis and management in this case?

   a. Resting energy expenditure likely is less than expected for a patient with normal renal function
   b. Maintenance of positive energy balance reduces protein catabolism and makes the management of renal failure easier
   c. Expected metabolic abnormalities include hyperkalemia, hypercalcemia, and metabolic alkalosis
   d. Nonoliguric renal failure usually is associated with a better outcome

COMMENT: Among patients with nonoliguric renal failure, treatment may differ little from that required for identical patients with normal renal function. Management of fluids, solutes, and nutrition usually is not affected by nonoliguric renal failure, although blood urea nitrogen level may be elevated. The extent of renal dysfunction is limited and almost always is reversible. Use of renal replacement therapies rarely is necessary. Acute renal failure can result in severe derangements in electrolyte and acid-base physiologic mechanisms. Of all electrolyte abnormalities that might occur, hyperkalemia is the most serious. Other electrolyte abnormalities, such as hyponatremia, hyperphosphatemia, hypocalcemia, and metabolic acidosis are common and must be monitored carefully.

The metabolic requirements of a patient with acute renal failure are those of a critically ill, hospitalized patient. Measurement of actual resting energy expenditure has shown that caloric requirements of patients with multiple organ failure that includes renal failure often are 50% greater than are those of healthy persons. Although acute renal failure can necessitate fluid restriction, providing adequate nutrition is an important aspect of treatment. Positive energy balance may make management of uremia and hyperkalemia less difficult. If adequate calories are provided, endogenous protein catabolism with resultant generation of urea and release of potassium can be avoided. Maintenance of positive energy balance with glucose and lipids should reduce protein catabolism, urea generation, and hyperkalemia.

ANSWER: b, d

REFERENCE: *Chapter 9—Critical Care: Application of Metabolic Economics to the Critically Ill Patient*

23. A patient needs renal replacement therapy. Which of the following statements is/are true concerning the differences between hemodialysis and continuous arteriovenous hemodialysis (CAVHD)?

a. Anticoagulation is not required for CAVHD
b. Hemodynamic instability is a particular problem with both techniques
c. Both techniques decrease serum urea nitrogen levels
d. Continuous arteriovenous hemodialysis will likely result in better removal of excessive volume

COMMENT: Table 9.6

ANSWER: c, d

REFERENCE: *Chapter 9—Critical Care: Application of Metabolic Economics to the Critically Ill Patient*

24. Which of the following statements is/are true concerning continuous arteriovenous hemofiltration (CAVH)?

a. The technique runs continuously
b. It is not associated with hemodynamic instability
c. Systemic heparin anticoagulation is necessary
d. Fluid balance and correction of electrolyte abnormalities takes several days

COMMENT: Continuous arteriovenous hemofiltration is an extracorporeal filtration technique that removes extracellular fluid across a synthetic membrane by means of a hydrostatic pressure gradient between the indwelling arterial and venous catheters. Arteriovenous access is accomplished by means of percutaneous cannulation of the femoral artery and vein with a low incidence of complications. Although full systemic anticoagulation is not necessary for CAVH, heparinization of the extracorporeal circuit is required. Continuous arteriovenous hemofiltration is run continuously for as many days as renal replacement is needed. Experience with CAVH has shown little or no hemodynamic instability with treatment of critically ill patients with renal failure. The stable nature of this therapy is attributed to a slow, continuous fluid and solute removal and to the fact that the membrane does not induce complement activation when in contact with blood. Fluid balance and serum electrolyte concentrations can be titrated to any level in a matter of hours by means of manipulation of the composition and rate of replacement solution. Solute clearance with CAVH is limited by the ultrafiltration and replacement fluid exchange rate. For patients with high urea generation rates, solute removal with CAVH may be inadequate, and variations of the technique can be used to enhance clearance.

ANSWER: a, b

REFERENCE: *Chapter 9—Critical Care: Application of Metabolic Economics to the Critically Ill Patient*

Table 9.6. COMPARISON OF RENAL REPLACEMENT THERAPIES

	Hemodialysis	Peritoneal dialysis	CAVH/CAVHD
Description	Rapid, intermittent	Slow, intermittent	Slow, continuous
Access	Arteriovenous or venovenous	Abdominal catheter	Arteriovenous
Anticoagulation	Required	Not required	Required
Solute removal	Excellent	Excellent	Good with standard CAVH; excellent with CAVHD
Fluid removal	Good to excellent	Good	Excellent
Hemodynamic instability	Marked	None	None
Risks of procedure	Hypotension, hypoxemia disequilibrium syndrome	Infection, peritonitis; intraabdominal adhesions; respiratory distress	Dehydration, hemorrhage, electrolyte imbalance
Overall appraisal	Useful for urgent removal of solutes or poisons	Contraindicated with abdominal operation	Allows great flexibility with fluid and electrolyte balance
	Hemodynamic instability limits use in intensive care patients	Useful in care of burn patients and when vascular access is poor	Solute removal enhanced with CAVHD

CAVH, continuous arteriovenous hemofiltration; CAVHD, continuous arteriovenous hemodialysis.

25. Which of the following statements is/are true concerning outcome among patients with acute renal failure?
    a. The mortality for ischemic acute tubular necrosis without other organ failure is approximately 6%
    b. Multiple organ failure complicated with acute renal failure is associated with mortality ranging from 50% to 90%
    c. Recovery of renal function after 6 weeks is unlikely
    d. There is no difference in survival between oliguric and nonoliguric renal failure

COMMENT: Survival of patients with acute renal failure is a function of successful management of the primary disease from which the renal failure was derived. The mortality for ischemic acute tubular necrosis without organ failure has been reported to be approximately 6%. In contrast, the mortality for multiple organ failure complicated by acute renal failure ranges from 50% to 90%. Among patients who survive the acute phase of illness, recovery of renal function after acute renal failure depends on the type and extent of injuries to the renal parenchyma. If renal function is not returned after 6 weeks, recovery is unlikely. Nonoliguric renal failure usually is limited in its extent and is almost always reversible.

ANSWER: a, b, c

REFERENCE: *Chapter 9—Critical Care: Application of Metabolic Economics to the Critically Ill Patient*

26. Which of the following statements meet(s) the criteria for organ failure?
    a. Bilirubin level greater than 5 mg/dL
    b. Creatinine level greater than 3 mg/dL
    c. Alveolar-arterial oxygen gradient greater than 300 mm Hg
    d. Glasgow Coma Scale score less than 10

COMMENT: Multiple organ failure is defined by dysfunction of two or more of the six vital organ systems—cardiovascular, respiratory, nervous, renal, liver, and host defense. A definition of organ system failure is included in Table 9.7.

ANSWER: a, b, c, d

REFERENCE: *Chapter 9—Critical Care: Multiple Organ Failure*

Table 9.7. **CRITERIA FOR ORGAN FAILURE**[a]

System	Criterion
Cardiovascular	Cardiac index <2.5 L/m² per min with left atrial pressure >10 mm Hg
	Inotropic or vasopressor drugs required to maintain adequate perfusion
Respiratory	Alveoloarterial O₂ gradient >300 mm Hg
Nervous	Glasgow coma score <10
Renal	Creatinine >3 mg/dL
Liver	Bilirubin >5 mg/dL
Host defenses	Positive blood culture
	Invasive tissue infection
	Anergic to common antigens

[a]Arbitrary definitions of the University of Michigan surgical intensive care unit.

27. Phases of multiple organ failure include:
    a. Generalized increased capillary permeability
    b. A hypermetabolic state
    c. Organ malfunction
    d. All of the above

COMMENT: Multiple organ failure progresses through the following well-defined clinical phases: Phase 1—generalized increased capillary permeability resulting in edema, weight gain, and intravenous volume replacement, and increased protein concentration in urine and lymph. Although the pulmonary microvasculature has been most thoroughly studied, it is apparent that the lung is simply the most obvious end organ in a generalized permeability defect. Phase 2—a hypermetabolic state with increased $\dot{V}o_2$ and a compensatory increase in oxygen delivery characterized by tachycardia and high cardiac output. This condition following systemic ischemia and reperfusion is similar to hypermetabolism following endotoxemia, localized sterile inflammation, and infusion of stress hormones, suggesting a common mechanism. Phase 3—organ malfunction due to localized edema and cellular injury, particularly in the kidney, liver, brain, and host defense system. Hemorrhagic shock predisposes to bacterial translocation and endotoxin absorption from the intestine. Phase 4—in the absence of systemic sepsis, organs may recover to normal or be irreversibly damaged, leading to a need for long-term support. If the phases of organ failure lead to systemic infection or irreversible tissue damage in the lung or brain, death of the entire organ is likely.

ANSWER: d

REFERENCE: *Chapter 9—Critical Care: Multiple Organ Failure*

28. Which of the following statements is/are true concerning the management of multiple system organ failure?
    a. Forced diuresis with negative fluid balance improves survival and relieves acute respiratory failure
    b. Titration of inotropic drugs on the basis of desired blood pressure optimizes results
    c. Nutritional support should be withheld for several days until the patient's condition stabilizes
    d. Continuous arteriovenous hemofiltration is preferred to intermittent hemodialysis for most critically ill patients
    e. Hepatic failure should be managed specifically with pharmacologic manipulation

COMMENT: The important principles in the management of multiple organ failure are to avoid further episodes of local or systemic ischemia and to keep the brain viable by means of pharmacologic or mechanical support of the failing organs until organ recovery occurs. Respiratory failure is managed by means of mechanical assistance for lung inflation and ventilation and by means of decreasing lung edema as much as possible. Airway intubation usually is needed. There is evidence that forced diuresis and negative fluid balance are associated with improved survival and relief of acute respiratory failure. Cardiac failure is managed with inotropic drugs. Although inotropic drugs usually are titrated to achieve a desired arterial blood pressure, it is more sensible to titrate inotropic agents to achieve a normal ratio of oxygen delivery to oxygen consumption. Monitoring of pulmonary arterial pressure and mixed venous saturation are essential for intelligent treatment of a patient with severe respiratory or cardiac failure. Adequate nutrition is important for recovery from organ failure. Renal failure is managed by means of mechanical substitution of renal function. Although hemodialysis and peritoneal dialysis can serve this purpose, each has a serious limitation in the treatment of a critically ill patient with multiple organ failure. Continuous arteriovenous hemofiltration and CAVHD are the methods of choice for renal replacement therapy. Hepatic failure often occurs as part of multiple organ failure syndrome but unfortunately there is no specific treatment.

ANSWER: a, d

REFERENCE: *Chapter 9—Critical Care: Multiple Organ Failure*

CHAPTER 10

FLUIDS, ELECTROLYTES, AND ACID–BASE BALANCE

1. Which of the following statements is/are true concerning total body water (TBW)?
   a. Total body water in men represents a higher percentage of body weight than it does in women
   b. In infants, water constitutes up to 80% of body weight
   c. Total body water content decreases with increasing age
   d. Total body water is equally distributed within the intracellular and extracellular compartments

COMMENT: The total volume of water within the body is called *total body water* (TBW). The relation between TBW and body weight is relatively consistent for any given person and depends on the amount of fat in the body. Because fat contains little water, TBW as a percentage of body weight decreases with increasing body fat. The estimated TBW in men is 60% of body weight, whereas in women, who typically have more adipose tissue, the average TBW is 50% of body weight. The percentage of body weight accounted for by water also varies with age. In infants, water constitutes approximately 80% of body weight. Throughout adult life, a gradual decrease in TBW content occurs because the amount of fat within the body usually increases with age. For obese patients, estimates of TBW should be decreased 10% to 20% whereas for lean patients, estimates should be increased approximately 10%. Total body water is distributed within the intracellular and extracellular compartments. Intracellular fluid makes up approximately two thirds of TBW, or 40% of body weight.

ANSWER: a, b, c

REFERENCE: *Chapter 10—Fluids, Electrolytes, and Acid–Base Balance: Total Body Water and Fluid Compartments*

2. Which of the following statements is/are correct concerning the body fluid compartments?
   a. Both the extracellular and intracellular components of TBW can be directly measured
   b. The intravascular space accounts for most extracellular fluid
   c. All water in the interstitial space is freely exchangeable
   d. Transcellular fluid, separated from other compartments by both endothelial and epithelial barriers, constitutes approximately 4% of TBW

COMMENT: Total body water is distributed within the intracellular and extracellular compartments. Intracellular fluid cannot be measured directly but is calculated as the difference between TBW and measured extracellular water. Extracellular fluid can be measured directly. The extracellular fluid compartment can be further simplified into the intravascular and interstitial spaces. The intravascular space, which accounts for 20% of extracellular fluid, contains the plasma volume, which is approximately 8% of TBW or 5% of body weight. The interstitial space extends from the blood vessels to the cells themselves and includes the complex ground substance that composes the acellular matrix of tissue. Although the water within the space is thought to be freely exchangeable, this water exists in two phases. The free phase contains water that is generally freely exchangeable and in a constant state of flux. The bound or gel phase is composed of water closely associated with glycosaminoglycans, mucopolysaccharides, and other matrix components. This water is much less freely exchangeable. An additional extracellular fluid compartment, the transcellular compartment, consists of water that is poorly exchangeable under normal circumstances. This fluid is separated from other compartments by both endothelial and epithelial barriers and includes cerebrospinal fluid, synovial fluid, water within cartilage and bone, fluids of the eye, and the lubricating fluids of the serous membranes. Together these fluids constitute approximately 4% of TBW.

ANSWER: d

REFERENCE: *Chapter 10—Fluids, Electrolytes, and Acid–Base Balance: Total Body Water and Fluid Compartments*

3. Which of the following statements is/are true concerning the osmotic activity of body fluids?
   a. Urea contributes to the osmolality of a solution but not its tonicity
   b. The osmolality of the body remains fairly constant at approximately 289 mOsm/kg water
   c. The two primary regulators of water balance are antidiuretic hormone and aldosterone
   d. Serum level of sodium is the most valuable laboratory indicator of abnormal TBW content

COMMENT: Body fluids are aqueous solutions composed primarily of water and contained in different compartments of the body. The movement of water from these compartments depends on a number of physical properties, the most important of which is osmosis. According to the principles of osmosis, if two solutions are separated by a semipermeable membrane, water moves across the membrane to equalize the concentration of the osmotically active particles. Osmotic activity across a semipermeable membrane is determined by the concentration of solutes on each side of the membrane. The body is capable of fine regulation of solute and water concentrations, so osmolality remains fairly constant at an average of 289 mOsm/kg water. In response to small changes in cell volume, osmoreceptors in the paraventricular and supraoptic nuclei of the hypothalamus send signals to the neuronal centers that control the two primary regulators of water balance—thirst and secretion of antidiuretic hormone.

Changes in TBW are reflected by changes in extracellular solute concentration. Because sodium is the primary extracellular cation and potassium is the predominant intracellular cation, the serum level of sodium approximates the sum of the exchangeable total body sodium and exchangeable total body potassium divided by TBW. Because total body solute content remains relatively stable over time, changes in TBW content result in inversely proportional changes in serum level of sodium. Thus abnormalities in serum level of sodium are the indication of abnormal TBW content. Unlike the impermeable solutes excluded from the intracellular space, such as sodium, permeable solutes such as urea can freely cross the cell membranes. Although urea contributes to the osmolality of a solution, it has no effect on tonicity because it distributes equally across membranes and as such does not contribute to the osmoles that affect cell volume.

ANSWER: a, b, d

REFERENCE: *Chapter 10—Fluids, Electrolytes, and Acid–Base Balance: Osmotic Activity of Body Fluids*

4. Which of the following is/are true concerning control of the volume of body water?
   a. Osmoreceptors and baroreceptors work equally to control fluid balance under normal conditions
   b. The cardiac atrium regulates volume only by means of its sympathetic and parasympathetic connections
   c. The kidney is the primary effector organ in controlling water balance
   d. The conversion of angiotensin I to angiotensin II depends on the amount of the enzyme renin available
   e. Nitric oxide plays a number of important roles in regulation of renal hemodynamics

COMMENT: Changes in volume are detected by both osmoreceptors, which detect changes in plasma osmolality, and baroreceptors, which are sensitive to changes in pressure. The osmoreceptors are responsible for day-to-day fine-tuning of volume. The baroreceptors contribute relatively little to control of fluid balance under normal conditions. Changes in effective circulating volume are sensed by the volume receptors of the intrathoracic capacitance vessels and atria, the pressure receptors of the aortic arch and carotid arteries, the intrarenal baroreceptors, and to a lesser extent, the hepatic and cerebrospinal volume receptors. These baroreceptors control volume by means of sympathetic and parasympathetic connections. The atria also appear to serve as endocrine organs capable of directing responses to volume changes with elaboration of the hormone atrial natriuretic peptide.

The main hormonal mediator of baroreceptor modulation of volume control is the renin-angiotensin system. The result of this complex system of receptors or messengers is a change in sodium and water balance mediated by the kidneys. It is through changes in sodium and water reabsorption that volume and pressure ultimately normalize. Renin is a proteolytic enzyme released in response to changes in arterial pressure, changes in delivery of sodium to the macula densa of the distal convoluted renal tubule, increases in β-adrenergic activity, and increases in cellular levels of cyclic adenosine monophosphate. Renin cleaves angiotensin I from circulating angiotensinogen. Angiotensinogen is abundant, so this reaction is enzyme dependent rather than substrate dependent. Angiotensin I is further cleaved to angiotensin II, which acts locally and systemically to increase vascular tone. Angiotensin II affects sodium reabsorption by decreasing renal plasma flow and the glomerular filtration coefficient. Finally, angiotensin II increases sodium reabsorption by means of direct tubular action and stimulation of aldosterone release from the adrenal cortex. The importance of nitric oxide and its many biologic functions is recognized. Nitric oxide participates in regulation of renal hemodynamics and renal handling of water and electrolytes.

ANSWER: c, d, e

REFERENCE: *Chapter 10—Fluids, Electrolytes, and Acid–Base Balance: Volume Control*

5. Which of the following statements is/are true concerning parenteral electrolyte solutions?
   a. Lactated Ringer's solution contains physiologic concentrations of all important electrolytes
   b. Glucose is added to hypotonic saline solutions to increase their tonicity
   c. Approximately one half of all exogenously administered albumin ends up in the extravascular space
   d. Normal saline solution provides excessive sodium and chloride, and the excess can cause body sodium overload

COMMENT: A number of electrolyte solutions can be used for parenteral administration. Lactated Ringer's solution is a physiologic solution containing many of the electrolytes found in plasma. The disadvantage of this solution is the relatively low sodium content (130 mEq/L) compared with plasma. Hyponatremia can occur with extended use of lactated Ringer's solution. Isotonic saline solution (0.9% or normal saline solution) contains 154 mEq of both sodium and chloride. The excess of both sodium and chloride can lead to electrolyte and acid-base disturbances. Infusion of large volumes of 0.9% saline solution can lead to total body sodium overload and hyperchloremia. The less-concentrated saline solutions are hypoosmotic and have excess free water. In addition, 0.2% saline solution is hypotonic with respect to plasma and can cause red blood cell lysis if rapidly infused. For this reason, 5% dextrose is added to these solutions to increase the tonicity.

Plasma expanders are commonly used to treat surgical patients. Plasma protein solutions such as 5% and 25% albumin act initially by increasing plasma oncotic pressure. Abnormalities in microvascular permeability, such as those found in the pulmonary circulation in adult respiratory distress syndrome, in regional circulatory bed burns or infections, and in the systemic circulation in sepsis, can cause extravasation of these proteins into the interstitial space. Approximately one half of all exogenously administered albumin ends up in the extravascular space. The half-life of exogenously administered albumin is approximately 11 days.

ANSWER: b, c, d

REFERENCE: *Chapter 10—Fluids, Electrolytes, and Acid–Base Balance: Fluid and Electrolyte Therapy*

6. An 11-year-old boy has experienced severe diarrhea for 10 days. He has decreased skin turgor, sunken eyes, orthostatic hypotension, and tachycardia. Which of the following statements may be true concerning diagnosis and treatment in this case?

   a. The hematocrit likely is elevated
   b. The blood urea nitrogen (BUN) may be elevated out of proportion to serum level of creatinine
   c. The serum level of sodium is elevated
   d. Fluid resuscitation should begin with D5/.2 normal saline because of the expected high serum sodium associated with excessive fluid loss

COMMENT: Chronic volume deficits may manifest as decreased skin turgor, weight loss, sunken eyes, hypothermia, oliguria, orthostatic hypotension, and tachycardia. Serum level of BUN and creatinine may be elevated with a high BUN to creatinine ratio. The hematocrit may be elevated as well. Plasma level of sodium is not an indicator of intravascular volume, and if the losses have been isotonic, plasma sodium concentration remains normal. Fluid resuscitation for hypovolemia is initiated with an isotonic solution such as lactated Ringer's solution. Urine flow in critically ill patients is monitored with an indwelling Foley catheter; the goal of a urine output of 0.5 mL/kg per hour is desirable.

ANSWER: a, b

REFERENCE: *Chapter 10—Fluids, Electrolytes, and Acid–Base Balance: Fluid and Electrolyte Therapy*

7. Which of the following statements is/are true concerning maintenance intravenous fluid therapy?

   a. The total daily water requirement for a 70-kg man is approximately 2500 mL/d
   b. Normal maintenance intravenous therapy requires administration of sodium, potassium, calcium, phosphate, and magnesium
   c. Fluid volume calculations for elderly patients generally are lower than for young patients
   d. A child requires less maintenance fluid per kilogram than does a larger person

COMMENT: Maintenance fluid replacement is aimed at replacing fluids normally lost during the course of a day. Calculation of maintenance fluid replacement does not include replacement of preexisting deficits or ongoing additional losses. Formulas for calculating maintenance fluid requirements adjust for differences in body weight and for changes in TBW content. A smaller or younger person who has a high percentage of TBW in relation to body weight requires more maintenance fluid per kilogram than does a larger person. The total daily water requirement for a 70-kg man is approximately 2500 mL/d. Because hypervolemia is poorly tolerated by older persons and by patients with cardiac disease, the volume calculated is generally diminished in this age group. Normal maintenance therapy requires administration of sodium and potassium. Replacement of calcium, phosphate, or magnesium generally is not necessary for patients who need short-term therapy. Critically ill patients, however, can have critical deficits in these electrolytes, which must be replaced.

ANSWER: a, c

REFERENCE: *Chapter 10—Fluids, Electrolytes, and Acid–Base Balance: Fluid and Electrolyte Therapy*

8. Which of the following statements is/are true concerning postoperative fluid treatment of a surgical patient?

    a. Standard formulas are available that essentially can direct therapy for all patients

    b. Isotonic solutions containing potassium should be used throughout the postoperative period

    c. Urine output should be maintained at a level greater than 0.5 mL/kg per hour

    d. A urine specific gravity greater than 1.012 may indicate the patient is dehydrated

COMMENT: Fluid therapy during the postoperative period should be tailored to each patient and depends on the adequacy of patient's volume status at the completion of the operative procedure as well as ongoing fluid losses. Maintenance fluid should be supplemented by replacement of the additional fluids needed to replace the ongoing third-space loss as well as losses from various tubes and drains. In general, isotonic solution should be used for volume resuscitation during the early postoperative period. It is best not to give potassium supplements during this period unless they are specifically required as indicated by serum electrolyte measurements. Monitoring fluid status during the postoperative period is best accomplished with careful monitoring of vital signs, urine output, and central venous pressure, if necessary. Urine output is maintained at a level greater than 0.5 mL/kg per hour. A urine specific gravity greater than 1.010 to 1.012 indicates that urine is being concentrated and the patient may not be receiving adequate hydration.

ANSWER: c, d

REFERENCE: *Chapter 10—Fluids, Electrolytes, and Acid–Base Balance: Fluid and Electrolyte Therapy*

9. Which of the following statements is/are true concerning abnormalities in serum level of sodium?

    a. The most common cause of hyponatremia is a deficit in total body sodium

    b. Hyponatremia can occur in situations of excessive solute

    c. Most surgical patients with hyponatremia are best treated with free water restriction

    d. Central nervous system effects are the predominant symptom of hypernatremia

    e. Hypernatremia should be rapidly corrected with free water administration

COMMENT: The most common cause of hyponatremia is an excess of free water rather than a deficit of total body sodium. Hyponatremia frequently occurs among postoperative or posttrauma patients because increased secretion of antidiuretic hormone acts on the collecting tubules of the kidney to increase free water reabsorption. Although hyponatremia most often results from an excess of free water, it can occur in the presence of excess solute. In this situation, TBW content is either normal or diminished, but plasma osmolality is increased. An example of this hyperosmolar-hyponatremic state is uncontrolled hyperglycemia. Excess of solute also may be caused by exogenous administration or ingestion of mannitol, ethanol, methanol, or ethylene glycol. Most surgical patients with hyponatremia are euvolemic or hypervolemic. Such patients, if they have no symptoms, are best treated by means of free water restriction, because free water overload is the cause of the condition.

Hypernatremia is a less common problem among surgical patients than is hyponatremia and usually is the result of excess free water loss associated with hypovolemia. Hypernatremia also can be caused by increased total body content of sodium, which usually is related to exogenous administration of sodium. The symptoms of hypernatremia are related to the hyperosmolar state. Central nervous system effects predominate because of cellular dehydration as water passes into the extracellular space. Once hypernatremia becomes symptomatic, it is associated with significant morbidity and mortality. Prompt management of hypernatremia is essential. Rapid correction of hypernatremia, however, is associated with high risk of cerebral edema and herniation. Because chronic hypernatremia is relatively well tolerated, there are few advantages to rapidly correcting the free water deficit. Moderate degrees of hypernatremia are tolerated well, and symptoms rarely develop unless serum sodium levels exceed 160 mEq/L. The development of symptoms also depends on the rapidity with which hypernatremia develops.

ANSWER: b, c, d

REFERENCE: *Chapter 10—Fluids, Electrolytes, and Acid–Base Balance: Concentration Changes in Body Fluids*

10. Which of the following statements is/are true concerning abnormalities in serum level of potassium?

    a. Hyperkalemia can occur in an otherwise normal surgical patient because of excessive intravenous administration of potassium

    b. The primary electrocardiographic (ECG) change associated with severe hyperkalemia is peaked T waves

    c. Temporary management of hyperkalemia includes administration of calcium, sodium bicarbonate, or glucose and insulin

    d. Alterations in membrane potentials reflected in cardiac and skeletal muscle are common results of both hypokalemia and hyperkalemia

    e. A reduction in serum level potassium of 1 mEq/L requires replacement of 40 mEq of potassium

COMMENT: Potassium is the most important intracellular cation and is a major determinant of intracellular osmolality. Because of the large differences between intracellular and extracellular potassium concentrations, a transmembrane potential is generated. Alterations in potassium concentration gradient (both hyperkalemia and hypokalemia) have profound effects on transmembrane potential and consequently on cellular function. This is especially true for cardiac, skeletal, and smooth muscle. Extracellular potassium concentration is primarily determined by renal excretion. Approximately 90% of ingested potassium is secreted in the urine. Hyperkalemia therefore rarely develops from excessive potassium intake in the absence of renal insufficiency, because the capacity for renal potassium excretion is large. Among surgical patients, diminished renal function is perhaps the most common problem leading to hyperkalemia. Both chronic and acute renal failure cause the deficit in potassium excretion. Hyperkalemia also can be associated with cellular disruption, as with crush injuries or lysis of erythrocytes in large hematomas or after massive blood transfusion.

The clinical manifestations of hyperkalemia are related primarily to membrane depolarization. The most life-threatening manifestations are related to the cardiac effects of membrane depolarization. Mild hyperkalemia results in peaked T waves on an ECG and can cause paresthesia and weakness. More severe forms of hyperkalemia cause flattened P waves, prolongation of the QRS complex, and deep S waves on an ECG. Ventricular fibrillation and cardiac arrest may follow. Severe hyperkalemia with ECG abnormalities necessitates urgent treatment. Rapid infusion of 10% to 20% calcium gluconate can reduce the effects of hyperkalemia on membrane potentials. Administration of sodium bicarbonate is another temporary measure. The increase in serum level of sodium antagonizes the effects of hyperkalemia on the membrane potential, whereas the increase in extracellular pH shifts potassium into the cells. Movement of potassium into the intracellular compartment can be achieved by giving insulin and glucose.

Hypokalemia usually is caused by depletion of total body potassium due to decreased potassium intake, increased extrarenal potassium losses, or increased renal potassium losses. Decreased serum potassium levels also can be caused by redistribution of potassium into the intracellular space. Symptoms of hypokalemia, like those of hyperkalemia, manifest as disturbances in membrane potentials. As potassium levels decrease to less than 2.5 mEq/L, muscle weakness is common. Primary management of hypokalemia is potassium replacement. The route and rate of potassium replacement depend on the presence and severity of symptoms. A decrease in serum potassium of 1 mEq/L represents a total body potassium deficiency of 100 to 200 mEq.

ANSWER: c, d

REFERENCE: *Chapter 10—Fluids, Electrolytes, and Acid–Base Balance: Compositional Changes*

11. Which of the following statements is/are true concerning abnormalities in calcium concentration?

   a. Parathyroid hormone affects calcium homeostasis only at the exchange of calcium between bone and extracellular fluid
   b. Approximately 45% of total plasma calcium is in the ionized state and is responsible for most physiologic actions
   c. Changes in plasma protein levels or pH can alter the proportion of calcium in the ionized state
   d. Intravenous administration of normal saline is the first step in management of hypercalcemia
   e. Classic signs of hypocalcemia include hyperactive deep tendon refluxes, the Chvostek sign, and the Trousseau sign

COMMENT: Calcium is a divalent cation found in abundance in the human body. Approximately 99% of total body calcium is located in bone in the form of hydroxyapatite crystals. Calcium homeostasis depends on the exchange of calcium between bone and extracellular fluid, renal excretion, and intestinal absorption. These three processes are controlled to a great extent by parathyroid hormone. In extracellular fluid, calcium exists in three forms: ionized calcium, nonionized calcium, and protein-bound calcium. Ionized calcium, which constitutes approximately 45% of total calcium, is responsible for most physiologic actions of calcium in the body, and its level is tightly controlled by regulatory mechanisms. Some nonionized calcium is complexed with nonprotein anions, including phosphate and citrate, and does not easily disassociate. These molecular forms make up only approximately 15% of total calcium present in plasma. Approximately 40% of extracellular nonionized calcium is bound to proteins, most being bound to albumin. Changes in plasma protein level or pH can alter the proportion of calcium in the ionized state.

The most common cause of hypercalcemia is primary hyperparathyroidism. Hypercalcemia also can be caused by malignant disease by means of metastasis to bone or autonomous tumor secretion of hormone-like substances that alter calcium homeostasis. Neuromuscular effects may be the earliest manifestations and include muscle fatigue, weakness, personality disorders, psychosis, confusion, and coma. Elevation of total serum calcium concentration to greater than 14 mg/dL necessitates prompt treatment to prevent serious and possibly lethal complications. Immediate measures are directed at maximizing renal excretion of calcium. Vigorous hydration with 0.9% saline solution to prompt diuresis should be the initial step in treatment. Addition of potassium to the resuscitation fluid and furosemide also can be used for treatment.

Serum calcium levels less than 8 mg/dL can be associated with symptoms and signs that are primary manifestations of neuromuscular abnormalities. These include muscle cramps, perioral tingling, paresthesia, laryngeal stridor, tetany, seizures, and psychotic behavior. Classic signs of hypocalcemia include hyperactive deep tendon reflexes, the Chvostek sign, and the Trousseau sign. Symptomatic hypocalcemia is best managed with intravenous infusion of calcium in the form of calcium gluconate or calcium chloride.

ANSWER: b, c, d, e

REFERENCE: *Chapter 10—Fluids, Electrolytes, and Acid–Base Balance: Compositional Changes*

12. Which of the following statements is/are true concerning alterations in serum level of magnesium?

    a. Renal failure is the primary cause of hypermagnesemia
    b. Hypomagnesemia can occur during prolonged periods of intravenous fluid replacement
    c. Symptoms of hypomagnesemia can mimic symptoms of hypocalcemia
    d. Intravenous administration of magnesium sulfate usually is the most efficient method of correction of magnesium deficiency

COMMENT: Renal failure is the primary cause of hypermagnesemia. Because of the ability of the kidneys to excrete large magnesium loads, hypermagnesemia rarely occurs if renal function remains normal. Because the kidneys can conserve magnesium well in states of magnesium depletion, hypomagnesemia rarely occurs as the result of poor intake alone. The combination of low intake and increased gastrointestinal loss can lead to hypomagnesemia. Prolonged periods of intravenous fluid replacement without magnesium replacement and long-term use of loop diuretics or other medications such as cyclosporine or aminoglycosides can also result in hypomagnesemia. Deficiencies of magnesium can cause signs and symptoms similar to those of hypocalcemia. Hypomagnesemia can be managed with oral administration of magnesium; however, large doses frequently cause diarrhea. Severe deficits therefore are best corrected by means of intravenous administration of magnesium sulfate at a dose of 50 to 100 mEq/d.

ANSWER: a, b, c, d

REFERENCE: *Chapter 10—Fluids, Electrolytes, and Acid–Base Balance: Compositional Changes*

13. Which of the following statements is/are true concerning the derangement of metabolic acidosis?

    a. An important acid in the body is sulfuric acid
    b. Excessive loss of bicarbonate can occur with intestinal or pancreatic fistula
    c. Ketoacidosis can occur with either hyperglycemia or hypoglycemia
    d. Lactic acidosis is present when serum lactate concentration is greater than 2 mEq/L
    e. Lactic acidosis can be associated with ethanol toxicity

COMMENT: Most clinically significant metabolic acidosis is related to the net loss of bicarbonate, which occurs when consumption due to loss or titration is greater than bicarbonate generation. Under normal circumstances of ingestion of the average amount of protein in the U.S. diet, approximately 70 mEq acid is generated daily. The main source of acid is sulfuric acid from the metabolism of sulfur-containing amino acids. Increased protein intake and tissue catabolism resulting in greater metabolism of sulfur-containing amino acids can lead to generation of increased amounts of sulfuric acid. This excess acid uses excess bicarbonate for neutralization. Diarrhea, intestinal or pancreatic fistula, and burns can cause metabolic acidosis because of loss of bicarbonate.

The two most common types of organic acidosis are ketoacidosis and lactic acidosis. The abnormality primarily responsible for ketoacidosis is deficiency of insulin whether primary, as in diabetic ketoacidosis, or secondary, as in association with hypoglycemia. Under normal conditions, a small amount of ketoacid is produced. During prolonged starvation, production of ketoacids increases to modest levels, providing an important source of energy to nonhepatic tissues, particularly the brain. In ketoacidosis, production of ketoacid is excessive because of insulin deficiency. In diabetic acidosis, insulin deficiency contributes to hyperglycemia by decreasing the metabolism of glucose by extrahepatic tissue and increasing hepatic production of glucose.

Lactic acidosis can be divided into type A, caused by tissue hypoxia, and type B, caused by other mechanisms. Hypoxia, the most common cause of lactic acidosis, impairs mitochondrial oxidation of nicotinamide adenine dinucleotide (NADH) to NAD that is necessary for glycolysis. Normal serum lactate concentration is less than 2 mEq/L. Lactate acidosis is caused by hypoxemia, usually as the result of increased production of lactate and decreased use, and serum lactate concentrations greater than 6 mEq/L. The most common cause of type B lactate acidosis is ethanol intoxication.

ANSWER: a, b, c, e

REFERENCE: *Chapter 10—Fluids, Electrolytes, and Acid-Base Balance: Acid-Base Disturbances; Metabolic Acidosis*

14. Which of the following statements is/are true concern renal tubular acidosis?

   a. Renal tubular acidosis is primarily caused by reduction in ammonia excretion
   b. The renal tubular defect in renal tubular acidosis can be at the distal or the proximal renal tubule
   c. In distal renal tubular acidosis associated with hyperkalemia, the defect involves increased tubular permeability with backleak of secreted sodium and potassium into the tubular cell
   d. Uremic acidosis occurs independently of protein intake

COMMENT: The impaired ability of the kidney to excrete acid and hence generate bicarbonate may be caused by a decrease in the number of functioning nephrons and is called *uremic acidosis* or *renal tubular acidosis*. Renal tubular acidosis, which can occur in both acute and chronic renal failure, is primarily caused by reduction in ammonia excretion secondary to a reduction in the number of functioning proximal tubular cells. A decrease in proximal tubular bicarbonate reabsorption contributes to the development of acidosis. Although the onset of uremic acidosis is related to declining renal function, its appearance can be influenced by diet-dependent protein and organic anion ingestion. Renal tubular acidosis can be classified as distal or proximal, depending on the primary site of the renal tubular defect leading to acidosis. In renal tubular acidosis with hyperkalemia, the mechanism is decreased luminal negativity secondary to impaired sodium reabsorption. In distal renal tubular acidosis with hypokalemia, mechanisms including increased tubular permeability with backleak of secreted hydrogen ion into the tubular cell and reduced hydrogen ion pump activity are proposed mechanisms.

ANSWER: a, b

REFERENCE: *Chapter 10—Fluids, Electrolytes, and Acid–Base Balance: Acid–Base Disturbances; Metabolic Acidosis*

15. Clinical manifestations of acute metabolic acidosis include:

   a. Decreased cardiac contractility
   b. Decreased catecholamine secretion
   c. Peripheral arteriolar dilatation
   d. Shift of the oxygen-hemoglobin disassociation curve to the left

COMMENT: The most important cardiovascular effects of acute metabolic acidosis are peripheral arteriolar dilatation, a decrease in cardiac contractility, and central venous constriction. These can cause cardiovascular collapse and pulmonary edema. Catecholamine secretion is stimulated by metabolic acidosis, and in mild cases, heart rate may be increased. In addition to these cardiovascular effects, metabolic acidosis can affect oxygen delivery by shifting the oxygen-hemoglobin disassociation curve to the right.

ANSWER: a, b, c

REFERENCE: *Chapter 10—Fluids, Electrolytes, and Acid–Base Balance: Acid–Base Disturbances; Metabolic Acidosis*

16. Which of the following statements is/are true concerning the compensatory mechanisms and management of metabolic acidosis?
    a. Maximal renal compensation for metabolic acidosis occurs before full respiratory compensation can occur
    b. All patients with lactic acidosis should receive prompt treatment with bicarbonate
    c. Potassium replacement is essential even in the face of normal or high serum potassium levels in the management of diabetic ketoacidosis
    d. Sodium bicarbonate administration should be simultaneous with volume resuscitation in the care of patients with hypoxia secondary to shock

COMMENT: The kidney is extremely sensitive to changes in serum bicarbonate concentration and responds by increasing net acid excretion primarily by increasing ammonia excretion. Maximal renal compensation requires 2 to 4 days. Delay in achieving maximal renal response to an increased acid load causes blood pH to decline, which stimulates hyperventilation. Although effective in promptly increasing blood pH, ventilatory compensation is only partial, and full respiration compensation requires 12 to 24 hours. The most important principle of management of mild to moderate acute metabolic acidosis is correction of the underlying cause. Among surgical and trauma patients, metabolic acidosis often is the result of hypoxia secondary to inadequate tissue perfusion and subsequent lactic acidosis. Volume or blood resuscitation alone may be enough to correct the acidosis. Attempts to correct acidosis with exogenous bicarbonate before correction of inadequate tissue perfusion usually are unsuccessful. The use of bicarbonate for the management of lactic acidosis is controversial at best. In several studies, the use of bicarbonate to treat patients with lactic acidosis did not improve clinical measurements or outcome. Correction of both acidosis and hypoglycemia of diabetic ketoacidosis is best achieved by the administration of insulin. Volume resuscitation also is required. Potassium replacement is essential, even in the face of normal or high serum levels of potassium, because hypokalemia develops as acidosis and hyperglycemia are corrected.

ANSWER: c

REFERENCE: *Chapter 10—Fluids, Electrolytes, and Acid–Base Balance: Acid–Base Disturbances; Metabolic Acidosis*

17. Which of the following statements is/are true concerning metabolic alkalosis?
    a. Either increased extracellular bicarbonate concentration or inhibited renal excretion of bicarbonate can cause metabolic alkalosis
    b. In metabolic alkalosis secondary to prolonged gastric outlet obstruction, urine pH usually is acidic
    c. Hypokalemia can lead to metabolic alkalosis
    d. The respiratory compensatory mechanisms for metabolic alkalosis are ineffective

COMMENT: Sustained metabolic alkalosis occurs only if extracellular bicarbonate concentration is increased and renal excretion of excess bicarbonate is inhibited. Neither alone is sufficient to result in metabolic alkalosis. Extracellular bicarbonate concentration is increased by numerous mechanisms. Loss of hydrochloric acid is the leading cause of metabolic alkalosis among surgical patients. External loss of gastric acid results in net gain in bicarbonate, which causes metabolic alkalosis. Although the kidney can excrete excess bicarbonate, this must be accompanied by excretion of sodium. Renal excretion of sodium is limited in the face of volume depletion, which also occurs with external losses of gastric secretion. As volume depletion progresses, sodium is conserved in exchange for hydrogen. Thus in metabolic alkalosis due to prolonged gastric outlet obstruction, the urine, although initially alkalotic, becomes paradoxically acidotic in prolonged or uncorrected cases. Hypokalemia and cellular exchange of potassium for hydrogen also can lead to metabolic alkalosis. Hypokalemia results in enhanced proximal tubular bicarbonate reabsorption and distal tubular acid secretion. The main compensatory mechanism in metabolic alkalosis is respiratory, because the presence of metabolic alkalosis implies renal dysfunction in either generating or failing to excrete increased amounts of bicarbonate. Hypoventilation is limited by the development of hypoxemia, which stimulates ventilation. Among the four major types of acid-base disorders, this compensatory mechanism is the least effective.

ANSWER: b, c, d

REFERENCE: *Chapter 10—Fluids, Electrolytes, and Acid–Base Balance: Acid–Base Disturbances; Metabolic Alkalosis*

18. Which of the following statements is/are true concerning the clinical presentation and management of severe metabolic alkalosis?
    a. In most cases clinical signs are obvious
    b. Correction of potassium and volume depletion corrects most cases of metabolic alkalosis
    c. Acetazolamide can enhance renal excretion of bicarbonate
    d. Acid replacement should be provided at a molar equivalent basis for excess serum bicarbonate

COMMENT: Clinical signs of metabolic alkalosis may not be prominent, because the condition usually develops relatively slowly. Correction of the underlying cause is the mainstay of management of this disorder. In general, correction of potassium and volume depletion corrects the metabolic alkalosis. Among patients without intravascular volume deficits, renal excretion of bicarbonate can be enhanced by means of administration of the carbonic acid anhydrase inhibitor acetazolamide. If renal excretion of bicarbonate cannot be increased because of underlying renal insufficiency or if metabolic alkalosis is severe, acid can be administered to directly titrate the excess extracellular bicarbonate. Acids that can be used include ammonium chloride, arginine hydrochloride, or dilute hydrochloric acid. Partial correction of alkalosis is the initial goal. A general guide is that 2.2 mEq/kg decreases serum bicarbonate by approximately 5 mEq/L.

ANSWER: b, c

REFERENCE: *Chapter 10—Fluids, Electrolytes, and Acid–Base Balance: Acid–Base Disturbances; Metabolic Alkalosis*

19. Which of the following statements is/are true concerning respiratory alkalosis?
    a. Exposure to high altitudes can result in respiratory alkalosis
    b. Renal compensation for respiratory alkalosis is obtained by means of increasing excretion of bicarbonate
    c. Symptoms of respiratory alkalosis can mimic those of hypocalcemia
    d. Management of acute respiratory alkalosis may involve a brown paper bag

COMMENT: A primary decrease in Pco_2 resulting in an increase in extracellular pH is called *respiratory alkalosis.* Hyperventilation and the ensuing decrease in Pco_2 may be secondary to hypoxia, reflux simulation from decreased pulmonary compliance, drugs, mechanical ventilation, and other causes. The two most common causes of hypoxia resulting in respiratory alkalosis are pulmonary disease and exposure to high altitudes. Renal compensation for respiratory alkalosis is not achieved by means of increasing excretion of bicarbonate but by decreasing net acid excretion, primarily through a reduction in ammonia excretion and increases in organic anion excretion. Chronic respiratory alkalosis is generally asymptomatic. Acute respiratory alkalosis can cause sensations of breathlessness, dizziness, and nervousness and can result in circumoral and extremity paresthesia, altered levels of consciousness, and tetany. These signs are related to decreased cerebral blood flow due to a decrease in Pco_2 and decreased ionized calcium concentration due to an increase in blood pH. Rebreathing, by means of breathing in and out of a paper bag, can temporarily relieve the symptoms of acute symptomatic respiratory alkalosis.

ANSWER: a, c, d

REFERENCE: *Chapter 10—Fluids, Electrolytes, and Acid–Base Balance: Acid–Base Disturbances; Respiratory Alkalosis*

20. Which of the following statements is/are true concerning respiratory acidosis?

    a. Respiratory acidosis is associated with chronic pulmonary disease far more commonly than is hypoxemia

    b. The initial buffering effect occurs at the cellular level

    c. Renal compensation occurs within 24 hours

    d. Correction of hypoxemia among patients with chronic lung disease can worsen respiratory acidosis

COMMENT: Respiratory acidosis, the decrease in extracellular pH due to a primary increase in P_{CO_2}, is caused by inadequate ventilation. Although pulmonary disease commonly causes hypoxemia, respiratory acidosis is far less common, because defusion of oxygen is more readily impaired than is diffusion of carbon dioxide. An increase in P_{CO_2} increases the level of carbonic acid (H_2CO_3) which disassociates into hydrogen and bicarbonate ions. Cellular exchange of sodium and potassium ions for hydrogen ions allows the reaction to continue in this direction with increased extracellular bicarbonate. This tissue buffering is accomplished within minutes. Persistently elevated P_{CO_2} also increases renal acid excretions. Full renal compensation occurs over 3 to 5 days. Management of chronic compensated respiratory acidosis can be complicated by accompanying hypoxemia. In chronic hypercapnia, the chemical chemoreceptors may be insensitive, and the accompanying hypoxemia can supply the main respiratory drive through stimulation of peripheral chemoreceptors. Among such patients, complete correction of hypoxemia can further depress respiration and worsen respiratory acidosis.

ANSWER: b, d

REFERENCE: *Chapter 10—Fluids, Electrolytes, and Acid–Base Balance: Acid–Base Disturbances; Respiratory Acidosis*

CHAPTER 11

TRAUMA

1. Which of the following statements is/are true concerning all traumatic deaths?

    a. Most trauma deaths are caused by complications such as sepsis and multiple organ failure

    b. Prevention is the most important strategy to reduce the number of early trauma deaths

    c. Training programs such as the advanced trauma life support course of the American College of Surgeons are critical in decreasing trauma-related deaths during the golden hour

    d. Massive hemorrhage and severe brain injury are the most frequent causes of death during the prehospital phase of care after injury

COMMENT: Trauma deaths occur at three traditionally recognized times after injury. Approximately one half of all trauma-related deaths occur within seconds or minutes of injury and are related to lacerations of the aorta, heart, brainstem, brain, and spinal cord. These injuries are best addressed with prevention strategies—either devices that prevent injury or laws that limit certain behavior patterns. The second mortality peak occurs within hours of injury and accounts for approximately 30% of deaths, one half of which are caused by hemorrhage and one half by central nervous system injuries. Important reductions in mortality during this period have resulted from the development of trauma systems, rapid prehospital transport times, and training of physicians in the care of injured patients during the first hour after trauma—the golden hour.

ANSWER: b, c, d

REFERENCE: *Chapter 11—Trauma: Introduction*

2. Which of the following statements is/are true regarding the epidemiologic aspects of trauma?
   a. The risk of dying of injury is equal for male and female victims
   b. Trauma is the third cause of death for all age groups, but the years of productive life lost (YPLL) index is higher after trauma than after cardiovascular disease or cancer
   c. Children rarely sustain fatal injuries
   d. Drinking and driving is the most important cause of fatal motor vehicle accidents

COMMENT: Persons younger than 45 years sustain almost 80% of all injuries and account for 75% of the total lifetime costs. Young men are at highest risk, not because of physiologic distinctions but because of the propensity to engage in high-risk activities. Overall, the risk of dying after injury among the male population is seven times higher than that among the female population. Traumatic deaths result in a higher number of YPLL than deaths associated with cancer and cardiovascular disease. This is because injuries are more prevalent among the younger population. The age-adjusted YPLL before 75 years of age in 1996 (per 100,000 population) was 1,919, 1,554, and 1,223 for injury, cancer, and heart disease, respectively. For each traumatic death there are an average of 36 YPLL, compared with 16 for cancer and 12 for cardiovascular disease. The leading causes of death among children are motor vehicle accidents, burns, drowning, falls, and poisoning. Injury to children leads to a large number of deaths, disabilities, days of missed school, medical costs, and missed workdays for parents. Alcohol ingestion is an important cause of fatal vehicular accidents. Although progress has been made in the prevention of drinking and driving, during 1997, 39% of all traffic deaths were alcohol related.

ANSWER: b, d

REFERENCE: *Chapter 11—Trauma: General Considerations; Epidemiology*

3. Which of the following statements is/are true?
   a. Injury severity is directly proportional to the amount of kinetic energy transferred to tissues
   b. Temporary cavitation occurs only after blunt trauma
   c. The biomechanics of blunt aortic rupture involve acceleration-deceleration forces
   d. Tensile strain is an important component of the mechanism of blunt pancreatic injury

COMMENT: The severity of any injury is directly proportional to the amount of kinetic energy transferred to the tissues, whether by a projectile or by blunt impact. Kinetic energy is a function of the mass of an object and its velocity. Cavitation occurs as tissue impacted by a moving body recoils from the point of impact, away from the object. This occurs after both blunt and penetrating trauma. Differential acceleration in the thorax makes the aorta the most common site of shear injury. Tensile strain causes injury by directly compressing the tissue. In the abdomen, the pancreas, liver, spleen, and occasionally the kidneys are subject to tensile strain injury, particularly after frontal impact.

ANSWER: a, c, d

REFERENCE: *Chapter 11—Trauma: General Considerations; Biomechanics of Injury*

4. Which of the following statements is/are correct regarding motor vehicle collisions?
   a. The restrained occupant of a vehicle receives less kinetic energy transfer than unrestrained occupants in a car accident
   b. In general, the kinetic energy transferred to the occupant of a vehicle is similar to that exerted on the vehicle itself
   c. The predictable injury patterns resulting from the down and under movement of unrestrained occupants of the front seat of a vehicle in a frontal impact are tibial plateau fractures, knee dislocations, femur fractures, hip dislocation, blunt chest and abdominal trauma, head injury, and cervical spinal injury
   d. Cervical spinal injuries caused by hyperextension of the neck are common after rear-impact collisions

COMMENT: An occupant of a vehicle receives kinetic energy transfer similar to that of the vehicle itself. In this regard, a description of vehicular damage can be useful for general categorization of patients. When an automobile collides with an object, passengers collide with the interior of the automobile, and the internal organs collide with the body wall or are sheared from anatomic attachment. With the down and under movement, the knees strike the dashboard, and the thighs absorb the primary energy transfer. Dislocated knees, fractured femurs, and posterior fracture dislocations of the hips are expected. After the knee impact, the upper part of the body flexes forward and moves up and over the steering wheel. The chest or abdomen undergoes impact with the steering wheel and the head hits the windshield. The head stops the forward momentum of the torso, and kinetic energy is absorbed by the cervical spine. Rear-impact collisions occur when stationary objects or slow-moving vehicles are struck from behind. The amount of kinetic energy generated depends on the difference between the velocities of the two vehicles rather than the sum as in forward collisions. After a rear impact, the vehicle and its occupants accelerate forward, and hyperextension of the cervical spine with injury can occur.

ANSWER: b, c, d

REFERENCE: *Chapter 11—Trauma: General Considerations; Motor Vehicle Collisions*

5. Which of the following statements is/are correct regarding restraint devices?
   a. A three-point seat belt is designed to allow the kinetic energy transferred by the impact to be absorbed by the pelvis and upper part of the chest
   b. Seat belt injuries usually are caused by improper use of the device
   c. The use of a lap belt only is associated with increased risk of compression injuries to intraabdominal organs, diaphragmatic rupture, and compression fractures of the lumbar spine.
   d. The use of diagonal shoulder straps without a lap belt is associated with blunt carotid injury and fractures of the clavicle and ribs

COMMENT: Properly used three-point restraints allow the kinetic energy transferred by the impact to be absorbed by the bony pelvis and chest. If improperly positioned, however, lap belts can rise above the pelvis and deliver the compression force to the soft tissues of the abdominal cavity or retroperitoneum. Common injuries when lap belts are incorrectly strapped above the anterior iliac crest include compression injuries to the intraabdominal organs (liver, pancreas, spleen, small bowel, large bowel), increased intraabdominal pressure and diaphragmatic rupture, and anterior compression of the lumbar spine. Diagonal shoulder straps should be worn in combination with lap belts to prevent forward motion of the trunk. Diagonal shoulder straps should not be worn alone because this can be associated with chest and neck injuries if the pelvis is not secured by the lap belt. Injuries associated with shoulder straps include carotid artery contusion with or without thrombosis and fractures of the clavicle and ribs.

ANSWER: a, b, c, d

REFERENCE: *Chapter 11—Trauma: General Considerations; Restraint Device Injury*

6. The response of the body to hemorrhage includes all of the following except:
   a. Increased adrenergic output with tachycardia, peripheral vasoconstriction, increased myocardial contractility, and pulmonary vasodilation
   b. Increased secretion of renin from decreased renal blood flow
   c. Aldosterone-mediated absorption of sodium in the renal tubules
   d. Increased serum glucose level

COMMENT: The body has both immediate and sustained responses to hemorrhage. The immediate response includes increased sympathetic activity from catecholamine release, causing tachycardia, peripheral and pulmonary vasoconstriction, increased myocardial contractility, and increased blood pressure. The sustained responses increase resorption of sodium and water in response to increased aldosterone release. The increases in renin secretion are caused by increased adrenergic activity and decreased renal blood flow. The stress hormone response with catecholamine, cortisol, and glucagon increases serum glucose concentration.

ANSWER: a

REFERENCE: *Chapter 11—Trauma: Patient Care Phase; Shock*

7. Which of the following statements is/are correct regarding biochemical assessment of the shock state?
   a. Serum lactate levels have been shown to correlate with injury severity scores and mortality
   b. The time interval for normalization of the arterial base deficit has prognostic significance
   c. Base deficit and lactate level are closely related and have been shown to correct rapidly with resuscitation
   d. Lactate level and base deficits are measured in routine blood gas analysis

COMMENT: Serum lactate level and base deficit have a near linear relation, and both have been shown valuable in assessing shock. Lactate level is a measured value but is not routinely obtained with many blood gas instruments. Base deficit is a calculated value obtained during blood gas analysis. Both base deficit and lactate level correct with resuscitation. The time interval to normalization has been shown to have prognostic significance. Base deficit values have been shown to correlate with anatomic and physiologic injury scores and mortality. The severity of the initial lactate value has been correlated to mortality risk but not to injury severity score.

ANSWER: b, c

REFERENCE: *Chapter 11—Trauma: Patient Care Phase; Shock*

8. Which of the following statements is/are correct concerning classification of hemorrhage?

a. Class II hemorrhage (15% to 30%) almost always is associated with decreased systolic blood pressure and the requirement for blood as part of the resuscitation

b. Class IV hemorrhage is uncompensated hemorrhagic shock and necessitates crystalloid and blood resuscitation and frequently surgical treatment

c. Class II and III hemorrhage may be associated with mental status changes

d. In Class I hemorrhage, the blood volume loss can be restored within 24 hours by means of transcapillary refill

COMMENT: Classification of hemorrhage is clinically useful.

ANSWER: b, c, d

REFERENCE: *Chapter 11—Trauma: Patient Care Phase; Shock*

9. A 32-year-old man has been involved in a motor vehicle accident and has undergone scoop and run transport, arriving at the hospital 10 minutes after trauma. The patient is not cyanotic and is breathing spontaneously. Blood pressure is 100/45 mm Hg, pulse rate is 120 beats/min, and there are no external signs of systemic trauma. Pupils are both 4 mm, round, and reactive. The patient opens his eyes when his name or a command to open his eyes is shouted at him. He makes incoherent sounds. When supraorbital pressure is applied, the right extremities extend, and the patient uses his left arm to grasp the hand applying the stimulus. The Glasgow Coma Scale (GCS) score is:

a. Total GCS score, 6; eye score, 2; verbal score, 2; motor score, 2

b. Total GCS score, 11; eye score, 3; verbal score, 3; motor score, 5

c. Total GCS score, 9; eye score, 2; verbal score, 2; motor score, 5

d. Total GCS score, 8; eye score, 3; verbal score, 3; motor score, 2

e. Total GCS score, 20; eye score, 2; verbal score, 3; motor score, 5

COMMENT: The GCS score is the standard nomenclature for describing level of consciousness. It consists of the sum of eye, verbal, and motor subscale scores with a range of 3 to 15. The eye scale ranges from 1 to 4 points for never open, open to pain, open to command, or open spontaneously. The verbal score ranges from 1 to 5 for no verbalization, garbled, inappropriate, confused, or oriented verbalization. The motor score ranges from 1 to 6 for no movement, decerebrate posturing, decorticate posturing, withdrawal from pain, localizes pain, or obeys commands. The motor scale is scored for the best response of any limb.

ANSWER: c

REFERENCE: *Chapter 11—Trauma: Definitive Care Phase; Head Injury*

10. A 22-year-old is man is found down and transported to the emergency department. Initial neurologic examination reveals no focal deficits. The pupils are equal, round, and reactive. The patient is not opening his eyes, not verbalizing, and localizing pain with all extremities (GCS score, 6). Vital signs have been normal since the patient was found. The following should be part of initial resuscitation in this case:

a. Intubation and mechanical ventilation targeting $Paco_2$ 30 mm Hg
b. Intubation and mechanical ventilation targeting $Paco_2$ 35 mm Hg
c. Restriction of fluids until computed tomography (CT) is performed
d. Administration of 0.25 g/kg mannitol as an intravenous bolus
e. Administration of intravenous sedation and analgesia

COMMENT: Resuscitation of patients with severe traumatic brain injury (GCS score, 8) must be based on full fluid resuscitation. Fluid restriction is no longer practiced; volumes are administered as for any trauma resuscitation. Isotonic fluids are used. Sedation and analgesia are administered. No specific treatment is directed at decreasing intracranial pressure (ICP) in the absence of signs of intracranial hypertension. When any of these signs is present, however, hyperventilation to a $Paco_2$ between 30 and 35 mm Hg is initiated, and mannitol is administered if intravascular volume is normal.

ANSWER: b, e

REFERENCE: *Chapter 11—Trauma: Definitive Care Phase; Head Injury*

11. The following are clinical signs of intracranial hypertension and should precipitate treatment aimed at lowering ICP:

a. Glasgow Coma Scale score of 8
b. Anisocoria
c. Extensor posturing
d. Pupils that are 7 mm bilaterally
e. Decreased responsiveness on the part of a patient with hypotension

COMMENT: Clinical signs of intracranial hypertension include abnormal pupillary findings (anisocoria, bilateral pupillary dilatation, nonreactivity of one or both pupils, or oval or irregular pupillary shape), flaccidity or decerebrate or decorticate motor posturing, or progressive neurologic deterioration not attributable to other causes, such as drugs, hypoxia, or hypotension. Only when signs of intracranial hypertension are evident is therapy to decrease ICP indicated.

ANSWER: b, c, d

REFERENCE: *Chapter 11—Trauma: Definitive Care Phase; Head Injury*

12. Hyperventilation is an important tool in the control of intracranial hypertension. Which of the following statements is/are true of hyperventilation?

    a. Hyperventilation decreases cerebral blood volume by inducing vasoconstriction
    b. When it is elected to use hyperventilation, a $Paco_2$ range of 25 to 30 mm Hg should be the target
    c. A $Paco_2$ of 45 mm Hg is satisfactory for a patient with a GCS score of 6 but no signs of herniation
    d. Iatrogenic ischemia is a risk of hyperventilation
    e. Jugular saturation monitoring can be a useful adjunct when hyperventilation is used to manage intracranial hypertension

COMMENT: Hyperventilation is used to manage intracranial hypertension when specific indicators are present before ICP monitoring or when intracranial hypertension is proved after an ICP monitor has been placed. Hyperventilation causes cerebral vasoconstriction. It decreases ICP by decreasing cerebral blood volume but with the attendant risk of a dangerous decrease in cerebral blood flow. In the absence of intracranial hypertension, moderate vasoconstriction is desired, so a $Paco_2$ at the lower end of eucapnia (e.g., 35 mm Hg) is the target. When ICP is definitely elevated and hyperventilation is used, the initial range of $Paco_2$ is 30 to 35 mm Hg. Values lower than that are considered extreme hyperventilation. The risk of iatrogenic cerebral ischemia often is addressed by means of monitoring the oxygen saturation of the jugular venous blood as it leaves the brain.

ANSWER: a, d, e

REFERENCE: *Chapter 11—Trauma: Definitive Care Phase; Head Injury*

13. A young patient is struck on the head with a bat and has a documented brief loss of consciousness. He reports a moderate headache, but there is no nausea or vomiting. Examination shows no abnormal neurologic signs. The following are appropriate methods of management:

    a. Observation with neurologic tests every 4 hours without further imaging
    b. Observation in an intensive care unit (ICU) with neurologic tests every hour without further imaging
    c. Discharge to family at home with a "head sheet"—a lists of symptom that necessitate immediate return to the hospital
    d. Discharge to family at home with a head sheet if CT findings are normal
    e. Discharge to family at home with a head sheet if skull radiographs are normal

COMMENT: The proper evaluation of mild head injury is critical because of the phenomenon of the patient who "talks and dies." If a patient loses consciousness or has any abnormal neurologic findings or behavior such as nausea and vomiting or perseverative questioning, there must be a high suspicion of intracranial abnormality. Close observation of patients with a history of loss of consciousness or brief posttraumatic amnesia and nothing else is acceptable as long as a reliable neurologic examinations can be performed no less than 1 hour apart. An alternative in the care of such patients is discharge to someone at home if a CT scan is completely normal. It is somewhat more controversial but still acceptable to discharge such a patient to someone at home if high-quality skull radiographs are read by a competent, experienced reader as completely normal. In the United States, however, it is highly recommended that CT be performed instead of skull radiographs. Any patient with more than a history of a brief loss of consciousness, mild headache, or a brief period of amnesia should undergo imaging and be admitted. A head sheet is not a substitute for any of the above measures.

ANSWER: b, d, e

REFERENCE: *Chapter 11—Trauma: Definitive Care Phase; Head Injury*

14. A 26-year-old man involved in a motor vehicle accident as an unrestrained passenger has epistaxis, pain, and swelling in the nasoethmoidal region. Which of the following statements is/are true?

a. The cribriform plate may be fractured
b. The nose should be packed anteriorly for initial control of epistaxis
c. Anterior and posterior nasal packs should be inserted for control of epistaxis
d. If clear fluid is draining from the nose, the lacrimal system has been disrupted

COMMENT: Nasoethmoidal fractures may be associated with injuries to the cribriform. plate, ethmoidal roof, lacrimal system, medial canthal tendons, and blood vessels of the nose. Signs and symptoms include cerebrospinal fluid rhinorrhea, anosmia due to olfactory tract damage, epistaxis, epiphora, and telecanthus. Nasal packing should be avoided in the management of nasoethmoidal and cribriform fractures because of the risk of intracranial injury.

ANSWER: a

REFERENCE: *Chapter 11—Trauma: Definitive Care Phase; Maxillofacial Injuries*

15. An orbital floor blow-out fracture is associated with which of the following findings?

a. Enophthalmos
b. Exophthalmos
c. Diplopia
d. Limitation of upward gaze

COMMENT: Fracture of the orbital floor—the most common type of orbital fracture—leads to herniation of the orbital contents into the maxillary sinus with resultant enophthalmos or hypophthalmos, entrapment of the inferior rectus or inferior oblique muscles, and even optic nerve or optic vessel injury.

ANSWER: a, c, d

REFERENCE: *Chapter 11—Trauma: Definitive Care Phase; Maxillofacial Injuries*

16. The most important factor(s) in ensuring successful management of mandibular fractures is/are:

a. Removing teeth in the fracture line
b. Completely immobilizing the bone fragments
c. Correcting any premorbid occlusal abnormalities
d. Eliminating contamination and infection

COMMENT: Successful healing of mandibular fractures depends on adequate immobilization of the bone fragments, elimination of contamination, and restoration of the patient's premorbid occlusion. Whenever possible, teeth should be saved.

ANSWER: b, d

REFERENCE: *Chapter 11—Trauma: Definitive Care Phase; Maxillofacial Injuries*

17. An 18-year-old patient with extensive maxillofacial trauma is in respiratory distress. A tracheotomy should be performed if:

a. Cervical spine injury is suspected
b. The mandible is also fractured
c. The patient also has severe epistaxis
d. Le Fort III fracture is present

COMMENT: When a patient needs airway intervention and support, tracheotomy is indicated whenever a stable airway cannot be ensured by means of spontaneous support or by means of oral or nasal endotracheal intubation without causing further damage. Whenever cervical spinal injury is suspected and oral or nasal intubation would necessitate manipulation of the cervical spine, tracheotomy should be performed with the patient in traction.

ANSWER: a

REFERENCE: *Chapter 11—Trauma: Definitive Care Phase; Maxillofacial Injuries*

18. A 70-year-old female victim of a motor vehicle accident struck her forehead on the dashboard. The resultant frontal sinus fracture should be repaired surgically to avoid:

a. Mucocele formation
b. Posttraumatic forehead deformity
c. Overlooking a dural tear
d. Such a fracture does not require surgical repair

COMMENT: Displaced frontal sinus fractures often are associated with tears of the frontal dura. If not managed surgically, they can cause mucocele formation, which can cause a mass effect on the frontal lobes and symptoms of severe sinusitis. Depressed frontal sinus fractures also are particularly disfiguring.

ANSWER: a, b, c

REFERENCE: *Chapter 11—Trauma: Definitive Care Phase; Maxillofacial Injuries*

19. Which of the following statements is/are true regarding penetrating neck trauma?

a. Wounds that penetrate the platysma muscle mandate hospital admission
b. All patients with penetrating neck trauma need a chest radiograph
c. Wounds of the posterior triangle rarely involve the esophagus or major vessels
d. Zone II injuries are the most common and carry the highest mortality
e. Expanding or large neck hematoma in zone II indicates a need for preoperative angiography

COMMENT: Wounds that do not penetrate the platysma are considered superficial and do not warrant extensive evaluation. Wounds that penetrate the platysma must be considered a serious surgical problem that mandates hospital admission and further evaluation. All patients with blunt or penetrating neck trauma should have a chest radiograph to rule out thoracic trauma. Patients in stable condition need soft-tissue neck radiographs to look for retropharyngeal hematoma, tracheal narrowing or deviation, retained missile fragments and pathways, and subcutaneous or retropharyngeal air.

ANSWER: a, b

REFERENCE: *Chapter 11—Trauma: Definitive Care Phase; Neck Injuries*

20. Cervical esophageal injuries:

a. Occur among 20% of patients with penetrating neck wounds
b. Are associated with a 25% mortality if the patient is not treated within 48 hours of the injury
c. Necessitate drainage only if associated with substantial tissue loss
d. Can manifest as crepitus or odynophagia
e. Can be ruled out with normal findings at esophagography

COMMENT: Because all reported deaths of cervical esophageal injuries are the result of a delayed or missed diagnosis, a particularly thorough search is warranted.

ANSWER: d

REFERENCE: *Chapter 11—Trauma: Definitive Care Phase; Neck Injuries*

21. Tension pneumothorax is most commonly associated with:

a. Stab wounds
b. Gunshot wounds
c. Positive pressure ventilation
d. Sucking chest wounds
e. Multiple rib fractures

COMMENT: Tension pneumothorax is a life-threatening complication of chest trauma and must be part of the differential diagnosis for any patient with hypotension. Tension pneumothorax occurs when intrathoracic pressure in a hemithorax is greater than atmospheric pressure. The result is a mediastinal shift and circulatory impairment. Tension pneumothorax is much more common among patients undergoing positive pressure ventilation and occurs infrequently among spontaneously breathing patients.

ANSWER: c

REFERENCE: *Chapter 11—Trauma: Definitive Care Phase; Chest Injuries*

22. The most important therapeutic goal for elderly patients with rib fractures is:

   a. To ensure adequate analgesia
   b. To provide mechanical stabilization of the chest wall
   c. To achieve vital capacity greater than 1 liter
   d. To use only colloid intravenous solutions
   e. To keep the patient intravascularly "dry"

COMMENT: Even a single rib fracture can be associated with considerable morbidity for elderly patients. To prevent pulmonary complications, it is essential that the patient be able to maintain good ventilatory mechanics and a strong cough. By far the most important goal is to ensure adequate analgesia.

ANSWER: a

REFERENCE: *Chapter 11—Trauma: Definitive Care Phase; Chest Injuries*

23. Successful management of penetrating chest trauma by means of tube thoracostomy is best indicated by:

   a. Chest radiograph showing good position of the tube
   b. Chest tube output less than 1,000 mL
   c. Absence of an air leak
   d. A chest radiograph showing full expansion of the lung and complete evacuation of hemothorax
   e. Improved breath sounds after tube placement

COMMENT: Approximately 85% of all penetrating chest injuries can be managed by means of tube thoracostomy alone, if chest drainage is effective. To achieve hemostasis, it is necessary to achieve full expansion of the lung and remove all blood and clot. If these goals are not met, failure of nonsurgical management is likely. A chest radiograph is the best way to make sure the chest tube is doing what it should.

ANSWER: d

REFERENCE: *Chapter 11—Trauma: Definitive Care Phase; Chest Injuries*

24. The morbidity associated with flail chest is primarily caused by:

   a. Mechanical instability of the chest wall
   b. The underlying pulmonary parenchymal injury
   c. Paradoxical chest wall motion and pendelluft
   d. Myocardial contusion
   e. Fluid overload

COMMENT: The pathophysiologic mechanism of flail chest has been misunderstood until fairly recently. It tended to focus on dysfunction of the ventilatory pump and instability of the chest wall. More recent experience has shown that the severity of the underlying lung injury is the main determinant of clinical course. All patients with flail chest need an aggressive approach to analgesia, and some may benefit from chest wall stabilization, but the need for long-term mechanical ventilation is largely determined by the degree of parenchymal injury.

ANSWER: b

REFERENCE: *Chapter 11—Trauma: Definitive Care Phase; Chest Injuries*

25. The best anatomic landmarks for placement of tube thoracostomy for trauma are:

   a. Second intercostal space, midclavicular line
   b. Tenth intercostal space, anterior axillary line
   c. Fifth interspace, posterior axillary line
   d. Midaxillary line at the level of the mid sternum
   e. Anterior axillary line at the level of the nipple or inframammary crease

COMMENT: The best landmarks for placement of tube thoracostomy are those that allow for the easiest, safest, and most reproducible approach. The anterior axillary line, just behind the pectoralis muscle, is the thinnest and anatomically simplest portion of the chest wall. It is necessary to stay anterior to the midline to avoid the long thoracic nerve. Choice of the inframammary crease should put the tube at approximately the level of the fifth interspace.

ANSWER: e

REFERENCE: *Chapter 11—Trauma: Definitive Care Phase; Chest Injuries*

26. Generally accepted indications for diagnostic peritoneal lavage in the care of trauma patients include which of the following?

    a. Gunshot wounds of the abdomen
    b. Lack of consciousness with signs of abdominal injury
    c. Multiple injuries and unexplained shock
    d. Awake and alert condition with reliable abdominal examination
    e. Possible intraabdominal injury, equivocal diagnostic findings, and the need for prolonged general anesthesia for nonabdominal injuries

COMMENT: Diagnostic peritoneal lavage is most commonly used in the care of patients who have sustained blunt abdominal trauma. When the patient has a mechanism of injury or physical findings that suggest the possibility of intraabdominal injury and does not have reliable physical findings, peritoneal lavage is indicated. Diagnostic peritoneal lavage also is indicated as a rapid means of ascertaining the presence of intraabdominal hemorrhage and determining the need for emergency operative intervention when there is hemodynamic instability and the possibility of intraabdominal injury. Prolonged anesthesia is a special circumstance during which the physical findings are not clear and is another indication for peritoneal lavage. When the equipment is available, a focused abdominal sonogram for trauma (FAST) is a reasonably reliable substitute for diagnostic peritoneal lavage.

ANSWER: b, c, e

REFERENCE: *Chapter 11—Trauma: Definitive Care Phase; Abdominal Injuries*

27. Indications for "damage control" laparotomy include which of the following?

    a. Disruption of the colon that cannot be repaired primarily
    b. Clinical or laboratory evidence of severe coagulopathy
    c. Hyperglycemia
    d. Severe parenchymal injury that can be controlled only with packing
    e. Hypothermia

COMMENT: Damage control laparotomy is an abbreviated approach to the management of intraabdominal injury. Definitive repair of injuries is delayed, and emphasis is placed on rapid control of hemorrhage and keeping the operating time as short as possible. In addition to the presence of devastating parenchymal injury that can be controlled only with packing, there are several physiologic indicators of the desirability of damage control laparotomy. These include profound coagulopathy and, by extension, hypothermia, because of the effects of body temperature on the ability of the patient to form clot.

ANSWER: b, d, e

REFERENCE: *Chapter 11—Trauma: Definitive Care Phase; Abdominal Injuries*

28. A 20-year-old man was the restrained passenger in a high-speed motor vehicle crash. On arrival in the emergency department, he has pain and tenderness in the left lower part of the chest and left upper quadrant of the abdomen. There is also left-shoulder pain but no tenderness. Blood pressure is 120/85 mm Hg and stable in the emergency department. Computed tomography of the abdomen shows severe disruption of the spleen without a blush sign and a moderate amount of free intraperitoneal fluid. Important factors in the decision about operative versus nonoperative management include which of the following?

a. Vital signs and hemodynamic stability
b. The presence of left shoulder pain
c. The amount of free fluid seen in the abdomen on CT scan
d. The presence of left rib fractures on a chest radiograph
e. The appearance of the spleen on a CT scan

COMMENT: Vital signs and hemodynamic stability, changes in hematocrit over time, and the need for blood transfusion are the major determinants of the appropriateness of nonoperative management of splenic injury. The presence of left-shoulder pain without associated left-shoulder tenderness to palpation is consistent with Kehr's sign (referred pain caused by diaphragmatic irritation due to a subdiaphragmatic process such as hematoma from a ruptured spleen) and is not in and of itself an indication for operative intervention. The amount of free fluid and the appearance of the spleen on a CT scan correlate poorly with the need for operative intervention. The presence of a splenic blush on a CT scan correlates with an increased likelihood of the need for operative intervention but is not an absolute indication for operative intervention.

ANSWER: a

REFERENCE: *Chapter 11—Trauma: Definitive Care Phase; Abdominal Injuries*

29. A 26-year-old man is involved in a motor vehicle crash. He is unconscious on arrival at the emergency department. During resuscitation and initial evaluation, which of the following is/are true concerning the diagnosis of possible pelvic fracture in this case?

a. Routine pelvic radiographs are not indicated
b. Pelvic inlet and outlet views often are needed for the assessment of pelvic fractures
c. The physical examination should not include iliac wing compression to assess pelvic instability
d. Computed tomography is the optimum method for initial evaluation of possible pelvic fractures

COMMENT: Routine pelvic radiographs are almost always indicated when there is major mechanical trauma and it is not possible to perform a reliable examination of a patient who has a blunted response to pain. Inlet and outlet views rarely are needed, because other imaging methods are available. Computed tomography is an excellent method for fracture imaging but not as the initial study. Iliac wing compression should rarely, if ever, be performed if a patient cannot respond to painful stimuli. Pelvic compression can exacerbate hemorrhage and is an unreliable method of physical assessment.

ANSWER: c

REFERENCE: *Chapter 11—Trauma: Definitive Care Phase; Retroperitoneal Injuries*

30. A 42-year-old woman injured in a major fall arrives with an initial blood pressure of 76/50 mm Hg and a heart rate of 132 beats/min. She reports abdominal and pelvic pain. She is awake and alert. After rapid initial administration of 2 L crystalloid, blood pressure increases to 84/58 mm Hg with a heart rate of 122 beats/min. Initial radiographs show a clear chest radiograph and type 11 pelvic fracture. Which of the following statements best represents the correct management plan for the patient?

a. Continue resuscitation. Perform diagnostic peritoneal lavage. If the result is grossly positive, transport the patient to the operating room. If the result is negative, consider placement of a pneumatic antishock garment. Perform arteriography and embolization

b. Continue resuscitation. Perform diagnostic peritoneal lavage. If the result is grossly positive, perform immediate pelvic-abdominal CT to confirm pelvic fracture hemorrhage. If the CT findings are abnormal, perform arteriography and embolization

c. Continue resuscitation. Obtain a CT scan. If the CT scan shows liver or spleen injury, pursue initial nonoperative management. Place a pelvic external fixator. Perform arteriography if evidence of continued hemorrhage is present

d. Continue resuscitation. Obtain a CT scan. If the CT scan shows liver or spleen injury, transport the patient to the operating room. If the CT scan shows pelvic hemorrhage, perform arteriography and embolization

e. Continue resuscitation. Apply pneumatic antishock garment and perform immediate diagnostic arteriography and embolization for fracture site hemorrhage

COMMENT: The patient is in an advanced state of hemorrhagic shock. Intraabdominal sources of hemorrhage must be immediately identified and treated. Computed tomography and arteriography are relatively contraindicated because of the time required and the severity of the shock state. Given a low incidence of false-positive results of diagnostic peritoneal lavage, a grossly positive result indicates life-threatening intraabdominal hemorrhage and mandates laparotomy.

ANSWER: a

REFERENCE: *Chapter 11—Trauma: Definitive Care Phase; Retroperitoneal Injuries*

31. A 52-year-old man struck by an automobile sustains abdominopelvic trauma and arrives at the emergency department in a state of shock. Diagnostic peritoneal lavage is performed, and the result is grossly positive. The patient is taken directly to the operating room for exploratory laparotomy. The spleen is found to be severely lacerated, necessitating splenectomy. The only abdominal or pelvic injury is a large retroperitoneal hematoma on the left that progresses into the pelvic retroperitoneum during the operation. The anesthesiologist notices that the urine is blood tinged. Which of the following represents the most appropriate management?

a. Complete the abdominal exploration and close. Obtain immediately postoperative CT scan to image the left kidney

b. Obtain an intraoperative intravenous pyelogram. If the findings are normal, complete the abdominal exploration and close

c. Perform renal exploration by mobilizing the kidney laterally through Gerota's fascia and reflecting it up on its pedicle

d. Perform renal exploration by exposing the midline aorta and identifying and controlling the left renal artery and vein

e. Perform intraoperative cystography to evaluate possible bladder rupture

COMMENT: Large retroperitoneal hematoma (perinephric) with expansion into the pelvis suggests severe renal injury. Although conservative management of many blunt renal injuries is possible, expanding hematoma is a relatively strong indication for exploration. Exploration is best and most safely accomplished by means of first obtaining vascular control of the proximal renal artery and vein.

ANSWER: d

REFERENCE: *Chapter 11—Trauma: Definitive Care Phase; Retroperitoneal Injuries*

32. A 21-year-old man has no sensation below the clavicles and cannot move his extremities after a rollover motor vehicle crash. He has hypotension and bradycardia. Which of the following statements is/are true?

   a. Intracavitary bleeding must be excluded before hypotension is ascribed to spinal shock
   b. Therapy with methylprednisolone must be initiated within 8 hours of injury
   c. Maintaining cord perfusion may help minimize secondary injury to the spinal cord
   d. Intubation is unlikely to be necessary in the care of this previously healthy patient
   e. Preservation of rectal tone and the bulbocavernosus reflex is indicative of an incomplete lesion

COMMENT: Hypotension after high spinal cord injury can be caused by interruption of descending sympathetic pathways that mediate vasomotor tone. Hemorrhage must be ruled out as the cause of hypotension for any trauma patient. Initial resuscitation should be performed with intravenous crystalloid. Once hemorrhage has been identified and controlled, spinal shock can be managed with a pure α-adrenergic agonist such as phenylephrine. Bradycardia is caused by unopposed vagal tone to the sinoatrial node and can be managed with atropine. Adequate perfusion of the spinal cord, maintained by means of supporting mean arterial pressure, may be important in minimizing secondary cord injury. Methylprednisolone, as an initial bolus of 30 mg/kg followed by a drip of 5.4 mg/kg per hour for the next 23 hours, is routine treatment of patients with spinal cord injury and neurologic deficit and should be initiated within 8 hours of injury. Respiratory failure caused by loss of function of abdominal wall, intercostal, and accessory muscles and by loss of diaphragmatic function is common among patients with cervical spinal injuries. Many patients with cervical spinal fractures need early intubation and mechanical ventilation. Incomplete lesions have a better prognosis for neurologic recovery and affect timing of spinal stabilization. Preservation of rectal tone, sacral sparing of sensation, and a preserved bulbocavernosus reflex are indicative of an incomplete lesion.

ANSWER: a, b, c, e

REFERENCE: *Chapter 11—Trauma: Definitive Care Phase; Orthopedic and Spinal Injuries*

33. A 50-year-old woman jumps from the midspan of a bridge over a waterway. She arrives at a trauma center with hypotension, tachycardia, and an unstable pelvis. Radiographs show a widened pubic symphysis and disruption of both sacroiliac joints. All of the following are true of this patient except:

   a. She is at high risk of serious associated injuries
   b. She has a 40% risk of mortality
   c. She has probably lost one or two units of blood because of the pelvic fracture
   d. She is an appropriate candidate for application of a pneumatic antishock garment
   e. She is an appropriate candidate for angiography and embolization of bleeding pelvic vessels

COMMENT: Disruption of the pelvic ring requires transmission of an enormous amount of force to the torso. Patients who sustain pelvic fractures are at high risk of serious associated injuries, especially intracranial and visceral trauma. Patients with pelvic fracture who have hypotension have a mortality as high as 40%. Symphyseal disruptions can result in loss of one to two units of blood. Disruption of the posterior elements of the pelvis can cause life-threatening hemorrhage. Patients in unstable condition benefit from application of a pneumatic antishock garment and emergency angiography of the pelvic vessels followed by therapeutic embolization.

ANSWER: c

REFERENCE: *Chapter 11—Trauma: Definitive Care Phase; Orthopedic and Spinal Injuries*

34. A man comes to the emergency department after sustaining a gunshot wound of the right lower leg. He states he was shot with a high-powered rifle during a drive-by shooting. Physical examination shows large entrance wound and exit wounds on the calf. There are no distal pulses. Radiographs show a shattered tibia and fibula. Which of the following statements is/are true?

a. The fracture is classified as a grade II open fracture
b. The patient needs irrigation and débridement of devitalized tissues within 12 hours of injury
c. The patient is a poor candidate for application of a external fixator
d. The patient will likely need vascular repair and possibly release of a lower leg compartment
e. The patient should be treated with oral antibiotics

COMMENT: Open fractures caused by high-velocity gunshot wounds are classified as grade III injuries. Because this patient has evidence of concomitant vascular injury, the fracture is classified as grade III-C. Open fractures require irrigation and débridement within 8 hours of injury to minimize risk of infection, osteomyelitis, and nonunion. Patients with grade III injuries should be treated with broad-spectrum parenteral antibiotics. Application of an external fixator is appropriate for severe open fractures, especially those with a large degree of soft-tissue damage. Timing of vascular repair and orthopedic repair should be individualized. Patients with vascular injury and severe fractures are at risk of compartment syndrome and should undergo fasciotomy if there is any question about elevated compartment pressures or ischemia-reperfusion injury.

ANSWER: d

REFERENCE: *Chapter 11—Trauma: Definitive Care Phase; Orthopedic and Spinal Injuries*

35. Two days after injury, a patient awaiting fixation of multiple long-bone fractures and a pelvic fracture has sudden onset of respiratory distress. Which of the following statements is/are true?

a. The patient may have a pulmonary embolism
b. Fat embolism syndrome may be developing
c. The patient is at high risk of pneumonia and acute respiratory distress syndrome
d. The pathophysiologic changes of fat embolism syndrome are caused by blockage of the pulmonary microcirculation by fat globules
e. Most patients with fat embolism syndrome have a fulminant course associated with respiratory failure, neurologic compromise, and scattered petechiae

COMMENT: Patients with multiple fractures managed with immobilization are at high risk of a multitude of complications, the most frequent being pulmonary. Trauma patients who are not receiving prophylaxis have an 8% incidence of deep venous thrombosis. When the patient is treated with either subcutaneous heparin or compression stockings, the incidence decreases to 3%. Fat embolism syndrome occurs among 5% to 10% of patients with multiple long-bone or concomitant pelvic fractures. Petechiae, respiratory failure, and varying degrees of neurologic impairment characterize the syndrome. Most patients do not have the typical fulminant course. The pathophysiologic mechanism involves an interaction between fat, platelets, and leukocytes that initiates an inflammatory response and results in endothelial damage, increased capillary permeability, and decreased levels of pulmonary surfactant.

ANSWER: a, b, c

REFERENCE: *Chapter 11—Trauma: Definitive Care Phase; Orthopedic and Spinal Injuries*

36. Which of the following statements is/are true regarding a patient with a mangled extremity?

   a. A variety of scoring systems can be used to predict the likelihood of amputation for a patient with a mangled extremity
   b. Scoring systems are reliable predictors of functional outcome
   c. Young patients who undergo primary amputation rarely return to productive lives
   d. Treatment decisions regarding a mangled extremity are complex and must involve a variety of subspecialists

COMMENT: Preservation of an extremity with severe soft-tissue and neurovascular injury may be technically feasible but imprudent. Patients often need numerous operations and ultimately may be left with a functionally useless limb. Young patients who undergo primary amputation often return to productive lives within 1 year. A variety of scoring systems can be used to predict the likelihood of amputation but not to predict functional outcome. Decisions regarding a mangled extremity are complex and require input from a number of specialists. The general trauma surgeon ought to coordinate this process, because he or she is cognizant of the effect of attempts at limb salvage on the overall resuscitation of the patient.

ANSWER: a, d

REFERENCE: *Chapter 11—Trauma: Definitive Care Phase; Orthopedic and Spinal Injuries*

37. An unrestrained 39-year-old woman crashes her 1970 pick-up truck into a tree at 50 miles per hour (80 km/h). Clinical and radiographic findings that suggest blunt thoracic injury include:

   a. Sternal fracture underlying a steering wheel imprint
   b. Widened mediastinum and altered aortic arch contour on chest radiograph
   c. First rib fracture
   d. Ruptured spleen

COMMENT: Thoracic aortic injury is caused by rapid deceleration, usually in a motor vehicle crash or a fall from great height. Injuries that can be survived are acute pseudoaneurysms resulting from transverse tears of the media and intima that leave the adventitia intact. These occur at the aortic isthmus between the ligamentum arteriosum and the left subclavian artery, a point of fixation resulting in a shearing force load in rapid deceleration. Urgent diagnostic evaluation is essential if successful repair is to be accomplished before complete rupture and exsanguinating hemorrhage occur.

Chest radiography is the best screening test for blunt thoracic aortic injury. Findings that suggest the need for further evaluation include widened superior mediastinum, loss of the aortic contour, tracheal or esophageal deviation to the right, depression of the left main stem bronchus, first rib fracture, sternal fracture, thoracic spine fracture, and multiple rib fractures on the left side. Although multiple injuries are common in rapid deceleration trauma, ruptured spleen is not a specific risk indicator for thoracic aortic injury.

Thoracic aortography is the standard in the diagnosis of blunt thoracic aortic injury. Spiral CT with rapid intravenous infusion of contrast medium has been reported effective in evaluation of this injury. Transesophageal echography has been suggested as an alternative to conventional aortography. Both of these modalities should be used carefully in centers with extensive experience.

ANSWER: a, b, c

REFERENCE: *Chapter 11—Trauma: Definitive Care Phase; Vascular Injuries*

38. A 14-year-old male skateboarder is struck by an automobile and sustains an open tibial plateau fracture of the right leg. Pulses are absent at the right ankle. Which of the following statements is/are true?

   a. Immediate arteriography should be performed
   b. Doppler signal characteristics alone do not indicate the absence of arterial occlusion
   c. An ankle-brachial ratio of 0.6 at Doppler pressure testing is abnormal
   d. Arteriography always should be performed in the angiography suite

COMMENT: Careful physical examination of the injured extremity is an essential first step in the diagnosis of vascular injury. Complete occlusion or arterial disruption results in distal ischemia and produces the classic physical findings of pain, pallor, pulse deficit, paresthesia, and diminished perfusion. After adequate fluid resuscitation has been completed, peripheral pulses should be palpable. Measurement of segmental arterial pressure by means of Doppler technique is a valuable adjunct in the examination of vascular trauma to the extremities. However, the presence of audible Doppler signals over an artery in an extremity does not rule out arterial injury or indicate adequate perfusion.

The use of a Doppler device for evaluation of extremities includes measurement of distal blood pressure. This is accomplished by means of placing the probe over the selected artery in the foot or at the wrist and slowly inflating a blood pressure cuff at the ankle or the forearm. The pressure at which Doppler signals cease indicates the perfusion pressure at the level of the blood pressure cuff. This pressure should be compared with the other extremity in upper extremity evaluation or with the highest upper extremity pressure in lower extremity evaluation. For a healthy and normovolemic person, the ankle-brachial index is 1.1. A ratio less than 0.9 or a 20-mm difference between extremities should arouse suspicion of serious arterial trauma. For hypovolemic patients, however, both lower extremity ankle-brachial indices frequently are diminished to as low as 0.75. Reevaluation after resuscitation is essential if both lower extremity indices are diminished. Doppler examination for acute venous disruption has not been evaluated and is likely to be unreliable.

Arteriography is indicated in the care of patients with suspected vascular trauma unless there is a clear indication for immediate surgical intervention, such as exsanguinating hemorrhage or clear signs of arterial occlusion for which the operative approach is straightforward. For example, patients with posterior dislocation of the knee or tibial plateau fracture and loss of distal pulses with signs of ischemia need immediate operative repair of the popliteal artery. In this instance, arteriography is both unnecessary and time consuming.

ANSWER: b, c

REFERENCE: *Chapter 11—Trauma: Definitive Care Phase; Vascular Injuries*

39. A 23-year-old male police officer sustains a shotgun injury to the medial aspect of the right leg. There is a wide area of pellet entrance wounds. There is a faintly palpable posterior tibial pulse, and the ankle-brachial ratio is 0.75. An arteriogram is obtained. Which of the following statements is/are true?

a. Any sign of arterial injury on the arteriogram necessitates immediate exploration
b. The first sign of compartment syndrome is loss of the distal pulse
c. A compartment pressure of 29 mm Hg is normal
d. The severity of a shotgun injury is inversely proportional to the distance of the victim from the barrel

COMMENT: The aggressive use of arteriography for suspected occult vascular trauma results in the detection of clinically insignificant lesions that can be managed nonoperatively. These include intimal irregularity, focal spasm with minimal narrowing, and small pseudoaneurysms. Although these lesions have been aggressively managed with operative therapy in the past, considerable evidence suggests that nonoperative therapy for some asymptomatic lesions is safe and effective. Surveillance for subsequent occlusion or hemorrhage is mandatory. Duplex scanning offers an accurate, noninvasive method to follow these lesions of the extremities. Operative therapy is indicated for thrombosis, for chronic symptoms of occlusive disease, and for failure of small pseudoaneurysms to undergo thrombosis.

Nonoperative therapy may be indicated for clinically insignificant lesions if the patient has multiple injuries. For these patients, development of extremity compartment syndrome is a devastating complication after arterial trauma. The syndrome is uncommon in the thigh and forearm but is frequent in the calf. The most sensitive sign of compartment syndrome is pain on passive stretch of the involved muscle. Although many devices are available to measure compartment pressures in the calf, many trauma surgeons are aggressive in use of four-compartment fasciotomy whenever there is extensive soft-tissue injury or skeletal trauma in the leg combined with vascular trauma or a history of prolonged ischemia. For any patient with lower-extremity trauma who has signs of pain or distal ischemia, the compartment pressure should be measured and fasciotomy performed as needed. Capillary perfusion requires 25 mm Hg. Compartment pressures are normally between 10 and 20 mm Hg. Persistent pressures greater than 25 mm Hg suggest the presence of compartment syndrome. An uncontrolled or unrecognized compartment syndrome produces nerve and muscle damage and prevents good functional recovery despite the patency of the vascular repair.

The severity of a shotgun wound is determined by the size of the shot, the amount of powder in the shell, and the proximity to the barrel. The severity of injury rapidly decreases as the distance from the barrel of the shotgun increases.

ANSWER: d

REFERENCE: *Chapter 11—Trauma: Definitive Care Phase; Vascular Injuries*

40. A 35-year-old woman is stabbed in the abdomen. She sustains through-and-through wounds of the stomach, pancreas, portal vein, and vena cava. Which of the following statements is/are true?

a. The inferior vena cava below the liver should be repaired because of a high risk of complications
b. Most of the oxygen supply to the liver comes from portal venous blood flow
c. The inferior vena cava above the liver can be ligated without serious consequences
d. The vena cava should be approached directly through the colonic mesentery

COMMENT: The vena cava, right renal hilum, and right iliac artery can be exposed by a Kocher maneuver combined with mobilization of the right colon. The portal area is best exposed by means of the combination of a Kocher maneuver and mobilization of the hepatic flexure of the colon from the underlying duodenum and head of the pancreas. Injuries to the vena cava or portal vein present management challenges because of the insidious nature of continuing blood loss, the difficulty of obtaining proximal and distal control, and the high risk of subsequent thrombosis. Ligation of these vessels should be performed only as a desperate measure for patients in unstable condition. Massive lower-extremity edema accompanies ligation of the infrarenal vena cava, and ligation above the renal veins always is fatal. Portal venous ligation should be avoided if at all possible. The portal vein provides 80% of the oxygen and nutrient blood flow to the liver. Direct suture and patch angioplasty are the most effective ways to repair injuries to the great veins. Mesenteric venous injury can be managed by means of ligation without serious complications.

ANSWER: a, b

REFERENCE: *Chapter 11—Trauma: Definitive Care Phase; Vascular Injuries*

41. Upper extremity vascular injury is characterized by the following:

a. High incidence of limb loss
b. Frequent need for fasciotomy
c. High incidence of concomitant nerve injury
d. Result of penetrating injuries in most instances

COMMENT: The most common sites of extremity arterial trauma are the brachial artery and the superficial femoral artery. Penetrating injuries are more common than are blunt injuries. If they do occur, blunt injuries usually are associated with severe fractures or dislocations. Supracondylar humeral fractures are associated with high risk of brachial artery injury. Concomitant peripheral nerve injuries occur among 60% of patients with vascular injuries in the extremities. The extensive collateral circulation and the smaller muscle mass in the arm make acute arterial occlusion in the arm less likely to cause limb-threatening ischemia than is occlusion in the leg. The priorities of prompt diagnosis and timely restoration of perfusion, however, are applicable to upper extremity arterial trauma. A possibly limb-threatening situation is caused by injury to the brachial artery proximal to the origin of the profunda brachii artery or by occlusion of both the ulnar and radial arteries; prompt arterial repair should be undertaken. In contrast, if isolated radial or ulnar arterial occlusion occurs, reconstruction is not needed if adequate flow into the hand through the remaining vessel can be documented. Fasciotomy in the forearm is rarely needed and is necessary only after prolonged delay in restoration of flow or if there is extensive soft-tissue injury.

ANSWER: c, d

REFERENCE: *Chapter 11—Trauma: Definitive Care Phase; Vascular Injuries*

42. A 5-year-old boy was climbing a tree and lost his balance. He is admitted to the hospital with a blood pressure of 100/70 mm Hg and a pulse rate of 100 beats/min. The initial hematocrit is 39%, and microscopic hematuria is detected. The initial CT scan is shown in Fig. 11.81. Appropriate treatment of this child includes which of the following?

a. Admission to the ICU
b. Diagnostic peritoneal lavage to look for blood
c. Immediate operation to remove the spleen
d. Serial physical examinations and blood draws for hematocrit
e. Drainage of the liver laceration

COMMENT: Nonoperative management of solid organ injuries (liver, spleen, or kidney) is the initial treatment of pediatric trauma patients. However, because some of these children still need an operation for continued or delayed bleeding, initial observation in the ICU is justified. The degree of injury to the organ should be documented with CT. There is no need for diagnostic peritoneal lavage if the patient is in stable condition, because the presence of blood does not dictate the need for operative therapy. A child treated nonoperatively needs continued reevaluation by a surgeon so that hemodynamic stability and the absence of intestinal injuries can be assured. Appropriate treatment of a child in stable condition with a solid organ injury includes 24- to 48-hour observation in an ICU, serial measurement of hematocrit and hemoglobin until these values stabilize, resumption of oral intake when ileus resolves, resumption of walking when the hematocrit and hemoglobin level are stable and hematuria has resolved, and discharge from the hospital when hematocrit and hemoglobin level are stable and the child is eating and walking. Contact sports should be avoided for at least 6 weeks or until a follow-up CT scan shows resolution of the injury.

ANSWER: a, d

REFERENCE: *Chapter 11—Trauma: Definitive Care Phase; Pediatric Trauma, Fig. 11.81*

43. A 4-year-old girl is struck by a car. She is unconscious at the scene but is awake and crying on admission to the hospital. The initial blood pressure is 60 mm Hg systolic, and the heart rate is 150 beats/min. Initial treatment of this child includes:

a. Immediate intubation
b. Insertion of an intraosseus infusion device
c. Fluid bolus of 10 mL/kg Ringer's lactate
d. Fluid bolus of 1,000 mL Ringer's lactate
e. Immediate transfusion of packed red blood cells at 10 mL/kg

COMMENT: Resuscitation of a child in a state of shock must be prompt and driven by a protocol. Because this child is awake and crying, the airway can be assumed to be adequate, at least for the time being. Of more immediate concern is the blood pressure because hypotension is a late sign of shock in a child, and once it develops, it must be reversed rapidly or death may result. Intravenous access can be established percutaneously in the upper or lower extremities, but if two attempts are unsuccessful, an intraosseus nail should be placed in children younger than 6 years and rapid fluid resuscitation initiated. Warmed Ringer's solution can be given as a bolus of 20 mL/kg and repeated twice, but if the child's condition cannot be stabilized, blood should be transfused at 10 mL/kg packed red cells, and operative therapy should be considered.

ANSWER: b

REFERENCE: *Chapter 11—Trauma: Definitive Care Phase; Pediatric Trauma*

44. A 1-year-old baby sustains head trauma in a "fall" from a countertop in her home. She is in a coma and brought in by means of private vehicle. Neither parent can give a clear description of the traumatic event. The child has equal but dilated pupils and shallow respirations. The initial CT scan is shown in Fig. 11.79. All of the following are appropriate steps in the treatment of this child except:

a. Rapid sequence intubation
b. Ventilation to maintain a P_{CO_2} of 35 mm Hg
c. Establishment of intravenous access
d. Notification of child protective services
e. Administration of mannitol at a dose of 1 g/kg

COMMENT: Serious head trauma is responsible for most deaths after pediatric trauma, and patients who survive can have permanent disabilities. When prevention of head trauma fails, secondary prevention measures must be aimed at avoidance of hypoxia and hypotension, which can worsen the outcome after brain injury. Intubation to avoid hypoxia and assurance of eucapnia (carbon dioxide approximately 35 mm Hg) are appropriate. Avoidance of hypotension begins with brisk fluid resuscitation. Neurosurgical consultation should be obtained immediately. Mannitol is contraindicated until hemodynamic stability is assured and should be used only with impending brain herniation or at the request of the neurosurgeon. Because the degree of injury is not consistent with the history obtained and because there is a discrepancy between the two parents' reports, it is the legal obligation of the treating physician to notify as soon as possible the agency responsible for child protection.

ANSWER: e

REFERENCE: *Chapter 11—Trauma: Definitive Care Phase; Pediatric Trauma*

45. A 10-year-old boy was riding in the back seat of a car that was struck broadside at an intersection. The paramedics state the child was restrained with a lap belt only. The child was awake and alert in transport but reported severe back pain and inability to move the lower extremities. Which of the following findings suggest(s) associated small-intestinal injury in this case?

a. The presence of hypotension and bradycardia
b. Fluid seen in the pelvis on abdominal CT scan
c. A seat-belt sign on the abdominal wall
d. Delayed development of vomiting, fever, and abdominal tenderness
e. Abnormal findings on a FAST

COMMENT: The presence of a Chance fracture of the lumbar spine associated with use of a lap belt without a harness always suggests associated intestinal injury. These injuries usually are fairly subtle at initial presentation and can manifest only as mild abdominal pain. The presence of a seat-belt mark on the abdominal wall also is highly suggestive of blunt force and intestinal injury. Evidence of fluid on an abdominal CT scan not associated with solid organ injury is another sign. The FAST is not sensitive for bowel injury, but diagnostic peritoneal lavage is. Delayed manifestations of intestinal injury among children include fever, leukocytosis, abdominal pain, nausea, vomiting, and abdominal distention.

ANSWER: b, c, d

REFERENCE: *Chapter 11—Trauma: Definitive Care Phase; Pediatric Trauma, Fig. 11.85*

46. Which of the following statements is/are true regarding injury prevention among children?

    a. Most childhood deaths occur in the hospital

    b. Most childhood injuries can be prevented with already existing methods

    c. The are no effective programs to reduce the incidence of violent death among children

    d. The most effective form of injury prevention is education

    e. Most physicians and parents are well educated about injury prevention

COMMENT: By far the most pediatric deaths occur outside the hospital. Thus only prevention is effective in decreasing the incidence of pediatric deaths after trauma. Analysis of injuries occurring among children has shown that most children were not using existing prevention devices when the injuries occurred. Examples of successful injury prevention devices include the use of helmets while riding a bicycle, the use of smoke detectors and fire-retardant sleepwear, and the development of a comprehensive community-based program to stem violent injuries. Most physicians and parents are poorly educated regarding the need for and the effectiveness of injury prevention, yet most pediatric injuries would be prevented with existing methods. Engineering devices that are automatic are the most effective forms of prevention because they are passive; that is, they protect without any form of active involvement of the parent or child.

ANSWER: b

REFERENCE: *Chapter 11—Trauma: Definitive Care Phase; Pediatric Trauma*

47. Which of the following statement is/are true regarding geriatric trauma?

    a. Although they are less frequently injured than younger persons, elderly patients are more likely to die when they are injured

    b. Geriatric patients who survive injury are more likely to have complications and permanent loss of independent function than are young patients

    c. One third of trauma care dollars are spent on the elderly

    d. Elderly patients' lengths of stay in the hospital average twice as long as those of similarly injured nongeriatric patients

COMMENT: All of these statements are true regarding geriatric trauma.

ANSWER: a, b, c, d

REFERENCE: *Chapter 11—Trauma: Definitive Care Phase; Geriatric Trauma*

48. Which of the following statements is/are true regarding geriatric falls?

    a. Falls are the third most frequent cause of accidental injury and death among the elderly

    b. Falls by the elderly usually occur on steps or level ground in and around the home

    c. Risk factors for geriatric falls include sensory impairment, neuromuscular disorders, unstable gait, dementia, lower-extremity weakness, postural hypotension, and the effects of medications or alcohol

    d. Approximately 75% of falls by the elderly are caused by an underlying medical problem

    e. Assessment after a fall that includes laboratory studies, electrocardiography, 24-hour Holter monitoring, and environmental evaluation by a nurse practitioner has been documented to result in decreased episodes of falling

COMMENT: Falls are the most common cause of accidental injury and death among the elderly. Unlike younger patients, who often fall from height, the elderly are more likely to fall on stairs or level ground in and around the home. Factors that contribute to the likelihood of falling include a variety of physiologic derangements and effects of medications. Underlying medical disorders cause 25% of falls. Assessment after a fall that includes total medical evaluation and assessment of the patient's home can decrease the risk of future falls for an individual patient.

ANSWER: b, c, e

REFERENCE: *Chapter 11—Trauma: Definitive Care Phase; Geriatric Trauma*

49. All of the following statements are true regarding the elderly and motor vehicle trauma except:
    a. Elderly patients are more likely to be involved in crashes in which alcohol plays a role
    b. Elderly patients are more likely to be involved in crashes that involve intersections, right-of-way judgments, traffic sign violations, and two-car incidents than are crashes involving younger drivers
    c. Crash patterns among the geriatric population probably relate in some measure to preexisting medical conditions, diminution of cognitive and motor skills, and to side effects of medications
    d. The aged are involved in crashes as pedestrians more frequently than any other group, including children
    e. Elderly patients have a higher death rate than do young pedestrian victims with comparable injuries

COMMENT: The pattern of crashes in which the elderly are most likely involved reflects underlying medical conditions, use of medications, and diminution of cognitive and motor skills. This accounts for a higher number of crashes related to errors in driving judgment than to risk-taking behavior. The elderly are much less likely to be involved in crashes involving alcohol. The elderly also are involved in pedestrian versus automobile crashes more frequently than is any other age group, including children. Elderly persons have higher mortality than do similarly injured younger patients.

ANSWER: a

REFERENCE: *Chapter 11—Trauma: Definitive Care Phase; Geriatric Trauma*

50. Age-associated changes in the cardiovascular system include:
    a. Decreased myocardial responsiveness to catecholamines
    b. Decreased contractility and stroke volume
    c. Increased myocardial compliance
    d. Decreased susceptibility to arrhythmia
    e. Atherosclerotic coronary artery disease

COMMENT: The aging cardiovascular system undergoes a variety of changes that make it less able to respond appropriately to physiologic stress. These include decreased stroke volume and contractility, decreased responsiveness to catecholamines, decreased myocardial compliance, increased susceptibility to arrhythmia, and coronary artery disease.

ANSWER: a, b, e

REFERENCE: *Chapter 11—Trauma: Definitive Care Phase; Geriatric Trauma*

51. Which of the following statements is/are true regarding physiologic changes that occur with aging?
    a. Changes in the respiratory system that accompany aging include decreased vital capacity and forced expiratory volume, increased functional residual capacity, decreased compliance, and decreased diffusion capacity
    b. The kidneys have decreased glomerular filtration rate and decreased excretory capacity because of loss of functional glomeruli
    c. The cause of osteoporosis is multifactorial; it includes increased bone resorption, loss of estrogenic hormones, diminished physical activity, and impaired calcium absorption by the intestine
    d. Body composition changes profoundly with aging; the changes include increased fat mass and decreased lean muscle mass, total body water, and bone density
    e. Although the number of T cells is unchanged with aging, activation and proliferation of T cells and their ability to produce cytokines are impaired

COMMENT: All of the above are physiologic changes associated with aging.

ANSWER: a, b, c, d, e

REFERENCE: *Chapter 11—Trauma: Definitive Care Phase; Geriatric Trauma*

52. Systemic inflammation, multiple organ dysfunction syndrome, and sepsis frequently follow major injury. Which of the following interventions has/have been shown to improve outcomes?

a. Early fixation of long-bone fractures
b. Goal-directed resuscitation to achieve specific oxygen delivery targets
c. Rapid restoration of tissue perfusion and correction of base deficit
d. Early use of total parenteral nutrition

COMMENT: Local effects of tissue injury stimulate the systemic inflammatory response. Early fracture fixation, débridement of devitalized tissue, and arrest of hemorrhage limit this response. Early and complete resuscitation limits the magnitude of the systemic response to ischemia and reperfusion. Markers of adequate tissue perfusion and correction of acidosis help to guide resuscitative management, whereas goal-directed therapy aimed at achieving specific values for oxygen delivery or utilization have yet to be proved. Nutritional support of an injured patient is crucial to good outcome. Early enteral nutrition has been shown to reduce risk of septic complications after injury.

ANSWER: a, c

REFERENCE: *Chapter 11—Trauma: Definitive Care Phase; Critical Care and Postinjury Management*

53. Immune function is modified after major injury. Which of the following statements is/are true?

a. Levels of circulating interleukin (IL-1) and IL-6 decrease immediately after major injury
b. After injury, early activation of polymorphonuclear neutrophilic leukocytes (PMNs) occurs
c. Defects in lymphocyte function after injury decrease CD3 and CD4 subpopulations
d. Immunologic defects associated with trauma are inevitable and cannot be manipulated by appropriate resuscitative intervention

COMMENT: The immunologic effects of trauma are global. The humoral response is primarily proinflammatory with elevations in levels of tumor necrosis factor, IL-1, and IL-6. Activation of PMNs has been observed after injury with increased adhesion molecule expression, margination, and exaggerated respiratory burst. Impairment of lymphocyte function and macrophage antigen results in increased risk of septic complications. Appropriate resuscitative care, including reversal of tissue ischemia and early enteral nutrition, can ameliorate this immunologic response.

ANSWER: b, c

REFERENCE: *Chapter 11—Trauma: Definitive Care Phase; Critical Care and Post Injury Management*

54. Complications after injury can be classified as disease related or provider related. Which of the following statements is/are true concerning complications after injury?

a. Identification of recurrent process errors forms the basis of continuous quality improvement (CQI) initiatives
b. Studies show that errors in the operating room are more common and lethal than are those made during resuscitation or critical care
c. Missed injuries are common but can be excluded with a careful secondary survey at admission
d. Errors in care can be reduced by standardizing care with practice guidelines and reducing variability

COMMENT: Errors made by providers and delays in care delivery result in adverse outcomes. Unduly complex care processes, such as those in ICUs, are particularly prone to error and result in lethal complications. In one study this type of error was more common than were lethal errors made during other phases of care. Recurrent process errors should be identified and route causes corrected with CQI initiatives. Missed injuries are common and may not be evident to either patient or physician at admission. A careful tertiary survey after admission helps identify these injuries, most of which are minor orthopedic injuries. Standard CQI practices aimed at reducing the complexity and variability of care processes decrease the number of errors and complications.

ANSWER: a, d

REFERENCE: *Chapter 11—Trauma: Definitive Care Phase; Critical Care and Postinjury Management*

55. Which of the following statements is/are true regarding maternal blood volume during pregnancy?

   a. Erythrocyte volume is much greater than plasma volume
   b. The plasma and erythrocyte volumes do not increase considerably until the third trimester
   c. Plasma and erythrocyte volumes expand most rapidly during the second trimester
   d. Almost 35% of maternal blood volume can be lost before signs of shock are observed

COMMENT: Maternal blood volume (plasma and erythrocytes) begins to increase during the first trimester but expands most rapidly during the second trimester, reaching approximately 45% above nonpregnant levels. The increase in plasma volume, which is proportionally greater than the enlarged erythrocyte volume, results in anemia of pregnancy. This physiologic hypervolemia masks volume loss and can give the clinician an unfounded sense of security about the hemodynamic stability. Almost 35% of the mother's blood volume can be lost before signs of shock are noticed.

ANSWER: c, d

REFERENCE: *Chapter 11—Trauma: Definitive Care Phase; Trauma in Pregnancy*

56. Which of the following statements is/are true regarding abruptio placentae?

   a. It can occur in the absence of obvious abdominal injury
   b. It usually manifests as vaginal bleeding
   c. It is associated with a 50% maternal mortality rate
   d. It is more common among patients who have hypertension or diabetes

COMMENT: Abruptio placentae is the most common cause of fetal death during maternal injury. It carries a 30% to 70% rate of fetal death and 1% maternal mortality rate. Abruptio placentae can occur in the absence of obvious abdominal injury, because maternal shock is a far greater stimulus for abruption than are the mechanical forces of trauma that disrupt the placenta. Abruptio placentae is more common in the presence of hypertension, diabetes mellitus, advanced age, multiparity, and maternal use of tobacco or cocaine.

ANSWER: a, b, d

REFERENCE: *Chapter 11—Trauma: Definitive Care Phase; Trauma in Pregnancy*

57. The indication(s) for cesarean section during celiotomy for trauma is/are as follows:

   a. Pregnancy near term
   b. Mechanical limitation for maternal organ repair
   c. Cervical spinal injury
   d. Perforated sigmoid colon

COMMENT: During celiotomy for trauma, the following are indications for cesarean section: maternal shock, pregnancy near term, threat to life from exsanguination (injury or disseminated intravascular coagulation), risk of fetal distress exceeding risk of prematurity, and unstable thoracolumbar spinal injury.

ANSWER: b

REFERENCE: *Chapter 11—Trauma: Definitive Care Phase; Trauma in Pregnancy*

58. Successful outcome of postmortem cesarean section is likely if the time between maternal death and delivery is:

   a. Less than 5 minutes
   b. Between 10 and 20 minutes
   c. Between 15 and 20 minutes
   d. No times have been estimated relative to fetal outcome

COMMENT: Successful outcome of postmortem cesarean section depends on the duration of the gestation and the time between maternal death and delivery. Under optimal conditions, at 26 to 28 weeks of gestation, there is approximately a 50% fetal survival rate. Therefore postmortem cesarean section is justified if the estimated gestational age is 26 to 28 weeks. If the time between maternal death and delivery is less than 5 minutes, the fetal prognosis is considered excellent. If the time since maternal death is approximately 20 minutes, fetal prognosis is poor. Uncertainty about time of maternal death is not a contraindication to this procedure.

ANSWER: a

REFERENCE: *Chapter 11—Trauma: Definitive Care Phase; Trauma in Pregnancy*

59. Which of the following statements is/are true regarding the physiologic alterations of pregnancy?

    a. A decrease in gastroesophageal sphincter competency can lead to a tendency toward aspiration and vomiting

    b. Cardiac output increases 40% to 50% but systemic vascular resistance and pulmonary vascular resistance decrease

    c. Both vital capacity and residual volume increase

    d. Although there is a significant increase in tidal volume, minute ventilation decreases almost one half

COMMENT: As pregnancy progresses, both diaphragmatic excursion and thoracic circumference increase; the result is larger tidal volumes. Associated with this change is an approximately 40% increase in minute ventilation. Although vital capacity stays approximately the same, there is an approximately 20% decrease in residual volume. The relaxant effect of progesterone and estrogen on smooth muscle diminishes esophageal sphincter competency; the result is an increased propensity toward vomiting. Throughout pregnancy, cardiac output increases as much as 50% above normal until approximately the 24th week of gestation, and then it plateaus. This increase in cardiac output is a result of a modest increase in heart rate and stroke volume related to the expanded blood volume and the direct inotropic effect of estrogen.

ANSWER: a, b

REFERENCE: *Chapter 11—Trauma: Definitive Care Phase; Trauma in Pregnancy*

60. Which of the following is/are recommended for management of frostbite?

    a. Moist heat

    b. Early amputation

    c. Padding and elevation

    d. Vasodilator and heparin

    e. Topical application of antimicrobial agent

COMMENT: Rapid rewarming is the goal achieved by immersing the tissue in a large water bath at 40°C (104°F to 108°F). The water should feel warm but not hot to a normal hand. The bath should be large enough to prevent rapid loss of heat, and the water temperature should be maintained.

ANSWER: a

REFERENCE: *Chapter 11—Trauma: Definitive Care Phase; Envenomation and Environmental Injuries*

61. Chilblain (chronic pernio) is:

    a. Caused by repeated and chronic exposure to a cold but nonfreezing environment

    b. Also known as trenchfoot

    c. Caused by chronic vasculitis likely related to hereditary protein C or S deficiency

    d. Characterized by pruritic, red, elevated lesions on the affected area

    e. Managed by means of elevation and rapid immersion rewarming

COMMENT: Cold injuries limited to the digits, extremities, or exposed surfaces are caused by either direct tissue freezing or by chronic exposure to an environment just above freezing (chilblain or pernio; trenchfoot). Chilblain describes local cold injury characterized by pruritic, red-purple papules, macules, plaques, or nodules on the skin.

ANSWER: a, d

REFERENCE: *Chapter 11—Trauma: Definitive Care Phase; Envenomation and Environmental Injuries*

62. Which of the following modalities is/are effective in restoring blood flow and minimizing tissue damage after frostbite?

    a. Sympathetic blockade

    b. Intraarterial vasodilating agents (reserpine, tolazoline)

    c. Calcium channel blockers (nifedipine)

    d. Heparin with or without thrombolytic therapy

    e. None of the above

    f. All of the above

COMMENT: Treatment with antiadrenergics (prazosin hydrochloride, 1 to 2 mg/d) or calcium channel blockers (nifedipine, 30 to 60 mg/d) and careful protection from further exposure often is helpful.

ANSWER: f

REFERENCE: *Chapter 11—Trauma: Definitive Care Phase; Envenomation and Environmental Injuries*

63. The transition zone of systemic hypothermia, in which the adaptive physiologic responses to heat loss are lost, occurs between what temperatures?

    a. 35°C and 33°C
    b. 33°C and 30°C
    c. 30°C and 27°C
    d. 27°C and 24°C

COMMENTS: The transition from a safe zone of hypothermia, in which physiologic adaptations to heat loss are working, to a danger zone of hypothermia, in which shivering is abolished, metabolism decreases, and heat loss is passively accepted, occurs between 33°C and 30°C.

ANSWER: b

REFERENCE: *Chapter 11—Trauma: Definitive Care Phase; Envenomation and Environmental Injuries*

64. The Severinghaus mathematical correction used to correct blood gas values for systemic hypothermia indicates that for each one-degree Celsius decrease in temperature, the change in P_{CO_2} and P_{O_2} is:

    a. P_{CO_2} decreases 4.4% and P_{O_2} decreases 7.2%
    b. P_{CO_2} increases 4.4% and O_2 decreases 7.2%
    c. P_{CO_2} decreases 7.2% and O_2 decreases 4.4%
    d. P_{CO_2} increases 7.2% and O_2 decreases 4.4%
    e. P_{CO_2} increases 4.4% and O_2 increases 7.2%

COMMENT: Perhaps the greatest controversy regarding the pulmonary effects of hypothermia revolves around the need to correct blood gas values to the patient's hypothermic body temperature. Arterial blood gas samples always are warmed to 37°C before the measurements are obtained. A nomogram of Severinghaus mathematical corrections is then used to estimate the blood gas values at the patient's actual body temperature. With each one-degree Celsius decrease in temperature, P_{CO_2} decreases 4.4%, and P_{O_2} decreases 7.2%. Thus, a blood gas sample evaluated at 37°C with a P_{CO_2} of 40 mm Hg and a P_{O_2} of 70 mm Hg for a patient with a body temperature of 32°C is reported as having a P_{CO_2} of 32 mm Hg and a P_{O_2} of 48 mm Hg after temperature correction.

ANSWER: a

REFERENCE: *Chapter 11—Trauma: Definitive Care Phase; Envenomation and Environmental Injuries*

65. For a trauma patient, severe hypothermia with an associated mortality greater than 50% is defined as a core body temperature less than:

    a. 36°C
    b. 34°C
    c. 32°C
    d. 30°C
    e. 28°C

COMMENT: Compared with other patient populations, the mortality associated with hypothermia among trauma victims is so high that some experts have proposed classifying it as a distinct form of hypothermia. The following zones of severity for injury hypothermia have been proposed:

Mild hypothermia: 36°C to 34°C (<96.8°F to 93.2°F)

Moderate hypothermia: 34°C to 32°C (<93.2°F to 89.6°F)

Severe hypothermia: <32°C (<89.6°F)

ANSWER: c

REFERENCE: *Chapter 11—Trauma: Definitive Care Phase; Envenomation and Environmental Injuries*

66. The heat deficit of a 70-kg man at 33°C is approximately:

    a. 58 kcal
    b. 280 kcal
    c. 70 kcal
    d. 140 kcal
    e. 232 kcal

COMMENT: Basal metabolic heat generation produces approximately 70 kcal/h, and shivering produces as much as 250 kcal/h. Given the specific heat of the body (0.083 kcal/kg per degree Celsius), 58 kcal is needed to increase the temperature of a 70-kg patient one degree Celsius.

ANSWER: e

REFERENCE: *Chapter 11—Trauma: Definitive Care Phase; Envenomation and Environmental Injuries*

CHAPTER 12

BURNS

1. A 19-year-old man sustains a 50% flame burn in an automobile accident. He is brought immediately to the trauma and burn center and undergoes prompt resuscitation and early surgery. Seven days later he has a moderate fever and a hyperdynamic circulation. There is no evidence of infection. The cause of this hypermetabolic response includes:

   a. A change in hypothalamic function with increased amounts of circulating counterregulatory hormones
   b. Bacterial contamination of open wounds
   c. Enhanced heat loss through evaporation of fluid through wounds
   d. High levels of circulating TNFα

COMMENT: Patients with large burns or other serious trauma routinely have a hypermetabolic response. The cause is not entirely understood, but it is likely to involve a combination of a number of factors, including a change in hypothalamic function with increase in glucagon, cortisol, and catecholamine levels; deficient gastrointestinal barrier function with translocation of bacteria and their byproducts; bacterial contamination of wounds with systemic release of bacterial products; and enhanced heat loss across wounds. Such patients commonly have a moderate fever, hyperdynamic circulation, and increased protein catabolism in the absence of infection. Although it can be difficult, it is important for the clinician to attempt to differentiate hypermetabolic response from evolving occult infection.

ANSWER: a, b, c

REFERENCE: *Chapter 12—Burns: Systemic Response to Burn Injury*

2. A 16-year-old boy and his 18-month-old cousin are injured in a house fire. The younger cousin was overcome by smoke and sustained a 50% flame burn and inhalation injury. The adolescent suffered burns of face and hands, totaling about 50% of the body surface, during a successful attempt to rescue the young cousin. Differences that can be expected between these two patients include all of the following except:

   a. Airway edema, should it occur, will be less imminently threatening to the adolescent
   b. The younger child can be expected to need more fluid per kilogram than the older child
   c. The younger child can be expected to need substantially more fluid because of the inhalation injury
   d. In the care of the younger child, fluid administration should be severely limited to avoid exacerbation of inhalation injury

COMMENT: The smaller airways of young children make mucosal edema more rapidly progress to airway obstruction. There are also perceived to be a number of differences in resuscitation requirements between young children and adolescents and adults. Infants and very young children may have a decreased ability to concentrate urine. It is therefore often recommended that they have a resuscitation target of 1 to 2 mL/kg per hour of urine rather than the usual 0.5 mL/kg per hour of urine. School-age and older children usually can be resuscitated with lower volumes of fluid. Inhalation injury has been documented in a number of studies to increase fluid resuscitation requirements as much as 50% over the predicted target. This is likely because of increased release of systemic mediators from the injured lung. Patients with inhalation injury should be maintained in a euvolemic state. Hypovolemia is not of benefit in the management of inhalation injury.

ANSWER: d

REFERENCE: *Chapter 12—Burns: Initial Evaluation; Systemic Initial Evaluation*

3. A 2-year-old child arrives in the emergency department with an extensive scald burn. Points of history that suggest abuse include all of the following except:

a. Differing histories from caregivers interviewed separately
b. Healed burns and bruises elsewhere on the child's body
c. An anxious affect demonstrated by the child
d. Evidence on examination that the burn occurred several hours before arrival in the emergency department

COMMENT: All burned children need evaluation for abuse or neglect, which is reported to occur among as many as 20% of patients in this age group admitted for burn care. It is an ethical and legal mandate that suspicious injuries be reported to the appropriate state agency. All children should be admitted to the hospital regardless of injury size to provide for their safety and allow for detailed evaluation. Points of history that suggest abuse include delayed presentation for medical care, conflicting histories from caregivers, and previous injuries. Suspicious burn patterns include those with sharply demarcated margins, those of uniform depth, the absence of splash marks in scald injuries, stocking or glove patterns or burn sparing of flexor surfaces, sparing of body parts in contact with porcelain, and deep localized contact injuries.

ANSWER: c

REFERENCE: *Chapter 12—Burns: Initial Evaluation; Injuries of Abuse*

4. A 12-year-old girl is referred to the burn unit for management of a progressive exfoliating disease. Clinical points that suggest a diagnosis of toxic epidermal necrolysis include all of the following except:

a. The absence of oral lesions
b. Intense erythema of the conjunctiva
c. Desquamating rash of the torso that appears to be progressing onto the extremities
d. Guaiac-positive stool

COMMENT: Toxic epidermal necrolysis is a variant of erythema multiforme major. The cause is unknown, but it is often traced to administration of a new drug. The histologic features are disruption of the dermal epidermal junction in all cutaneous and mucosal surfaces. The degree of cutaneous and mucous membrane involvement varies. Often the most serious morbidity is related to the visceral wound. Treatment is prevention of wound desiccation and superinfection with topical antimicrobial agents and biologic dressings while awaiting spontaneous healing. Nutritional and respiratory support is essential. The patients are prone to septic episodes because of the loss of the epidermal barrier from the skin and viscera.

ANSWER: a

REFERENCE: *Chapter 12—Burns: Initial Evaluation; Systemic Initial Evaluation*

5. A 30-year-old woman is extricated unconscious from a burning house. Although covered with soot, she has sustained no burn. She is spontaneously coughing up large amounts of carbonaceous material, and progressive stridor develops. An endotracheal tube is inserted, and bronchoscopic findings confirm the presence of an inhalation injury. Physiologic aberrations that can be expected over the next few days include all of the following except:

a. Upper airway edema and bronchospasm
b. Small-airway occlusion
c. Loss of lung volume from decreased chest wall compliance
d. Pulmonary infection

COMMENT: Inhalation injury is a leading cause of mortality in burn units. Five physiologic aberrations are common. These include upper airway obstruction due to progressive edema; reactive bronchospasm from aerosolized irritants; small-airway occlusion due to edema, sloughing of endobronchial debris, and loss of ciliary clearing; and microatelectasis due to loss of surfactant and alveolar edema. The clinical consequences of these physiologic changes include airway obstruction, which is managed with endotracheal intubation; bronchospasm, which is managed with β-agonists; ventilation-perfusion mismatch, which is managed with adjusted ventilatory support; and obstruction of small airways with pulmonary infection, which is managed with pulmonary toilet and antibiotics. It is often not possible to predict the degree of subsequent pulmonary dysfunction for patients with inhalation injury, because these changes evolve gradually. It is quite common for pulmonary function to be normal or near normal in the first few days after injury and subsequently deteriorate. If there is an overlying chest wall burn, decreased chest wall compliance can decrease lung volume.

ANSWER: c

REFERENCE: *Chapter 12—Burns: Selected Critical Care Issues; Inhalation Injury and Respiratory Failure*

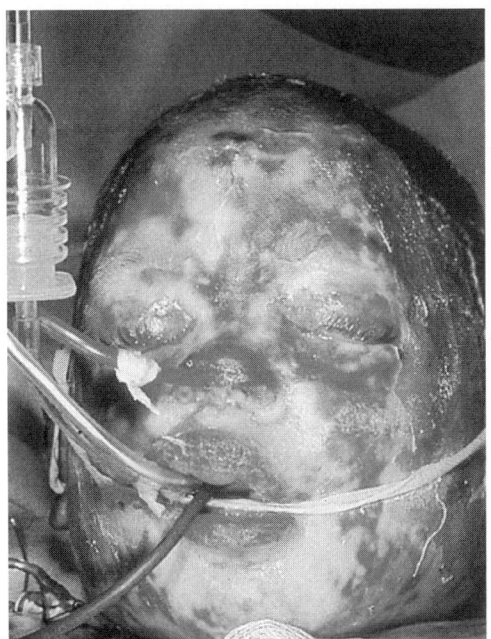

Figure 12.3

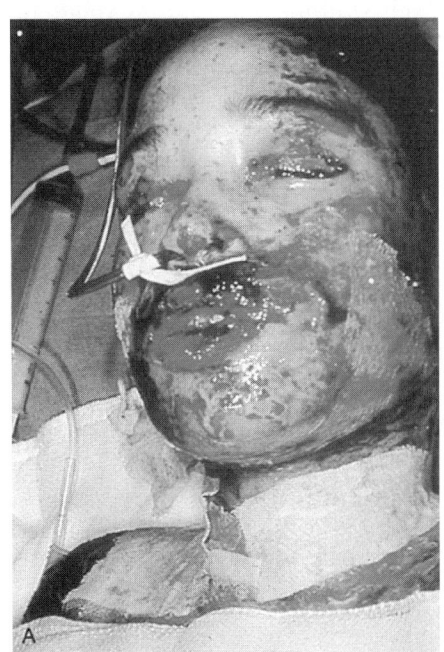

Figure 12.8A

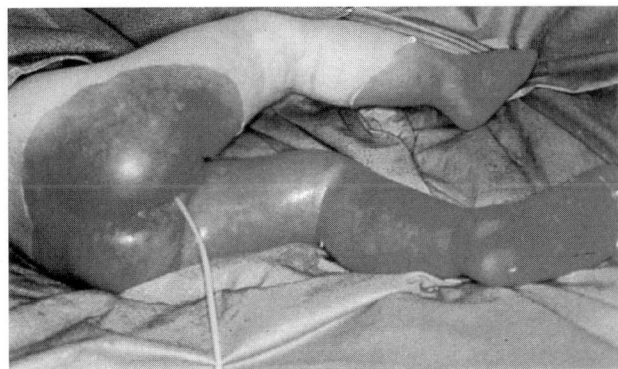

Figure 12.13

CHAPTER 13

ANESTHESIOLOGY AND PAIN MANAGEMENT

1. Muscle relaxants are a class of anesthetic agents used to prevent movement and facilitate surgical exposure. Which of the following statements is/are true concerning the use of muscle relaxants in surgical procedures?

a. Succinylcholine produces rapid obvious muscle fasciculations

b. Pancuronium can be reversed by increasing acetylcholine concentration with an anticholinesterase inhibitor (neostigmine)

c. Prolonged periods of muscle relaxation for patients requiring prolonged ventilation should be used in conjunction with analgesics and amnesic agents

d. The best clinical test for complete reversal of neuromuscular blockade is the ability of the patient to produce a large negative inspiratory force

COMMENT: Neuromuscular blocking agents can be classified as depolarizing or nondepolarizing inhibitors of the neurotransmitter acetylcholine at the neuromuscular junction. The only noncompetitive inhibitor used clinically is succinylcholine. This drug rapidly binds to the neuromuscular junction and produces depolarization, clinically apparent as fine muscle fasciculations occurring approximately 60 seconds after injection. All other clinically useful muscle relaxants are called *competitive inhibitors* and do cause depolarization when they attach to the neuromuscular junction. Because these agents compete with acetylcholine, the block produced is in direct proportion to the concentration of the agent relative to the concentration of acetylcholine. If the concentration ratio is low enough, competitive relaxants can be "reversed" if the concentration of acetylcholine is artificially elevated. An increase in acetylcholine concentration can be achieved with a drug that blocks metabolism of anticholinesterase (neostigmine).

Nondepolarizing relaxants are frequently used in the care of critically ill patients who are difficult to treat otherwise during prolonged periods of mechanical ventilation. It is imperative that these drugs be given in conjunction with analgesics and amnesic agents, because neuromuscular blocking agents have no analgesic or amnestic properties and only prevent motion of voluntary muscles. Patients therefore can be totally aware and in pain and unable to communicate. All muscles of the body do not have equal sensitivity to muscle relaxants. The diaphragm is resistant to neuromuscular blockade, whereas the neck and pharyngeal muscles that support the airway are most sensitive. It is possible for a patient with an endotracheal tube to spontaneously breathe and even to produce a large negative inspiratory force and yet have complete airway obstruction when the tube is removed because of effects of residual muscle relaxants on upper airway muscles. The definitive clinical test for complete reversal of neuromuscular blockade is the ability of the patient to sustain a head lift from the bed for 5 seconds.

ANSWER: a, b, c

REFERENCE: *Chapter 13—Anesthesiology and Pain Management: Anesthetic Agents and Their Physiologic Effects*

2. Narcotics are commonly used in the administration of general anesthesia. Which of the following statements is/are true concerning this class of agents?
   a. Narcotics have profound analgesic and amnestic properties
   b. Narcotics can cause hypotension through direct myocardial depressive effects
   c. Naloxone should be used routinely for the reversal of narcotic analgesia
   d. Patients with acute injuries and hypovolemia are at high risk for decreases in blood pressure with the use of narcotic analgesics
   e. Propofol is a new intravenous short-acting narcotic used frequently in the outpatient setting

COMMENT: Narcotics and synthetic analogues belong in the class of drugs called *opioids.* Narcotics produce profound analgesia and respiratory depression. They have no amnesic properties, no myocardial depressive effects, and no muscle relaxant properties. Narcotics can cause marked hemodynamic effects indirectly through the release of histamine or blunting of sympathetic vascular tone due to analgesic properties. Acutely injured patients may be hypovolemic and in pain and have a high sympathetic tone and peripheral resistance. Therefore such patients can have a dramatic decrease in systemic blood pressure with minimal doses of opioids. All opioids can be reversed with naloxone. Naloxone reversal, however, can be dangerous because the agent instantly reverses not only the analgesic effects of the opioid but also the analgesic effects of native opioids. Naloxone treatment has been associated with acute pulmonary edema and myocardial ischemia and should not be used electively to reverse the effects of narcotics. Propofol is a lipid-soluble substitute isopropyl phenol nonnarcotic agent that produces rapid induction of anesthesia followed by awakening in 4 to 8 minutes.

ANSWER: d

REFERENCE: *Chapter 13—Anesthesiology and Pain Management: Anesthetic Agents and Their Physiologic Effects*

3. Local anesthetics are essential agents used in current surgical practice. Which of the following statements is/are true concerning the use of local anesthetic agents?
   a. Complications due to excessive plasma concentration can result only from inadvertent intravascular injection of the agent
   b. Bupivacaine has a slow onset but a long duration
   c. The addition of epinephrine to a local anesthetic agent lowers the toxicity and increases the duration of local anesthesia
   d. Hypotension that occurs when a local anesthetic is administered in the form of a spinal epidural block is the result of myocardial depression

COMMENT: Local anesthetics constitute a class of drugs that produce temporary blockage of nerve conduction by binding to neuronal sodium channels. Adverse consequences associated with the use of local anesthetics fall into three categories: acute central nervous system toxicity due to excessive plasma concentration, hemodynamic and respiratory consequences due to excessive conduction block of the sympathetic or motor nerves, and allergic reactions. Whenever a local anesthetic is injected, there can be unintentional intravascular injection or an overdose of the drug due to rapid uptake from the tissues. Both can cause seizures. Complications can be minimized by means of aspiration before injection to avoid intravascular injection and limiting the doses to the safe range. When local anesthetics are administered for a spinal or epidural block, progressive blockade of the sympathetic nervous system produces systemic vasodilation. If the block travels along the thoracolumbar region, sympathetic blockade results in marked systemic vasodilation and bradycardia with resultant hypotension.

Local anesthetics are divided into two groups: esters and amides. The more commonly used agents, the amides, include lidocaine and bupivacaine. Lidocaine has a fast onset of action but a short duration, whereas bupivacaine has a slower onset but lasts 4 to 12 hours. Addition of epinephrine (100 µg) decreases the toxicity and increases the duration of a local anesthetic.

ANSWER: b, c

REFERENCE: *Chapter 13—Anesthesiology and Pain Management: Anesthetic Agents and Their Physiologic Effects*

4. General anesthesia is not without risks. Which of the following statements is/are true concerning the risk associated with general anesthesia?

a. Current estimates for mortality due to anesthesia alone are 1:10,000
b. Human error accounts for 50% to 75% of anesthetic-related deaths
c. Most anesthetic-related deaths are associated with overdose of analgesic agents
d. The most common problems associated with adverse anesthetic outcomes are related to the airway

COMMENT: Anesthetic agents effectively obtund or completely block nearly all physiologic protective mechanisms; therefore, there is associated risk even without a surgical procedure. With the advent of newer agents and monitoring techniques, it is estimated the mortality due to anesthesia alone has decreased from approximately 1:10,000 in the 1950s to as low as 1:100,000 or less for healthy persons today. It has been estimated that 50% to 75% of anesthetic-related deaths are caused by human error and are preventable. The most common problems associated with adverse outcomes are related to the airway: inadequate ventilation, unrecognized esophageal intubation, unrecognized extubation, and unrecognized disconnection from a ventilator.

ANSWER: b, d

REFERENCE: *Chapter 13—Anesthesiology and Pain Management: Risks Associated with Anesthesia*

5. A 65-year-old man with a history of coronary artery disease and recent myocardial infarction needs elective colon resection for a nonobstructing neoplasm. Which of the following statements is/are true concerning the risks of general anesthetic for this patient?

a. The age of the infarct has no effect on perioperative risk of reinfarction
b. The incidence of reinfarction appears to stabilize after 6 months
c. Invasive hemodynamic monitoring has no effect on perioperative reinfarction rate
d. Reinfarction has minimal effect on mortality
e. Perioperative infarction most frequently occurs more than 72 hours after an operation

COMMENT: A history of myocardial infarction is an important risk factor for general anesthesia. Large retrospective studies have shown that the incidence of reinfarction is related to the time elapsed since the previous myocardial infarction. The incidence of reinfarction appears to stabilize at approximately 1% after 6 months, the highest rate of reinfarction occurring in the first 3 months after infarction. The mortality from reinfarction among patients undergoing noncardiac surgery has been reported to be 20% to 50%. Death usually occurs within the first 48 hours after an operation. Invasive hemodynamic monitoring with pulmonary arterial catheters and aggressive pharmacologic intervention has been found to decrease reinfarction rates.

ANSWER: b, d

REFERENCE: *Chapter 13—Anesthesiology and Pain Management: Risks Associated with Anesthesia*

6. Which of the following factors adversely affects the risk of perioperative cardiac complications and reinfarction for the patient in *7*?

    a. More than five premature ventricular beats per minute on an electrocardiographic rhythm strip
    b. The anesthetic technique used
    c. Withdrawal of medical therapy with β-blockers and topical nitrates
    d. Length of surgical procedure less than 3 hours
    e. Known three-vessel coronary artery disease

COMMENT: The incidence of reinfarction increases among patients undergoing intrathoracic or intraabdominal procedures that last longer than 3 hours. Site of surgery and anesthetic technique have not been shown to change the incidence of reinfarction if the procedure lasts less than 3 hours. Patients with known three-vessel or left main coronary artery disease are at increased risk. Those who have undergone previous coronary artery bypass grafting are at substantially decreased risk of reinfarction. Prophylactic therapy with β-blockers, calcium channel agents, and nitrates has not proved beneficial; however, withdrawal of these agents has been associated with perioperative ischemia, myocardial infarction, and death. Congestive heart failure is the single most important predictor of postoperative cardiac morbidity. Rhythm disturbances, particularly frequent premature ventricular beats (more than 5 beats/min), are independently associated with increased risk of perioperative cardiac complications.

ANSWER: a, c, e

REFERENCE: *Chapter 13—Anesthesiology and Pain Management: Risks Associated with Anesthesia*

7. Anesthetic techniques used in the care of patients with severe pulmonary disease include:

    a. Intubation at a deep level of anesthesia
    b. Choice of an anesthetic agent that produces bronchodilation
    c. The use of epidural analgesia for postoperative pain control
    d. Perioperative use of intermittent positive pressure breathing

COMMENT: Patients with severe pulmonary diseases need special anesthetic techniques. Obstructive pulmonary disease can be either chronic (COPD) or acute (asthma). In either case, the reversible component of obstruction should be reversed before elective surgery. In operations on patients with reactive airway disease, the endotracheal tube can induce severe bronchospasm. Even when a patient has received good preoperative care, reactive bronchospasm can complicate induction of and emergence from anesthesia. The principal method used to prevent or diminish this "foreign body"–induced bronchospasm is intubation at a deep level of anesthesia, when reflexes are blunted. The classic method of treating a patient with severe asthma is to induce anesthesia with an agent that produces bronchodilation and to ventilate the patient with an inhalation agent until deep anesthesia is achieved before laryngoscopy and intubation. The tube should be removed while the patient is spontaneously ventilating, but with the inhalation agent still in effect, to bring the patient to consciousness while ventilation is provided by mask.

Because of the possible adverse effects of systemic narcotics on respiratory drive, the use of epidural narcotics and local anesthetics for postoperative pain control has become popular. These techniques allow earlier removal of the tube and, for patients undergoing intrathoracic and upper abdominal operations, helps restore pulmonary function toward preoperative values. Preoperative use of intermittent positive pressure breathing has not been found to decrease the incidence of postoperative pulmonary complications.

ANSWER: a, b, c

REFERENCE: *Chapter 13—Anesthesiology and Pain Management: Risks Associated with Anesthesia*

8. Over the last decade, the routine use of invasive and noninvasive monitoring devices has been instituted for the administration of most anesthetics. Which of the following statements is/are true concerning monitoring of a surgical patient?

a. A pulse oximeter reading reflect changes in Pao_2 only below 80 mm Hg
b. Monitoring of end tidal carbon dioxide reflects changes in ventilation but not cardiac output
c. Intermittent, noninvasive systemic blood pressure monitoring with an oscillometric blood pressure cuff has essentially replaced clinical measurement by means of auscultation
d. Pulmonary arterial catheter monitoring is generally reserved for critically ill patients with serious left ventricular dysfunction

COMMENT: Pulse oximetry continuously, noninvasively, and inexpensively provides arterial hemoglobin saturation and peripheral pulse values. It must be remembered, however, that a pulse oximeter measures oxygen saturation, not arterial oxygen tension (o_2). The Pao_2 must decrease to less than 80 mm Hg before any significant change in oxygen saturation occurs. End tidal carbon dioxide monitoring reflects metabolism (production of carbon dioxide, circulation (blood flow to the lungs), and ventilation (respiratory rate in an intact ventilatory circuit). It can be used as a surveillance monitor for both the respiratory circuit and the cardiovascular system. Any acute decrease in cardiac output decreases output to the lung and increases alveolar dead space, causing an acute decrease in end tidal carbon dioxide.

Hemodynamic stability can be monitored with a variety of methods, the most basic of which is measurement of systemic arterial blood pressure. Intermittent, noninvasive measurement of systemic blood pressure with an oscillometric blood pressure cuff has become the standard in the operating room. The accuracy equals that of clinical measurement by means of auscultation. When tighter control is required for patients with severe hypertension or heart disease or for patients who may have acute blood loss, invasive arterial monitoring is used. For patients with left ventricular dysfunction who are undergoing extended surgical procedures with marked fluid shifts and possible blood loss, central venous pressure monitoring frequently is used. Pulmonary arterial catheter monitoring is reserved for more critically ill patients and for those with severe left ventricular dysfunction.

ANSWER: a, c, d

REFERENCE: *Chapter 13—Anesthesiology and Pain Management: Monitoring the Surgical Patient*

9. Correct statements concerning complications in the postanesthesia care unit include which of the following?

a. The use of nitrous oxide has been well documented to increase the incidence of postoperative nausea
b. Perioperative myocardial ischemia usually is easily diagnosed in the early postoperative period
c. Hypothermia has a deleterious effect on drug metabolism and therefore delays recovery from anesthesia
d. The serotonin antagonist ondansetron holds promise as the superior antiemetic agent in the perioperative period

COMMENT: Twenty-four percent of patients have a complication in the postanesthesia care unit. Nausea, vomiting, and airway problems cause 70% of these complications. Problems with maintenance of airway support are by far the most common respiratory complication. Hypothermia has a deleterious effect on altering drug metabolism and delaying recovery. Nausea and vomiting are rarely unifactorial and cause considerable discomfort. There is little evidence to favor one anesthetic or anesthetic technique over another. Nitrous oxide does not appear to increase the incidence of nausea in well documented studies. The new serotonin antagonist ondansetron has been shown in several studies to be superior to other agents as a perioperative antiemetic agent.

Perioperative myocardial ischemia is an extremely important complication but is difficult to recognize. Diagnosis is complicated because only 10% to 30% of patients with documented myocardial infarction have pain and postoperative electrocardiographic changes often are nonspecific. Caregivers must therefore look for secondary indications of ongoing ischemia, such as hypotension, arrhythmia, elevated filling pressures, or postoperative oliguria.

ANSWER: c, d

REFERENCE: *Chapter 13—Anesthesiology and Pain Management: Common Problems in the Postoperative Period*

10. Patient-controlled analgesia (PCA) is a commonly used technique for postoperative analgesia. Which of the following statements is/are true concerning the use of PCA?

    a. Satisfactory pain relief is provided with administration of higher narcotic doses
    b. The technique cannot be used in the care of semiconscious or uncooperative patients
    c. Patient-controlled analgesia is as safe as conventional intramuscular administration of pain medication
    d. Excessive administration of narcotic medication can be limited with a lockout duration that controls administration of the narcotic

COMMENT: The technique of PCA is based on evidence that small intravenous bolus doses of narcotics on demand can improve pain relief at the same or less total narcotic dose. The system requires some degree of sophistication and a conscious patient who has been instructed in the technique. Numerous studies have demonstrated that PCA is as safe as conventional intramuscular medication. The patient can be restricted from receiving excessive agents by means of setting a lockout interval duration of several minutes during which a dose of narcotic cannot be successfully administered. The total hourly dose also can be limited.

ANSWER: b, c, d

REFERENCE: *Chapter 13—Anesthesiology and Pain Management: Postoperative Acute Pain Management*

11. During an airway examination, the patient opens his mouth and the uvula is partially seen. This is called:

    a. Mallampati I
    b. Mallampati II
    c. Mallampati III
    d. Mallampati IV
    e. Mallampati V

COMMENT: The preprocedure evaluation should include a review of current medications and coexisting disease and a brief physical examination, including evaluation of the airway. It is important to determine how difficult it may be to obtain control of the airway if apnea should occur. Although there is no absolute standard for predicting difficult intubation, a simple four-step examination helps to determine the likelihood. First, the patient should have a normal mouth opening. Second, the patient should have normal neck flexion and extension. Third, the physician should be able to fit three finger widths under the patient's chin between the thyroid cartilage and the mentum. Finally, when the patient opens his or her mouth and is asked to stick out the tongue, the airway can be classified depending on whether the uvula can be completely seen (Mallampati class I), only partly seen (class II), not seen with only the hard and soft palate visible (class III), or only hard palate visible (class IV). This classification is roughly predictive of progressive difficulty in intubation due to difficulty in visualizing the larynx.

ANSWER: b

REFERENCE: *Chapter 13—Anesthesiology and Pain Management*

12. A patient in an intensive care unit is recovering from acute respiratory distress syndrome. To manage ventilation, the patient has been relaxed with a nondepolarizing muscle relaxant (atracurium). To reverse the effects of atracurium, the following should be administered:

a. Neostigmine 1 mg/kg with 7 μg/kg of glycopyrrolate
b. Neostigmine in incremental doses until muscle tone returns plus 7 mg/kg glycopyrrolate
c. Neostigmine 0.05 mg/kg plus 7 mg glycopyrrolate
d. Neostigmine 10 mg plus 0.5 mg glycopyrrolate
e. None of the above

COMMENT: Clinically useful muscle relaxants include competitive inhibitors, which do not cause depolarization when they attach at the neuromuscular junction. Because these agents compete with acetylcholine, the block produced is in direct proportion to the concentration of the agent relative to the concentration of acetylcholine. If the concentration ratio is low enough, competitive relaxants can be reversed if the concentration of acetylcholine is artificially elevated. Acetylcholine concentration can be increased with a drug that blocks its metabolism, an anticholinesterase (neostigmine) (Table 13.1). The neuromuscular blocking agent is still present, but motor function returns if the acetylcholine concentration is high enough to out-compete the blocking agent. There is a ceiling to which anticholinesterase drugs can elevate acetylcholine; therefore high levels of nondepolarizing relaxants cannot be reversed. Reversing neuromuscular relaxants is not analogous to using naloxone to reverse the effects of opioids. The reversal agent neostigmine does not compete or combine with the relaxant.

There are systemic consequences to increasing the plasma concentration of acetylcholine. Acetylcholine is the predominant neurotransmitter in the preganglionic sympathetic and parasympathetic nervous systems and in the postganglionic parasympathetic nervous system. For this reason, an anticholinergic drug (atropine or glycopyrrolate) must be given with the anticholinesterase to prevent the undesirable effects of a generalized acetylcholine overdose.

REFERENCE: *Chapter 13—Anesthesiology and Pain Management*

TABLE 13.1. ANTAGONISM OF NONDEPOLARIZING NEUROMUSCULAR BLOCKADE

Dose	Time to peak effect (min)	Dose	Use with
Anticholinesterases			
Edrophonium	1–2	0.5–1.0 mg/kg	—
Neostigmine	3–5	0.04–0.07 mg/kg	—
Pyridostigmine	10–12	0.2–0.3 mg/kg	—
Anticholinergics			
Glycopyrrolate	—	0.008 mg/kg (0.5–0.6 mg/70 kg)	Neostigmine
Atropine	—	0.007–0.02 mg/kg (0.05–1.5 mg/70 kg)	Pyridostigmine Edrophonium
			Neostigmine

13. A patient using a ventilator in an intensive care unit is treated with a nondepolarizing muscle relaxant, and ventilator use is discontinued the next day. To ensure that the patient does not have residual neuromuscular blockade, the following can be done:

a. Measure negative inspiratory force and ensure that it is greater than −25 cm water
b. Ensure that the patient can maintain an adequate minute ventilation with a spontaneous respiratory rate less than 25 per minute
c. Obtain a nerve stimulator and see that the patient has four twitches with the twitch monitor
d. Test to see whether the patient can lift the head off the bed for more than 5 seconds
e. None of the above

COMMENT: All muscles in the body are not equally sensitive to muscle relaxants. The diaphragm is most resistant to neuromuscular blockade, and the neck and pharyngeal muscles that support the airway are most sensitive. It is possible for a patient with an endotracheal tube to spontaneously ventilate and even to produce a large negative inspiratory effort and yet develop complete airway obstruction when the tube is removed because of the effects of residual muscle relaxant on the upper airway muscles. The definitive clinical test for complete reversal of neuromuscular blockade is the patient's ability to sustain a head lift from the bed for 5 seconds.

ANSWER: d

REFERENCE: *Chapter 13—Anesthesiology and Pain Management*

14. During a minor surgical procedure performed with intravenous sedation, the patient reports pain when the surgical incision is extended. What should be done?

a. Titrate a small amount of narcotic, such as 50 μg fentanyl
b. Titrate a small amount of a short-acting benzodiazepine, such as 1 mg midazolam
c. Slowly titrate in a combination of fentanyl and midazolam
d. Infiltrate the incision site with 1% lidocaine
e. None of the above

COMMENT: A variety of minor surgical procedures can be accomplished safely and comfortably with anesthesia provided by infiltration of local anesthetics (most commonly 1% lidocaine) and mild sedation or anxiolysis with an intravenous benzodiazepine. All intravenous benzodiazepines, narcotics, and other intravenous anesthetics produce apnea if given in a high enough dose. Because there is substantial patient to patient variability in response to a given dose, it is important that intravenous anxiolytics be given slowly in small, incremental doses to achieve a safe sedated state. Another important factor is that anesthesia is provided by means of infiltration of the local anesthetic and not by means of intravenous sedation. Intravenous agents, including narcotics, cannot overcome the pain of a surgical incision. If large doses of narcotics are given for this purpose, once the surgical stimulus ends, the patient can quickly become apneic. The duration of respiratory depression for even short-acting narcotics is much longer than the painful stimulus of the incision.

ANSWER: d

REFERENCE: *Chapter 13—Anesthesiology and Pain Management*

15. Which of the following sedative agents can be injected solely without risk of apnea?
    a. Propofol
    b. Ketamine
    c. Midazolam
    d. Fentanyl
    e. None of the above

COMMENT: When opioids are titrated intravenously, patients first become apneic because of the respiratory depressive effect (shifting the carbon dioxide response curve), but they still breathe on command. As the dose increases, patients become apneic and unresponsive.

Propofol is a lipid-soluble substituted isopropyl phenol that produces rapid induction of anesthesia in 30 seconds followed by awakening in 4 to 8 minutes. Intravenous propofol can effectively produce total anesthesia, including amnesia, analgesia, and some degree of muscle relaxation. Propofol has important roles in intensive care units when used as a continuous infusion sedative at dosages of 25 to 50 mg/kg per minute. When the infusion is discontinued, the patient becomes alert within minutes. Propofol can produce substantial hypotension when intravenous induction doses are administered.

Ketamine is a phencyclidine derivative that produces anesthesia characterized by dissociation between the thalamus and limbic systems. Induction of anesthesia is achieved within 60 seconds after intravenous injection of 1 to 2 mg/kg or within 2 to 4 minutes of intramuscular injection of 5 to 10 mg/kg. Patients appear to be in a cataleptic state in which their eyes remain open with a slow nystagmic gaze. The drug produces intense amnesia and analgesia but has been associated with unpleasant visual and auditory hallucinations that can progress to delirium. At low doses, patients continue to spontaneously breathe but cannot be expected to protect the airway should vomiting occur. At higher doses, ketamine acts as a respiratory depressant and produces complete apnea.

Benzodiazepines are the primary class of agents used as amnesics and anxiolytics. The prototype drug, diazepam, has been more recently replaced by its water-soluble analogue of shorter duration, midazolam. Benzodiazepines produce anxiolysis and some degree of amnesia but have no analgesic properties. Midazolam is always used intraoperatively in conjunction with an opioid or inhalation agent. Midazolam can be used in combination with the short-acting opioid fentanyl to produce conscious sedation for minor procedures. Benzodiazepines can produce apnea and have synergistic effects with narcotics. Very small doses of midazolam and fentanyl can quickly cause unconsciousness and apnea.

ANSWER: e

REFERENCE: *Chapter 13—Anesthesiology and Pain Management*

CHAPTER 14

TUMOR BIOLOGY

1. Examples of histologic conditions that demonstrate metaplasia include:
   a. Barrett's esophagus
   b. Keloid formation
   c. Wound healing by granulation
   d. Second degree thermal injury to skin

COMMENT: Metaplasia involves abnormal transformation of one fully differentiated, adult tissue into another kind of differentiated tissue. Metaplasia involves acquired transformation rather than an abnormality in initial development, which is more accurately described as *heterotypia* or *heteroplasia*. Metaplastic transformation can involve reprogramming of epithelial stem cells to a new differentiation pathway and in some circumstances can be considered a premalignant condition. Examples of metaplastic conditions associated with increased risk of future neoplasia include glandular metaplasia of the esophagus (Barrett's esophagus), intestinal metaplasia of the stomach, and ductal metaplasia of the exocrine pancreas.

ANSWER: a

REFERENCE: *Chapter 14—Tumor Biology: Carcinogenesis and the Spectrum of Neoplasia*

2. Recent investigation suggests that malignant transformation usually exhibits which of the following characteristics?
   a. Rapid growth of cells transformed by the occurrence of isolated defects in membrane growth receptors
   b. Progressive accumulation of acquired genetic defects over a period of years
   c. Defects in autonomic nervous system regulation
   d. Combined effects of inherited and acquired genetic defects

COMMENT: A large body of evidence suggests that malignant transformation is a multistep process, now recognized as the stepwise accumulation of genetic and epigenetic events required for neoplastic growth. This process likely explains the age-dependent nature of the incidence of tumor among humans and the sequential appearance of histologic intermediates in the development of frank malignant growth. A sequence of events defined for several tumor suppressor genes is frequently called *loss of heterozygosity.* This term was coined because the inherited presence of one mutant and one wild-type allele is initially manifested by the appearance of heterozygosity when DNA is analyzed by restriction fragment length polymorphism. A "second hit" involving loss of the wild-type allele eliminates this heterozygous condition, effectively resulting in a reduction to homozygosity with only the mutated form of the gene remaining.

Through analysis of the molecular events associated with various stages in the colonic adenoma-carcinoma sequence, the requirement for various genetic mutations during the stages of tumor progression can be clarified. The earliest histologic event in colorectal carcinogenesis involves formation of small, benign adenomas consisting primarily of hyperplastic epithelium. This process is accelerated in patients with inherited inactivation of the adenomatous polyposis coli (*APC*) gene, implying that loss of *APC* function influences early events in this multistep pathway. Although small adenomas frequently harbor only wild-type copies of the K-*ras* protooncogene, 50% of adenomas exceeding 1 cm in greatest dimension have activating K-*ras* mutations. The implication is that this genetic event may be required for adenoma progression. Later events observed during conversion to carcinoma in situ and fully invasive cancer include allelic loss at the 18q21 chromosome locus, which contains the *DCC* (deleted in colon cancer) gene, and loss of heterozygosity at 17p13, the site of the p53 tumor suppressor gene. The requirement for multiple rate-limiting molecular events in the process of malignant transformation explains why sporadic neoplasia typically occurs with increasing age, whereas persons who inherit mutations in these genes tend to have early-onset neoplasia.

ANSWER: b, d

REFERENCE: *Chapter 14—Tumor Biology: Multistep Models of Carcinogenesis*

3. In the United States, the most common cause of cancer-related death is:
   a. Lung cancer
   b. Pancreatic cancer
   c. Bladder cancer
   d. Breast cancer

COMMENT: In the United States 52.4% of all cancer deaths occur among men. For both men and women, lung cancer is the single most common cause of cancer death, followed by prostate cancer among men and breast cancer among women. For both sexes, colorectal and pancreatic cancer represent the third and fourth most common causes of cancer death. These common neoplasms account for a sizable fraction of all cancer deaths. For men, lung cancer, prostate cancer, and colorectal cancer account for 54% of all cancer deaths, whereas cancers of the lung, breast, colon, and rectum account for one half of all cancer deaths among women.

ANSWER: a

REFERENCE: *Chapter 14—Tumor Biology: Cancer Epidemiology*

4. Infectious agents have been postulated to have a role in oncogenesis among humans. For which of the following malignant tumors does evidence exist linking viruses to human disease?

    a. Hepatocellular cancer
    b. Gastric cancer
    c. Hodgkin's disease
    d. Cervical cancer

COMMENT: Among biologic agents, several human DNA tumor viruses have been causally implicated in human neoplasia. The hepatitis B and hepatitis C viruses have been strongly linked to development of hepatocellular cancer, primarily by indirectly provoking cellular proliferation in response to immune-mediated injury. Similarly, infection with specific high-risk types of human papilloma viruses (e.g., HPV-16, HPV-18, HPV-33) is associated with squamous cell carcinoma of the anogenital tract, including carcinoma of the uterine cervix, carcinoma of the anus, and vulvar carcinoma. In the case of Epstein-Barr virus, latent infection is associated with numerous malignant tumors, including Burkitt's lymphoma, Hodgkin's disease, T-cell malignant tumors, and squamous tumor of the oropharynx. Attention has been placed on the ability of bacterial pathogens to act as cancer-causing agents. Primary among these, *Helicobacter pylori* infection has been implicated not only in the causation of gastric mucosa–associated lymphoid tissue (MALT) lymphoma but also in initiating the sequence of events that may cause intestinal-type gastric adenocarcinoma.

ANSWER: a, c, d

REFERENCE: *Chapter 14—Tumor Biology: Cancer Etiology*

5. Evidence suggests that the risk of which of the following cutaneous malignancies increases with acute solar exposure with resultant sunburn?

    a. Squamous cell cancer
    b. Basal cell cancer
    c. Melanoma
    d. Kaposi's sarcoma

COMMENT: With respect to ultraviolet radiation, similar mechanisms of carcinogenesis have been observed. Solar ultraviolet radiation is a potent inducer of DNA damage, often in the form of pyrimidine dimers. These DNA lesions appear to lead directly to mutation in a number of cancer-related genes, including *ras* oncogenes and the p53 tumor suppressor gene. Inherited syndromes associated with deficiencies in pyrimidine dimer repair, such as xeroderma pigmentosum, are associated with an increased risk of skin cancer. Acute and chronic ultraviolet injury also can lead to recognition of altered skin antigens by suppressor T lymphocytes, perhaps leading to decreased immune surveillance of malignant cells. Unequivocal evidence confirms ultraviolet radiation as a primary cause of basal cell and squamous cell skin cancer, the two most common forms of malignant growth among humans. Although the relation between melanoma and ultraviolet light is complex, a large body of evidence suggests that although long-term low-level exposure to the sun may be a predisposing factor to squamous and basal cell carcinoma, melanoma risk is specifically enhanced by acute episodes of sunburn, especially early in life. Unlike the known contribution of ionizing and ultraviolet radiation to cancer risk, the role of other forms of physical energy, including low-frequency electric and magnetic fields, remains uncertain.

ANSWER: c

REFERENCE: *Chapter 14—Tumor Biology: Cancer Etiology*

6. The risk of breast cancer among women is increased by which of the following factors?
   a. Obesity
   b. Nulliparity
   c. Multiple pregnancies
   d. Low-fiber diet

COMMENT: Several studies have shown apparent hormone-related risk factors for breast cancer among women. In general, factors that increase cumulative estrogen exposure increase risk of breast cancer. These factors include early menarche, late menopause, obesity, and nulliparity or late age at first pregnancy. In the case of obesity, adipose tissue is a rich source of aromatase enzyme activity, which leads to increased peripheral conversion of androstenedione to estrone and estradiol. Although data conflict somewhat, results of several studies have suggested that prolonged treatment with higher-dose postmenopausal replacement estrogen is associated with moderate increases in risk of breast cancer. Together these factors have generated considerable interest in the role of hormonal manipulation as a means of chemoprevention among patients at high risk. The incidence of several other tumor types may be similarly influenced by hormonal factors, including endometrial cancer, ovarian cancer, and prostate cancer.

ANSWER: a, b

REFERENCE: *Chapter 14—Tumor Biology: Cancer Etiology*

7. Genetic defects associated with the development of colorectal cancer have been studied extensively. The gene most commonly mutated in sporadic colorectal cancer is:
   a. *BRAC*
   b. *APC*
   c. *Rb*
   d. Notch

COMMENT: One of the earliest steps in the development of colorectal cancer is the loss of function of the tumor suppressor gene *APC*, which is considered a gatekeeper gene in colorectal cancer. This gene was first identified as the gene responsible for familial adenomatosis coli (FAP) by means of demonstration of cosegregation of mutant alleles in affected kindreds. More than 70% of sporadic colorectal cancers are believed to involve somatic mutations in *APC*. Further support for the role of *APC* in the development of polyps and colorectal cancer stems from the studies of a mouse genetic model for FAP known as Min (multiple intestinal neoplasia). Mutations among Min mice, like those among many patients with FAP, cause premature truncation of *APC* protein and development of multiple adenomatous polyps and cancer of the intestine.

ANSWER: b

REFERENCE: *Chapter 14—Tumor Biology: Tumor Initiation and Progression in Colorectal Cancer*

8. Studies involving patients taking nonsteroidal anti-inflammatory drugs (NSAIDs) have had the unexpected finding that the patients had a lower than expected incidence of which of the following cancers?

   a. Gastric cancer
   b. Breast cancer
   c. Colorectal cancer
   d. Hepatocellular cancer

COMMENT: Studies of large numbers of patients taking aspirin or NSAIDs for various indications have revealed lower incidence of colorectal cancer among these patients than among patients not taking these agents. It is known that NSAIDs block activity of the enzyme cyclooxygenase (COX), which is involved in the production of prostaglandins. Further investigation has revealed two forms of this enzyme. Cyclooxygenase-1 is constitutively expressed and thought to be involved in decreasing inflammation. Cyclooxygenase-2 is an inducible form of the enzyme and has found to be elevated in colorectal adenoma and carcinoma. The mechanism of reduction of colorectal cancer risk by NSAIDs is thought to be primarily from inhibition of COX-2. Therefore, selective COX-2 inhibitors have been developed. In addition to their most frequent use in reducing inflammation, these agents are being used in clinical trials of the treatment of patients at increased risk of colorectal cancer from FAP. The recommendation for more widespread use of COX-2 inhibitors in the chemoprevention of colorectal cancer will depend on the results of these trials.

ANSWER: c

REFERENCE: *Chapter 14—Tumor Biology: Cyclooxygenases and Carcinogenesis*

CHAPTER 15

HUMAN GENE THERAPY

1. Human gene therapy requires the transfer of genetic information to targeted cells. A common experimental approach has been to use viruses as the agents of transfer, so-called *vectors.* Which of the following viruses have been used in gene transfer?

   a. Oncoretroviruses
   b. Adenoviruses
   c. Adeno-associated viruses
   d. Pox viruses
   e. Herpesviruses

COMMENT: Five types of viruses have been used as gene therapy vectors in clinical trials: oncoretroviruses, adenoviruses, adeno-associated viruses, poxviruses, and herpesviruses. Other viruses being explored as potential vectors in animal models include alphaviruses, baculoviruses, lentiviruses, and Epstein-Barr virus. All viruses have certain common elements. The viral genome is enclosed in a protein coat called a *capsid.* Depending on the type of virus, the genome can be surrounded by an outer lipoprotein membrane called an *envelope.* In enveloped viruses, the envelope and its glycoproteins mediate attachment and entrance to the host cell, whereas in nonenveloped viruses, the capsid proteins adopt these functions. The tropism of a virus can therefore be altered through changes in the envelope or the capsid proteins. Both of these techniques are commonly used in the development of gene therapy vectors. One of the most common manipulations is called *pseudotyping*—replacement of the envelope gene of a virus with that of another virus to change its tropism and infectivity.

ANSWER: a, b, c, d, e

REFERENCE: *Chapter 15—Human Gene Therapy: Viral Vectors*

2. Retroviruses have proved to be dependable agents for transfer of genetic material for gene therapy experiments. However, all retroviruses have a common feature that limits their utility. What is that feature?

a. Need for introduction by intranasal installation
b. Induction of polycythemia
c. Ability to transduce only cells undergoing division
d. Induction of inflammatory reaction, which limits repetitive administration

COMMENT: The most important shortcoming of retroviruses is that they can transduce only cells that are actively dividing. This is because the retrovirus preintegration complex cannot traverse the nuclear membrane except when the membrane is fragmented during mitosis. Retroviruses therefore are suitable only for transducing cells that can be grown ex vivo in culture or dividing cells in vivo. This limits the range of applications for which retroviruses are suitable. Use of cytokines and other techniques, such as partial hepatectomy, have been used to make otherwise nondividing cell types more susceptible to transformation by oncoretroviruses. Another liability of retroviruses is that they are labile in the human circulation because of rapid inactivation by complement. This imposes limits their use in vivo.

ANSWER: c

REFERENCE: *Chapter 15—Human Gene Therapy: Retroviral Vectors*

3. Adenovirus vectors do not require cell division to transduce target tissues. This feature has made them attractive agents for gene therapy trials. However, adenoviral vectors have limitations due to:

a. Induction of systemic inflammatory responses
b. Need for intraperitoneal injection
c. Occurrence of symptoms resembling Parkinson's disease in some recipients
d. Induction of hyperglycemia

COMMENT: First-generation adenovirus vectors can transduce cells effectively and can achieve high initial levels of expression. Because they produce low levels of viral proteins from the other early and late gene regions, however, they elicit a cellular immune response, limit the duration of transgene expression, and result in destruction of the transduced cells. Immunogenicity is the primary disadvantage of adenoviral vectors, limits the duration of transgene expression, and precludes readministration of the vector. Although this does not prevent the use of adenoviral vectors in protocols designed to kill transduced cells, it is problematic for many other types of gene therapy in which prolonged expression of a transgene is desired.

ANSWER: a

REFERENCE: *Chapter 15—Human Gene Therapy: Adenovirus*

4. Nonviral means to introduce genetic material have been used in gene therapy experiments. Potentially useful vectors include

   a. Liposomes
   b. Naked DNA
   c. Transformed *Helicobacter pylori* organisms
   d. Naked mRNA

COMMENT: Nonviral systems include liposomes, naked DNA, and DNA-protein complexes and have several advantages over viral vector systems. Nonviral vectors are theoretically safer than viral vectors because there is no danger of replication or competent virus contamination. Nonviral systems also are largely nonimmunogenic and can be readministered if needed. Nonviral vectors can carry a larger transgene than most viral vectors. Retroviruses and adenoviruses, the two most commonly used viral vectors in clinical trials, have a transgene capacity of no greater than 8 kb, whereas liposomes and DNA-protein complexes can deliver DNA cosmids of up to 50 kb. Production of nonviral vectors is easier than production of viral vectors, in large part because the former are prepared in vitro, eliminating the need for packaging cell lines. The primary disadvantage of nonviral vectors is low efficiency of gene transfer, which limits their utility for many applications.

ANSWER: a, b

REFERENCE: *Chapter 15—Human Gene Therapy: Nonviral Vectors*

CHAPTER 16

TRANSPLANTATION AND IMMUNOLOGY

1. T lymphocytes are divided into two main subclasses: CD4$^+$ and CD8$^+$. Which of the following statements is/are true concerning these classes of T cells?

   a. CD4$^+$ T-cells are restricted to recognizing antigens of the class II major histocompatibility complex (MHC)
   b. CD8$^+$ T cells perform primarily cytotoxic functions
   c. CD4$^+$CD8$^+$ double-positive cells are well-differentiated mature cells
   d. CD4$^+$ T cells also perform suppressor functions

COMMENT: T cells are divided into two main subclasses: CD4$^+$ and CD8$^+$. CD4$^+$CD8$^+$ double-positive cells usually are immature T cells or thymocytes, whereas the fully differentiated T cell usually is single positive. Because of molecular interactions, CD4$^+$ T cells are restricted to recognizing antigens in the context of the class II MHC and usually perform roles related to B-cell help, T-cell help, and inflammatory responses, such as delayed and contact hypersensitivity. CD8$^+$ T cells are restricted to class I MHC and perform cytotoxic functions. Experimental studies have shown that both CD4$^+$ and CD8$^+$ T cells can act as suppressor T cells.

ANSWER: a, b, d

REFERENCE: *Chapter 16—Transplantation and Immunology: Transplant Immunology Initiation of the Immune Response*

2. Which of the following statements is/are true concerning clinical syndromes of rejection?

   a. Hyperacute rejection occurs with kidney, heart, liver, and lung transplantation
   b. The histologic characteristics of acute rejection include lymphocyte infiltration accompanied by plasma cells, eosinophils, or neutrophils
   c. Vascular atherosclerosis and obliteration are characteristic of chronic rejection
   d. Transplantation across major ABO incompatibility results in hyperacute rejection of a renal or cardiac transplant

COMMENT: Hyperacute rejection is the result of binding of preformed antibody to the allograft at the time of revascularization in the operating room. Complement is activated, and the result is endothelial cell destruction, vascular leak, recruitment of platelets and neutrophils, thrombosis of vessels, and destruction of the graft in minutes to hours. Kidney, heart, pancreas, and lung allografts all are susceptible to hyperacute rejection; however, liver grafts are relatively resistant to this process and often are transplanted across antibody differences and even across an ABO difference. Acute rejection usually occurs days to weeks after transplantation and is initiated by T cell–dependent immunity characterized microscopically by lymphocytic infiltration accompanied by plasma cells, eosinophils, and a few mast cells or neutrophils. Chronic rejection usually occurs months to years after transplantation. It is characterized by loss of normal histologic structure, fibrosis, and atherosclerosis. Chronic rejection is the main cause of graft failure and death in all types of organ transplantation.

ANSWER: b, d

REFERENCE: *Chapter 16—Transplantation and Immunology: Transplant Immunology; Effector Mechanisms of the Immune Response*

3. The term *tolerance* refers to responses including long-term graft acceptance without the need for chronic immunosuppression. T and B lymphocytes can be tolerant or unresponsive to antigen in a variety of specific ways. Which of the following is/are (a) mechanism(s) of tolerance?

   a. Clonal abortion
   b. Clonal deletion
   c. Clonal anergy
   d. Suppression

COMMENT: Clonal abortion is the developmental process whereby nascent T-cell and B-cell clones, which recognize autoantigen with high affinity, are eliminated. Clonal deletion can encompass the processes of clonal abortion but it also refers to elimination of mature T-cell and B-cell clones. Clonal anergy is a state in which the potential relative-reactive clones and their receptors are physically present but do not respond to antigen. Suppression generally refers to an active process in which a leukocyte or its soluble products inhibit the development or effector function of immune lymphocytes.

ANSWER: a, b, c, d

REFERENCE: *Chapter 16—Transplantation and Immunology: Transplant Immunology; Regulation of the Immune Response*

4. Which of the following statements is/are true concerning currently approved immunosuppressant agents?

   a. Azathioprine is useful in the management of acute rejection
   b. Methylprednisolone is particularly useful in immunosuppression because it has lesser toxicity than does prednisone
   c. Cyclosporine blocks transcription of several early T-cell activation genes
   d. FK-506 is both more potent and less toxic than is cyclosporine
   e. The monoclonal antibody OKT3 interferes with T-cell antigen recognition function

COMMENT: The most important principle of immunosuppression is to induce prophylaxis of rejection with high doses of drugs at the time of allografting. The dosages of the drugs are decreased within days to weeks to less toxic maintenance levels. The antimetabolite azathioprine interferes with nucleic acid metabolism, inhibits proliferation and clonal expansion of activated lymphocytes, and eliminates alloantigen-specific immune responses. This agent is used during induction immunosuppression and for maintenance immunosuppression but has little role in the management of acute rejection. Glucocorticoids are the mainstays of almost all immunosuppressive regimens. All glucocorticoids have similar immunosuppressive actions, and none is more effective than any other at equipotent doses. Complications and side effects are equivalent at all equipotent doses. Cyclosporine inhibits the rotamase activity of cyclophilin. Therefore the main immunosuppressive activity of cyclosporine is to block transcription of several early T-cell activation genes. The macrolide antibiotic FK-506 is 10 to 100 times more potent than cyclosporine on a molar basis but it also is associated with a number of serious and similar toxicities. Antibodies are given for only short periods for prophylaxis of rejection and to manage acute rejection. There are two major types of antibody preparations—polyclonal antibodies such as antilymphocyte or antithymocyte globulin and monoclonal antibodies. OKT3 is used for both induction and management of rejection and is the most efficacious agent for the management of rejection.

ANSWER: c, e

REFERENCE: *Chapter 16—Transplantation and Immunology: Transplantation and Immunology; Regulation of the Immune Response*

5. Numerous toxicities and adverse effects are associated with immunosuppression. Which of the following statements is/are true concerning complications of immunosuppression?

   a. Transplant recipients are susceptible mainly to infections with unusual organisms (fungus, virus, atypical bacteria)
   b. Immunosuppressive agents can blunt the inflammatory response to infection and cause late presentation of infection
   c. Development of malignant disease appears primarily caused by direct mitogenic effects of the agent
   d. Lymphoma is the most common malignant tumor among transplant recipients
   e. Graft-versus-host disease is a progressive condition and is extremely difficult to manage

COMMENT: The most obvious complication of immunosuppression is infection. As immunosuppression becomes stronger and more effective, the recipient's ability to resist infection diminishes. Transplant recipients are susceptible to both typical bacterial infections (upper urinary tract infection, pneumonia, wound infection) and infections with unusual organisms (fungi, viruses, atypical bacteria). Immunosuppressive agents block the inflammatory response to infection so that the signs and symptoms are subtle or manifest late in the infectious process.

Another complication in allograft recipients is malignant disease. The immunosuppressive drugs do not appear to be directly mitogenic or transforming but rather probably suppress immune mechanisms that keep transformed cells in check. Squamous cell carcinoma of the exposed area of the skin is by far the most common malignant tumor. Lymphoma is the next most common tumor; it is 10 to 100 times more common among transplant recipients than among the general population. The tumor usually is non-Hodgkin's B-cell lymphoma and often is related to malignant transformation by Epstein-Barr virus.

Another complication of organ allografting is graft-vs-host disease. This disease usually is self-limited as donor cells stimulated by the host alloantigen are eliminated by immunosuppression or host antidonor responses.

ANSWER: b

REFERENCE: *Chapter 16—Transplantation and Immunology: Transplant Immunology; Regulation of the Immune Response*

6. Current clinical protocols determine a limited number of variables and parameters for matching and allocation of donor organs to potential recipients. Which of the following statements is/are true concerning aspects of immunity important for clinical transplantation?

   a. HLA matching is important for renal, pancreatic, and hepatic transplantation
   b. A cross-matching assay shows whether there are preformed antibodies in the recipient's serum that will react with antigens on the cell surface of the potential donor's lymphocytes
   c. A patient with a history of multiple transfusions or previous transplantation has a high panel reactive antibody (PRA)
   d. A normal heterozygous person with a complete donor-recipient match has a four-antigen match

COMMENT: ABO compatibility is required for successful transplantation. The central position of the MHC in immune regulation suggests that HLA matching also is important for allografting. Data prove that HLA matching is important for renal and pancreatic transplantation. Data also show that HLA matching is not important for hepatic transplantation and does not affect graft survival. The main loci typed are HLA-A, HLA-B, and HLA-DR. For a normal, completely heterozygous person this results in six antigens typed, and a complete donor-recipient match is called a *six-antigen match*. An important test for graft compatibility is cross-matching. The results of this assay show whether preformed antibodies are present in the potential recipient's serum that will react with antigens on the cell surface of the potential donor's lymphocytes. A positive cross-match means that such antibodies are present and that hyperacute rejection will occur if transplantation is performed. Another important test that reflects the presence of host antidonor antibodies is the PRA. Most patients on transplantation lists send serum samples to the transplantation center on a regular basis. These samples are tested against a panel of typing cells of known HLA specificities. Most persons should have no anti-HLA antibodies and have a low PRA value (zero to 5%). Patients who have received transfusions, are pregnant, have undergone previous transplantation, or have an autoimmune disorder that induces a large number of antibodies may have a high PRA value (50% to 99%). The presence of a very high PRA value suggests a patient is likely to have a positive cross-match.

ANSWER: b, c

REFERENCE: *Chapter 16—Transplantation and Immunology: Transplant Immunology; Regulation of the Immune Response*

7. Which of the following characteristics or conditions excludes someone as a suitable cadaveric organ donor?

   a. Active systemic bacterial infection
   b. Primary malignant tumor of the central nervous system
   c. Age older than 65 years
   d. History of cholecystectomy if the liver is being donated

COMMENT: The characteristics of a suitable cadaveric organ donor can be divided into those that are general and those that are organ specific. The general attributes of an acceptable organ donor include establishment of a diagnosis of brain death, previously good general health, and relative hemodynamic stability from the time of the advanced precipitating brain death until organ procurement is complete. As experience has been gained with donors considerably less than ideal, it has become apparent that arbitrarily defined chronologic age limits for organ donors are unnecessary.

Active systemic infection is an absolute contraindication to organ donation. Documented positive blood cultures for known systemic infection that has not been completely eradicated exclude the potential organ donor because of risk of transmission of infection to an immunosuppressed recipient. All potential organ donors, whether or not they are considered at high risk, should be tested for HIV infection as well as hepatitis B and C virus infection. Cancer, treated or not, has long been considered to contravene in organ donation. The only exception has been a primary malignant tumor of the central nervous system.

The condition of particular organs in great measure dictates individual suitability for transplantation. Preexisting hepatic disease usually can be identified before organ procurement. A history of hepatitis or cirrhosis of any kind precludes donation. Although calculous biliary tract disease appears to be a contraindication to hepatic procurement, previous cholecystectomy for uncomplicated cholelithiasis is not an absolute contraindication to liver donation.

ANSWER: a

REFERENCE: *Chapter 16—Transplantation and Immunology: Organ Preservation; Contemporary Clinical Practice*

8. Which of the following statements is/are true concerning techniques for multiple organ procurement and preservation?

a. The liver and pancreas usually are removed en bloc and separated in a bench procedure
b. Renal allograft function is improved with use of machine perfusion
c. University of Wisconsin (UW) cold storage solution is favored in most programs for hepatic and pancreatic transplantation
d. Cardiac allografts have the shortest limit of cold ischemia

COMMENT: The complexity of multiple organ procurement involves the coordination of at least two teams—thoracic and abdominal. The liver and pancreas usually are removed en bloc with the organs separated as a bench procedure; the celiac axis is retained for the liver. The kidneys also are removed en bloc. Studies indicate that posttransplantation renal allograft function is similar whether simple hypothermia or the more cumbersome technique of machine perfusion is used. For decades, the primary solution used for cold storage preservation of kidneys was Euro-Collins solution. A new solution, UW solution, has been developed with ingredients designed to provide high-energy phosphate precursors, hydrogen ion buffering capacity, and antioxidant properties. Although the advantage over Euro-Collins solution for kidneys is unclear, UW solution is used for preservation by nearly all programs in which hepatic and pancreatic transplantation is performed. Both organs can be stored reliably for 24 hours. Kidneys can generally be safely stored for 36 to 48 hours before transplantation. Cardiac preservation has changed relatively little in recent years. Hyperkalemic crystalloid cardioplegia solution is used at 4°C, and 4 hours is generally the accepted limit of cold ischemia. The current limit of cold ischemia for small bowel is approximately 12 hours.

ANSWER: a, c, d

REFERENCE: *Chapter 16—Transplantation and Immunology: Organ Preservation; Contemporary Clinical Practice*

9. A 30-year-old woman has chronic renal failure as a secondary consequence of diabetes mellitus. She is approaching dialysis, and her 35-year-old brother offers to donate a kidney. The patient is blood type A. In the course of the evaluation of the brother, which of the following factors would preclude living-related donation of a kidney?

a. Polycystic renal disease
b. History of renal stone
c. Blood type B
d. Blood type A

COMMENT: Evaluation of a possible living kidney donor begins with assessment of ABO blood type, histocompatibility testing, and determination of a cytotoxic cross-match result. The latter is a test for preformed antidonor antibody directed at relevant HLA-A, HLA-B, and HLA-DR gene products. This test result must be negative for transplantation to proceed. Careful medical and psychosocial screening is performed to find inherited renal disease, such as polycystic kidney disease, which precludes donation, or other evidence of renal dysfunction. A history of passage of a renal stone is not necessarily a contraindication to donation. General good health is a prerequisite. If the findings at physical examination are normal, screening with a chest radiograph, electrocardiogram, survey blood work, and urinalysis is completed.

ANSWER: a, c

REFERENCE: *Chapter 16—Transplantation and Immunology: Renal transplantation; Recipient Assessment*

10. A 45-year-old man with end-stage renal disease secondary to diabetes mellitus undergoes cadaveric renal transplantation. The graft is a three-antigen match, and the initial recovery is uncomplicated. The recipient serum creatinine concentration decreases to 0.9 mg/dL. Six weeks after the operation, the patient reports fever and malaise. The serum creatinine concentration is 1.5 mg/dL. In addition to acute rejection, the differential diagnosis should include:

a. Posttransplantation immunoproliferative disease
b. Herpes virus infection
c. Wound infection
d. Hyperacute rejection

COMMENT: Infection and neoplasia are the two primary categories of posttransplantation complication specifically attributable to the need for maintenance of an immunosuppressed state. Almost all recipients of renal transplants have an infection at some point. Early infections tend to be associated with the surgical procedure, involving the wound, perinephric space, or bladder. Pneumonia may be related to intraoperative intubation and mechanical ventilation. Approximately 4 to 6 weeks after transplantation, viral infections first start to appear. Cytomegalovirus infection is common, especially if a seronegative recipient receives an organ from a seropositive donor. Prophylactic antiviral regimens have been devised for such high-risk combinations, but cytomegalovirus disease can still occur. This herpesvirus infection manifests as fever, malaise, anorexia, and diminished renal allograft function. Extrarenal manifestations include interstitial pneumonitis, myocarditis, gastrointestinal involvement, and cerebritis. Antiviral therapy with ganciclovir is generally effective, although treatment must be given for 3 to 4 weeks and recurrence is possible, particularly among children.

ANSWER: b

REFERENCE: *Chapter 16—Transplantation and Immunology: Renal Transplantation; Complications*

11. Long-term survivors after renal transplantation are at an increased risk of neoplasia relative to control populations. Which of the following neoplasms has/have been associated with the posttransplantation state?

a. Cervical cancer
b. Squamous cell skin cancer
c. Melanoma
d. Lymphoma

COMMENT: The incidence of neoplasia is considerably higher among renal transplant recipients than among the general population. It has been estimated that cancer develops in approximately 4% of recipients. This figure underestimates the true incidence, because longer graft and patient survival times seem to be associated with continuing cumulative risk. The most common malignant tumor after renal transplantation is skin cancer, primarily squamous cell carcinoma. Transplant recipients are at higher risk of nodal spread and multiple tumors than are persons who are not immunosuppressed.

Posttransplantation lymphoproliferative disease can develop in association with Epstein-Barr virus infection. It is thought that B-cell transformation occurs under the influence of this virus. Initially, polyclonal proliferation occurs, but full B-cell lymphoma can develop if the condition is not arrested by reduction or cessation of immunosuppression. Progression to oligoclonal or monoclonal disease requires institution of chemotherapy. Cervical carcinoma in situ occurs at a rate 14 times higher than for the general population, and there is a 100-fold increase in the incidences of vulvar and anal carcinoma. The progression of epithelial carcinoma does not appear to be affected by reduction or even cessation of immunosuppressive drugs.

ANSWER: a, b, d

REFERENCE: *Chapter 16—Transplantation and Immunology: Renal Transplantation; Long-term Complications and Outcome*

12. Increases in serum creatinine values and diminished urine output soon after renal transplantation are the hallmarks of acute rejection. The differential diagnosis of decreased renal function also includes:

a. Cyclosporine toxicity
b. Transplant arterial stenosis
c. Ureteral stenosis
d. Cytomegalovirus infection

COMMENT: Acute rejection typically occurs 1 week to 3 months after transplantation. Decreased allograft function with increasing serum creatinine values and diminished urine output are hallmarks of rejection. Additional signs and symptoms, such as low-grade fever, allograft tenderness, and hypertension may suggest the diagnosis. It is important to confirm the suspicion of allograft rejection with percutaneous biopsy whenever possible, because several other diagnoses can have similar findings. These include cyclosporine or tacrolimus nephrotoxicity, ureteral obstruction, infection, transplant renal arterial stenosis, and recurrence of the underlying renal disease.

Acute allograft rejection usually is managed first by means of increasing immunosuppression. Pulse glucocorticoids (4 to 8 mg/kg methylprednisolone daily for 3 days) reverses one half to two thirds of first rejection episodes. Episodes with a more prominent vascular component and those unresponsive to glucocorticoids are managed with anti–T-cell antibody. The most common agent is murine monoclonal antibody directed against the CD3 receptor. A 7 to 10 day course of treatment reverses as many as 94% of steroid-resistant rejection episodes. Alternatives include equine or rabbit polyclonal antilymphocyte preparations.

ANSWER: a, b, c, d

REFERENCE: *Chapter 16—Transplantation and Immunology: Renal Transplantation; Rejection*

13. Which of the following patients would be a candidate for liver transplantation?

a. A 48-year-old man with end-stage liver disease secondary to non-A, non-B hepatitis
b. A 35-year-old man with primary sclerosing cholangitis, ulcerative colitis, and end-stage liver disease
c. A 22-year-old woman with fulminant hepatic failure secondary to acetaminophen overdose
d. A 4-year-old child with congenital biliary atresia after failure of a Kasai procedure
e. A 48-year-old patient with alcoholic cirrhosis and a 2.5-cm central, unresectable hepatoma

COMMENT: In the absence of contraindications, almost any disease resulting in liver failure is amenable to liver transplantation. Primary sclerosing cholangitis is a common indication for transplantation because there is no other effective treatment. The common association with inflammatory bowel disease can somewhat complicate the timing of the procedure; however, in general, hepatic transplantation does not affect the outcome of ulcerative colitis. Non-A, non-B hepatitis is the most common form of hepatitis leading to liver transplantation. Viral hepatitis does recur in the transplanted liver, but it usually follows an indolent course. Biliary atresia is by far the most common indication for hepatic transplantation among pediatric patients. Recommended treatment includes construction of a portoenterostomy (Kasai procedure), if this can be done before the infant is 3 months of age. After this point, success rates diminish markedly. For patients without a satisfactory course, multiple revisions of the portoenterostomy should be avoided to facilitate subsequent transplantation. The most common causes of fulminant hepatic failure are non-A, non-B hepatitis, hepatitis B, and various drug toxicities. In the latter group, acetaminophen toxicity is particularly prominent. Primary malignant tumor of the liver, most often hepatoma, sometimes is an indication for transplantation, but the results usually are worse than in the management of other diseases because of recurrence. Transplantation is justified in the occasional case in which the tumor is central but relatively small, if the patient is otherwise healthy, and if there is no evidence of extrahepatic disease after exhaustive evaluation.

ANSWER: a, b, c, d, e

REFERENCE: *Chapter 16—Transplantation and Immunology: Hepatic Transplantation; Indications for Hepatic Transplantation*

14. Which of the following statements is/are correct concerning postoperative complications after hepatic transplantation?

    a. Primary nonfunction occurs among 5% to 10% of transplanted livers in the immediate postoperative period
    b. Biliary leak, although a common complication, usually is of minimal clinical importance
    c. Portal venous thrombosis occurs much more commonly than does hepatic arterial thrombosis
    d. If postoperative bleeding is encountered, immediate return to the operating room is indicated

COMMENT: Primary nonfunction of the allograft occurs after 5% to 10% of liver transplantation procedures. Most cases of nonfunction are related to inadequate tissue preservation or occult organ dysfunction in the donor, but a sizable percentage can be caused by immunologic mechanisms. In the worst-case scenario, the patient does not regain consciousness, coagulopathy ensues, and multiple organ failure develops. Liver enzyme values show hepatocellular injury with aspartate aminotransferase and alanine aminotransferase values in the range of 5,000 to 10,000 U/L and little bile production. Hepatic arterial thrombosis occurs among 5% of adults who undergo hepatic transplantation and as many as 25% of children. Postoperative venous thrombosis is much less common than hepatic artery thrombosis, occurring in 2% to 3% of cases. Laparotomy to control postoperative bleeding is required in 15% of cases. In about one half of reoperations, a specific bleeding point is identified. The survival rate is higher in these cases than in those in which diffuse bleeding is encountered, presumably because the latter circumstance usually is associated with poor allograft function and resultant coagulopathy. If profuse bleeding occurs after hepatic transplantation, a common and sensible policy is to provide transfusions until hypothermia and coagulopathy are corrected with subsequent (1 to 3 days) evacuation of blood from the peritoneal cavity. Biliary leakage is a feared complication with a high (50%) mortality. The high mortality may be the result of a concomitant hepatic arterial thrombosis and infection of the leaked bile or of difficulty of bile duct repair in the area of inflamed tissue.

ANSWER: a

REFERENCE: *Chapter 16—Transplantation and Immunology: Hepatic Transplantation; Postoperative Complications*

15. For patients who survive cardiac transplantation for 1 year, the most common cause of death is:

    a. Acute rejection of the graft
    b. Gastrointestinal hemorrhage
    c. Allograft vasculopathy
    d. Rupture of aortic aneurysm

COMMENT: Among patients who survive beyond the first year, the primary limit to long-term survival is cardiac allograft vasculopathy. Widely presumed to be a consequence of "chronic rejection," this process has an incidence of approximately 5% per year. Cardiac allograft vasculopathy can cause progressive insufficiency of coronary flow, myocardial infarction, and death. In contrast to the usual pattern of focal proximal lesions in conventional atherosclerosis, coronary arteries are diffusely involved, and conventional revascularization techniques are not feasible. New immunosuppressive or antiproliferative agents may prevent this process. Research has drawn attention to the importance of donor stress associated with brain death and ischemia-reperfusion injury in the incidence and severity of cardiac allograft vasculopathy in animal models.

ANSWER: c

REFERENCE: *Chapter 16—Transplantation and Immunology: Cardiac Transplantation; Results*

16. Which of the following statements is/are true concerning the results of lung transplantation?

 a. The 1-year survival rate after single-lung transplantation is considerably better than after bilateral transplantation
 b. The worst survival is among patients with pulmonary hypertension
 c. Patients with cystic fibrosis have markedly poorer results than do patients with emphysema
 d. Infection is a common cause of mortality in both the early and the late posttransplantation period

COMMENT: Since the first successful lung transplantation, more than 3,000 transplantation procedures have been performed. The overall 1-year actuarial survival rate after lung transplantation is approximately 70% (single lung, 70%; bilateral lung, 74%). Two years after transplantation, the survival rate decreases to 63%. Patients with emphysema have the best survival rate at 1 and 2 years, and those with pulmonary hypertension have the worst (77% versus 61%). Patients with cystic fibrosis do almost as well as the group with emphysema (72%). The survival rate continues to decrease at 3 years with an overall survival rate of 57%, which decreases to 51% at 4 years and 46% at 5 years. Causes of recipient death can be categorized according to the time frame in which they occur. Early death (less than 90 days after transplantation) most commonly results from bacterial infection. Infection also accounts for approximately one third of late deaths (more than 90 days) after transplantation. A similar percentage results from manifestations of chronic rejection and obliterative bronchiolitis.

ANSWER: b, d

REFERENCE: *Chapter 16—Transplantation and Immunology: Pulmonary Transplantation; Results*

17. Which of the following statements is/are true concerning physiologic changes after lung transplantation?

 a. Among patients with pulmonary hypertension, changes in right ventricular function and pulmonary arterial pressure take weeks to months to resolve
 b. In single-lung transplantation, changes in pulmonary function occur almost immediately after transplantation
 c. Patients who undergo double-lung transplantation have better pulmonary function results and better exercise capabilities than do patients who undergo single-lung transplantation
 d. After single-lung transplantation, ventilation-perfusion mismatch persists and carbon dioxide retention occurs

COMMENT: Single-lung transplantation in the care of patients with pulmonary hypertension has been particularly illustrative of the potential for reversal of right ventricular dysfunction. As soon as the lung is implanted, the morphologic features of the right ventricle change markedly, as assessed with transesophageal echocardiography. The intraventricular septum, previously bulging into the left ventricle, immediately assumes the normal position. An increase in contractility of the right ventricle occurs with a substantial decrease in dilatation. Pulmonary arterial pressure immediately decreases and is essentially normal by the time the patient leaves the operating room.

One would also expect marked ventilation-perfusion mismatch to occur with ventilation to the native lung occurring preferentially because the native lung is much more compliant. Conversely, perfusion should preferentially go to the newly transplanted lung because of lower pulmonary vascular resistance. Despite this occurrence, patients who undergo this operation do well from a functional standpoint. By 3 months after transplantation, the ventilation-perfusion mismatch narrows. Despite this mismatch, patients do not have carbon dioxide retention. From a clinical standpoint, improvement in pulmonary function occurs almost immediately after transplantation. The measurement most often used is FEV_1, and marked improvement is seen within 2 weeks. The FEV_1 essentially triples and then remains fairly stable. Improvement after bilateral lung transplantation is slightly better. Although patients who receive two lungs may do better on pulmonary function tests, this benefit is not translated to considerably better exercise capability.

ANSWER: b

REFERENCE: *Chapter 16—Transplantation and Immunology: Pulmonary Transplantation; Posttransplantation Physiology*

18. Type 1 diabetes mellitus and type 2 diabetes mellitus can be differentiated on clinical grounds. Factors consistent with type 1 diabetes mellitus include:

    a. History of ketoacidosis
    b. Onset before 14 years of age
    c. Strong family history of the disease
    d. Glucose-stimulated C-peptide level less than 30 ng/mL

COMMENT: For most patients referred for pancreatic transplantation, it is not difficult to determine on clinical grounds whether the candidate has type 1 (insulin-dependent) diabetes mellitus. It is uncertain whether patients with type 2 (non-insulin-dependent) diabetes mellitus will benefit from pancreatic transplantation. However, the pathophysiologic features of type 2 diabetes mellitus include peripheral insulin resistance and elevated peripheral insulin levels; therefore addition of a transplanted pancreas may not be of benefit. Despite this, there are some reports of successful pancreatic transplantation for type 2 diabetes mellitus.

Type 1 diabetes is characterized by juvenile onset, no history of obesity, a history of episodes of ketoacidosis, and no strong family history. If a transplantation candidate has an uncertain clinical history, measurement of serum C peptide level after oral administration of 100 g glucose can confirm the diagnosis of insulinopenic type 1 diabetes mellitus.

ANSWER: a, b, d

REFERENCE: *Chapter 16—Transplantation and Immunology: Pancreatic and Islet Transplantation; Classification and Pathophysiology*

19. Indications for pancreas transplantation include:

    a. Severe, labile diabetes caused by lack of compliance with the prescribed insulin regimen
    b. Severe autonomic neuropathy
    c. Type 1 diabetes with diabetic nephropathy but without other forms of secondary diabetic complications
    d. New-onset type 1 diabetes in a teenager

COMMENT: In most cases, the indications for pancreatic transplantation are not difficult to determine for any given candidate. Most candidates have marked secondary complications, including diabetic retinopathy, peripheral and autonomic neuropathy, end-stage renal disease, and a history of labile diabetes. Labile diabetes is an indication for transplantation; however, if the patient is noncompliant with the insulin regimen, he or she will not likely comply with the immunosuppression regimen and should not undergo transplantation. Patients with newly diagnosed type 1 diabetes mellitus should be treated medically. This is particularly true because for unknown reasons secondary complications do not develop before puberty.

ANSWER: b, c

REFERENCE: *Chapter 16—Transplantation and Immunology: Pancreatic and Islet Transplantation; Pancreatic Transplantation*

20. Donor factors that should exclude pancreatic procurement and transplantation include:

a. Donor blood glucose concentration of 400 mg/dL
b. Donor serum amylase concentration of 770 U/L
c. Donor age 6 years and weight 19 kg
d. Donor history of alcohol consumption

COMMENT: Few exclusion criteria automatically prevent procurement of a pancreas. Most centers do not use donors younger than 8 years and lighter than 30 kg because the pancreas is difficult to reconstruct and the thrombosis rate is high. After 55 years of age, the β cell mass begins to decline, so this has been a maximum age in many centers. Donor alcohol abuse can cause chronic pancreatitis, but this can be determined at the time of procurement by means of visual inspection of the pancreas. Exclusion of a donor because of past alcohol use should not be automatic. Abnormal donor glucose and amylase levels are the most common reasons that inexperienced surgeons reject a donor pancreas. Neither of these factors has ever been shown to affect outcome.

ANSWER: c

REFERENCE: *Chapter 16—Transplantation and Immunology: Pancreatic and Islet Transplantation; Organ Procurement*

21. Proof of benefit of pancreatic transplantation comes from demonstrated effect in arrest or reversal of all secondary complications except:

a. Diabetic nephropathy
b. Diabetic retinopathy
c. Diabetic peripheral neuropathy
d. Diabetic autonomic neuropathy

COMMENT: Studies conducted after pancreatic transplantation have shown that successful transplantation is beneficial in the arrest and reversal of peripheral and autonomic neuropathy and prevention and reversal of nephropathy. Short-term studies of retinopathy have not shown benefit. Long-term study of patients in the Diabetes Control and Complications Trial showed prevention of retinopathy and slowing of progression of retinopathy. It is likely that similar long-term studies of recipients of pancreatic transplants would show an effect on retinopathy.

ANSWER: b

REFERENCE: *Chapter 16—Transplantation and Immunology: Pancreatic and Islet Transplantation; Effects of Pancreatic Transplantation on Secondary Complications*

22. Barriers to successful islet transplantation include all of the following except :

a. Nonspecific immunity
b. Recurrent autoimmunity
c. Inability to isolate a sufficient number of human islets from the whole pancreas
d. Inordinate vulnerability of islets to rejection compared with the whole pancreas

COMMENT: The development of successful islet transplantation has been hampered by obstacles unique to islet transplantation. Until recently, the yield from islet isolation from the whole pancreas was very low. It is now possible to reverse diabetes in a human with the islets from a single human pancreas. There is no evidence in either humans or rodent models that islets are more sensitive to rejection than the whole pancreas. Islets, however, appear to be peculiarly sensitive to the effects of nonspecific immunity mediated by cytokines and nitric oxide. Similarly, islets are peculiarly sensitive to recurrent autoimmunity.

ANSWER: c, d

REFERENCE: *Chapter 16—Transplantation and Immunology: Pancreatic and Islet Transplantation; Barriers to Successful Islet Transplantation*

CHAPTER 17

EVIDENCE-BASED SURGERY

1. Which of the following definitions is/are true concerning clinical outcome measurements?

    a. Postoperative mortality refers to death within the hospital after an operation
    b. Relative risk reduction is the reduction of adverse clinical outcomes due to progression disease, achieved by a treatment
    c. The absolute risk reduction is the difference in event rates between control and treatment groups
    d. The number needed to be treated is the number of patients necessary in a study to reach statistical significance

COMMENT: The most commonly used clinical measures of the consequences of surgical therapy are mortality, gains in life expectancy, relative risk and relative risk reduction, absolute risk reduction, and number needed to be treated. Mortality is the most reliably measured clinical outcome. It is most meaningfully expressed as the proportion of deaths from a particular cause over a defined time interval and most reliably measured from death certificates. Postoperative mortality usually refers to death within 30 days after a procedure. However, because patients today commonly have hospital stays that are far shorter than one month, care must be taken to differentiate between in-hospital versus postoperative mortality. The relative risk is the ratio of probabilities of adverse outcomes in two treatments being compared. Alternatively, retrospective study designs commonly measure odds ratios rather than relative risk. Relative risk reduction is the reduction of adverse clinical outcomes due to the progression of disease, achieved by a treatment. It is expressed in the difference in event rates between the control and treatment groups, divided by the event rate in the control group. Relative risk reduction does not reflect the magnitude of the risk without therapy, and thus it overestimates or underestimates the effect of therapy when adverse events in untreated patients are very rare or very common, respectively. The absolute risk reduction is the difference in event rates between the control and treatment groups. Last, the number needed to be treated is the number of patients who must be treated to prevent one adverse event.

ANSWER: b, c

REFERENCE: *Chapter 17—Evidence-based Surgery: Clinical Outcomes Measurement*

2. Patient reported outcomes have been used with increased frequency in the area of evidence-based surgery. Which of the following statements is/are true concerning such outcomes?

    a. Quality of life assessment can be either generic or disease-specific
    b. Psychometric measures are based on the patient's rating of his or her health on a continuum
    c. Patients' satisfaction refers to patient's subjective evaluation of their health care
    d. Utility measures refer to the value placed by the individual on a particular health state

COMMENT: Surgical studies have increasingly examined patient-reported outcome measures such as patient-reported health status or health-related quality of life, including functioning and well-being as reported by patients, and patients satisfaction with health care. Quality of life is a broad concept that encompasses a person's experience and assessment of aspects of life. Health-related quality of life encompasses several dimensions of health status that are directly experienced by the person, including physical functioning, psychological well-being, cognitive functioning, social and role functioning, and general health perceptions. There are two basic approaches to quality of life assessment: generic and disease specific. Generic instruments are designed for use across different diseases, treatments, settings, and patient groups. The major advantage is they can be used in any population and allow comparisons of the relative impact of various health interventions. Disease-specific measures focus on dimensions of health related to a particular disease, population, symptom, or problem and may be more responsive to a change in the patient's condition than a generic instrument. Health profiles attempt to measure multiple important dimensions of health-related quality of life. Descriptive or psychometric measures are based on the patient's reporting or ratings of his or her health state on a continuum. Utility measures, derived from economic and decision theory, refer to the value placed by the individual on a particular health state. Patient satisfaction refers to patients' subjective evaluation of their health care. Patient ratings of care reflect what they think is important about the quality of care, including the doctor–patient relationship and their perception of the accuracy of diagnosis and therapy

ANSWER: a, b, c, d

REFERENCE: *Chapter 17—Evidence-based Surgery: Patient-reported Outcomes Measurements*

3. Which of the following statements is/are true concerning randomized clinical trials?

a. Randomized clinical trials are generally accepted as the definitive approach for assessing the efficacy of a new treatment
b. There is little information to be gained on the natural history of a disease while conducting a randomized clinical trial
c. Randomized clinical trials can be applied to essentially all new therapies
d. A randomized clinical trial is the most ethical way to assess the treatment of a clinical problem

COMMENT: Randomized clinical trials have many strengths and weaknesses. First, randomized clinical trials are generally accepted as the definitive approach for assessing the efficacy of a new treatment. The process of randomization, when properly implemented, provides the means by which the myriad factors that may influence the results of a trial are equally distributed between the experimental treatment group and the usual care one. A second strength is ability to provide information on the natural history of a disease during both usual care and the experimental treatment. There are also several weaknesses in the randomized clinical trial. The cost of such studies are usually considerable. It is impossible to subject all new therapies to a randomized clinical trial evaluation in part because of those costs. Such studies also require considerable time, both for recruitment and, frequently, to obtain the outcomes of interest. There are also instances in which undertaking a randomized trial is simply not ethical, such as withholding a known appropriate treatment to assess another experimental therapy. Finally, randomized clinical trials are not based on random samples of the population of patients. Investigators in a given trial may seek to exclude all but a very specific subset of patients with a particular disease. It is therefore often difficult for the results of a randomized clinical trial to be generalized to the population of patients with a particular disease.

ANSWER: a

REFERENCE: *Chapter 17—Evidence-based Surgery: Methodologic Considerations*

4. The value of a study in directing care is based on the strength of the clinical evidence. Which of the following statements is/are true concerning the United States Preventive Services Task Force classification of levels of evidence?

a. The highest quality level of evidence comes from a randomized, controlled trial
b. A well-designed controlled trial has the same level of evidence whether or not randomization is included
c. Level III evidence is generally drawn from clinical descriptive studies and/or case reports
d. Level IV quality of evidence is considered the strongest level in this classification

COMMENT: Table 17.1.

ANSWER: a, c

REFERENCE: *Chapter 17—Evidence-based Surgery: Methodologic Considerations*

Table 17.1. UNITED STATES PREVENTIVE SERVICES TASK FORCE CLASSIFICATION OF LEVELS OF EVIDENCE

Level	Quality of Evidence
I	Evidence obtained from at least one properly conducted randomized, controlled trial
II-1	Evidence obtained from well designed controlled trials without randomization
II-2	Evidence obtained from well designed cohort or case-control analytic studies, preferably from more than one center or research group
II-3	Evidence obtained from several time series with or without intervention, or dramatic result in uncontrolled experiments
III	Opinions of respected authorities based on clinical experiences, descriptive studies and case reports, or reports of expert committees

5. The quality of a measurement is determined by reliability and validity and is an important factor that can affect the quality of evidence. Which of the following statements is/are true concerning these qualities?

a. Reliability refers to a measure's consistency or repeatability
b. A reliable measurement is consistent regardless of the observer
c. Validity is a function of reliability
d. A reliable measurement is always valid

COMMENT: Reliability refers to a measure's consistency or repeatability; that is, does it give the same result repeatedly when the same thing is measured? Reliability is often measured by the following: Test-retest repeatability is the repeated use of the same measure on the same subject, yielding the same value results, when the property measured is something that should be stable over the time between the two measurements and interrated reliability provides consistency of results when several observers or judges obtain the information or make judgments. Validity refers to whether a measure reflects what is intended to measure (i.e., accuracy). Validity is a function of reliability: unreliable measures cannot be valid. However, reliable measures may lack validity because of built-in sources of bias.

ANSWER: a, b, c

REFERENCE: *Chapter 17—Evidence-based Surgery: Methodologic Considerations*

6. Which of the following would be considered a major database source?

a. Medical records
b. Patient-based surveys
c. Surgeon's opinions
d. Administrative databases

COMMENT: There are three major sources of databases for most medical and surgical effectiveness research: administrative databases, medical records, and patient-based surveys. Administrative databases, large claims files collected for billing purposes, are very useful for outcomes studies of a descriptive nature such as exploring variations in treatment patterns. Medical records offer a rich source of information about patients and their care. In general, medical charts document patients' histories, chief complaints, presenting symptoms, physical examinations, clinical assessments and diagnoses, diagnostic laboratory results, procedures, medications, in-hospital responses to therapy, clinical courses, and discharge plans. Patient surveys can obtain information unavailable in either the administrative files or the medical records. Survey instruments can be designed to capture subjective information such as a perception of quality, satisfaction, personal preferences, or utility.

ANSWER: a, b, d

REFERENCE: *Chapter 17—Evidence-based Surgery: Methodologic Considerations*

TWO

SURGICAL PRACTICE

Section A
HEAD AND NECK

CHAPTER 18

HEAD AND NECK

1. Recognized risk factors for cancer of the upper aerodigestive tract include:
   a. Tobacco smoking
   b. Alcohol consumption
   c. Epstein-Barr virus infection
   d. Tobacco chewing

COMMENT: The best-recognized carcinogens are tobacco use and alcohol consumption. These behaviors account for approximately 80% of all cases of cancer of the upper aerodigestive tract, and users of these drugs have a 15-fold greater increase of development of squamous cell carcinoma than do nonsmokers and nondrinkers. Aside from smoking and drinking, other, less-recognized risk factors for malignant tumors of the head and neck exist, and these should be included in the complete history. They include (a) exposure to ultraviolet and ionizing radiation, exposure to neoprene inorganic arsenics, burns, and riboflavin deficiency for skin cancers; (b) exposure to wood dust, leather manufacturing, nickel refining, radium dial painting, thorotrast, and mustard gas for nose and paranasal sinus cancer; (c) ingestion of nitrosamine or salted fish, Epstein-Barr virus types II and III infection, and vitamin deficiency for nasopharyngeal carcinoma; (d) betel nut chewing, snuff use, tobacco chewing, reverse smoking, syphilis, vitamin B and riboflavin deficiencies, and chronic irritation for oral carcinoma; (e) exposure to asbestos, coke ovens, or wood dust and riboflavin deficiency for laryngeal and hypopharyngeal carcinoma; (f) radiation exposure, iodine deficiency, and genetic inheritance for thyroid cancer; and (g) radiation exposure and Inuit heritage for salivary gland neoplasms.

ANSWER: a, b, c, d

REFERENCE: *Chapter 18—Head and Neck: Diagnostic Evaluation*

2. A 45-year-old man reports severe throat pain and inability to swallow because of pain and fever. Physical examination reveals a temperature of 103°F (39.4°C), hoarseness, and erythema and swelling of the supraglottis. Appropriate initial therapy includes:

a. Intravenous penicillin
b. Intravenous steroids
c. Humidified air
d. Tracheostomy
e. Oral ampicillin

COMMENT: An important consideration in the evaluation of a patient with a sore throat is not to miss an occult supraglottitis. This condition often is misdiagnosed as pharyngitis; however, suspicion should be heightened when the patient states that the sore throat is lower than usual or that there is impressive odynophagia and hoarseness, which rarely accompany uncomplicated pharyngitis. Since the universal institution of *Haemophilus influenzae* B vaccine, the epidemiologic characteristics of epiglottitis and supraglottitis have changed. More cases are being diagnosed among adults than among children, and the dominant organism has shifted from *Haemophilus* to *Staphylococcus aureus* and *Streptococcus pyogenes*. The disease usually is more indolent among adults than among children. If there is rapid onset of symptoms (less than 4 hours) accompanied by a high fever (more than 102.5°F [39.2°C]) and a white blood cell count greater than 20,000/dL, the airway should be secured immediately, because rapid airway compromise is likely. If these criteria are not met, adults can typically be treated with intravenous augmented penicillin therapy, humidification, and steroid therapy in an intensive care unit. The acute phase of inflammation responds to therapy within 48 to 72 hours.

ANSWER: a, b, c

REFERENCE: *Chapter 18—Head and Neck: Infectious Processes; Pharyngitis*

3. A 60-year-old woman has a painless mass in the right cheek that has been present for 2 months. Physical examination shows a painless, immobile mass associated with the right parotid gland. Findings at examination of the cranial nerves are normal. No adenopathy is found. Results of routine laboratory tests and a chest radiograph are within normal limits. Appropriate initial therapy includes:

a. Superficial parotidectomy
b. Superficial parotidectomy with ipsilateral neck dissection
c. Fine-needle aspiration of the mass
d. Total parotidectomy with seventh cranial nerve reconstruction

COMMENT: The salivary glands are divided into the major salivary glands (parotid, submandibular, and sublingual glands) and the minor salivary glands (several thousand glands distributed through the upper aerodigestive tract). Approximately 80% of salivary gland neoplasms originate in the parotid gland, 10% to 15% in the submandibular gland, and the others in the sublingual and minor salivary glands. Approximately 80% of parotid neoplasms are benign, and approximately 50% of submandibular neoplasms are benign. Fewer than 40% of sublingual and minor salivary lesions are benign. Malignant tumors often are asymptomatic, but signs and symptoms indicative of malignant growth include rapid tumor enlargement, pain, trismus, and facial or other cranial nerve paralyses. An essential diagnostic test is fine-needle aspiration, which has 95% sensitivity for salivary gland neoplasms. Any patient with a mass in the salivary glands should undergo fine-needle aspiration for histologic diagnosis and surgical planning.

ANSWER: c

REFERENCE: *Chapter 18—Head and Neck: Salivary Gland Neoplasms*

4. The most common histologic type of malignant tumor of the head and neck is:
   a. Adenocarcinoma
   b. Squamous cell cancer
   c. Melanoma
   d. Sarcoma

COMMENT: The neoplasm most commonly affecting the head and neck is squamous cell carcinoma. More than 90% of head and neck cancers are of this histologic type. The incidence of synchronous primary tumors varies from 2.5% to as high as 25%. A synchronous tumor rate of 5% to 15% is highest among patients with tumors of the hypopharynx. Tumors of the digestive tract, that is, oral cavity, oropharynx, or hypopharynx, tend to have second primary lesions in other regions of the digestive tract. Conversely, laryngeal lesions tend to have second primary tumors in other portions of the respiratory tract, predominantly the lungs and main stem bronchi.

ANSWER: b

REFERENCE: *Chapter 18—Head and Neck: Treatment by Site*

5. A 56-year-old man with a long history of smoking has new-onset hoarseness. Laryngoscopic examination reveals a tumor involving the right vocal cord with fixation of the vocal cord. Biopsy shows invasive squamous cell carcinoma. Appropriate initial treatment includes:
   a. Cisplatin, 5-fluorouracil, and radiation therapy
   b. Radiation therapy alone
   c. Laryngectomy and bilateral neck dissection
   d. Laser ablation of vocal cord tumor

COMMENT: Results of a landmark study of advanced laryngeal cancer conducted by the Department of Veterans Affairs changed the management of advanced laryngeal tumor. In this seminal study, induction chemotherapy (cisplatin and 5-fluorouracil) was combined with radiation therapy as an alternative to traditional laryngectomy with radiation therapy in the treatment of patients with advanced squamous carcinoma of the larynx. Analysis after a median 60-month follow-up period showed the larynx was preserved in 66% of surviving patients without a decrease in survival rate. The estimated survival rate for the two groups was similar at 53% and 56%. A 10-year follow-up study on this same study population showed no significant difference in overall survival rate. Thirty percent of patients in the surgery arm were alive, as were 25% of patients in the chemotherapy arm. According to the results of this study, patients with stage III and IV laryngeal cancer typically are treated with induction chemotherapy and radiation therapy in an effort to preserve the larynx. Surgery is reserved for patients who do not respond to chemotherapy or those with recurrences after completion of treatment.

ANSWER: a

REFERENCE: *Chapter 18—Head and Neck: Treatment by Site; Larynx*

Section B
ESOPHAGUS

CHAPTER 19

ESOPHAGUS: ANATOMY, PHYSIOLOGY, AND GASTROESOPHAGEAL REFLUX DISEASE

1. Which of the following statements is/are true concerning the surgical anatomy of the esophagus?

   a. Surgical exposure of the cervical esophagus is best gained through the right side of the neck

   b. Spontaneous esophageal perforation tends to be associated with leakage into the left chest

   c. Access to the entire thoracic esophagus can be obtained only through the left side of the chest

   d. The lower esophageal sphincter (LES) can be recognized distinctly by means of inspection of the gastroesophageal junction

COMMENT: Detailed knowledge of the relations of the esophagus is essential for the surgeon to identify the site and importance of lesions with indirect studies such as endoscopy, contrast radiography, and computed tomography (CT) as well as for safe performance of surgical procedures. The cervical esophagus is approximately 5 cm long. It begins at the level of C6 and extends to the lower border of T1, curving slightly to the left in its descent. Although the surgical approach to this portion of the esophagus can be from either side of the neck through an incision along the anterior border of the sternocleidomastoid muscle, the left side is chosen if possible. Above the level of the tracheal bifurcation, the esophagus moves to the right of the descending aorta. It then moves to the left, passes behind the tracheal bifurcation and the left main bronchus, and descends to the diaphragm. In the lower third, the esophagus courses anteriorly and to the left to pass through the diaphragmatic hiatus. The lower part of the esophagus is covered only by flimsy mediastinal pleura on the left, and this portion is most commonly the site of spontaneous perforation in Boerhaave's syndrome. In general, the lower part of the esophagus is most easily approached through the left side of the chest, but access to the supraaortic esophagus is restricted. Thus left thoracotomy is most useful for performing procedures involving the lower part of the esophagus. However, access to the entire thoracic esophagus can be obtained only from the right side of the chest. This incision, however, limits access to intraabdominal organs by the position of the liver and therefore normally necessitates a separate upper abdominal incision.

The abdominal esophagus begins where the esophagus enters the abdomen through the diaphragmatic hiatus. It is surrounded by a fibroelastic membrane, the phrenoesophageal ligament, which arises from the subdiaphragmatic fascia. The lower limit of the pharyngoesophageal membrane anteriorly is marked by a prominent fat pad, which corresponds to the gastroesophageal junction. The LES is a zone of high pressure 3 to 5 cm long at the lower end of the esophagus. Although the LES does not correspond to any macroscopic anatomic structure, its function appears to be related to the microscopic architecture of the muscle fibers.

ANSWER: b

REFERENCE: *Chapter 19—Esophagus: Anatomy, Physiology, and Gastroesophageal Reflux Disease; Anatomy*

2. Which of the following statements is/are true concerning the blood supply and lymphatic drainage of the esophagus?

   a. The thoracic esophagus receives no direct branches from the aorta, allowing the technique of transhiatal (blunt) esophagectomy
   b. Bleeding esophageal varices are most prominent in the midesophagus
   c. Lymphatic drainage of the lower third of the esophagus goes entirely to the abdominal lymphatic system
   d. Nodal involvement in esophageal cancer is common even if the tumor is limited to the level of the submucosa

COMMENT: The blood supply and venous drainage of the esophagus are largely segmental. The inferior thyroid artery provides the main blood supply to the cervical portion of the esophagus. The thoracic portion of the esophagus receives its blood supply from two sources: branches from two or three bronchial arteries provide the proximal arterial supply, and branches directly from the aorta supply the more distal thoracic esophagus. Intrathoracic mobilization of the esophagus during antireflux procedures often necessitate ligation of these branches. The venous plexus in the submucosa collects capillary blood and delivers it into a periesophageal venous plexus. The left gastric vein or coronary vein provides the principal collateral in portal hypertension when esophageal varices develop. The submucosal veins become much more superficial in the most distal esophagus, 1 to 2 cm above the gastroesophageal junction, and are consequently the most common site of bleeding in portal hypertension.

The lymphatic vessels of the esophagus form a rich submucosal network that drains into regional lymph nodes in the periesophageal connective tissue. There is thus little barrier to longitudinal spread of cancer in the esophagus. Lymphatic drainage from the upper two thirds of the esophagus usually is cephalic, but drainage from the lower one third is in both directions. Although lymphatic metastasis in the esophagus generally involves the regional lymph nodes in proximity, nodal involvement can occur several centimeters away from the primary lesion because of the rich intramural lymphatic anastomotic channels. When carcinoma is limited to the mucosa, the incidence of lymphatic metastasis is low, but once the lesion enters the submucosa, the incidence increases to 60%.

ANSWER: d

REFERENCE: *Chapter 19—Esophagus: Anatomy, Physiology, and Gastroesophageal Reflux Disease; Anatomy*

3. A 57-year-old male undergoes a transhiatal esophagectomy for Barrett's carcinoma. His postoperative course is uncomplicated, but on postoperative day five, the patient is noted to have an episode of aspiration during his first attempts to swallow liquids. Which of the following statements is/are true concerning the reasons behind this problem?

   a. His anastomosis is likely strictured
   b. There is likely a leak at his anastomosis at the neck
   c. The patient likely has delayed gastric emptying due to the vagotomy associated with the procedure
   d. Injury to the right and/or left recurrent laryngeal nerves may have occurred during the resection resulting in cricopharyngeal sphincter dysfunction

COMMENT: The innervation of the cricopharyngeal sphincter and cervical portion of the esophagus is from both the right and left recurrent laryngeal nerves. These nerves, arising from the vegus, travel dorsally around the subclavion artery on the right and the arch of the aorta on the left. They give off branches to both the esophagus and trachea as they ascend in the tracheoesophageal grove. The nerves may be injured during dissection of the upper esophagus in the neck, or during the mediastinal dissection during transhiatal esophagectomy. Although much attention has been given to the vocal chord dysfunction that accompanies recurrent laryngeal nerve damage, it is also clear that cricopharyngeal sphincter dysfunction and motility problems of the cervical esophagus can result from injury to these nerves. Serious episodes of aspiration following recurrent nerve injury are caused not only by cricopharyngeal dysfunction, but also inability to close the glottis during swallowing and loss of the protection afforded by effective coughing.

ANSWER: d

REFERENCE: *Chapter 19—Esophagus: Anatomy, Physiology, and Gastroesophageal Reflux Disease; Anatomy*

4. Which of the following statements is/are true concerning the process of swallowing and esophageal transit of food?
   a. A bolus of food is advanced into the upper esophagus via both peristalsis and an existing pressure gradient
   b. Movement of the food bolus from the esophagus into the stomach involves both peristalsis and a negative pressure gradient.
   c. Swallowing can be either voluntary or a reflex
   d. Neuromuscular diseases affecting cervical esophageal compliance can result in dysphagia

COMMENT: During swallowing, the pressure in the pressure in the hypopharyx arises abruptly to at least 60 mmHg as a consequence of the backward movement of the tongue and contraction of posterior pharyngeal constrictors. A sizable pressure difference develops between the hypopharyngeal pressure and the less than atmospheric mid-esophageal or intrathoracic pressure. This pressure gradient speeds the movement of food from the hypopharynx into the esophagus when the cricopharyngeous or upper esophageal sphincter relaxes. The bolus is both propelled by peristaltic contraction of the posterior pharyngeal constrictors and sucked into the esophagus by the negative pressure. Critical to the bolus being received is the compliance of the cervical esophagus: when compliance is lost because of muscle disease, dysphagia can result.

Swallowing can be started at will, or it can be elicited as a reflex by the stimulation of areas in the mouth of pharynx, among them the anterior and posterior tonsillar pillars in the posterior lateral walls of the hypopharynx.

Pharyngeal activity in swallowing initiates the esophageal phase. Owing to the helical arrangement of its circular muscles, the body of the esophagus functions as a worm drive propulsive pump and is responsible for transmitting a bolus of food into the stomach. The esophageal phase of swallowing represents work done by the esophagus during alimentation to move the food into the stomach over a gradient of 12 mm Hg from a negative-pressure environment (intrathoracic pressure of -6 mmHg) to a positive-pressure environment (intraabdominal pressure of 6 mm Hg). Effective and controlled smooth-muscle function in the lower third of the esophagus is therefore important in pumping food across this gradient.

ANSWER: a, c, d

REFERENCE: *Chapter 19—Esophagus: Anatomy, Physiology, and Gastroesophageal Reflux Disease; Physiology*

5. Which of the following statements is/are true concerning esophageal peristaltic activity?
   a. A sleeve resection in the esophagus generally disrupts peristalsis and leads to ineffective swallowing
   b. The propulsive force of the esophagus is relatively strong
   c. Consecutive swallows are not followed by individual peristaltic waves
   d. Esophageal distension results in an esophageal contractual wave
   e. A large hiatal hernia can disrupt esophageal peristalsis

COMMENT: The peak of a primary peristaltic contraction initiated by a swallow (primary peristalsis) moves down the esophagus at a rate of 2 to 4 cm/s and reaches the distal esophagus about 9 seconds after swallowing starts. Consecutive swallows produce similar primary peristaltic waves, but when the act of swallowing is rapidly repeated, the esophagus remains relaxes and peristaltic wave occurs only after the last movement of the pharynx. Progress of the wave through the esophagus is maintained by sequential activation of esophageal muscles initiated by efferent vagal nerve fibers arising in the swallowing center.

Continuity of esophageal muscle is not necessary for sequential activation if the nerves are intact. If the muscles, not the nerves, are cut transversely, the pressure wave begins distally below the cut as it dies out at the proximal end above the cut. For this reason, a sleeve resection of the esophagus can be performed without destroying its normal function. Afferent impulses from the receptors within the esophageal wall are not essential for progress of the coordinated wave. Afferent nerves, however, do travel to the swallowing center from the esophagus, because if the esophagus is distended at any point, a contractual wave begins with a forceful closure of the upper esophageal sphincter and sweeps down the esophagus.

Despite the rather powerful occlusive pressure, the propulsive force of the esophagus is relatively feeble. Orderly contractions of muscular wall and anchoring the esophagus at its inferior end are necessary for efficient aboral propulsion to occur. Loss of the inferior anchor, as happens with a large hiatal hernia, can lead to inefficient propulsion.

ANSWER: b, e

REFERENCE: *Chapter 19—Esophagus: Anatomy, Physiology, and Gastroesophageal Reflux Disease; Physiology*

6. The lower esophageal sphincter
   a. Is clearly visible grossly in humans
   b. Actively remains closed to prevent reflux of gastric contents into the esophagus
   c. Has intrinsic myogenic tone that is modulated by neural and hormonal mechanisms.
   d. Increases its pressure in response to gastrin and motilin
   e. Decreases its pressure in response to calcium channel blockers, caffeine, theophallin, and diazepam

COMMENT: The lower esophageal sphincter provides a pressure barrier between the esophagus and stomach. Although an anatomically distinct lower esophageal sphincter has been difficult to identify, microdissection studies show that it in humans, the sphincter-like function is related to the architecture of the muscle fibers at the junction of the esophageal tube with the gastric pouch. The sphincter actively remains closed to prevent reflux of gastric contents into the esophagus and opens by relaxation that coincides with a pharyngeal swallow. The lower esophageal returns to its resting level after the peristaltic wave has passed through the esophagus. Consequently, gastric juice that may flow back through the open valve during swallow is returned to the stomach. The lower esophageal sphincter has intrinsic myogenic tone that is modulated by neural and hormonal mechanisms. The α-adrenergic neurotransmitters or beta blockers stimulate the lower esophageal sphincter and alpha blockers and beta stimulants decreases pressure. The hormones gastrin and motilin have been shown to increase lower esophageal sphincter pressure: cholecystokinin, estrogen, glucagon, progesterone, somatostatin, and secretin decrease lower esophageal sphincter pressure. Some pharmacologic agents, such as antacids, cholinergic agonists, metoclopromide are known to increase lower esophageal sphincter pressure. Anticholinegics, barbiturates, calcium channel blockers, caffeine, diazepam, and theophylline decrease lower esophageal sphincter pressure. Peppermint, chocolate, coffee, ethanol, and fat are all associated with deceased lower esophageal sphincter pressure and may be responsible for esophageal symptoms during a sumptuous meal.

ANSWER: b, c, d, e

REFERENCE: *Chapter 19—Esophagus: Anatomy, Physiology, and Gastroesophageal Reflux Disease; Physiology*

7. Which of the following statements is/are true concerning the clinical presentation of patients with gastroesophageal reflux disease (GERD)?
   a. The severity of clinical symptoms correlates nicely with the severity of the underlying esophagitis
   b. The symptom of regurgitation of gastric contents is well controlled with proton pump inhibitors
   c. The diagnosis of GERD can be made very accurately in almost all patients based on symptoms
   d. Although dysphagia may be present in patients with GERD, investigation should be made to rule out a more serious underlying disorder such as esophageal carcinoma

COMMENT: The common complaints in patients with GERD are heartburn, regurgitation, and occasionally dysphagia. The diagnosis of GERD based on symptoms alone, however, is correct in approximately two-thirds of patients because the symptoms are not specific for gastroesophageal reflux and can be caused by other diseases. This fact underscores the need for objective diagnosis before surgical treatment is undertaken. It is also well recognized that the severity of symptoms is not necessarily related to the severity of the underlying disease. Regurgitation is the spontaneous return of gastric contents to the area proximal to the gastroesophageal junction. The symptom is typically worse when the patient lies down, at night, or after a meal. Patients commonly compensate by not eating late at night and by sleeping particularly upright with several pillows or in a chair. This symptom is often less effectively relieved than heartburn by the use of antisecretory agents. Dysphagia is present in up to 40% of patients with GERD. It is generally manifested as the sensation of food hanging up in the lower esophagus rather than difficulty transferring the bolus from the mouth to the esophageal inlet. Classically, dysphagia is limited to solid food with the normal passage of liquids. The presence of dysphagia may also be the sign of a more serious underlying disease such as esophageal carcinoma. This symptom therefore should be investigated promptly and thoroughly.

ANSWER: d

REFERENCE: *Chapter 19—Esophagus: Anatomy, Physiology, and Gastroesophageal Reflux Disease; Gastroesophageal Reflux Disease*

8. The common denominator for virtually all episodes of gastroesophageal reflux is the loss of the normal high-pressure zone of the gastroesophageal junction and the loss of the resistance to the reflux of gastric juice from the stomach to the esophagus. Which of the following statements is/are true concerning the pathophysiology involving the GE junction.

  a. The loss of the high-pressure zone is permanent in essentially all patients with GERD
  b. A permanently defective sphincter is a signal that surgical therapy is likely to be needed for consistent and long-term control of symptoms
  c. Activities that produce a pressure gradient across the diaphragm such as coughing, sniffing or straining can precipitate reflux
  d. Esophageal mucosal damage caused by repetitive exposure to gastric juice results in inflammatory injury of the underlying muscle leading to a permanently defective high-pressure zone or sphincter

COMMENT: In humans, a zone of high-pressure can be identified at the junction of the esophagus and the stomach. This lower esophageal sphincter provides a barrier between the esophagus and the stomach that normally prevents gastric contents from entering the stomach. The common denominator for virtually all episodes of gastroesophageal reflux is the loss of the normal high-pressure zone and resistance it imposes to the flow of gastric juice from the environment of higher pressure, the stomach, to an environment of lower pressure, the esophagus. In severe disease, the high-pressure zone is usually permanently obliterated or reduced. In early disease or normal subjects, loss of the high-pressure zone is usually transient.

For the clinician, the finding of a permanently defective sphincter has several implications. Foremost, it almost always associated with esophageal mucosal injury and predicts that the patient's symptoms would be difficult to control with medical therapy. It is a signal that surgical therapy is likely to be needed for consistent and long-term control of symptoms. It is now accepted that when the sphincter is permanently defective, the condition is irreversible, even with the associated esophagitis is healed. Mucosal damage, caused by repetitive exposure to gastric juice, results in an inflammatory injury of the underlying muscle. This leads to a permanently defective high-pressure zone or sphincter caused initially by the loss of abdominal length and eventually the loss of pressure and overall length. Subsequent inflammation of the esophagus also results in the loss clearance ability and prolonged esophageal exposure to gastric juice. This signals the presence of advanced disease and places the patient at risk for Barrett's metaplasia, stricture, and aspiration. In normal subjects, almost all episodes of reflux are precipitated by belching, which remains an important but decreasing cause of reflux as the grade of esophagitis worsens. Activities that produce a pressure gradient across the diaphragm, such as coughing, sniffing, or straining, become increasingly important in precipitating reflux as the disease, graded according to the severity as the esophagitis progresses. In patients with severe esophagitis, episodes of acid reflux occur spontaneously which suggests that the sphincter is defective in the resting state and that the barrier is permanently lost.

ANSWER: b, c, d

REFERENCE: Chapter 19—Esophagus: Anatomy, Physiology, and Gastroesophageal Reflux Disease; Gastroesophageal Reflux Disease

9. Which of the following statements is/are true concerning the pathophysiology of GERD?

   a. Repeated exposure of the lower esophagus to gastric juice results in a transformation of squamous epithelium to columnar epithelium.
   b. A patient may compensate for the symptoms of GERD by increasing swallowing, which ultimately may complicate the process.
   c. A Schatzki's ring is usually seen in the mid-esophagus and is usually associated with significant obstructive symptoms.
   d. The development of intestinal metaplasia in the cardiac type mucosa can set the stage for malignant degeneration and the development of a squamous cell carcinoma of the lower esophagus

COMMENT: An incompetent esophageal sphincter leads to exposure of the lower esophagus to gastric juice. Repeated exposure causes inflammation of the squamous epithelium, and the development of columnar epithelium. The development of intestinal metaplasia in the cardiac type mucosa can set the stage for the malignant degeneration and the developments of a "Barrett's" cancer (adenocarcinoma). In order to compensate for the symptoms of reflux, the patient begins to have an increase in swallowing, which allows saliva to bathe the injured mucosa and alleviates the discomfort induced by exposure to gastric acid. Increased swallowing, however, results in aerophagia, bloating, and repetitive belching. The distension induced by aerophagia leads to further exposure of the terminal squamous epithelium, repetitive injury, and the development of cardiac-type mucosa. This process can also lead to the development of a fibroidic mucosal ring at the squamous columnar junction (Schatzki's ring). Although often impressive on radiologic examination, a Schatzki's ring seldom leads to significant obstructive symptoms.

ANSWER: a, b

REFERENCE: *Chapter 19—Esophagus: Anatomy, Physiology, and Gastroesophageal Reflux Disease; Gastroesophageal Reflux Disease*

10. Barrett's esophagus can complicate advanced GERD. Which of the following statements is/are true concerning Barrett's esophagus?

   a. Factors predisposing to the development of Barrett's esophagus include early onset of GERD, an abnormal lower esophageal sphincter physiology, and reflux of mixed gastric and duodenal contents into the esophagus
   b. Prospective studies have demonstrated the progression of non-dysplastic Barrett's epithelium to low- and high-grade dysplasia and ultimately carcinoma
   c. The prevalence of dysplasia in patients presenting with Barrett's esophagus ranges from 33%–50%
   d. Prospective studies suggest that 1% of patients with Barrett's esophagus progress to adenocarcinoma per year

COMMENT: Traditionally, Barrett's esophagus was identified by the presence of any columnar mucosa extending at least 3cm into the esophagus. Recent data indicating a specialized intestinal-type epithelium is the only tissue predisposing the malignant degeneration, coupled with the finding of similar risk for malignancy in segments of intestinal metaplasia 3 cm long, have resulted in the diagnosis of Barrett's esophagus being given to endoscopically visible tissue of any length demonstrated to have intestinal metaplasia on histology. The hallmark of intestinal metaplasia is the presence of goblet cells. Factors predisposing to the development of Barrett's esophagus include early onset of GERD, abnormal lower esophageal sphincter and esophageal body physiology, and reflux of mixed gastric and duodenal contents into the esophagus. The prevalence of dysplasia in patients presenting with Barrett's esophagus ranges from 15% to 25%. Few prospective studies have documented the progression of non-dysplastic Barrett's epithelium to low- or high-grade dysplasia. Those data suggest that 5%–10% of patients progress to dysplasia per year and 1% to adenocarcinoma.

ANSWER: a, b, d

REFERENCE: *Chapter 19—Esophagus: Anatomy, Physiology, and Gastroesophageal Reflux Disease; Barrett's Esophagus*

11. Which of the following statements is/are true concerning the treatment of Barrett's esophagus?

    a. Patients with Barrett's esophagus indefinite for dysplasia can be managed with proton pump inhibitors indefinitely
    b. Follow-up of patients with low-grade dysplasia after surgery is simplified
    c. It is often possible to distinguish between high-grade dysplasia and invasive carcinoma
    d. Patients with high-grade dysplasia should have a total esophagectomy

COMMENT: Once identified, Barrett's esophagus complicated by dysplasia should be treated aggressively. Patients, whose specimens are indefinite for dysplasia, should be treated with an aggressive medical regimen, consisting of proton pump inhibitor therapy for three months and then undergo a second biopsy. It is important that the esophagitis be healed with proton pump inhibitors before the presence or absence of dysplasia is determined. The presence of severe inflammation makes the microscopic interpretation of dysplasia difficult. Patients with low-grade dysplasia should be treated with either aggressive medical therapy or anti-reflux surgery. Surveillance follow-up, however, following anti-reflux surgery may be difficult because biopsies within the wrap may be difficult for the inexperienced to perform. High-grade dysplasia should be confirmed by two pathologists knowledgeable in gastrointestinal pathophysiology. Corroboration of dysplasia is important before any consideration of esophagectomy. Most would agree that it is the standard of care to proceed with a total esophagectomy in patients with high-grade dysplasia. On average 45%–50% of these patients harbor invasive cancer when the specimen is removed. It is not possible with present technology, including endoscopic ultrasound, to differentiate between patients who do and do not harbor a cancer. Furthermore, the esophageal adenocarcinoma associated with high-grade dysplasia identified with surveillance endoscopy is highly curable with 5-year survival rates approaching 90%.

ANSWER: c, d

REFERENCE: *Chapter 19—Esophagus: Anatomy, Physiology, and Gastroesophageal Reflux Disease; Barrett's Esophagus*

12. Which of the following statements is/are true concerning the medical treatment of gastroesophageal reflux disease?

    a. Acid suppression therapy may provide symptomatic improvement but yet allow progression of disease
    b. A course of medical therapy usually results in long-term effective relief of symptoms
    c. The presence of either mucosal damage or Barrett's esophagus will predict a high risk of medical failure
    d. Gastric acid suppression is usually effective therapy regardless of the extent of esophagitis

COMMENT: The mainstay of medical therapy of GERD is acid suppression. Patients with persistent symptoms should be given hydrogen-potassium proton pump inhibitors. These usually are effective in normal doses and these agents can effectively reduce gastric acid by 80%–90%. This usually heals mild esophagitis, but healing may occur in only ¾ of patients with severe esophagitis. It is important to realize in patients who reflux a combination of gastric and duodenal juice, inadequate acid suppression therapy may provide symptomatic improvement while still allowing mixed reflux to occur. This can result in an environment conducive to persistent mucosal damage in an asymptomatic patient. Unfortunately, within 6 months of discontinuation of any form of medical therapy for GERD, 80% of patients experience a recurrence of symptoms. Patients presenting for the first time with symptoms suggestive of gastroesophageal reflux may be given initial therapy with H2 blockers. Failure of H2 blockers to control symptoms, or the immediate return of symptoms after cessation of treatment, suggests either that the diagnosis is incorrect or that the patient has a relatively severe disease. Endoscopic examination at this stage of the evaluation provides the opportunity for assessing the severity of mucosal damage and determining whether Barrett's esophagus is present. Both these findings at initial endoscopy predict a high risk of medical failure.

ANSWER: a, c

REFERENCE: *Chapter 19—Esophagus: Anatomy, Physiology, and Gastroesophageal Reflux Disease; Treatment of Gastroesophageal Reflux Disease*

13. Prior to surgical therapy of GERD, objective documentation is indicative. Which of the following statements is/are true concerning the evaluation of patients with gastroesophageal reflux?

    a. 24-hour pH monitoring has the highest sensitivity and specificity of all tests currently available
    b. Acid exposure is considered to occur with a pH less than 2 on pH monitoring
    c. With modern techniques, radiographic evaluation of patients with GERD is not necessary
    d. Assessment of the esophageal body is important in determining the type of operation

COMMENT: The success of surgical therapy of GERD is directly proportional to the degree of certainty of the diagnosis. Careful evaluation is therefore appropriate in patients in which surgery will be considered. Endoscopic visualization of the esophagus is a critical part of the preoperative evaluation of a patient with GERD. It is the main aim to detect complications of gastroesophageal reflux, the presence of which often influence the therapeutic decisions. 24-hour ambulatory pH monitoring is currently considered the gold standard for the diagnosis of GERD because it has the highest sensitivity and specificity of all tests available. The units used to express the esophageal exposure to gastric juice are (a) cumulative time the esophageal pH is below a certain threshold; (b) frequency of reflux episodes below a chosen threshold; (c) the duration of the episodes. Most centers use a pH of 4 as the threshold. Radiographic assessment of the anatomy of the esophagus and the stomach is one of the most important parts of the preoperative evaluation. Critical issues are assessed, including the presence of esophageal shortening, the size reducibility of a hiatal hernia, and the propulsive function of the esophagus with both liquids and solids. The presence of poor esophageal body function, in addition to the likelihood of relieving regurgitation, dysphagia, and respiratory symptoms after surgery, may influence the decision to perform a partial rather than a complete fundoplication. The function of the esophageal body is best assessed with esophageal manometrics.

ANSWER: a, d

REFERENCE: *Chapter 19—Esophagus: Anatomy, Physiology, and Gastroesophageal Reflux Disease; Treatment of Gastroesophageal Reflux Disease*

14. Laparoscopic fundoplication should include which of the following:

    a. Crural dissection and identification and preservation of both vagi
    b. Circumferential dissection of the esophagus
    c. Fundus mobilization by division of the short gastric vessels
    d. Constructing the fundoplication by grasping the anterior portion of the stomach and pulling it behind the esophagus

COMMENT: The successful performance of a laparoscopic fundoplication includes crural dissection and identification and preservation of both vagi, including the hepatic branch of the anterior vegus. In addition a large left hepatic artery arising from the left gastric artery is present in up to 25% of patients and should also be identified and avoided. The esophagus should be circumferentially dissected and both crura identified and closed posteriorly behind the esophagus. The fundus is mobilized and the short gastrics are divided. This permits better visualization of the procedure and ensures that the repair is constructed with the posterior portion of the fundus. The Harmonic scalpel facilitates the performance of this process. Finally, a short, loose fundoplication is created by enveloping the lower esophagus with the anterior and posterior walls of the fundus. The most common error in constructing a fundoplication is to grasp the anterior portion of the stomach and pull it behind the esophagus. This results in the twisting of the gastric fundus around the esophagus. Rather, the esophagus should be enveloped by an untwisted fundus before suturing.

ANSWER: a, b, c

REFERENCE: *Chapter 19—Esophagus: Anatomy, Physiology, and Gastroesophageal Reflux Disease; Laparoscopicness in Fundoplication*

15. Which of the statements is/are true concerning the results and complications of laparoscopic anti-reflux surgery?

   a. The average reported postoperative complication rate is less than 10%

   b. The rate of conversion to a open procedure is greater than 10%

   c. Successful relief of symptoms occurs in over 90% of patients

   d. Temporary dysphagia is common, but usually improves with time

   e. Laparoscopic surgery is the most cost-effective treatment of disease requiring long-term therapy

COMMENT: The average postoperative complication rate following laparoscopic anti-reflux surgery is 8% (range 2%–13%) and a rate of conversion to an open procedure is 2% (range 1%–10%). Mortality is uncommon. Reports document the ability of laparoscopic fundoplication to relieve typical reflux symptoms (heartburn, regurgitation, and dysphagia) in more than 90% of patients in a follow-up interval approaching three years in some series. These results are comparable to those obtained in the modern era of open fundoplication. Temporary dysphagia is common after surgery and generally resolves within three months. Dysphagia persistent beyond three months occurs usually in less than 10% of patients. Three cost-utility analysis of long-term medical therapy versus laparoscopic fundoplication for GERD have been performed. All three studies concluded that laparoscopic surgery is the most cost-effective treatment of patients likely to require life long therapy.

ANSWER: a, c, d, e

REFERENCE: *Chapter 19—Esophagus: Anatomy, Physiology, and Gastroesophageal Reflux Disease; Treatment of Gastroesophageal Reflux Disease*

CHAPTER 20

TUMORS, INJURIES, AND MISCELLANEOUS CONDITIONS OF THE ESOPHAGUS

1. Benign tumors of the esophagus are rare, constituting less than 1% of esophageal neoplasms. Which of the following statements is/are true concerning benign esophageal neoplasms?

   a. Most esophageal polyps are located just above the gastroesophageal junction

   b. Malignant degeneration of leiomyoma of the esophagus is a frequent occurrence

   c. Asymptomatic leiomyoma can be followed with barium esophagograms and endoscopic ultrasonography

   d. Most cases of leiomyoma of the esophagus necessitate esophagectomy

COMMENT: Leiomyoma is the most common benign intramural esophageal tumor and characteristically occurs among patients 20 to 50 years of age. More than 80% of cases of esophageal leiomyoma occur in the middle and lower thirds of the esophagus. Tumors less than 5 cm in diameter rarely cause symptoms. When the lesion is larger than this, dysphagia, retrosternal pressure, and pain are the common complaints. Bleeding more often occurs with the malignant form of the tumor, leiomyosarcoma. Malignant degeneration of leiomyoma is exceedingly rare. Asymptomatic leiomyoma or one discovered incidentally at barium swallow examination can be safely followed with periodic barium esophagrams and endoscopic ultrasonography.

Although excision of the esophageal mass provides the only definitive tissue diagnosis, the characteristic radiographic appearance, slow growth rate, low risk of malignant degeneration, and the ability to follow leiomyoma with endoscopic ultrasonography justify conservative management. Tumors that are symptomatic or larger than 5 cm in diameter should be excised. Tumors of the middle third of the esophagus are approached through right thoracotomy, whereas those in the distal third are approached through left thoracotomy. Once the esophagus is encircled and the tumor located, the overlying longitudinal muscle is split in the direction of its fibers. The tumor is then gently dissected away from the contiguous underlying submucosa and adjacent muscle. When enucleation of the tumor is complete, the longitudinal esophageal muscle is reapproximated, although a large extramucosal defect can be left without complication. Giant leiomyoma of the cardia and adjacent stomach may require esophageal resection for removal. When resection is complete, leiomyoma almost never recurs.

Benign polyps of the esophagus are rare and typically arise in the cervical esophagus. Most occur among older men and are frequently attached to the cricoid cartilage. The histologic composition is fibrovascular tissue with varying amounts of associated fat.

ANSWER: c

REFERENCE: *Chapter 20—Tumors, Injuries, and Miscellaneous Conditions of the Esophagus: Benign Esophageal Tumors and Cysts*

2. Esophageal cysts arise as outpouchings of the embryonic foregut. Which of the following statements is/are true concerning esophageal cysts?

a. The cysts are lined by goblet cells with intestinal metaplasia
b. Most esophageal cysts cause symptoms in the first year of life
c. An asymptomatic esophageal cyst can be managed conservatively
d. The diagnosis of esophageal cyst is usually made radiographically

COMMENT: In the embryonic stages, the esophagus is lined by simple columnar ciliated epithelium, which eventually is replaced by stratified squamous epithelium. An esophageal cyst therefore can contain both of these types of epithelium as well as fat and smooth muscle. The esophageal duplication cyst is a variation of the foregut cyst, extends along the length of the thoracic esophagus, and is lined by squamous epithelium. More than 60% of esophageal cysts cause either respiratory or esophageal symptoms in the first year of life. Those located in the upper third of the esophagus tend to present in infancy; lower-third cysts may be asymptomatic initially and manifest later in childhood. Adults have dysphagia, choking, and retrosternal pain when previously asymptomatic cysts enlarge as the result of bleeding or infection. The diagnosis of esophageal cyst usually can be made on the basis of atypical radiographic appearance. Evidence on posteroanterior and lateral chest radiographs, barium esophagrams, and in some cases computed tomographic scans confirms the diagnosis for almost all patients. Because esophageal cysts have a predilection for bleeding, ulceration, perforation, and infection, excision usually is recommended, usually by means of extramucosal resection, which causes little morbidity.

ANSWER: b, d

REFERENCE: *Chapter 20—Tumors, Injuries, and Miscellaneous Conditions of the Esophagus: Benign Esophageal Tumors and Cysts*

3. Which of the following statements is/are true concerning the pathologic mechanism of squamous cell carcinoma of the esophagus?

    a. Carcinoma in situ typically progresses to invasive squamous cell carcinoma in 2 to 4 years
    b. The most common location of this tumor is the distal one third of the esophagus
    c. It tends to be multifocal
    d. The fungating and ulcerative forms occur with equal frequency
    e. Lymph node metastasis is present in 75% of patients at initial diagnosis

COMMENT: Esophageal carcinoma occurs over a spectrum that ranges from the early lesion (carcinoma in situ), which is limited to the mucosa, to the more advanced form, in which the tumor penetrates the muscle layers of the esophagus and beyond. Carcinoma in situ typically is found in patients 40 to 50 years of age and gradually progresses to invasive squamous cell carcinoma over 2 to 4 years. Using the arbitrary division of the esophagus, 8% of squamous cell carcinomas occur in the cervical esophagus, 55% in the upper and midthoracic segments, and 37% in the lower thoracic segment, which extends to the gastroesophageal junction. Sixty percent of squamous cell carcinomas of the esophagus are fungating intraluminal growths, 25% are ulcerative lesions associated with extensive infiltration of the adjacent esophageal wall, and 15% are infiltrating. Esophageal carcinoma tends to be multifocal. A patient who survives therapy for one carcinoma has at least twice the risk of development of a second primary esophageal neoplasm than does the healthy population.

Esophageal carcinoma is notorious for its aggressive biologic behavior. Mediastinal, supraclavicular, or celiac lymph node metastasis is present in at least 75% of patients with esophageal cancer at initial diagnosis. When lymph node metastases are present, the 5-year survival is only 3%, compared with 42% when there is no lymph node spread.

ANSWER: a, c, e

REFERENCE: *Chapter 20—Tumors, Injuries, and Miscellaneous Conditions of the Esophagus: Malignant Esophageal Tumors; Squamous Cell Carcinoma*

4. The incidence of adenocarcinoma of the esophagus is increasing rapidly, which is largely the result of the growing prevalence of adenocarcinoma arising in Barrett's mucosa. Which of the following statements is/are true concerning esophageal adenocarcinoma associated with Barrett's mucosa?

    a. Patients with Barrett's mucosa are 5 to 10 times more likely to have adenocarcinoma than is the general population
    b. The diagnosis of Barrett's mucosa depends on histologic documentation of columnar mucosa extending at least 2 cm above the anatomic esophageal junction
    c. Barrett's mucosa with intestinal metaplasia is the type most often associated with adenocarcinoma
    d. Esophageal adenocarcinoma has a better prognosis than does squamous cell carcinoma
    e. The diagnosis of severe dysplasia of Barrett's mucosa warrants surveillance esophagoscopy and biopsy every 6 months

COMMENT: It is estimated that patients with Barrett's esophagus are 40 times more likely to have adenocarcinoma than is the general population. The true incidence of Barrett's esophagus in the general population is unknown, but it is estimated that adenocarcinoma occurs among as many as 8% to 15% of patients with columnar epithelium–lined esophagus. Until recently, the diagnosis of Barrett's mucosa required documentation of columnar epithelium extending into the esophagus at least 2 cm above the anatomic esophagogastric junction. Barrett's mucosa now is defined as a change in the esophageal epithelium of any length that can be seen endoscopically and that is confirmed to have intestinal metaplasia (with goblet cells) at biopsy. Of the three histologic patterns of Barrett's mucosa, the specialized or intestinal type of metaplasia has the greatest association with carcinoma. Dysplasia occurs to varying degrees in Barrett's mucosa and is clearly a premalignant lesion. Severe dysplasia usually is associated with carcinoma in situ and mandates therapy, by means of esophagectomy, when possible. As is true of squamous cell carcinoma, esophageal adenocarcinoma has an aggressive biologic behavior characterized by frequent transmural invasion and lymphatic spread.

ANSWER: c

REFERENCE: *Chapter 20—Tumors, Injuries, and Miscellaneous Conditions of the Esophagus: Malignant Esophageal Tumors; Adenocarcinoma*

5. Which of the following statements is/are correct concerning diagnostic studies for esophageal carcinoma?

    a. Computed tomography (CT) of the chest and upper abdomen is useful for both staging and predicting resectability

    b. Esophagoscopy is unnecessary for adult patients with dysphagia with normal findings at barium esophagography

    c. Bronchoscopy should be performed for all patients with carcinoma of the upper and middle thirds of the esophagus

    d. Bone and brain scans should be obtained routinely to rule out distant metastasis

    e. Endoscopic ultrasonography is a potentially sensitive examination for the staging of esophageal cancer

COMMENT: An adult patient with new-onset dysphagia needs both barium esophagography and esophagoscopy to rule out carcinoma. The barium swallow examination should be performed first. Tumors of the cervical esophagus are difficult to identify at barium swallow examination, and carcinoma of the cardia can be confused with achalasia or esophageal spasm. Nevertheless, a barium swallow examination localizes obvious pathologic changes in the esophagus in preparation for esophagoscopy. It also allows the endoscopist to predict the level at which the tumor is located and the area that requires the most careful examination. Computed tomography of the chest and upper abdomen is the standard radiographic technique for staging of esophageal carcinoma. Esophageal wall thickness, regional adenopathy, or pulmonary, liver, adrenal, or distant nodal metastasis can be identified. Although CT is suggested to have a role in evaluation of the resectability of esophageal carcinoma, it is particularly limited in its ability to show invasion of the gastric cardia or aortic invasion.

Contiguity of the esophageal tumor with the aorta or spine is not synonymous with invasion. A bone scan is not warranted unless the patient has specific symptoms that suggest bone metastasis. Routine brain scans are not indicated because brain metastasis from carcinoma of the esophagus is uncommon. Bronchoscopy should be performed on patients with carcinoma of the upper and middle thirds of the esophagus to exclude invasion of the posterior membranous trachea or main stem bronchi, which precludes safe esophagectomy. Endoscopic ultrasonography is being used with increasing frequency as an adjunct to the standard radiologic and endoscopic assessment of esophageal disease. It offers the potential for more sensitive staging of esophageal carcinoma by showing the depth of invasion and the presence of abnormal mediastinal adenopathy.

ANSWER: c, e

REFERENCE: *Chapter 20—Tumors, Injuries, and Miscellaneous Conditions of the Esophagus: Diagnostic Investigations*

6. Which of the following conditions is/are associated with the development of esophageal carcinoma?

    a. Caustic esophageal stricture

    b. Achalasia of the esophagus

    c. Plummer-Vinson syndrome

    d. Esophageal diverticula

COMMENT: Chronic irritation of the esophageal mucosa by a variety of noxious stimuli (alcohol, tobacco, hot foods and liquids) eventually may lead to the development of esophageal carcinoma. A variety of other esophageal lesions have a recognized premalignant nature. A patient who survives the initial injury long enough to have a caustic esophageal stricture has a 1,000-fold higher risk of carcinoma than does with the normal population. Ten percent to 12% of patients with achalasia of the esophagus observed 15 years or more have esophageal carcinoma. This is thought to be related to the irritating effects of the fermenting intraesophageal contents on the adjacent esophageal mucosa. Plummer-Vinson syndrome is a premalignant esophageal condition. Patients with this syndrome are typically elderly women who have cervical dysphagia associated with an esophageal web and iron deficiency anemia. Approximately 10% of patients eventually have squamous cell carcinoma of the hypopharynx, oral cavity, or esophagus. There have been isolated reports of esophageal carcinoma found incidentally within esophageal diverticula, presumably as the result of the irritating effects on the mucosa of stagnant, putrefying food within the pouch. Esophageal diverticula are therefore regarded as premalignant esophageal lesions, although this occurrence is extremely rare.

ANSWER: a, b, c, d

REFERENCE: *Chapter 20—Tumors, Injuries, and Miscellaneous Conditions of the Esophagus: Premalignant Esophageal Lesions*

7. Which of the following statements is/are true concerning nonresectional therapy for esophageal carcinoma?

    a. Radiation therapy can be associated with 5-year survival rates equal to those of surgery

    b. Esophageal intubation to provide palliation for esophageal cancer is associated with minimal morbidity and mortality

    c. Endoscopic laser fulguration is successful in relieving dysphagia for as many as 75% of patients

    d. There is little or no role for surgical bypass for unresectable carcinoma of the esophagus

COMMENT: Therapy for esophageal carcinoma is influenced by the knowledge that in most of these patients, local tumor invasion or distant metastatic disease precludes cure. Although squamous cell carcinoma is generally regarded as a radiosensitive and therefore potentially curable tumor, radiation therapy has not achieved cure for most patients. Although "curative" supervoltage radiation techniques have been used, the average 5-year survival after such treatment is 6% to 10% in most series. This is somewhat poorer than 5-year survival rates after resection, which usually range from 10% to 15%.

A variety of endoesophageal tubes have been used for palliation in the care of patients with esophageal carcinoma. These tubes are divided into two types—pulsion tubes, which are pushed through the tumor with the aid of an esophagoscope, and traction or pull-through tubes, which are pulled into place by means of downward traction through a gastrostomy. As are many conceptually simple procedures, implementation in the clinical setting is difficult. Transoral esophageal intubation is associated with an overall mortality of 14% and a complication rate of 25%, the latter due to perforation of the esophagus, migration of the tubes, or obstruction of the tubes by food or tumor overgrowth. Expandable intraesophageal metallic stents placed endoscopically have been used for palliative treatment of patients with resectable esophageal carcinoma. Endoscopic laser fulguration of esophageal carcinoma has been used to achieve temporary relief of esophageal obstruction in patients with unresectable tumors. Several sessions usually are needed to resect sufficient tumor to achieve an adequate lumen, but functional success with restoration of a comfortable volume can be achieved in 75% to 80% of cases. Although a variety of surgical procedures, such as substernal gastric or colonic bypass, have been developed for palliative internal bypass of unresectable esophageal carcinoma, the average survival of only 4 to 6 months among such patients and the mortality rates of these procedures, as high as 25%, do not justify their use.

ANSWER: c, d

REFERENCE: *Chapter 20—Tumors, Injuries, and Miscellaneous Conditions of the Esophagus: Treatment of Esophageal Cancer*

8. Which of the following statements is/are correct concerning the options for resection of esophageal carcinoma?

    a. Reflux esophagitis seldom occurs after esophagectomy and intrathoracic esophagogastric anastomosis because of the limited life expectancy of these patients

    b. Transhiatal esophagectomy, although conceptually sound, is not technically possible for most patients with esophageal carcinoma

    c. Transhiatal esophagectomy is associated with lower long-term survival rates than is standard transthoracic esophagectomy

    d. Long-term survival after radical transthoracic esophagectomy with en bloc dissection of contiguous lymph node–bearing tissues is comparable with that after transhiatal esophagectomy

COMMENT: For most patients with localized esophageal carcinoma, resection provides the most effective and reliable palliation of dysphagia. The traditional surgical approach to distal esophageal carcinoma has been a left thoracoabdominal incision. Tumors involving the midesophagus have been resected either through a thoracoabdominal incision or separate thoracic and abdominal incisions. High thoracic esophagogastric anastomosis is performed. The most important disadvantages of this technique are the necessity for thoracotomy on debilitated patients with esophageal obstruction and the disastrous complications—mediastinitis and sepsis associated with intrathoracic esophageal anastomotic leak. Although operative mortality rates have improved, the operation can still be associated with high morbidity and mortality. Another disadvantage of standard intrathoracic esophagogastric anastomosis is inadequate long-term relief of dysphagia either because of tumor recurrence at the anastomotic suture line or because of development of reflux esophagitis above the anastomosis. Although it has been long taught that patients with esophageal carcinoma do not live long enough to have reflux esophagitis after a low intrathoracic esophagogastric anastomosis, this is clearly not the case. Development of reflux in these patients can produce not only severe pyrosis and reflux symptoms but also dysphagia from benign stenosis.

The technique of transhiatal esophagectomy without thoracotomy has been popularized as an operation that minimizes the factors responsible for poor results of traditional transthoracic esophageal resection and reconstruction. If the surgeon is experienced, transhiatal esophagectomy without thoracotomy is possible for more than 95% of patients with carcinoma. The survival data are comparable to those in most series of transthoracic resection. The results usually show decreased postoperative morbidity and mortality. Although radical transthoracic esophagectomy with en bloc dissection of contiguous lymph node–bearing tissue conceptually appears to offer a better "cancer operation" than does transhiatal esophagectomy with no formal lymphnode dissection, current survival results are not statistically different. These data suggest that survival after resection for esophageal carcinoma is more a function of the extent and stage of the tumor than the size of the specimen or the number of lymph nodes removed.

ANSWER: d

REFERENCE: *Chapter 20—Tumors, Injuries, and Miscellaneous Conditions of the Esophagus: Resection*

9. In an effort to improve survival after esophageal resection, trials of multimodality therapy with chemotherapy and radiation before esophagectomy have been completed. Which of the following statements is/are true concerning such treatment?

a. Multimodality therapy is indicated in the management of esophageal squamous cell carcinoma but not of adenocarcinoma
b. A complete response—no residual tumor in the resected specimen—is achieved by approximately 25% of patients treated with chemoradiation therapy
c. Operative mortality is considerably greater among patients who have undergone chemoradiation therapy than it is among patients treated with single-modality therapy
d. The encouraging results obtained with nonrandomized (phase II) trials have been borne out in subsequent prospective, randomized trials

COMMENT: Combined preoperative chemotherapy and radiation therapy before transhiatal esophagectomy for carcinoma has provided encouraging survival statistics in several nonrandomized phase II trials. Treatment has typically consisted of 3 to 4 weeks of preoperative chemotherapy with cisplatin and 5-fluorouracil and concurrent radiation therapy in the range of 40 to 50 Gy. Although hematologic toxicity and radiation esophagitis are common and preoperative deaths due to bone marrow suppression can occur, there has been no statistically significant increase in perioperative mortality compared with that among patients with no preoperative therapy. Approximately 25% to 30% of patients have no remaining tumor in the resected esophagus (T0N0 status, or complete response) after preoperative chemoradiation, and for these patients, there may be survival benefit. However, despite the encouraging reports of phase II trials, the few published reports of prospective, randomized controlled trials comparing chemoradiation therapy and esophagectomy with surgery alone have generally not shown significant overall survival benefit. At present, chemoradiation therapy before esophagectomy for cancer should be considered investigational.

ANSWER: b

REFERENCE: *Chapter 20—Tumors, Injuries, and Miscellaneous Conditions of the Esophagus: Treatment of Esophageal Cancer; Multimodality Therapy*

10. Which of the following statements is/are true concerning corrosive injury to the esophagus?

   a. Alkaline injury is more destructive than is acid injury
   b. Acid ingestion is not injurious to the stomach because of its normal acidic pH
   c. Ingested caustic agents rapidly pass through the esophagus and stomach into the small intestine
   d. Unless perforation occurs, clinical manifestations resolve quickly, and there is initial clinical improvement
   e. Children are less likely to form a late esophageal stricture than are adults

COMMENT: Caustic injury occurs among two broad categories of patients—children younger than 5 years who accidentally swallow these agents and adults who are attempting suicide. The most common agents responsible for caustic esophageal injuries are alkalis, acids, bleach, and detergent. Ingestion of detergent and bleach almost always causes only mild esophageal irritation that heals without serious adverse sequelae. Acids and alkalis can have devastating effects, which range from acute multiple organ necrosis and perforation to chronic esophageal and gastric strictures. Alkalis are more destructive, producing liquefaction necrosis, which almost ensures deep penetration. Acids usually cause coagulation necrosis, which in part limits the depth of injury. Liquid alkali preparations have prolonged contact with the mucosa of the esophagus and stomach because of their high viscosity. Ingested acids typically pass through the esophagus quickly and produce major gastric injury with relative sparing of the esophagus. In response to either ingested acid or alkali, reflex pyloric spasm occurs, and these agents pool in the gastric antrum.

The clinical manifestations of caustic ingestion are directly related to the amount and character of the agent ingested. When esophageal or gastric perforation results from caustic ingestion, patients have progressive severe sepsis and hypovolemic shock until appropriate resuscitative measures are instituted. In the absence of gastric or esophageal perforation, the acute clinical manifestations typically resolve within days and clinical improvement lasts for weeks. After this, symptoms due to either esophageal or gastric stricture begin. Most adults who ingest liquid alkali have severe esophageal and usually gastric injury that results in stricture formation. Children, who usually have more limited exposure from accidental ingestion, are less likely to have severe injuries.

ANSWER: a, d, e

REFERENCE: *Chapter 20—Tumors, Injuries, and Miscellaneous Conditions of the Esophagus: Caustic Injury*

11. Which of the following statements is/are correct concerning treatment of a patient with a caustic esophageal or gastric injury?

   a. Corticosteroids should be administered immediately
   b. Endoscopic examination of the entire esophagus and stomach should be performed as soon as possible
   c. When patients need operative intervention, exploration is best performed through the abdomen
   d. If organ resection is indicated, restoration of alimentary continuity should be deferred until the patient has recovered from the acute insult
   e. For patients with esophageal stricture after second- and third-degree burns, dilation therapy should be instituted as soon as possible after injury

COMMENT: Acute caustic ingestion is an indication for hospitalization. Initial management centers on stabilizing the patient's condition and assessing the severity of injury. Oral intake should be withheld and hypovolemia corrected with intravenous fluids. Careful observation for evidence of airway obstruction is mandatory. Broad-spectrum antibiotics are indicated once the diagnosis of substantial esophageal injury has been established to diminish the risk of pulmonary infection from aspiration as well as bacterial invasion through the damaged esophageal wall. Although corticosteroids have been advocated in the acute phase of caustic ingestion to minimize subsequent stricture formation, the efficacy has not been established. Because steroids can mask signs of sepsis and visceral perforation and impair healing, use of these agents to manage caustic esophageal injury can be deleterious and therefore is not recommended.

Contrast esophagography is the best way to make the diagnosis of esophageal perforation and should be performed if the diagnosis is suspected at the time of admission or in subsequent follow-up evaluation. Esophagoscopy should be performed soon after admission to establish whether serious esophageal injury has occurred and to allow grading of the severity of injury. Although it once was taught that an endoscope should not be advanced beyond the first burned area, complete examination of the esophagus and stomach is now recommended, especially if severe burns are not detected proximally. The use of a pediatric endoscope and adequate sedation can allow this procedure to be accomplished safely.

When ingestion of a caustic liquid necessitates operative intervention, exploration is best performed through the abdomen. This approach allows assessment of the injury to the intraabdominal organs and resection of areas of full-thickness gastric necrosis. Although only the lower esophagus is well visualized through the diaphragmatic hiatus, if esophageal resection is needed, transhiatal esophagectomy without thoracotomy is readily performed with the addition of a cervical incision. When esophageal and gastric resection is needed after acute caustic injury, restoration of alimentary continuity should be deferred until the patient has recovered from the acute insult. Cervical esophagostomy and insertion of an enteral feeding tube should be performed. Esophageal stricture formation almost always occurs after second- and third-degree burns. Dilation therapy has been the traditional therapy for chronic caustic esophageal strictures. It is important that dilation not be instituted until at least 6 to 8 weeks after the injury, when reepithelialization is complete, to minimize the risk of perforation.

ANSWER: b, c, d

REFERENCE: *Chapter 20—Tumors, Injuries, and Miscellaneous Conditions of the Esophagus: Caustic Injury*

12. A 54-year-old woman has epigastric and low retrosternal pain within 30 minutes of balloon dilation for achalasia. Which of the following statements is/are true concerning diagnosis and management in this case?

    a. Normal chest radiographic findings rule out esophageal perforation
    b. Barium should never be used in a contrast study being performed for the diagnosis of esophageal perforation
    c. Conservative, nonoperative treatment may be indicated
    d. If operative intervention is needed, the proper procedure is a transthoracic primary repair of the perforation combined with esophagomyotomy and partial fundoplication

COMMENT: It is axiomatic that pain or fever after esophageal instrumentation or operation is indicative of esophageal perforation until proved otherwise. It is an indication for immediate contrast esophagography. Because the morbidity and mortality associated with esophageal perforation are directly related to the time between diagnosis of the injury and repair or drainage, an aggressive attitude toward diagnosis of the perforation must be adopted. When the diagnosis is considered, a water-soluble contrast agent should be administered. If the results of this study are normal, dilute barium should be administered. Barium is relatively inert, and the fear of barium extravasating in the mediastinum through the site of injury and producing severe reactive mediastinitis is unfounded. A chest radiograph can help confirm the diagnosis by means of depicting air in the soft tissues of the neck or mediastinum or a hydrothorax or pneumothorax. Normal chest radiographic findings, however, do not rule out esophageal perforation.

Although most esophageal perforations necessitate operative intervention, selected patients can be treated nonoperatively with cessation of oral intake, administration of antibiotics, and intravenous hydration until the disruption heals or the small contained cavity begins to decrease in size. The types of injuries often amenable to such nonoperative management are cervical esophageal tears caused by esophagoscopy; intramural dissection occuring during dilation of a stricture or pneumatic dilation for achalasia, and asymptomatic esophageal anastomotic disruption discovered on a routine postoperative contrast study. Perforations complicating pneumatic dilation for achalasia occur among 4% to 6% of patients, and most are small and well managed medically with antibiotics and intravenous fluids. If operation is needed for repair of the perforation, the correct procedure is a transthoracic primary closure of the tear through a left thoracotomy combined with esophagomyotomy and nonobstructing partial (Belsey) fundoplication.

ANSWER: c, d

REFERENCE: *Chapter 20—Tumors, Injuries, and Miscellaneous Conditions of the Esophagus: Esophageal Perforation*

13. Which of the following statements is/are true concerning infectious esophagitis?

    a. *Candida albicans* is not normally found in the mouth but results from the overgrowth of this fungus in patients treated with broad-spectrum antibiotics
    b. Candidal esophagitis usually is self-limited and is seldom associated with chronic problems
    c. Systemic therapy is seldom indicated
    d. Small ulcers on the barium esophagram of a transplant recipient who reports dysphagia and odynophagia are likely caused by infection with herpes simplex virus

COMMENT: Chronic debilitation, immunosuppression, and prolonged use of antibiotics predispose to the development of infectious esophagitis. *Candida albicans* is the most common cause. *Candida albicans* is a fungus that normally is a commensal inhabitant of the mouth, oropharynx, and gastrointestinal tract. This fungus can become pathogenic in patients who are severely debilitated or immunosuppressed. The spread of broad-spectrum antibiotics, immunosuppression of organ transplant recipients, and the wide use of chemotherapeutic agents have resulted in a large number of cases of monilial esophagitis. As the disease progresses, transmural invasion of the esophageal wall occurs. Although the esophagitis can be controlled with antifungal therapy, if the patient survives the underlying illness, chronic stricture formation can occur after healing. Minimally suppressed patients with mild monilial esophagitis should receive oral nystatin suspension as primary treatment. Patients with greater degrees of immunosuppression or those with severe cases of esophagitis need high doses of fluconazole and ketoconazole. Intravenous fluconazole or amphotericin B is used to treat patients with granulocytopenia.

Viral esophagitis is the second most common cause of infectious esophagitis. Infection with herpes simplex virus is the most common infection among immunosuppressed transplant recipients. Viral esophagitis produces characteristic mucosal ulceration, dysphagia, and odynophagia. The esophageal ulcers are characteristically small (less than 1.5 cm in diameter). The diagnosis is established endoscopically by means of biopsy, brushings, and washings for cytologic and histologic examination and viral culture. The infection usually responds well to treatment with acyclovir.

ANSWER: d

REFERENCE: *Chapter 20—Tumors, Injuries, and Miscellaneous Conditions of the Esophagus: Infectious Esophagitis*

14. Which of the following statements is/are true concerning esophageal diverticula?

    a. A Zenker's diverticulum characteristically occurs in patients 70 years and older
    b. Mediastinal granulomatous disease can result in midesophageal traction diverticulum, which is usually asymptomatic
    c. An epiphrenic diverticulum to the right of the esophagus should be approached through left thoracotomy
    d. Minimally symptomatic epiphrenic diverticula smaller than 3 cm require no treatment

COMMENT: An esophageal diverticulum is an epithelium-lined mucosal pouch that protrudes from the esophageal lumen. Most esophageal diverticula are acquired and occur predominantly among adults. Pharyngoesophageal (Zenker's) diverticulum is the most common esophageal diverticulum and typically occurs in patients 30 to 50 years of age. Mediastinal granulomatous disease (e.g., tuberculosis or histoplasmosis) is the most common cause of midesophageal traction diverticulum. This type of diverticulum is much smaller than a pulsion diverticulum and has a characteristic blunt tapered tip that points toward the adjacent subcarinal or peribronchial lymph nodes to which it adheres. It is typically diagnosed as an incidental finding on a barium esophagram and is almost always asymptomatic. No specific treatment is indicated.

Epiphrenic or supradiaphragmatic diverticulum occurs within the distal 10 cm of the thoracic esophagus as a pulsion diverticulum that arises because of abnormally elevated intraluminal esophageal pressure. Although many patients have no symptoms when the diverticula are found on barium esophagrams, others have symptoms of the frequently associated esophageal conditions—hiatal hernia, diffuse esophageal spasm, achalasia, reflux esophagitis, and carcinoma. Pouches smaller than 3 cm and causing few or no symptoms require no treatment. Severe dysphagia, chest pain, or an anatomically dependent or enlarging pouch are indications for repair. The surgical approach to an epiphrenic diverticula is through left sixth or seventh interspace posterolateral thoracotomy. This is the case even for diverticula to the right of the esophagus. The correct operation is staple resection of the pouch and concomitant long esophagomyotomy 180 degrees away from the diverticulum resection site combined with partial (240 degrees) Belsey fundoplication.

ANSWER: b, c, d

REFERENCE: *Chapter 20—Tumors, Injuries, and Miscellaneous Conditions of the Esophagus: Diverticula*

15. Which of the following statements is/are true concerning tracheoesophageal fistula?
    a. Most acquired tracheoesophageal fistulas are caused by malignant disease
    b. Water-soluble contrast esophagography should be performed for diagnosis
    c. Malignant tracheoesophageal fistula can be managed effectively with an endoscopically inserted prosthesis or a covered expandable metallic stent
    d. A benign tracheoesophageal fistula caused by endotracheal intubation injury often necessitates thoracotomy for repair

COMMENT: Ninety percent of acquired fistulas between the esophagus and tracheobronchial tree in adults are caused by malignant disease. Tracheoesophageal fistula complicates the course of disease among approximately 5% of patients with esophageal carcinoma. Nearly 80% of patients with malignant tracheoesophageal fistula die within 3 months of the onset of symptoms. Among 85% of these patients, the cause of death is aspiration pneumonia, not distant metastatic disease. For the most part, malignant tracheoesophageal fistula represents incurable disease for which resection carries high mortality and is seldom indicated. Palliative relief of recurrent aspiration is the aim of therapy. Effective occlusion of the fistula can be achieved by means of insertion of one of a variety of available endoesophageal endoprostheses. These tubes are placed into the esophagus with the aid of an esophagoscope and can occlude the esophageal side of the fistula sufficiently to allow swallowing of liquids without aspiration into the tracheobronchial tree. Expandable metal stents have been used successfully in the management of malignant tracheoesophageal fistula.

Nonmalignant fistula is caused by erosion by contiguous infected subcarinal mediastinal lymph nodes; trauma; late sequelae of chronic midesophageal traction diverticulum; or erosion by an endotracheal or tracheostomy tube cuff in a patient who needs prolonged ventilatory support. Small fistulas, such as those caused by endotracheal intubation injury, are approached through a cervical collar or oblique incision anterior to the sternocleidomastoid muscle. Although such cuff injuries usually produce circumferential tracheal damage that necessitates tracheal resection, this procedure also can be performed through a cervical collar incision.

ANSWER: a, c

REFERENCE: *Chapter 20—Tumors, Injuries, and Miscellaneous Conditions of the Esophagus: Acquired Tracheoesophageal Fistulas*

CHAPTER 21

GASTRIC ANATOMY AND PHYSIOLOGY

1. Which of the following statements is/are true regarding the arterial blood supply to the stomach?
    a. The right gastric artery, a branch of the superior mesenteric artery, supplies the gastric antrum
    b. Because of rich intramural collateral vessels, gastric viability may be preserved after ligation of all but one major artery
    c. In cases of celiac arterial occlusion, gastric viability is maintained collaterally through pancreaticoduodenal arcades
    d. The left gastroepiploic artery is a branch of the celiac trunk

COMMENT: The stomach is an extremely well-vascularized organ. It is supplied by five major arterial distributions and protected from ischemia by rich intramural and extramural collateral vessels. The left gastric artery and right gastric artery, derived from the celiac distribution, supply the lesser curvature of the stomach. The right gastroepiploic artery, derived from the gastroduodenal artery, and the left gastroepiploic artery, from the splenic artery, traverse the greater curvature. The area adjacent to the spleen receives numerous short gastric arterial branches. In instances of celiac arterial occlusion, the superior mesenteric artery supplies the stomach collaterally through the pancreaticoduodenal arcades, which connect with the gastroduodenal artery. The stomach can be widely mobilized for use in reconstructive procedures, for example, during transhiatal esophagectomy. Advantage is taken of the abundant blood supply and collaterals of the stomach during mobilization. Gastric viability usually is preserved if one major arterial supply is preserved.

ANSWER: b, c

REFERENCE: *Chapter 21—Gastric Anatomy and Physiology: Gross Anatomy*

2. Which of the following statements is/are true regarding the vagus nerves?

   a. The right and left vagus nerves are derived from a nerve plexus inferior to the tracheal bifurcation

   b. The posterior vagus nerve is closely applied to the intrathoracic esophagus

   c. The anterior vagus supplies a hepatic division that passes to the right in the lesser omentum

   d. Approximately 90% of vagal fibers are afferent, transmitting information from the gastrointestinal tract to the central nervous system

   e. The vagus nerves transmit gastroduodenal pain sensations associated with peptic ulceration

COMMENT: The left and right vagus nerves are formed from a periesophageal nerve plexus between the tracheal bifurcation and the diaphragm. As the nerves pass through the esophageal hiatus, the anterior vagus is closely applied to the esophagus, and the posterior vagus nerve is intermediate in position between the esophagus and the aorta. The anterior vagus nerve supplies the hepatic division, which provides parasympathetic innervation to the liver and biliary tract. The hepatic division usually is easily seen in the thin gastrohepatic omentum and is constant in location. The hepatic division is a useful anatomic landmark in vagotomy. The posterior vagus nerve supplies fibers to the celiac division. After giving off hepatic and celiac divisions, both anterior and posterior vagus nerves supply branches to the gastric wall. Only 10% of vagal fibers are efferent, secretomotor fibers; almost 90% are afferent. Sensations of gastric pain are carried in sympathetic fibers, and vagotomy does not alter perception of painful gastric conditions or stimuli.

ANSWER: a, c, d

REFERENCE: *Chapter 21—Gastric Anatomy and Physiology: Gross Anatomy*

3. Important stimulants of gastrin release from endocrine cells in the antrum include:

   a. Acidification of the antral lumen

   b. Small peptide fragments and amino acids from luminal proteolysis

   c. Locally released somatostatin

   d. Dietary fat

COMMENT: Gastrin is processed to 34- and 17-amino-acid forms in endocrine cells in the gastric antrum. In addition to well-recognized stimulatory actions on gastric acid secretion, gastrin promotes mucosal growth of the gastric fundus and small intestine. The most important stimulant of gastrin release is a meal. Small peptide fragments and amino acids that result from intragastric proteolysis are the food components that stimulate gastrin release. Ingested fats and carbohydrates have no significant effect. In this regard, intraluminal pH strongly affects gastrin secretion. If intragastric pH is maintained above 3 after ingestion of a meal, gastrin release is strongly potentiated. Pernicious anemia and atrophic gastritis, which produce chronic achlorhydria, are associated with fasting hypergastrinemia and an exaggerated gastrin meal response. Conversely, antral acidification strongly inhibits gastrin secretion. Locally released somatostatin mediates the effects of luminal acidification and inhibits gastrin secretion.

ANSWER: b

REFERENCE: *Chapter 21—Gastric Anatomy and Physiology: Gastric Peptides*

4. At a cellular level, the major stimulant(s) of acid secretion by the gastric parietal cell is/are:

a. Histamine
b. Prostaglandin E_2
c. Acetylcholine
d. Gastrin
e. Norepinephrine

COMMENT: The three major stimulants of acid secretion by parietal cells are acetylcholine, gastrin, and histamine. Acetylcholine is released from cholinergic nerve endings close to parietal cells and binds to muscarinic receptors. Cholinergic stimulation of parietal cells is coupled with hydrolysis of membrane-associated lipids (phosphatidylinositides) and leads to increases in intracellular calcium. Histamine is released from mast cells in the lamina propria and reaches parietal cells by means of diffusion. Histamine occupies H_2 receptors, which can be selectively blocked by agents such as cimetidine. Histamine stimulation of parietal cell acid secretion is mediated by a cyclic adenosine monophosphate–dependent pathway. Gastrin is delivered to the fundic mucosa by the systemic circulation from its source in the antrum and duodenum. Like acetylcholine, gastrin increases membrane phosphoinositol turnover and increases intracellular calcium. Activation of parietal cells by acetylcholine, gastrin, or histamine can be blocked by somatostatin. Local release of somatostatin is physiologically important in modulating postprandial gastric acid secretion. Prostaglandin E_2 and its synthetic derivatives are potent inhibitors of histamine-stimulated acid secretion.

ANSWER: a, c, d

REFERENCE: *Chapter 21—Gastric Anatomy and Physiology: Gastric Acid Secretion*

5. Which of the following statements is/are true regarding human gastric acid secretion?

a. Fasting acid secretion, normally 2 to 5 mEq/h, is the result of ambient vagal tone and histamine secretion
b. Truncal vagotomy decreases basal secretion 80%
c. Administration of a histamine H_2 receptor antagonist can decrease basal acid secretion 80%
d. Fasting acid secretion, normally 5 to 10 mEq/h, is stimulated by circulating levels of gastrin

COMMENT: Both vagal tone and locally secreted histamine are presumed to be the determinants of basal acid secretion in humans. Gastrin does not have a role in basal acid secretion in healthy persons. Parietal cell activation and the resultant acid secretory response to a combination of agonists are greater than the sum of the responses to the agents used singly. This increase in responsiveness is called *potentiation.* Potentiating interactions are most apparent when the stimulants have different second-messenger systems, for example, acetylcholine and histamine. Conversely, blockade of receptors to one stimulant also blocks responsiveness to the other agonist. Because of this interaction, blockade of histamine receptors by agents such as cimetidine decreases responsiveness to acetylcholine. Blockade of acetylcholine release by means of vagotomy decreases responsiveness to histamine secreted by gastric mast cells. Both vagotomy and histamine H_2 receptor antagonists decrease basal acid secretion approximately 80%.

ANSWER: a, b, c

REFERENCE: *Chapter 21—Gastric Anatomy and Physiology: Regulation of Acid Secretion*

6. As a meal is emptied from the stomach, gastric acid secretion gradually returns to baseline. Which of the following statements correctly characterize(s) control of gastric acid secretion?

a. In humans, the most important inhibitory influence on gastrin release is exposure of the gastric mucosa to luminal acid
b. Acidification of the antral lumen causes reciprocal increases in somatostatin release and decreases in gastrin secretion
c. Antral distention stimulates gastric acid secretion
d. Acidification of the duodenal bulb inhibits gastric acid secretion
e. Exposure of the duodenum to hyperosmolar solutions inhibits acid secretion

COMMENT: Inhibitory regulation of gastric acid secretion is accomplished by central nervous system, gastric, and small-intestinal mechanisms. In humans, the most clearly established gastric inhibitory influence is suppression of gastrin release by exposure of the antral mucosa to luminal acid. Antral acidification causes release of gastric mucosal somatostatin, which is linked reciprocally to decreases in gastrin secretion. Antral distention inhibits gastric acid secretion. The inhibitory phase of gastric acid secretion begins with entrance of the products of digestion into the proximal duodenum. Acidification of the duodenal bulb and exposure of the duodenum to hyperosmolar solutions and those containing fat potently inhibit acid secretion.

ANSWER: a, b, d, e

REFERENCE: *Chapter 21—Gastric Anatomy and Physiology: Regulation of Acid Secretion*

7. Which of the following statements is/are correct regarding intrinsic factor?

a. Intrinsic factor is produced in chief cells located in the gastric fundus
b. Total gastrectomy is followed by folate deficiency caused by vitamin malabsorption due to intrinsic factor deficiency
c. Secretion intrinsic factor, like that of acid, is stimulated by gastrin, histamine, and acetylcholine
d. Intrinsic factor deficiency accompanies antral gastritis caused by *Helicobacter pylori* infection

COMMENT: The gastric mucosa is the site of production of intrinsic factor, which is a necessary cofactor for absorption of vitamin B_{12} by the ileal mucosa. Total gastrectomy and atrophic gastritis involving the proximal oxyntic mucosa are regularly followed by vitamin B_{12} deficiency, which manifests as pernicious anemia. Acid-secreting parietal cells are the site of synthesis of intrinsic factor. Like acid secretion, intrinsic factor secretion is stimulated by gastrin, histamine, and acetylcholine.

ANSWER: c

REFERENCE: *Chapter 21—Gastric Anatomy and Physiology: Intrinsic Factor*

8. It is widely agreed that the gastric mucosa secretes bicarbonate in addition to acid. Gastric secretion of bicarbonate is correctly characterized by which of the following statements?

    a. Bicarbonate is secreted by chief cells within gastric crypts
    b. Gastric bicarbonate secretion is stimulated by acetylcholine
    c. Gastric bicarbonate secretion during fasting results in luminal pH greater than 6 in healthy persons
    d. Prostaglandin E_2 is a potent stimulant of gastric bicarbonate secretion

COMMENT: The gastric cells responsible for bicarbonate secretion are believed to be surface mucous cells that face the gastric lumen between crypts. Although the total amount of gastric bicarbonate secreted is only a small fraction of total acid secretion, pH close to neutrality is maintained near the mucosal surface while bulk luminal pH is highly acidic. Cholinergic agonists, vagal stimulation, and sham feeding all increase gastric bicarbonate secretion. Prostaglandin E_2 and its synthetic derivatives are potent stimulants of bicarbonate secretion. Indomethacin and other drugs that inhibit prostaglandin formation decrease mucosal bicarbonate secretion.

ANSWER: b, d

REFERENCE: *Chapter 21—Gastric Anatomy and Physiology: Gastric Bicarbonate Secretion*

9. Gastric mucosal blood flow is regulated by neural, hormonal, and locally active influences. Which of the following statements correctly characterize(s) gastric blood flow?

    a. Stimulation of sympathetic nerves supplying the stomach is followed by gastric mucosal hyperemia and increased total gastric blood flow
    b. Vagal nerve stimulation is accompanied by decreased gastric mucosal blood flow
    c. Stimulants that increase acid secretion increase mucosal blood flow
    d. In humans, prostaglandins increase mucosal blood flow at doses that inhibit gastric acid secretion

COMMENT: Because the gastric mucosa is metabolically highly active, control of gastric mucosal blood flow is of great physiologic significance. Almost all stimuli that increase acid secretion also increase gastric blood flow. A large number of gastrointestinal hormones stimulate gastric blood flow, most because of their ability to increase acid secretion. Thus gastrin is a potent stimulant of blood flow, in proportion to its ability to increase acid secretion. Vagal nerve stimulation has the net effect of increasing mucosal and total gastric blood flow; sympathetic nerve stimulation is accompanied by opposite effects. Prostaglandins are important endogenous regulators of gastric blood flow. Prostaglandins of the E class increase blood flow at doses that suppress acid secretion. Inhibition of cyclooxygenase activity by indomethacin causes a reduction in resting gastric blood flow.

ANSWER: c, d

REFERENCE: *Chapter 21—Gastric Anatomy and Physiology: Gastric Blood Flow*

10. Which of the following statements correctly characterize(s) gastric motor activity associated with ingestion of a meal?

    a. Ingested gastric volumes are accommodated with little increase in pressure by reflex relaxation of the proximal stomach
    b. Receptive gastric accommodation is unaffected by proximal gastric vagotomy
    c. In humans, liquid emptying occurs more quickly than does solid emptying
    d. Gastric emptying of liquids is not affected by proximal gastric vagotomy

COMMENT: With ingestion of a meal, increasing gastric volumes are accommodated with little increase in intragastric pressure by relaxation of the proximal stomach. This process, called *receptive relaxation,* is mediated by a reflex carried by the vagal nerve. After the meal has been ingested, the proximal stomach is the predominant determinant of the rate of gastric emptying of liquids due to the gastroduodenal pressure gradient generated by proximal gastric contractions. Liquid emptying occurs more rapidly than does emptying of solids, in part because liquids are not subject to the sieving actions of the pylorus. Truncal and proximal gastric vagotomy abolish receptive relaxation. After vagotomy, an increased gastroduodenal pressure gradient occurs and correlates with accelerated liquid emptying. Emptying of solids usually is not greatly altered by proximal gastric vagotomy.

ANSWER: a, c

REFERENCE: *Chapter 21—Gastric Anatomy and Physiology: Gastric Motility*

CHAPTER 22

DUODENAL ULCER

1. *Helicobacter pylori* has been investigated as a possible etiologic agent in duodenal ulceration. Which of the following statements is/are correct regarding *H. pylori* infection among humans?

    a. *H. pylori* can be isolated from the antral gastric mucosa of nearly 100% of patients with active duodenal ulceration but only 1% to 2% of healthy volunteers
    b. *H. pylori* organisms have cell surface receptors that bind to small-intestinal mucous cells
    c. Therapeutic regimens for duodenal ulcer that eliminate the organism are associated with lower ulcer recurrence rates than those in which the organism persists
    d. The incidence of infection with the organism among healthy persons increases with age
    e. Antral gastritis is associated with development of duodenal ulcer

COMMENT: *Helicobacter pylori* has received enormous investigative attention as a possible infectious cause of peptic ulceration. The evidence that *H. pylori* causes ulcers is substantial but largely inferential. Antral gastritis is nearly always present in patients with duodenal ulceration. *Helicobacter pylori* infection of the antral mucosa is believed to cause gastritis. Although normal small-intestinal cells do not allow *H. pylori* binding, areas of gastric metaplasia usually are present in the duodenal mucosa immediately surrounding the ulcer. Resolution of gastritis follows eradication of the organism. Bactericidal drug regimens are associated with lower rates of ulcer recurrence than are those that have no antibacterial actions. It is clear, however, that not all patients with *H. pylori* infection eventually have ulceration. One half of patients with dyspepsia but no ulceration have evidence of *H. pylori* infection, and 20% of healthy volunteers harbor the organism. The incidence of infection increases with age in the population without symptoms.

ANSWER: d, e

REFERENCE: *Chapter 22—Duodenal Ulcer: Pathophysiology*

2. Development of duodenal ulceration depends on gastric acid secretion. Which of the following statements correctly characterize(s) acid secretion in patients with duodenal ulcer?

a. Patients with duodenal ulcer have decreased basal acid secretion

b. Maximal acid output of histamine averages 40 mEq/h in patients with duodenal ulcer, twice that of healthy persons

c. Tissue gastrin levels on average are one half of normal values among patients with active ulceration

d. Exogenously administered somatostatin is ineffective in suppressing acid secretion among patients with active ulceration

COMMENT: Formation of duodenal ulcer depends on gastric secretion of acid and pepsin. As a group, patients with duodenal ulcer have greater capacity for gastric acid secretion than do healthy persons. This is manifest by increased basal acid secretion, increased acid response to meal ingestion, and increased responsiveness to histamine stimulation. Evidence links abnormalities in secretion of the hormone gastrin with increased acid secretion. Increased secretion of gastrin is a consequence of antral infection with *H. pylori*.

ANSWER: b

REFERENCE: *Chapter 22—Duodenal Ulcer: Pathophysiology*

3. A 40-year-old man undergoes therapy for acute duodenal ulceration with 400 mg cimetidine twice a day and has resolution of symptoms within 6 weeks. The medication is continued as a nocturnal maintenance dose at the end of a 3-month treatment course. Recurrent symptoms develop 6 months after the initial diagnosis and endoscopic examination reveals recurrent ulceration. Biopsy of the antral mucosa shows moderate gastritis and the presence of *H. pylori*. Medical management designed to eradicate *H. pylori* and heal ulceration should include which of the following agents?

a. Cimetidine

b. Bismuth subcitrate

c. Amoxicillin

d. Metronidazole

e. Vancomycin

COMMENT: The observation that *H. pylori* infection has an important role in ulcer pathogenesis has led to the development of antimicrobial therapy for ulceration. Most successful regimens are based on a bismuth compound (colloidal bismuth subsalicylate or colloidal bismuth subcitrate) plus metronidazole alone or in combination with amoxicillin or tetracycline. Bismuth compounds act locally and achieve gastric concentrations greater than the minimum inhibitory concentration for 90% of *H. pylori* isolates. Metronidazole is secreted into the stomach at high concentration, and the in vivo activity of metronidazole is not diminished by gastric acidity. Triple therapy with bismuth, metronidazole, and tetracycline or amoxicillin eradicates *H. pylori* in 90% of cases. Ranitidine produces no eradication. Inclusion of a histamine H_2 receptor antagonist or omeprazole has been reported to increase the efficacy of antimicrobial therapy. Antimicrobial therapy has been recommended for peptic ulcer disease resistant to conventional therapy, including ulcers that relapse during maintenance therapy and those that do not heal despite histamine H_2 receptor antagonist or omeprazole therapy.

ANSWER: a, b, c, d

REFERENCE: *Chapter 22—Duodenal Ulcer: Drug Treatment of Ulcer Disease*

4. A 45-year-old man undergoes proximal gastric vagotomy to manage intractable duodenal ulceration. What physiologic alterations can be anticipated as a consequence of the operation?

   a. Reduction of basal acid secretion by approximately 25%
   b. Accelerated gastric emptying of liquids
   c. Accelerated gastric emptying of solids
   d. Fasting hypergastrinemia
   e. Postprandial hyperinsulinemia

COMMENT: Division of cholinergic vagal fibers directly affects parietal cell acid secretion by reducing stimulatory input. Basal acid secretion is diminished approximately 80%, and maximal acid output in response to pentagastrin stimulation is reduced approximately 70%. Fasting hypergastrinemia and an exaggerated gastrin response to meal ingestion occur because of loss of feedback inhibition of gastrin release and gastrin cell hyperplasia. Release of pancreatic polypeptide, secretin, and cholecystokinin may be decreased. Proximal gastric vagotomy accelerates gastric emptying of liquids owing to a loss of receptive relaxation. Gastric emptying of solids usually is not affected by proximal gastric vagotomy.

ANSWER: b, d

REFERENCE: *Chapter 22—Duodenal Ulcer: Operative Treatment of Ulcer Disease*

5. Which of the following statements is/are correct regarding postoperative rates of recurrent ulcer and dumping?

   a. Truncal vagotomy with antrectomy is associated with persistent dumping in 10% to 15% of patients
   b. Recurrent ulceration after truncal vagotomy and pyloroplasty occurs among 25% of patients within 10 years of the operation
   c. Patients who undergo proximal gastric vagotomy have a 10% to 15% risk of recurrent ulcer and an approximately 1% risk of persistent dumping
   d. Recurrent ulceration occurs among 5% of patients who undergo truncal vagotomy and antrectomy

COMMENT: Surgical recommendations for management of peptic ulceration should be based on safety, freedom from long-term postoperative symptoms, and avoidance of recurrent ulceration. Proximal gastric vagotomy has an operative mortality less than 1% and a risk of persistent dumping symptoms of approximately 1%. The low incidence of postoperative symptoms is associated with a relatively high risk of recurrent ulceration, estimated to be 10% to 15% 5 years postoperatively. After truncal vagotomy and pyloroplasty, dumping is initially present in 10% of patients and is persistent or severe in 1%. Recurrent ulceration occurs among 10% of patients who undergo truncal vagotomy and pyloroplasty. Truncal vagotomy with antrectomy is associated with the lowest risk of recurrent ulceration, 1% to 2%, but the greatest incidence of postoperative dumping symptoms, 10% to 15%.

ANSWER: a, c

REFERENCE: *Chapter 22—Duodenal Ulcer: Operative Treatment of Ulcer Disease*

6. A 50-year-old man with a 2-year history of duodenal ulceration has sudden, severe epigastric pain 4 hours before evaluation. Physical examination reveals a temperature of 101°F (38.4°C), pulse 80 beats/min, blood pressure 125/90 mm Hg, diminished bowel sounds, and abdominal muscular rigidity. An upright chest radiograph shows pneumoperitoneum. At laparotomy, an anterior perforation in the first portion of the duodenum is found. Optimal treatment would include:

a. Omental patch of the perforation followed by truncal vagotomy and antrectomy after 8 weeks
b. Omental patch of the perforation followed by truncal vagotomy and pyloroplasty after 8 weeks
c. Omental patch of the perforation followed by long-term administration of cimetidine
d. Omental patch of the perforation and proximal gastric vagotomy
e. Omental patch of the perforation only

COMMENT: Simple omental patching of a perforation in the treatment of patients with chronic ulcer disease does not yield satisfactory long-term results. As many as 80% of patients so treated have recurrent ulceration, and 10% have secondary complications. A definitive ulcer operation should be performed during the initial laparotomy if the following circumstances apply: (a) there has been no preoperative shock, (b) the perforation has been present for less than 48 hours, and (c) no life-threatening medical comorbidity exists. Omental patching of the perforation combined with proximal gastric vagotomy is a preferred approach because it combines safety, freedom from disabling postoperative symptoms, and a low rate of recurrent ulceration. In an alternative, newer approach omental patching of the perforation is followed by postoperative treatment with omeprazole and clarithromycin if the patient has *H. pylori* infection.

ANSWER: d

REFERENCE: *Chapter 22—Duodenal Ulcer: Operative Treatment of Ulcer Disease*

7. A 42-year-old man with a recently diagnosed duodenal ulcer has melena and near-syncope. After fluid resuscitation, upper gastrointestinal endoscopy is performed. During the examination, a 1-cm ulcer is found in the proximal duodenum. A fresh clot is observed within the ulcer, and blood is oozing around the clot. Optimal therapy would consist of which of the following?

a. Angiographic embolization of the gastroduodenal artery
b. Irrigation of the clot followed by endoscopic application of a heat probe
c. Transfusion and intravenous administration of cimetidine
d. Angiographic infusion of vasopressin into the gastroduodenal artery
e. Transfusion and oral omeprazole

COMMENT: The ability to visualize bleeding duodenal ulcers endoscopically has led to attempts to control hemorrhage endoscopically. Thermal coagulation can be achieved by means of bipolar electrocoagulation or direct application of heat through a probe. A National Institutes of Health consensus development conference has recommended endoscopic hemostatic therapy in the treatment of selected patients. Hematemesis, age older than 60 years, and serious medical comorbidity are clinical features that mandate endoscopic therapy. Rebleeding during hospitalization and the endoscopic findings of visible vessel, oozing, or bleeding associated with an adherent clot are other indications for endoscopic hemostasis. Operative intervention is appropriate for massive hemorrhage leading to shock or cardiovascular instability, prolonged blood loss necessitating continuation of transfusion, recurrent bleeding during medical therapy or after endoscopic therapy, and recurrent hemorrhage necessitating hospitalization. Operative therapy should consist of duodenotomy with direct ligation of the bleeding vessel within the ulcer base followed by a procedure to permanently reduce acid production.

ANSWER: b

REFERENCE: *Chapter 22—Duodenal Ulcer: Hemorrhage*

8. Which of the following statements is/are correct with regard to pyloric obstruction secondary to peptic ulceration?

    a. Pyloric obstruction is suggested by hypochloremic hyponatremic alkalosis
    b. Pyloric obstruction is suggested by hypochloremic hypokalemic alkalosis
    c. Approximately 80% of patients with benign gastric outlet obstruction obtain permanent relief of symptoms with endoscopically directed balloon dilatation
    d. The lifetime risk of pyloric obstruction among patients with peptic ulcer is 40%

COMMENT: Repeated episodes of ulceration and healing can lead to scarring and pyloric stenosis. The lifetime risk of this complication approximates 10%. Gastric outlet obstruction is characterized by the development of hypochloremic hypokalemic alkalosis due to loss of hydrochloric acid through vomiting and renal compensatory mechanisms that conserve hydrogen ion at the expense of secreted potassium. Although 85% of cases of pyloric stenosis are technically amenable to balloon dilation, fewer than 1 in 3 patients achieve permanent relief of symptoms by this means.

ANSWER: b

REFERENCE: *Chapter 22—Duodenal Ulcer: Obstruction*

9. A 50-year-old patient underwent truncal vagotomy and antrectomy with Billroth II reconstruction 2 years ago. The patient now has recurrent postprandial pain, nausea, and vomiting. Endoscopic examination reveals bile in the stomach; endoscopic biopsy shows histologic evidence of moderately severe gastritis. No other endoscopic abnormalities are found. Appropriate therapy could include:

    a. Octreotide administration
    b. Conversion of Billroth II gastrojejunostomy to Billroth I gastroduodenostomy
    c. Conversion of Billroth II gastrojejunostomy to Roux-en-Y gastrojejunostomy
    d. Roux-en-Y hepatojejunostomy

COMMENT: Symptoms related to bile reflux gastritis occur transiently among 10% to 20% of patients after truncal vagotomy and resection or drainage. Symptoms persist in only 1% to 2%. No completely satisfactory solution to bile reflux gastritis exists. Medicinal and dietary treatments have not proved beneficial. Operative diversion of biliary secretions from the gastric mucosa by means of Roux-en-Y gastrojejunostomy with an intestinal limb of 50 to 60 cm has been widely reported. The procedure eliminates bilious vomiting in nearly 100% of patients, but pain persists in as many as 30%, and 20% have delayed gastric emptying as a result of the procedure.

ANSWER: c

REFERENCE: *Chapter 22—Duodenal Ulcer: Alkaline Reflux Gastritis*

10. Which of the following clinical circumstances has/have been identified as predisposing factors for the development of stress ulceration?

   a. Intraperitoneal sepsis
   b. Hemorrhagic shock
   c. Isolated tibial fracture
   d. Second-degree burn of 50% of the body surface area
   e. Acute respiratory distress syndrome

COMMENT: Several risk factors or predisposing clinical conditions have been identified for stress ulceration. Specific risk factors include acute respiratory distress syndrome, multiple trauma, severe burn of more than 35% of the body surface area, oliguric renal failure, large transfusion requirements, hepatic dysfunction, hypotension, prolonged surgical procedures, and sepsis from any source. A direct correlation has been shown between acute upper gastrointestinal hemorrhage and the severity of critical illness.

ANSWER: a, b, d, e

REFERENCE: *Chapter 22—Duodenal Ulcer: Stress Gastritis*

11. A 35-year-old male smoker is involved in a house fire and receives a burn of 45% of body surface area. One half of the burned surface appears to be third degree. On the third postburn day, the patient has bloody drainage from a nasogastric tube and a decrease of 5% in hematocrit. Appropriate management includes which of the following?

   a. Urgent upper gastrointestinal radiographic contrast study to delineate the site of bleeding
   b. Immediate selective arteriography through the left gastric artery to diagnose and manage presumed stress ulceration
   c. Urgent esophagogastroduodenoscopy to identify the cause of bleeding
   d. Urgent intravenous infusion of vasopressin at 0.2 to 0.4 IU/min

COMMENT: Patients who have sustained a major thermal burn of 35% or more of total body surface area are at a predictably high risk of development of gastric erosions and hemorrhage. Endoscopic studies have shown that gastric erosions are present in 93% of these patients, whereas the occurrence of severe acute upper gastrointestinal hemorrhage among severely burned patients is 25% to 50%. At least 60% of patients at risk have stress erosions within 1 to 2 days after the precipitating event. Painless upper gastrointestinal bleeding may be the only clinical sign. The onset of hemorrhage often is delayed, usually occurring 3 to 10 days after the onset of the primary disease.

Esophagogastroduodenoscopy is the best diagnostic modality to confirm the diagnosis and to differentiate stress erosion from other sources of upper gastrointestinal hemorrhage. Identification of the bleeding source is correct in more than 90% of instances. If endoscopy does not provide enough information for diagnosis, visceral angiography through selective catheterization of the left gastric or splenic vessels may provide information regarding the primary vessel supplying the bleeding site. Barium examinations usually are of little value because of the superficial nature of stress erosion. Such an examination can be detrimental because it interferes with the interpretation of arteriographic findings.

ANSWER: c

REFERENCE: *Chapter 22—Duodenal Ulcer: Stress Gastritis*

12. Agents found to have an efficacy greater than 90% for prophylactic treatment of stress ulceration include which of the following?

    a. Antacids
    b. Histamine H$_2$ receptor antagonists
    c. Sucralfate
    d. Misoprostol

COMMENT: Hourly administration of antacid (30 to 60 mL) through a nasogastric tube to maintain gastric luminal fluid pH above 3.5 has proved to be effective prophylaxis. In a study involving 100 seriously ill patients randomly assigned to receive placebo or antacid prophylaxis, bleeding was detected in 25% of patients given no prophylaxis, compared with 4% of patients given antacids through a nasogastric tube. In a review of data derived from 16 prospective trials, when overt bleeding manifested by melena, hematemesis, or transfusion requirement was used as the minimum criterion, there was no significant difference in risk of bleeding when antacids and cimetidine were compared.

Continuous infusions of any of the histamine H$_2$ receptor antagonists provides more consistent maintenance of an intraluminal gastric pH greater than 3.5 than do the standard intermittent-infusion regimens. Advantages of continuous infusion of these agents include a potential reduction in toxicity, decreased pharmacy costs and nursing duties, and possible enhancement of therapeutic benefit. Results of controlled trials suggest that sucralfate, 1 g every 6 hours, may be as effective prophylactically as antacids or cimetidine. Among 100 critically ill patients, bleeding occurred in 6% of patients receiving antacids or cimetidine; none of the 34 patients treated with sucralfate had bleeding.

Given exogenously, natural or synthetic prostaglandins of the E, F, and I series inhibit gastric acid secretion. One group compared the efficacy of 15(R)-15 dimethyl prostaglandin E$_2$ given at antisecretory doses with that of antacids and found that stress-related bleeding occurred among 50% of patients given the synthetic prostaglandin derivative and among only 14% of patients receiving antacids.

ANSWER: a, b, c

REFERENCE: *Chapter 22—Duodenal Ulcer: Stress Gastritis*

13. A 25-year-old man is involved in an automobile accident. The resultant injuries include bilateral closed fractures of the femur, left pulmonary contusion, and closed head injury. Four days after injury, profuse upper gastrointestinal hemorrhage begins. Endoscopic examination reveals an area of confluent ulceration with bleeding in the gastric fundus. Endoscopic hemostasis fails. Appropriate immediate management includes:

    a. Lavage of gastric contents with iced saline solution
    b. Urgent total gastrectomy
    c. Selective arterial infusion of vasopressin through the left gastric artery
    d. Insertion of a Sengstaken-Blakemore balloon

COMMENT: Initial efforts to control gastric hemorrhage consist of gastric lavage with warmed saline solution. Lavage fragments existing clots, removes pooled blood, and reduces fibrinolysis at bleeding sites. More than 80% of patients with upper gastrointestinal hemorrhage stop bleeding with this approach. Use of antacids for definitive management of acute active stress bleeding is largely unsuccessful. Administration of histamine H$_2$ receptor blocking agents once active gastrointestinal bleeding has begun also usually is ineffective as a definitive form of therapy.

The endoscope has become the preferred therapeutic as well as diagnostic instrument because it has electrocauterization and laser photocoagulation capabilities. If endoscopic therapy fails, angiography is an additional way to control bleeding by means of selective infusion of vasopressin into the splanchnic circulation through the left gastric artery. Vasopressin is administered by means of continuous infusion through the catheter at a rate of 0.2 to 0.4 IU/min for a maximum of 48 to 72 hours.

Approximately 10% to 20% of patients with acute stress ulcers continue to bleed or have recurrent bleeding despite these measures. For these patients, total gastrectomy has a mortality ranging from 17% to 100%. In general, operative mortality rates for acute stress-induced hemorrhage range from 30% to 60% regardless of the surgical procedure undertaken.

ANSWER: c

REFERENCE: *Chapter 22—Duodenal Ulcer: Stress Gastritis*

14. With regard to benign gastric ulceration, the most common location of disease is which of the following?
    a. Along the greater curvature
    b. Immediately distal to the esophagogastric junction along the lesser curvature
    c. In the area of the incisura angularis along the lesser curvature
    d. Within the gastric antrum

COMMENT: Gastric ulcers can occur anywhere in the stomach, although they usually occur on the lesser curvature near the incisura angularis. Approximately 60% of ulcers are located at or slightly above the angularis. Fifteen percent to 23% of gastric ulcers are within the gastric antrum, and 10% are high on the lesser curvature. Only 5% of gastric ulcers are found on the greater curvature. In addition, 97% of all gastric ulcers occur within 2 cm of the junctional zone between fundic and antral mucosa. Gastric ulcers appear at different distances from the pyloric sphincter because the antrum extends for variable (2 to 16 cm) distances from the pylorus. It is interesting that with increasing age, this junctional zone moves proximally along the lesser curvature, as does the incidence of gastric ulcer.

ANSWER: c

REFERENCE: *Chapter 22—Duodenal Ulcer: Stress Gastritis*

15. Type I gastric ulcers are located in the gastric body, usually along the lesser curvature. Which of the following statements correctly characterize(s) type I gastric ulcers?
    a. Normal to low acid secretion
    b. Associated duodenal ulceration
    c. High frequency of blood group A
    d. Frequent association with hypergastrinemia

COMMENT: Gastric ulcers are divided into categories based on their location and gastric acid secretory status. A type I gastric ulcer is an ulcer in the body of the stomach, usually along the lesser curvature, associated with large volumes of secretion with a low to normal acid output. Type I ulcers are not associated with duodenal, pyloric, or prepyloric mucosal abnormalities. A slight predominance of patients with blood group A have this type of gastric ulcer. Type II gastric ulcer is located in the body of the stomach in combination with a duodenal ulcer. These patients usually are acid hypersecretors. Approximately 23% to 25% of gastric ulcers are type II. Type III gastric ulcers are characterized as prepyloric and account for approximately 23% of lesions. Patients with this lesion are typically acid hypersecretors. Type IV gastric ulcers occur high on the lesser curvature near the gastroesophageal junction. In the United States, the incidence of type IV gastric ulcer is less than 10%.

ANSWER: a, c

REFERENCE: *Chapter 22—Duodenal Ulcer: Stress Gastritis*

16. A 45-year-old man has epigastric pain that worsens with ingestion of food. The findings at physical examination are normal. Results of upper abdominal ultrasonography are unremarkable. Contrast radiography reveals a 2-cm ulcer in the gastric fundus along the lesser curvature. Therapy with omeprazole 20 mg per day is begun, but symptoms persist 3 weeks later. Appropriate management includes which of the following?

a. Increase in omeprazole dose to 40 mg/d
b. Addition of sucralfate 1 g every 8 hours
c. Addition of cimetidine 200 mg twice a day
d. Esophagogastroduodenoscopy with biopsy of ulcer

COMMENT: Approximately 5% of ulcers that appear radiographically benign are malignant. Gastroscopy is the most reliable method of differentiating benign and malignant gastric ulcers. The accuracy is more than 97% if multiple biopsies and brushings for cytologic examination are performed. Clinical features that prompt early endoscopic evaluation include considerable weight loss, symptoms of gastric outlet obstruction, palpable abdominal mass, and positive stool Hemoccult result or blood loss anemia. Endoscopic features that suggest the presence of a malignant tumor include an exophytic mass, abnormal or disrupted mucosal folds, necrotic ulcer crater, bleeding from the edge of the ulcer crater, stepwise depression of the ulcer edge, heaped-up margins, or small extensions of the ulcer that blur a portion of the ulcer wall. If initial biopsies do not show malignant cells but the endoscopic appearance strongly suggests that carcinoma underlies the ulcer, another endoscopic examination with deeper biopsies should be undertaken.

ANSWER: d

REFERENCE: *Chapter 22—Duodenal Ulcer: Stress Gastritis*

17. A 52-year-old woman is hospitalized with acute upper gastrointestinal hemorrhage. Endoscopic examination reveals a 2.5-cm ulcer in the area of the incisura angularis. The other endoscopic findings are normal. Continued bleeding necessitates therapy. Optimal therapy consists of which of the following?

a. Gastrotomy with oversewing of the bleeding site
b. Distal gastrectomy including the area of ulceration
c. Proximal gastric vagotomy and oversewing of the bleeding ulcer
d. Truncal vagotomy, pyloroplasty, and oversewing of the bleeding ulcer

COMMENT: A distinction should be made among the different types of gastric ulcer in selecting the most appropriate operative procedure, because treatment varies according to location, coexistent duodenal ulcer disease, and acid secretory status. The best elective operation for type I benign gastric ulcer is distal gastrectomy with gastroduodenal anastomosis. Gastrojejunostomy is an acceptable alternative. The ulcer should be included in the antrectomy specimen. The operative mortality rate associated with this procedure is 2% to 3%, the recurrence rate is 3%, and good to excellent clinical results can be anticipated for more than 90% of patients. The addition of truncal vagotomy does not appear to diminish the recurrence rate. Definitive management of hemorrhage is a procedure designed to control bleeding and to prevent recurrent ulceration. Antrectomy, which includes the ulcer with gastroduodenostomy, is considered the best procedure for surgical management of this complication. The quoted operative mortality rates in this setting range from 10% to 40%.

ANSWER: b

REFERENCE: *Chapter 22—Duodenal Ulcer: Gastric Ulcer*

CHAPTER 23

MORBID OBESITY

1. Severe obesity is associated with a large number of associated problems that form the basis of the term *morbid obesity*. Documented causes of excess mortality among severely obese patients include:

    a. Coronary artery disease
    b. Hypertension
    c. Adult-onset diabetes mellitus
    d. Obesity hypoventilation and sleep apnea
    e. Pulmonary embolization

COMMENT: Morbid obesity is arbitrarily defined as 100 pounds (45 kg) above ideal body weight as defined by actuarial tables. Premature death is much more common among severely obese persons. Morbidly obese men 25 to 34 years of age have a 12-fold higher mortality than do men of normal weight. Causes of early death include coronary artery disease, hypertension, impaired ventricular function, diabetes mellitus, sleep apnea and other hypoventilation syndromes, pulmonary embolization, and necrotizing soft-tissue infection.

ANSWER: a, b, c, d, e

REFERENCE: *Chapter 23—Morbid Obesity*

2. Jejunoileal bypass was formerly performed as a weight reduction procedure. The operation was abandoned because of the development of serious long-term complications associated with the procedure. Which of the following statements correctly characterize(s) results after jejunoileal bypass?

    a. Kidney stones occur with increased frequency because of increased absorption of pyruvate from the colon
    b. The most serious complication of jejunoileal bypass is development of cirrhosis due to protein-calorie malnutrition
    c. Bacterial overgrowth in the bypassed segment can be managed with oral vancomycin
    d. Rapid weight loss after jejunoileal bypass is associated with development of gallstones

COMMENT: Jejunoileal bypass is associated with a number of early and late complications. Malabsorption of bile salts coupled with rapid weight loss greatly increases risk of gallstone development. Multiple kidney stones are caused by excessive absorption of oxalate from the colon, where oxalate is ordinarily chelated with calcium. Malabsorption results in severe diarrhea, electrolyte abnormalities, metabolic acidosis, and anemia. Bacterial overgrowth in the bypassed intestinal segment coupled with protein malabsorption is postulated to be responsible for development of cirrhosis, the most serious complication of jejunoileal bypass. Bacterial overgrowth can be temporarily suppressed by metronidazole. Development of hepatic dysfunction is an indication for reversal of the bypass.

ANSWER: b, d

REFERENCE: *Chapter 23—Morbid Obesity: Jejunoileal Bypass*

3. Which of the following statements regarding gastroplasty and gastric bypass for morbid obesity is/are correct?

   a. Horizontal gastroplasty techniques that rely on a single horizontal application of a stapling device are associated with a 40% to 70% rate of inability to decrease weight
   b. Gastric bypass is followed by progressive weight loss over 36 months
   c. Gastric bypass is unsuccessful for weight loss among 10% to 15% of patients
   d. With three superimposed applications of a stapling device, dehiscence of the gastric bypass staple line occurs in less than 2% of cases

COMMENT: Horizontal gastroplasty includes (a) single application of a 90-mm stapling device without suture reinforcement of the stoma between upper and lower gastric pouches or (b) double application of staples with either a central or lateral polypropylene-reinforced stoma. The failure rate (loss of less than 40% of excess weight) for horizontal gastroplasty ranges from 40% to 70%. Vertical banded gastroplasty is a procedure in which a stapled opening is made in the stomach with the stapling device 5 cm from the cardioesophageal junction. Two applications of a 90-mm stapling device are made between this opening and the angle of His. A 1.5 cm by 5 cm strip of polypropylene mesh is wrapped around the stoma on the lesser curvature and sutured to itself.

Gastric bypass can be performed with placement of staples in a vertical or horizontal direction. The vertical direction is preferred because there is less risk of gastric pouch devascularization or splenic injury. With three superimposed applications of a 90-mm stapler, the incidence of staple line disruption has been less than 2%. Roux-en-Y gastric bypass results in markedly better weight loss than does vertical banded gastroplasty. Although gastric bypass is unsuccessful for 10% to 15% of patients, weight loss seems to remain stable for most patients 5 years or more after surgery.

ANSWER: a, c, d

REFERENCE: *Chapter 23—Morbid Obesity: Overview of Gastric Surgery for Morbid Obesity*

4. Which of the following statements is correct with regard to gastric bypass for obesity?

   a. Rapid weight loss after successful gastric bypass for obesity is associated with increased risk of cholelithiasis
   b. Marginal ulcer develops among 25% of patients who undergo gastric bypass
   c. Vitamin B_{12} deficiency is a complication of gastric bypass caused by gastric mucosal atrophy
   d. Anastomotic leak after gastric bypass often is heralded by bradycardia

COMMENT: The most serious complication after gastric bypass for obesity is anastomotic dehiscence. Leak is presumed to be caused by gastric necrosis due to ischemia from staple line application or ligation of the short gastric vessels. Patients may have little pain; tachycardia, tachypnea, and fever may be the only manifestations. Findings at physical examinations of morbidly obese patients with peritonitis are unreliable. Marginal ulcers occur among only 10% or fewer of patients who undergo gastric bypass and respond to histamine H_2 receptor antagonists. In rare instances, polyneuropathy has occurred after gastric bypass, usually in association with intractable vomiting and protein-calorie malnutrition. Vitamin B_{12} deficiency can occur after gastric bypass owing to decreased acid digestion of vitamin B_{12} in food. Monthly B_{12} supplementation should be routine. Cholelithiasis occurs among approximately one third of morbidly obese patients, and gallstone formation is accelerated in the early postoperative period by the effects of rapid weight loss.

ANSWER: a

REFERENCE: *Chapter 23—Morbid Obesity: Complications of Gastric Surgery*

CHAPTER 24

GASTRIC NEOPLASMS

1. Which of the following conditions is considered to increase the risk of gastric cancer?

   a. Pernicious anemia
   b. Previous partial gastrectomy
   c. Gastric hyperplastic polyps
   d. Gastric adenomatous polyps

COMMENT: The risk of gastric cancer is greater in stomachs that harbor adenomatous polyps. The risk of cancer has been estimated at 10% to 20% and is greatest for polyps more than 2 cm in diameter. Hyperplastic polyps, although common in the normal population, do not have malignant potential. The incidence of malignant gastric tumors increases among persons with chronic gastritis associated with pernicious anemia. When pernicious anemia has been present for 5 years, the risk of malignant gastric disease is twice that among age-matched controls. Increased risk of gastric carcinoids also exists among patients with pernicious anemia, presumably because of the effects of long-standing hypergastrinemia. A 3-fold increased risk of gastric cancer also exists among patients that have previously undergone partial gastric resection. Postgastrectomy cancer is a long-term concern; increased incidence of malignancy is not observed until 15 years postoperatively.

ANSWER: a, b, d

REFERENCE: *Chapter 24—Gastric Neoplasms: Premalignant Lesions*

2. A 55-year-old man is evaluated because of symptoms of epigastric pain and anorexia. Findings at physical examination are normal except for guaiac-positive stool. Upper endoscopic examination reveals a 1.5-cm ulcer along the lesser curvature of the stomach proximal to the incisura angularis. Optimal management consists of which of the following?

   a. Sucralfate 1 g four times a day for 8 weeks
   b. Endoscopic biopsy of the ulcer rim
   c. Endoscopic cauterization of the ulcer base
   d. Endoscopic biopsy of the ulcer base
   e. Misoprostol 400 mg twice a day for 8 weeks

COMMENT: The symptoms produced by gastric cancer and benign gastric ulcer are nonspecific and often similar. Pain is present in 70% of patients with gastric cancer and usually is constant, nonradiating, and not improved by food ingestion. Findings at physical examination usually are normal if the patient has early gastric cancer. One third of patients have guaiac-positive stool. Fiberoptic endoscopy is the definitive diagnostic method. Although the endoscopic appearance of gastric ulcers can suggest benign or malignant origins, definite distinction can be made only with gastric biopsy. Accurate diagnosis of gastric cancer can be made in 95% of cases if multiple biopsy specimens are obtained from the ulcer rim. Biopsy of the ulcer base more frequently reveals necrotic material.

ANSWER: b

REFERENCE: *Chapter 24—Gastric Neoplasms: Clinical Features*

3. A patient with gastric adenocarcinoma undergoes subtotal gastrectomy. Pathologic examination reveals that the tumor penetrates to the serosa. Regional lymph nodes are not involved. Distant metastatic lesions are not detected. What is the correct tumor stage and 5-year survival rate?

    a. Stage I, 90% 5-year survival rate
    b. Stage II, 45% 5-year survival rate
    c. Stage III, 15% 5-year survival rate
    d. Stage II, 15% 5-year survival rate
    e. Stage III, 2% 5-year survival rate

COMMENT: For early lesions of the antrum or middle stomach, distal subtotal gastrectomy including 80% of the stomach provides satisfactory 5-year survival without increases in operative morbidity. Proximal gastric lesions or larger lesions of the middle part of the stomach may necessitate total gastrectomy or esophagogastrectomy to encompass the tumor. Regardless of the extent of gastric resection, patients with more advanced tumors fare poorly because of the increased likelihood of lymphatic and hematogenous spread. The TNM system is shown in Table 24.2. The 5-year survival for patients with stage I disease (in situ carcinoma) is close to that of the normal population. For patients with disease in stage II, the 5-year survival rate approximates 45%, whereas 15% of patients with stage III disease survive 5 years. The long-term survival rate with systemic metastasis is negligible.

ANSWER: b

REFERENCE: *Chapter 24—Gastric Neoplasms: Curative Treatment*

Table 24.2. TNM CLASSIFICATION FOR STAGING OF GASTRIC CANCER

TNM DEFINITIONS
Primary Tumor

T1	Tumor confined to the mucosa
T2	Tumor involves the mucosa and submucosa and extends to but does not penetrate the serosa
T3	Tumor penetrates the serosa with or without invasion of adjacent structures
T4	Diffuse involvement on gastric wall without obvious boundaries (linitis plastica)

Regional Lymph Node Involvement

N0	No nodal metastasis
N1	Metastasis to perigastric lymph nodes in immediate vicinity of tumor
N2	Metastasis to lymph nodes distant from primary tumor or along both curvatures of the stomach

Distant Metastasis

M0	No distant metastasis
M1	Metastasis beyond regional lymph nodes

STAGE GROUPING

Stage I	T1, N0, M0
Stage II	T2–3, N0, M0
Stage III	T1–3, N1–3, M0
Stage IV	Tumor unresectable or metastatic

4. With regard to operative management of gastric carcinoma, which of the following statements is/are correct?

    a. Resection margins of 2 cm are necessary to prevent recurrence due to intramural metastasis
    b. Prophylactic splenectomy has been shown to improve outcome among similarly staged patients
    c. Extended lymphadenectomy that includes nodes along the aorta and esophagus has not been shown to improve survival in North American trials
    d. Long-term survival is rare if adjacent organs must be resected to achieve local control

COMMENT: In gastric cancer, microscopic involvement of the resection margin by tumor cells is associated with a poor prognosis. Unlike colon cancer, gastric cancer frequently has extensive intramural spread. Results of retrospective studies suggest that a line of resection 6 cm from the tumor mass is necessary to ensure a low rate of anastomotic recurrence.

The value of extended lymphadenectomy in the management of gastric adenocarcinoma is controversial. The largest favorable experience has been reported in Japan, where retrospective studies have shown improvement of approximately 10%, stage for stage, for patients with advanced disease. The benefits of extensive lymphadenectomy have not been confirmed in western countries.

Histologically positive lymph nodes are frequently present in the splenic hilum and along the splenic artery, and routine splenectomy has been practiced in some centers. Prophylactic splenectomy has not been found to improve outcome for similarly staged patients. Resection of adjacent organs may be needed for local control if direct invasion has occurred. In this circumstance, operative morbidity is increased, and long-term survival is rare.

ANSWER: c, d

REFERENCE: *Chapter 24—Gastric Neoplasms: Curative Treatment*

5. Which of the following statements regarding gastric leiomyosarcoma is/are correct?

   a. Leiomyosarcoma occurs with peak frequency in the second and third decades of life

   b. The primary histologic indicator of aggressive behavior is the number of mitoses per microscopic field

   c. Leiomyosarcoma usually is radiosensitive

   d. Lymphadenectomy is not indicated during resection because metastasis usually is hematogenous

COMMENT: Leiomyosarcoma occurs with equal frequency in both sexes in the sixth and seventh decades of life. The tumor frequently has prominent extraluminal growth and attains large size before causing symptoms. Leiomyosarcoma must be differentiated from its benign counterpart, leiomyoma. At gross inspection, the tumors are firm, grayish-white masses; a pseudocapsule separating tumor from normal smooth muscle sometimes is present. When the tumors reach a large size, central necrosis is common. Leiomyosarcoma usually is graded histologically; the frequency of mitotic figures is the main indicator of aggressive behavior. Lesions with more than 5 to 10 mitoses per 10 high-power fields have increased metastasis.

Intraperitoneal sarcomatosis is frequent, as is local recurrence after resection. Metastasis occurs by the hematogenous route, and thus hepatic involvement is common. Lymphatic metastasis occurs among fewer than 10% of patients. Negative surgical margins must be ensured histologically, but lymphadenectomy is not indicated because of the low frequency of lymphatic metastasis. Leiomyosarcoma is not radiosensitive, and chemotherapy has not been shown to improve survival.

ANSWER: b, d

REFERENCE: *Chapter 24—Gastric Neoplasms: Gastric Sarcomas*

6. Which of the following statements characterizing gastric lymphoma is/are correct?

   a. More than one half of gastrointestinal lymphomas occur in the stomach

   b. The peak incidence of gastric lymphoma is in the second and third decades of life

   c. Endoscopic biopsy provides enough information for a diagnosis in 90% of cases

   d. Gastric perforation occurs among 40% of patients treated with cytolytic agents instead of gastrectomy

COMMENT: The stomach is the site of more than one half of gastrointestinal lymphomas and is the most common organ involved in extranodal lymphoma. Gastric lymphoma is distinctly uncommon among children and young adults. The peak incidence is in the sixth and seventh decades of life. Radiologic findings are similar to those of adenocarcinoma. Endoscopic examination has become the diagnostic method of choice. Endoscopic biopsy combined with endoscopic brush cytologic examination provides a diagnosis in approximately 90% of cases. When gastric lymphoma is first diagnosed by endoscopic means, evidence of systemic disease should be sought. Computed tomography of the chest and abdomen to detect lymphadenopathy, lymphangiography, bone marrow biopsy, and biopsy of enlarged peripheral lymph nodes may be appropriate.

A multimodality program is used in most centers to manage primary gastric lymphomas. Gastrectomy is the first step in the therapeutic strategy. Increasing numbers of patients are treated with chemoradiation therapy alone. The risk of hemorrhage or perforation frequently alluded to in the past has probably been overstated. The risk of perforation if primary gastric lymphoma is managed with cytolytic agents and not resected approximates 5%.

ANSWER: a, c

REFERENCE: *Chapter 24—Gastric Neoplasms: Gastric Lymphoma*

Section D
SMALL INTESTINE

CHAPTER 25

ANATOMY AND PHYSIOLOGY OF THE SMALL INTESTINE

1. The small intestine contains an intrinsic nervous system that regulates motility. The aggregation of neurons, located between the circular and longitudinal layers of smooth muscle, that most directly regulates motility is the:

   a. Myenteric plexus
   b. Submucous plexus
   c. Celiac ganglion
   d. Superior mesenteric ganglion

COMMENT: The small intestine contains a complex, intrinsic nervous system called the *enteric nervous system* (ENS). The ENS is a network of approximately 10 to 100 million neurons with cell bodies within the bowel wall that contain as many neurons as does the spinal cord. The ENS is distinct from the autonomic nervous system and is unique in its ability to mediate reflex activity even when isolated from the central nervous system. The ENS contains two major plexuses, the myenteric (Auerbach's) plexus, located between the longitudinal and circular muscle layers, and the submucous (Meissner's) plexus. Enteric neurons have extensive connections with each other, intestinal smooth-muscle cells, epithelial cells, endocrine cells, extrinsic neurons, and the vasculature. Through these connections, the ENS provides neural control of all gastrointestinal functions, including motility, blood flow, secretion, and absorption. The chemical mediators in the ENS were initially thought to be limited to neurotransmitters such as acetylcholine and serotonin. Subsequent research has added purines to the list, such as adenosine triphosphate, and peptides, such as vasoactive intestinal peptide, somatostatin, and substance P. Nitric oxide also has been identified as a neurotransmitter in the ENS. More than 20 candidate neurotransmitters have been identified in enteric neurons.

ANSWER: a

REFERENCE: *Chapter 25—Anatomy and Physiology of the Small Intestine: Innervation*

2. A patient undergoes a contrast radiography small bowel for evaluation of intestinal pseudoobstruction. The normal transit time from the stomach to the cecum is:

   a. 30 to 60 minutes
   b. 1 to 2 hours
   c. 2 to 4 hours
   d. 10 hours

COMMENT: In healthy humans, the mean transit time in the small intestine documented with scintigraphic studies is 221 ± 49 minutes with a range of 131 to 322 minutes. The composition of the meal affects the rate of occurrence and propagation of contractions during the postprandial period. Frequency of contraction is greatest with meals containing glucose and least after meals high in fat. Therefore, transit is regulated to optimize absorption of nutrients.

ANSWER: c

REFERENCE: *Chapter 25—Anatomy and Physiology of the Small Intestine: Physiology; Motility*

3. The amount of water normally excreted in stool is:

   a. 100 mL/d
   b. 500 mL/d
   c. 1 L/d
   d. 2 L/d

COMMENT: The intestine has a remarkable ability to absorb and secrete large quantities of fluid. Absorption of water is a net result of fluxes into and out of the intestinal lumen. Approximately 8 to 10 L of fluid is presented to the small intestine each day, of which 1 to 2 L of water is oral intake. An additional 5 to 10 L of fluid is in the form of salivary (1 to 2 L), gastric (2 to 3 L), biliary (0.5 L), pancreatic (1 to 2 L), and intestinal secretions (1 L). Eighty percent of this fluid is absorbed in the small intestine. The colon absorbs most of the remaining fluid, and a small amount (0.1 L) is excreted in the stool. The balance between intestinal absorption and secretion of water is tightly regulated so that there is normally net absorption of fluid. Alterations in this fine balance due to either impaired absorption or augmented secretion can result in overall net secretion of water and diarrhea.

ANSWER: a

REFERENCE: *Chapter 25—Anatomy and Physiology of the Small Intestine: Digestion and Absorption; Absorption of Water and Electrolytes*

4. Orally ingested nutrients absorbed without involvement of intestinal lymphatics include:

   a. Cholesterol
   b. Long-chain fatty acids
   c. Short-chain fatty acids
   d. Fat-soluble vitamins

COMMENT: Short-chain fatty acids (fewer than 8 carbon atoms) are water soluble and enter and exit the enterocyte by means of simple diffusion and are taken up into the portal circulation without entering lymphatic vessels. Medium-chain triglycerides (6 to 14 carbon atoms) are absorbed into the enterocytes by means of both simple diffusion and the same absorptive process used by long-chain triglycerides. These fatty acids are not reassembled into complex lipid but enter the portal circulation directly as free fatty acids.

ANSWER: c

REFERENCE: *Chapter 25—Anatomy and Physiology of the Small Intestine: Digestion and Absorption; Lipid Digestion and Absorption*

5. Octreotide is a clinically useful peptide derived from:

   a. Secretin
   b. Somatostatin
   c. Gastrin
   d. Insulin

COMMENT: Somatostatin is synthesized and secreted from both neurons and endocrine cells (D cells) present in small quantities throughout the intestinal mucosa. Most of the biologic effects of somatostatin are inhibitory. Somatostatin inhibits biliary, gastric, and pancreatic secretion and release of a broad range of gastrointestinal hormones. Somatostatin also inhibits motility, presumably by means of inhibiting cholinergic neurons. The peptide decreases splanchnic and portal blood flow. A long-acting cyclic analogue of somatostatin, octreotide, is a useful clinical therapeutic agent in the treatment of patients with gastrointestinal hormone–secreting tumors, carcinoid syndrome, and enterocutaneous and pancreatic fistula.

ANSWER: b

REFERENCE: *Chapter 25—Anatomy and Physiology of the Small Intestine: Immunology; Endocrine Function*

CHAPTER 26

ILEUS AND BOWEL OBSTRUCTION

1. Which of the following statements is/are true concerning the pathophysiologic mechanism of small-bowel obstruction?

   a. Most of gas seen on plain abdominal radiographs is produced by gas-forming microorganisms
   b. Elevation of luminal pressure contributes to fluid accumulation in the small bowel in closed-loop but not open-loop small-bowel obstruction
   c. Intestinal blood flow initially increases to the bowel wall in early bowel obstruction
   d. In the face of obstruction, myoelectrical activity of the bowel is consistently increased

COMMENT: When a loop of bowel is obstructed, intestinal gas and fluid accumulate. Approximately 80% of the gas seen on plain abdominal radiographs is attributable to swallowed air. In the setting of acute pain and anxiety, patients with intestinal obstruction may swallow excessive amounts of air. Fluid accumulates intraluminally with open- or closed-loop small-intestinal obstruction because of a number of factors. Experimental studies and clinical investigations have shown that elevation of luminal pressures to higher than 20 cm water inhibits absorption and stimulates secretion of salt and water into the lumen proximal to an obstruction. In closed-loop obstruction, luminal pressures can exceed 50 cm water and can account for a substantial proportion of an accumulation of luminal fluid. In simple, open-loop obstruction, distention of the lumen by gas rarely leads to a luminal pressure higher than 8 to 12 cm water. Thus in open-loop obstruction, the contributions of high luminal pressure to hypersecretion may not be important. In response to heightened luminal pressure, total blood flow to the bowel may initially increase. Subsequently, however, blood flow to the bowel is compromised as luminal pressure increases, bacteria invade, and inflammation leads to edema within the bowel wall.

Accumulation of gas and fluid in the obstructed lumen changes myoelectrical function in the intestine proximal and distal to the obstructed segment. In response to distention, the obstructed segment itself can dilate, a process known as *receptive relaxation.* At sites proximal and distal to the obstruction, changes in myoelectrical activity are time dependent. There may be initial, intense periods of activity and peristalsis. Myoelectrical activity then is diminished and the interdigestive migrating myoelectrical complex is replaced by ineffectual and seemingly disorganized clusters of contractions.

ANSWER: b, c

REFERENCE: *Chapter 26—Ileus and Bowel Obstruction: Pathophysiology of Intestinal Obstruction*

2. A 45-year-old man with a history of previous right hemicolectomy for colon cancer has colicky abdominal pain that has become constant over the last few hours. He has marked abdominal distention and has had only minimal vomiting of a feculent material. His abdomen is diffusely tender. A radiograph of the abdomen shows multiple air fluid levels with dilatation of some loops to greater than 3 cm in diameter. The most likely diagnosis is:

a. Proximal small-bowel obstruction
b. Distal small-bowel obstruction
c. Acute appendicitis
d. Closed-loop small-bowel obstruction

COMMENT: Differentiating the various types of bowel obstruction can be difficult with the history, physical findings, and radiographic studies. The patient described has intermittent to constant pain with low-volume feculent vomiting. Distention is marked and progressive, and tenderness is diffuse. This scenario most likely fits open-loop distal small-bowel obstruction. The feculent vomiting suggests distal rather than proximal obstruction. The lack of severe pain and signs of peritoneal irritation suggest that closed-loop obstruction is unlikely. Colonic obstruction with an incompetent ileocecal valve would be another alternative to consider if gas in the colon had been seen on the radiograph.

ANSWER: b

REFERENCE: *Chapter 26—Ileus and Bowel Obstruction: Clinical Presentation and Differential Diagnosis*

3. Which of the following statements is/are true concerning laboratory tests that might be obtained for the patient discussed in question 2?

   a. The presence of a white blood cell count greater than 15,000/μL would be highly suggestive of closed-loop obstruction
   b. Metabolic acidosis mandates emergency exploration
   c. An elevation of the blood urea nitrogen level suggests underlying renal dysfunction
   d. There is no rapidly available test to differentiate tissue necrosis from simple bowel obstruction

COMMENT: There have been multiple attempts to use common clinical laboratory test criteria to identify the likelihood that obstruction is associated with strangulation. In most cases of simple obstruction, laboratory studies do not play a direct role in diagnosis but are helpful in understanding the extent of complications such as dehydration and fluid and electrolyte abnormalities. Elevation of the white blood cell count along with fever, tachycardia, and localized abdominal tenderness is one of the cardinal signs of risk of strangulation. However, such an elevation is nonspecific. Metabolic acidosis also may be associated with intestinal ischemia and be evidence of dehydration and fluid loss. Elevation of blood urea nitrogen level and other electrolyte abnormalities also represents fluid loss and dehydration. No noninvasive rapid laboratory tests can provide information to suggest that tissue necrosis is imminent.

ANSWER: d

REFERENCE: *Chapter 26—Ileus and Bowel Obstruction: Clinical Presentation and Differential Diagnosis*

4. The patient discussed in question 2 is admitted to the hospital and after 24 hours still has distention with no evidence of resolution. Which of the following radiographic studies would be considered appropriate at this time?

   a. Contrast enema
   b. Enteroclysis study with dilute barium
   c. Computed tomography with oral administration of dilute barium contrast medium
   d. None of the above

COMMENT: Contrast studies such as those listed above can provide specific localization at the point of obstruction and information about the nature of the underlying lesion. When obstruction of the small intestine is not resolving progressively, small-bowel follow-through is indicated to confirm the presence and location of the obstruction. The history of right hemicolectomy also may allow reflux through the colon to define the ileocolonic anastomosis and define the site of obstruction in a retrograde manner. The potential benefits of computed tomography include defining the obstruction and perhaps the nature of the lesion and defining any other evidence of abdominal disease such as metastases, ascites, or parenchymal liver abnormalities that might be present in a patient with a previous neoplasm. Although none of these tests is contraindicated, lack of improvement in this case likely mandates an operation and makes contrast studies unnecessary. There would appear to be no evidence of strangulation or perforation; therefore there are no contraindications to these studies.

ANSWER: a, b, c, d

REFERENCE: *Chapter 26—Ileus and Bowel Obstruction: Mechanical Obstruction of the Intestine; Radiographs and Imaging*

5. Initial treatment of the patient in question 2 should consist of:

   a. Fluid resuscitation with D5 half normal saline solution with 40 mEq of potassium chloride per liter

   b. Placement of an indwelling urinary catheter

   c. Nasogastric decompression with a nasogastric tube

   d. Immediate surgery

   e. Initiation of administration of broad-spectrum antibiotics at admission

COMMENT: The principles of treatment of a patient with small-bowel obstruction include initial fluid resuscitation and restriction of oral intake. The optimal fluid for resuscitation of this patient with a distal small-bowel obstruction would likely be Ringer's lactate or normal saline solution. Because gastric secretion is a small component of the fluid loss, potassium replacement is likely not particularly important. An indwelling urinary catheter should be placed to monitor the urine output to reflect fluid status. Invasive hemodynamic monitoring with a central line probably is unnecessary unless concerns are raised about cardiac status. Nasogastric decompression is indicated in all but mild cases. The nasogastric tube prevents distal passage of swallowed air, minimizes the discomfort of reflux of intestinal contents, and eliminates vomiting. There appears to be no clinical evidence suggesting the need for urgent operation; therefore resuscitation before surgery is of optimal importance in the care of this patient.

It has been well established that perioperatively administered antibiotics reduce wound infection and abdominal sepsis rates among patients undergoing operations to relieve intestinal obstruction, simple or strangulated. Once the decision has been made to proceed with surgery, broad-spectrum antibiotics that cover gram-negative aerobes and anaerobes should be given. The use of antibiotics to treat patients who have not been committed to operation has not been evaluated systematically. Giving antibiotics to patients who are being observed can obscure the underlying process and delay optimal therapy.

ANSWER: b, c

REFERENCE: *Chapter 26—Ileus and Bowel Obstruction: Mechanical Obstruction of the Intestine; General Considerations and Management of a Patient with Bowel Obstruction*

6. For the patient described in question 2, which of the following statements is/are true concerning the possible cause of bowel obstruction?

   a. Simple obstruction caused by an adhesion is most likely to resolve nonoperatively

   b. It is most likely that the obstruction is caused by recurrent malignant disease

   c. A history of colon cancer makes carcinomatosis the most likely diagnosis

   d. Lower abdominal procedures are more likely to result in obstructive adhesions than are upper abdominal procedures

COMMENT: Peritoneal adhesions account for more than one half of cases of small-bowel obstruction. Lower abdominal procedures such as appendectomy, hysterectomy, and abdominoperineal resection are common precursor operations to account for obstruction, although adhesions may follow any abdominal procedure, including cholecystectomy, gastrectomy, and abdominal vascular procedures. Simple adhesive obstruction is differentiated from other forms of obstruction by the capability to resolve without surgical intervention. In recent surveys, as many as 80% of episodes of small-bowel obstruction due to adhesions were found to resolve nonoperatively. The likelihood that obstruction is caused by a recurrent malignant tumor relates to several factors, including the origin of the primary tumor, the stage of the primary tumor, and the designation of original surgery as curative or palliative. Gastric and pancreatic cancers often manifest as or are subsequently complicated by peritoneal carcinomatosis and subsequent obstruction. With respect to colon and rectal carcinoma, as many as 50% of cases that manifest as obstruction after resection of the primary tumor may be caused by adhesions and not by recurrent malignant disease.

ANSWER: a, d

REFERENCE: *Chapter 26—Ileus and Bowel Obstruction: Mechanical Obstruction of the Intestine; Specific Types of Bowel Obstruction*

7. Which of the following statements is/are true concerning the cause of intestinal obstruction?

a. In the United States, peritoneal adhesions account for more than one half of the cases of small-bowel obstruction

b. A leading cause of bowel obstruction is early postoperative adhesions

c. Bowel obstruction cannot occur with a Richter's hernia

d. Ninety percent of cases of intussusception among adults are associated with a pathologic process, most commonly a tumor

COMMENT: Peritoneal adhesions account for more than one half of cases of small-bowel obstruction in the United States. Obstruction immediately after abdominal operations, however, is uncommon, occurring among only 1% of patients in the 4 weeks after laparotomy. Hernias of all types are second only to adhesions as the most frequent cause of obstruction. External hernias such as inguinal or femoral hernias can manifest as symptoms of obstruction. Femoral hernias are particularly prone to incarceration and bowel necrosis because of the small size of the hernia inlet. An important consideration is the Richter's hernia. In this variant, only a portion of the bowel wall is incarcerated. These most frequently occur in association with femoral or inguinal hernia. Complete obstruction can occur if more than one half to two thirds of the bowel circumference is incarcerated. Approximately 5% of cases of intussusception occur among adults. Intussusception occurs when one segment of bowel telescopes into an adjacent segment. The result is obstruction and ischemic injury to the intussuscepting segment. Ninety percent of adult cases are associated with pathologic processes. Tumors, benign and malignant, can act as a lead point against the intussusception in more than 65% of cases among adults.

ANSWER: a, d

REFERENCE: *Chapter 26—Ileus and Bowel Obstruction: Mechanical Obstruction of the Intestine; Specific Types of Bowel Obstruction*

8. An 82-year-old female nursing home resident is admitted with massive abdominal distention and constant abdominal pain with diffuse tenderness. An abdominal radiograph shows a massively distended loop of colon with a characteristic bent-inner-tube appearance. Treatment of this patient should include:

a. Urgent laparotomy because of massive colonic distention

b. An attempt at endoscopic decompression with a flexible sigmoidoscope

c. Elective laparotomy and sigmoid resection if endoscopic decompression is successful

d. If resected bowel is found at urgent laparotomy, colonic resection with primary anastomosis

COMMENT: The most common site of volvulus is the sigmoid colon, which accounts for 65% of cases. The preferred method and management involve endoscopic decompression. This conservative approach resolves the volvulus in 85% to 90% of cases, and elective resection of the redundant segment can be planned. After endoscopic decompression, the rate of recurrence of the volvulus is greater than 60% if sigmoid resection is not performed. If the patient has peritoneal findings, sepsis, and shock, rapid resuscitation followed by urgent resection and colostomy is warranted.

ANSWER: b, c

REFERENCE: *Chapter 26—Ileus and Bowel Obstruction: Mechanical Obstruction of the Intestine; Specific Types of Bowel Obstruction*

9. Which of the following statements is/are true concerning postoperative ileus?

  a. The use of intravenous patient-controlled analgesia has no effect on return of small-bowel motor activity
  b. The presence of peritonitis at the time of the original operation delays the return of normal bowel function
  c. The routine use of metoclopramide hastens the return of small-intestinal motor activity
  d. Contrast radiographic studies have no role in differentiating early postoperative bowel obstruction from normal ileus

COMMENT: The term *ileus* reflects the underlying alterations in motility of the gastrointestinal tract that lead to functional obstruction. From a practical standpoint, ileus represents the interval between abdominal exploration and the reappearance of flatus and bowel movements. Differentiating normal postoperative ileus and the prolonged course of paralytic ileus is based primarily on the time since operation and the clinical circumstances. Besides the location of the previous operation (upper abdominal, lower abdominal, pelvic), the nature of the previous operation and the findings may contribute. Peritonitis or spillage of noxious material increases the delay of return of normal bowel function. Differentiating paralytic ileus from mechanical obstruction often is difficult. Abdominal radiographs in the evaluation of postoperative ileus should reveal gas in segments of both the small and large bowel. Upper gastrointestinal contrast radiography or computed tomography can be helpful. Early postoperative obstruction is uncommon and is particularly rare for upper abdominal surgery. Most cases occur after operations on the colon, particularly abdominoperineal resection. There has been little success in the use of prokinetic agents to shorten recovery times after lower abdominal procedures. Recovery after postoperative ileus can take longer with intravenous patient-controlled analgesia than with intramuscular administration of narcotics.

ANSWER: b

REFERENCE: *Chapter 26—Ileus and Bowel Obstruction: Ileus and Pseudoobstruction; Ileus*

10. A 75-year-old woman is hospitalized after a fall in which she sustained a hip fracture. Several days after a surgical procedure to manage the fracture, progressive, painless abdominal distention is noticed. Which of the following statements is/are true concerning diagnosis and management in this case?

  a. Colonic distention with a cecal diameter greater than 12 cm in an indication for an urgent operation
  b. Endoscopic decompression can be attempted but seldom is successful
  c. After successful colonoscopic decompression, recurrence is unlikely
  d. A rectal tube generally is not successful primary treatment

COMMENT: Acute pseudoobstruction of the colon, known as Ogilvie's syndrome, is paralytic ileus of the large bowel characterized by rapidly progressive abdominal distention, often without associated pain. Plane radiographs of the abdomen may reveal air in the small bowel and distention of discrete segments of the colon (cecum or transverse colon) or the entire abdominal colon. Distention can become impressive. Often in chronic cases, distention in excess of 15 cm can be observed without evidence of colonic perforation or wall ischemia. Major risk factors for the development of Ogilvie's syndrome include severe blunt trauma, orthopedic trauma or procedures, acute cardiac events or coronary bypass surgery, acute neurologic events or neurosurgical procedures, and acute metabolic derangements. Initial management includes resuscitation and correction of the underlying metabolic and electrolyte abnormalities. A nasogastric tube is indicated if the patient is vomiting and prevents swallowed air from passing distally. If distention is painless and the patient has no signs of toxicity or bowel ischemia, expectant management can be successful in about 50% of cases. If distention worsens so that the cecal diameter increases beyond 10 to 12 cm or if it persists for more than 48 hours, colonoscopy is recommended. Endoscopic decompression is successful in 60% to 90% of cases, but colonic distention can recur in as many as 40% of cases. Rectal tubes are ineffective in managing distention of the proximal colon; however, such tubes can be useful after colonoscopy.

ANSWER: d

REFERENCE: *Chapter 26—Ileus and Bowel Obstruction: Ileus and Pseudoobstruction; Colonic Pseudoobstruction*

11. The most prominent initial symptom of closed-loop obstruction of the small intestine is:
    a. Abdominal pain
    b. Obstipation
    c. Abdominal distention
    d. Abdominal tenderness
    e. Blood in the stool

COMMENT: In closed-loop obstruction, the earliest symptom is pain caused by traction on the mesentery and distention within the closed loop. Peritonitis and abdominal tenderness appear only when the loop of intestine becomes necrotic. Proximal loops have not had a chance to distend, and distal loops may not have emptied themselves of gas and stool. Pain out of proportion to physical findings is a worrisome clinical feature. The differential diagnosis includes intestinal ischemia from thrombosis or embolus and retroperitoneal irritation (pancreatitis or rupture of an abdominal aortic aneurysm).

ANSWER: a

REFERENCE: *Chapter 26—Ileus and Bowel Obstruction: Mechanical Obstruction of the Intestine; Complications of Bowel Obstruction*

12. The one laboratory test that can allow diagnosis of impending strangulation of closed-loop obstruction is:
    a. Detection of metabolic acidosis (arterial pH less than 7.35)
    b. Doppler ultrasound examination of intestinal wall and mesenteric vascular system
    c. Computed tomography
    d. Measurement of serum level of amylase
    e. None of the above

COMMENT: No reliable laboratory test or imaging study allows identification of dead bowel, much less that the intestine is about to die. Close observation of the patient is the earliest means of determining that the bowel has become necrotic.

ANSWER: e

REFERENCE: *Chapter 26—Ileus and Bowel Obstruction: Mechanical Obstruction of the Intestine; Complications of Bowel Obstruction*

13. Twenty-four hours after onset of complete, open-loop obstruction of the mid-ileum, abdominal distention from gas is observed. The accumulation of gas is largely caused by:
    a. Bacterial fermentation of stagnant small-intestinal secretions
    b. Bacterial fermentation of stagnant mucus and feces in the large bowel
    c. Mismatch of carbon dioxide extrusion and absorption in obstructed bowel
    d. Distal propulsion of swallowed air
    e. All of the above

COMMENT: Eighty percent of accumulated gas is swallowed air. Fermentation of succus entericus by enteric flora cannot occur early in the course of small-bowel obstruction because it takes about a day before the enteric flora overgrows normal small intestine. This observation explains why patients with closed-loop obstruction often have no gas in the closed loop, even 24 hours after onset of obstruction.

ANSWER: d

REFERENCE: *Chapter 26—Ileus and Bowel Obstruction: Mechanical Obstruction of the Intestine; Complications of Bowel Obstruction*

14. The most prominent symptom(s) and/or sign(s) of acute sigmoid volvulus is/are:
    a. Periumbilical abdominal pain
    b. Lower abdominal pain
    c. Abdominal distention
    d. Obstipation
    e. Flatulence

COMMENT: The most common symptom is pain, and the most common sign is distention from accumulation of colonic gas. The pain is in the lower midabdomen and is consistent with the origin of pain afferents in the hindgut. Periumbilical pain is associated with midgut structures, such as the appendix and small intestine and is not prominent unless the small intestine is acutely obstructed. Flatulence ceases with sigmoid volvulus, but small amounts of mucus and stool distal to the loop can pass for several hours after the onset of symptoms.

ANSWER: b, c

REFERENCE: *Chapter 26—Ileus and Bowel Obstruction: Specific Types of Obstruction; Volvulus*

15. Which of the following medications is/are contraindicated in treatment of a patient with complete mechanical small-bowel obstruction:

    a. Morphine
    b. Bethanechol
    c. Neostigmine
    d. Erythromycin
    e. All of the above

COMMENT: Although currently controversial, use of narcotics is not recommended for pain control unless it has been determined that the patient is to undergo surgery. Narcotics can mask changes in physical findings. Bethanechol has no role in the management of ileus or mechanical obstruction; erythromycin can be useful in cases of ileus or pseudoobstruction. Neostigmine can be helpful in management of colonic pseudoobstruction, but has no role in therapy for mechanical obstruction of the small or large intestine.

ANSWER: e

REFERENCE: *Chapter 26—Ileus and Bowel Obstruction: Mechanical Obstruction of the Intestine; Complications of Bowel Obstruction*

16. Specific lesions predisposing to intestinal intussusception in adults include:

    a. None—most intussusceptions are idiopathic
    b. Ileocolic anastomosis
    c. Tumors of the small bowel (carcinoid, leiomyoma, metastatic melanoma)
    d. Intestinal tubes
    e. Lymphoma

COMMENT: Any tumor, primary or metastatic, of the small intestine can provide a lead point for intussusception of the small intestine. Any foreign body, such as a surgically placed tube, can provide a lead point as well. Because of its base in the mesentery and usually large size, lymphoma would be an unusual cause. Among children, most cases of intussusception are idiopathic; among adults, most cases have an identifiable cause.

ANSWER: b, c, d

REFERENCE: *Chapter 26—Ileus and Bowel Obstruction: General Considerations in the Management of the Patient with Bowel Obstruction*

17. Which of the following pharmacologic agents predispose(s) to prolongation of ileus after abdominal surgery?

    a. Intravenous narcotics
    b. Oral narcotics
    c. Sympatholytic agents
    d. Anticholinergics
    e. Haloperidol

COMMENT: Many medications, particularly narcotics, anticholinergics, and antipsychotic or antidepressive medications can prolong ileus. A search for other factors such as sepsis and metabolic or electrolyte abnormalities should be undertaken when ileus is prolonged. Sympatholytic agents such as neostigmine probably do not prolong ileus, but it is unclear whether they hasten its resolution as in colonic pseudoobstruction.

REFERENCE: *Chapter 26—Ileus and Bowel Obstruction: Ileus and Pseudoobstruction; Ileus, Management*

CHAPTER 27

CROHN'S DISEASE

1. The most common site of intestinal involvement in Crohn's disease is:

    a. Rectum
    b. Duodenum
    c. Ileum
    d. Stomach
    e. Transverse colon

COMMENT: The gross and microscopic features of Crohn's disease can occur in any segment of the gastrointestinal tract. The disease tends to be discontinuous and segmental, affecting isolated segments of the gastrointestinal tract. The terminal ileum with or without some involvement of the cecum is the most common site of disease and represents approximately 60% of cases. Crohn's disease limited to the colon occurs in 15% to 20% of cases. Ten percent of cases involve the proximal small bowel, and approximately 15% of patients have a pattern of multiple sites of disease. Perianal manifestations of Crohn's disease, including perianal fistula, abscess, and stenosis, occur among approximately one third of patients with Crohn's disease. In half of these cases, perianal disease occurs simultaneously with active disease elsewhere in the gastrointestinal tract.

ANSWER: c

REFERENCE: *Chapter 27—Crohn's Disease: Pathology*

2. Crohn's disease is associated with a number of extraintestinal manifestations. Extraintestinal problems not affected by therapy for intestinal disease include:

a. Sclerosing cholangitis
b. Episcleritis
c. Ankylosing spondylitis
d. Erythema nodosum

COMMENT: Crohn's disease is associated with a variety of extraintestinal manifestations. They include dermatologic, ocular, hepatobiliary, and joint disorders. Dermatologic disorders that occur with Crohn's disease include erythema nodosum and pyoderma gangrenosum. Ocular manifestations of Crohn's disease include uveitis and episcleritis. Ankylosing spondylitis, sacral ileitis, and a seronegative peripheral polyarthropathy are associated with Crohn's disease. Patients with Crohn's disease are at risk of primary sclerosing cholangitis, but this serious complication is less common with Crohn's disease than with ulcerative colitis. Crohn's disease–associated peripheral arthritis, uveitis, episcleritis, erythema nodosum, and possibly pyoderma gangrenosum parallel the activity of intestinal disease and typically regress with successful medical management or complete surgical resection of the affected segments of bowel. Ankylosing spondylitis and primary sclerosing cholangitis do not correlate with bowel disease activity, and thus the clinical course is not attenuated by surgical resection of intestinal Crohn's disease.

ANSWER: a, c

REFERENCE: *Chapter 27—Crohn's Disease: Clinical Features; Extraintestinal Disease*

3. A 25-year-old woman has right lower quadrant pain, anorexia, and leukocytosis. Appendectomy is recommended. At operation, the appendix appears normal, and additional exploration is undertaken. Features consistent with Crohn's disease include:

a. Thickening of the bowel wall
b. Serosal hyperemia
c. Mesenteric thickening
d. Encroachment of mesenteric fat on bowel wall

COMMENT: In most cases, the areas affected by Crohn's disease are readily apparent—the bowel wall is thick and indurated. Serosal hyperemia with a corkscrew appearance of the serosal vessels is typical. Areas of disease also show encroachment of the mesentery fat along the serosal surface of the bowel, often called *fat wrapping* or *creeping fat*. The mesentery of grossly diseased bowel often is massively thickened and stiff. Serosal manifestations of less severe disease are subtle and can be difficult to identify. Mild Crohn's disease typically has some degree of induration of the mesenteric bowel wall that can be detected with palpation.

ANSWER: a, b, c, d

REFERENCE: *Chapter 27—Crohn's Disease: Surgical Treatment of Crohn's Disease; Abdominal Exploration*

4. The patient in question 3 undergoes appendectomy. The presumed intraoperative diagnosis is Crohn's ileitis. After operative recovery, the most appropriate test to confirm the diagnosis is:

a. Esophagogastroduodenoscopy
b. Computed tomography (CT) of the abdomen
c. Colonoscopy
d. Barium enema

COMMENT: The colon and rectum are best evaluated with colonoscopy. Colonoscopy allows visualization of the mucosal disease and provides the opportunity for histologic evaluation with mucosal biopsy. In many cases, the colonoscope can also enter the terminal ileum for evaluation. Characteristics of Crohn's disease seen with colonoscopy include aphthoid ulcer, discrete serpiginous ulcerations that usually track along the long axis of the bowel, diseased mucosa separated by skip areas of normal mucosa, rectal sparing, and strictures.

ANSWER: c

REFERENCE: *Chapter 27—Crohn's Disease: Diagnosis; Colonoscopy*

5. A 46-year-old man with a known 10-year history of ileal Crohn's disease has a 3-day history of worsening lower abdominal pain, obstipation, and fever. Physical examination reveals a temperature of 102.5°F (39.2°C), hypogastric tenderness, and muscular guarding. The most appropriate test to evaluate for the possibility of abscess formation associated with Crohn's disease is:

   a. Radiographic enema examination with administration of water-soluble contrast medium
   b. Barium enema radiographic examination
   c. Computed tomography
   d. Barium small-bowel contrast study

COMMENT: The most typical CT finding of uncomplicated Crohn's disease is thickening of the bowel wall. The presence of such thickening correlates with disease activity and tends to dissipate with successful medical management. The CT findings of uncomplicated Crohn's disease are nonspecific. Routine abdominal CT does not assist in confirming the diagnosis of Crohn's disease. Computed tomography can be useful in identifying the complications associated with Crohn's disease. When an abscess or inflammatory mass is suspected, CT of the abdomen and pelvis should be performed. Most abscesses related to Crohn's disease are readily detectable with CT. Computed tomography allows assessment of possible ureteral obstruction due to compression by a retroperitoneal inflammatory mass. Computed tomography also can assist in the diagnosis of enterovesical fistula because of the presence of air within the urinary bladder.

ANSWER: c

REFERENCE: *Chapter 27—Crohn's Disease: Diagnosis; CT Scans*

6. For the patient in question 5, CT of the abdomen reveals an inflammatory mass involving the distal ileum. An abscess is not identified. The patient undergoes a 10-day regimen of bowel rest, intravenous nutritional support, and intravenous administration of steroids. Symptomatic resolution is incomplete. Bowel resection is recommended. The extent of bowel resected is determined by:

   a. Results of intraoperative frozen section examination of resection margins that have no granuloma
   b. Normal bowel at intraoperative visual inspection
   c. Results of intraoperative frozen section examination of resection margins that have granuloma but no submucosal inflammatory infiltrate
   d. A margin of 5 cm beyond grossly inflamed bowel

COMMENT: Small-bowel resection is the most common surgical procedure in the management of Crohn's disease of the small intestine. For many years the optimal extent of resection to provide the lowest risk of recurrence has been a subject of controversy. It was once thought that wide resection with generous margins of normal bowel combined with radical mesenteric excision would result in lower recurrence rates. The accumulated clinical data do not support the need for wide or radical resection for Crohn's disease. Resection should be wide enough to encompass the limits of gross disease. Wider resection offers no benefit in terms of decreasing the risk of recurrence, even when the mucosal resection margins have microscopic features of Crohn's disease. The extent of mesenteric resection does not affect the rate of recurrent disease. It is now generally accepted that resection to grossly normal intestinal margins is sufficient. Frozen section to exclude microscopic disease at the resection margins is not warranted because microscopically positive margins do not adversely affect long-term results.

ANSWER: b

REFERENCE: *Chapter 27—Crohn's Disease: Surgical Treatment of Crohn's Disease; Resection*

7. A 35-year-old patient with long-standing ileal Crohn's disease has symptoms of urinary tract infection and states that gas is passed during urination. Pelvic CT shows thickening of the ileal bowel wall and mesentery and gas within the bladder. Appropriate treatment includes:

a. Small-bowel resection
b. Partial cystectomy
c. Azathioprine
d. Life-long administration of trimethoprim and sulfamethoxazole

COMMENT: Most surgeons and gastroenterologists agree that the effects of chronic urinary tract infection on renal function in addition to symptoms of the primary ileal Crohn's disease are indications for an operation. As with other Crohn's fistulas, the surgical treatment is based on resection of the diseased segment of intestine with extirpation of the fistula track. With ileovesical fistulas, the connection to the bladder is most commonly located at the dome and débridement and primary closure can be affected without endangering the trigone. Partial cystectomy usually is not necessary.

ANSWER: a

REFERENCE: *Chapter 27—Crohn's Disease: Management of Complicated Crohn's Disease; Enteric Fistulas*

8. A young patient undergoes ileocecal resection for Crohn's disease complicated by obstruction. The site at highest risk of recurrence of Crohn's disease is:

a. Rectum
b. Colon distal to the anastomosis
c. Ileum proximal to the anastomosis
d. Sigmoid colon

COMMENT: Ileocecal or ileocolonic disease is managed similarly to disease limited to the terminal ileum. Resection to grossly normal margins with primary anastomosis is often the best surgical option. The long-term clinical course of terminal ileal disease with limited involvement of the proximal colon is similar to the clinical course of Crohn's disease involving only terminal ileum. Disease tends to recur at the anastomosis and preanastomotic ileum. The risk of recurrent disease affecting the distal colon or rectum is low, and the long-term risk of requiring a permanent stoma is low.

ANSWER: c

REFERENCE: *Chapter 27—Crohn's Disease: Crohn's Disease of the Colon*

9. The most common long-term complication of surgery for Crohn's is the risk of recurrent disease. The need for reoperation because of recurrent disease within 10 years approximates:

a. 10%
b. 33%
c. 66%
d. 95%

COMMENT: Reported crude and cumulative recurrence rates vary greatly. The rate of detection of endoscopic evidence of recurrence has been reported to vary from 28% to 73% 1 year and 77% to 85% 3 years after ileal resection. In most instances, endoscopically detected recurrence is minor and asymptomatic and therefore not of great clinical significance. The rate of recurrence of symptomatic Crohn's disease is approximately 60% 5 years postoperatively, and the recurrence rate increases such that 20 years postoperatively 75% to 95% of patients have symptomatic recurrences. The long-term risk of recurrence of Crohn's symptoms is high. Reports vary, but the percentage of patients who need reoperation to manage recurrent disease is approximately 20% at 5 years, 33% at 10 years, and 50% at 20 years.

ANSWER: b

REFERENCE: *Chapter 27—Crohn's Disease: Long-term Morbidity and Recurrence of Disease*

10. Patients who undergo operative therapy for Crohn's disease are at risk of symptomatic recurrence. The likelihood of recurrence can be decreased by:

a. Cigarette smoking
b. Long-term administration of nonsteroidal antiinflammatory drugs (NSAIDs)
c. Diet low in saturated fats
d. Long-term administration of 5-aminosalicylic acid (5-ASA)

COMMENT: Many putative risk factors for recurrence have been studied. The cumulative literature has validated few as true risk factors for postsurgical recurrence of disease. There is a growing body of evidence that indicates smoking can increase the risk of recurrence. There is some evidence to indicate that the use of NSAIDs also can promote recurrence of disease. All patients with Crohn's disease should be strongly advised to refrain from smoking cigarettes or taking NSAIDs. It does not appear as if diet has any influence on the likelihood of recurrence. Results of recent trials have indicated that the recurrence rate can be diminished with postoperative maintenance therapy. The most common maintenance therapies are controlled-release 5-ASA and 6-mercaptopurine. Maintenance with 5-ASA is associated with few side effects but requires up to 12 pills per day and is expensive. 6-Mercaptopurine is less expensive and is taken once a day, but it is associated with risk of bone marrow suppression. Patients taking 6-mercaptopurine maintenance need periodic blood cell counts.

ANSWER: d

REFERENCE: *Chapter 27—Crohn's Disease: Long-term Morbidity and Recurrence of Disease*

CHAPTER 28

SMALL INTESTINAL NEOPLASMS

1. The most common histologic type of small-intestinal malignancy is:

a. Non-Hodgkin's lymphoma
b. Adenocarcinoma
c. Carcinoid tumor
d. Gastrointestinal stromal tumor

COMMENT: Adenocarcinoma accounts for 30% to 50% of small-bowel tumors, making it the most common primary malignant tumor. Like adenoma, sporadic adenocarcinoma has a predilection for the duodenum with a marked decrease in frequency moving axially along the small bowel. Approximately 80% of tumors are located in the duodenum or proximal jejunum. Most studies show a slight male predominance. There are several risk factors for the development of adenocarcinoma. Malignant transformation of villous and tubulovillous adenoma is likely the most important and occurs predominantly in the periampullary region of the duodenum. Crohn's disease increases the risk as much as 100-fold and is a predisposing factor for cancer in the more distal small bowel in regions of dysplasia.

ANSWER: b

REFERENCE: *Chapter 28—Small Intestinal Neoplasms: Adenocarcinoma*

2. The most common site of gastrointestinal non-Hodgkin's lymphoma is the stomach. Gastric lymphoma is followed in frequency by lymphoma of the:

a. Duodenum
b. Rectum
c. Cecum
d. Ileum

COMMENT: Non-Hodgkin's lymphoma of the gastrointestinal tract represents 4% to 20% of all cases of non-Hodgkin's lymphoma. The gastrointestinal tract is the most common extranodal site. The stomach harbors the most lymphomas, followed by the small bowel and the colon. Twenty-five percent to 35% of cases of gastrointestinal non-Hodgkin's lymphoma occur within the small bowel. The distribution pattern is marked by relative sparing of the duodenum and equal frequency in the jejunum and ileum.

ANSWER: d

REFERENCE: *Chapter 28—Small Intestinal Neoplasms: Non-Hodgkin's Lymphoma*

3. The sites at which gastrointestinal carcinoids occur, in order of decreasing frequency, are:

a. Rectum, ileum, appendix
b. Appendix, ileum, rectum
c. Stomach, ileum, rectum
d. Stomach, duodenum, jejunum

COMMENT: Carcinoids are indolent malignant neuroendocrine tumors that arise from the enterochromaffin cells at the base of the crypts of Lieberkuhn. These cells are part of the amine precursor uptake and decarboxylation (APUD) system and can secrete peptides responsible for the carcinoid syndrome. Although 80% of carcinoids arise in the gastrointestinal tract, 10% of primary carcinoids occur in the bronchus or lung. Other sites, such as the ovaries, testicles, pancreas, and kidney, are far less common. Within the gastrointestinal tract, carcinoids are most often identified in the appendix, followed by the small bowel, which harbors approximately 30% of all gastrointestinal carcinoids. Almost one half of these arise in the distal 2 feet (0.6 m) of ileum.

ANSWER: b

REFERENCE: *Chapter 28—Small Intestinal Neoplasms*

4. A 50-year-old man has symptoms of partial small-intestinal obstruction. Computed tomographic (CT) evaluation reveals a mass in the distal ileum. The patient undergoes ileocecal resection. Histologic examination of the resected specimen shows a carcinoid tumor. Recovery is uncomplicated. Appropriate postoperative examination includes:

a. Computed tomography of the chest
b. Colonoscopy
c. Bone scan
d. None of the above

COMMENT: Unlike in the appendix, where multicentricity is rare, carcinoids of the small bowel are multiple 30% to 40% of the time. In addition, 30% to 50% of small bowel carcinoids are associated with second primary malignant tumors, most frequently of the breast and colon. Gastrointestinal carcinoids can elicit a marked desmoplastic reaction. The mesentery of the small bowel becomes fibrotic and foreshortened; the result is kinking of the bowel or even intestinal ischemia as a result of sclerosis of the mesenteric blood vessels. This finding is readily identified on CT scans and is sometimes associated with calcifications while the small bowel appears fixed and angulated.

ANSWER: b

REFERENCE: *Chapter 28—Small Intestinal Neoplasms: Non-Hodgkin's Lymphoma*

5. A 52-year-old woman has midabdominal pain. The surgical and medical histories are normal, and the review of systems shows otherwise normal findings. An abdominal CT scan is obtained to evaluate the symptoms. The scan shows a 7-cm rounded mass in association with the mid small bowel. The mass center is of mixed density, suggesting intralesional hemorrhage. The radiologic diagnosis is gastrointestinal stromal tumor. Appropriate operative therapy includes:

a. Wide local excision
b. Wide local excision and mesenteric adenectomy
c. Enucleation of the lesion
d. Wide local excision and omentectomy

COMMENT: At operation, wide local excision of the primary tumor is the most important goal. Lymph-node metastasis is rare, so wide mesenteric resection is not necessary. Benign leiomyoma can be difficult to differentiate from leiomyosarcoma at operation, and there are reports of late liver metastasis from presumed benign leiomyoma. Therefore wide excision should be performed, even for benign-appearing lesions.

Histologic differentiation between benign and malignant stromal tumors is difficult. No method has proved reliable. The strongest predictors of malignant behavior are size greater than 5 cm in diameter and mitotic count greater than five per high-power field, although their relevance as independent predictors has been questioned. Until better molecular biologic markers are available, tumor size and mitotic count together provide the best guidelines for postresection follow-up evaluation. Although reported in the literature, no consistent benefit of adjuvant therapy has been found, and surgical resection has provided the only long-term cures.

ANSWER: a

REFERENCE: *Chapter 28—Small Intestinal Neoplasms: Gastrointestinal Stromal Sarcomas*

Section E
PANCREAS

CHAPTER 29

PANCREATIC ANATOMY AND PHYSIOLOGY

1. Pancreas divisum results from incomplete fusion of the ventral pancreatic duct with the dorsal pancreatic duct during embryologic development. Which of the following statements correctly describe(s) pancreas divisum?

a. The body and tail of the pancreas drain through an accessory ampulla distal to the ampulla of Vater. The uncinate process drains through the ampulla of Vater
b. The entire pancreatic ductal system drains through the ampulla of Vater
c. The entire pancreatic ductal system drains through an accessory ampulla proximal to the ampulla of Vater
d. The body and tail of the pancreas are absent. The uncinate process drains through the ampulla of Vater

COMMENT: In 90% of persons, the main pancreatic duct, or duct of Wirsung, runs the entire length of the pancreas and joins the common bile duct to empty into the duodenum at the ampulla of Vater. The pancreatic duct is 2 to 3.5 mm in diameter and contains 20 secondary branches, which drain the tail, body, and uncinate process. The drainage of the lesser duct, or duct of Santorini, is variable. The lesser duct commonly drains the superior portion of the head of the pancreas. It empties separately into the second portion of the duodenum through the lesser papilla located 2 cm proximal to the ampulla of Vater. Pancreas divisum results from incomplete fusion of the ventral pancreatic duct with the dorsal duct during fetal development and is present in 5% of persons. In this anomaly, the lesser duct drains the entire pancreas through an accessory ampulla proximal to the ampulla of Vater. Inadequacy of this pattern of drainage can cause chronic pain.

ANSWER: c

REFERENCE: *Chapter 29—Pancreatic Anatomy and Physiology: Pancreatic Ducts*

2. Which of the following statements is/are correct with regard to the blood supply of the pancreas?

   a. The inferior pancreaticoduodenal artery, a branch of the celiac artery, divides into anterior and posterior branches to supply the pancreatic head
   b. The body and tail of the pancreas are supplied by branches of the splenic artery
   c. The superior pancreaticoduodenal artery is a branch of the gastroduodenal artery
   d. The body and tail of the pancreas are supplied by branches derived from the left renal artery

COMMENT: The pancreas receives its blood supply from a variety of major arterial sources. In the head of the pancreas, there are arcades in the anterior and posterior surfaces, which generally form collaterals. These arcades arise from branches of the gastroduodenal and superior mesenteric arteries. Immediately distal to the first portion of the duodenum, the gastroduodenal artery becomes the superior pancreaticoduodenal artery, which divides into anterior and posterior branches. The inferior pancreaticoduodenal artery is the first branch of the superior mesenteric artery and divides into anterior and posterior branches.

The body and tail of the pancreas are supplied by the splenic artery. The splenic artery arises from the celiac trunk and courses along the superior surface of the pancreas to the spleen. Approximately ten branches of the splenic artery supply the body and tail of the pancreas.

ANSWER: b, c

REFERENCE: *Chapter 29—Pancreatic Anatomy and Physiology: Arterial Supply*

3. In the performance of a pancreatoduodenectomy (Whipple procedure), the superior mesenteric vein is an important landmark. Which of the following statements is/are true with regard to the superior mesenteric vein?

   a. Small venous branches enter the superior mesenteric vein anteriorly as it courses beneath the neck of the pancreas
   b. The superior mesenteric vein joins the splenic vein at the superior border of the pancreas to form the portal vein
   c. Small venous branches enter the superior mesenteric vein laterally as it courses beneath the neck of the pancreas
   d. The course of the superior mesenteric vein is anterior to the neck of the pancreas

COMMENT: The venous drainage of the pancreas and duodenum follows the arterial supply. The anterior and posterior venous arcades drain the head; the body and tail drain into the splenic vein. All venous effluent from the pancreas ultimately drains into the portal vein, which is formed by the confluence of the superior mesenteric vein and the splenic vein at the superior border of the pancreas. The anterior and posterior venous arcades in the head of the pancreas drain directly into the suprapancreatic portal vein. The anteroinferior pancreaticoduodenal arcades drain with the right gastroepiploic vein to form a common venous trunk with the right colic vein. This trunk is known as the *gastrocolic trunk* and enters the superior mesenteric vein at the inferior border of the neck of the pancreas. The posteroinferior venous arcade empties directly into the superior mesenteric vein. The veins of the head drain laterally into the superior mesenteric and portal veins. No venous tributaries enter the superior mesenteric vein anteriorly. For this reason, it is safe to dissect the neck of the pancreas directly anterior to the superior mesenteric and portal veins when performing a pancreatoduodenectomy.

ANSWER: b, c

REFERENCE: *Chapter 29—Pancreatic Anatomy and Physiology: Venous Drainage*

4. The islets of Langerhans contain four major types of endocrine cells that secrete which of the following hormones?
   a. Insulin, somatostatin, glucagon, secretin
   b. Insulin, somatostatin, cholecystokinin, pancreatic polypeptide
   c. Insulin, somatostatin, glucagon, pancreatic polypeptide
   d. Insulin, secretin, glucagon, cholecystokinin

COMMENT: Within the pancreas are small nests of cells responsible for the secretion of hormones that control glucose homeostasis. These nests are called *islets of Langerhans* and constitute 2% of the pancreatic mass. The islets contain an average of 2,900 cells and range in diameter from 40 to 900 μm. The islets are composed of four major cell types—alpha (A), beta (B), delta (D), and PP or F cells, which secrete glucagon, insulin, somatostatin, and pancreatic polypeptide, respectively. The B cells are centrally located within the islet and constitute 70% of the islet mass, whereas the PP, A, and D cells are located at the periphery of the islet. They constitute approximately 15%, 10%, and 5% of the islet cell mass, respectively.

ANSWER: c

REFERENCE: *Chapter 29—Pancreatic Anatomy and Physiology: Endocrine Structure*

5. With regard to the control of pancreatic exocrine function, which of the following statements is/are correct?
   a. Cholecystokinin, a hormone released from the duodenal mucosa, is the predominant stimulus for pancreatic enzyme secretion
   b. Gastrin is a major stimulant for pancreatic bicarbonate secretion
   c. Secretin is released from the duodenum with mucosal acidification and stimulates pancreatic bicarbonate secretion
   d. Acetylcholine, released from pancreatic nerves, stimulates enzyme secretion

COMMENT: Enzyme secretion is regulated primarily through hormonal and neural factors. The enteric hormone cholecystokinin, released from endocrine cells in the duodenal mucosa, is the predominant regulator and stimulates acinar cells through specific membrane-bound receptors. Acetylcholine strongly stimulates acinar cells when released from postganglionic fibers of the pancreatic plexus and acts in synergy with cholecystokinin to potentiate enzyme secretion. Secretin weakly stimulates acinar cell secretion and potentiates the effect of cholecystokinin on the acinar cells. Bicarbonate is formed from carbonic acid by the enzyme carbonic anhydrase. Secretin, the main stimulant of bicarbonate secretion, is released from the duodenal mucosa in response to a duodenal luminal pH less than 3.0. Cholecystokinin only weakly stimulates bicarbonate secretion, whereas it potentiates secretin-stimulated bicarbonate secretion. Gastrin and acetylcholine are weak stimulants of bicarbonate secretion.

ANSWER: a, c, d

REFERENCE: *Chapter 29—Pancreatic Anatomy and Physiology: Exocrine Function*

6. Orally administered glucose provokes a greater insulin response than does an equivalent amount of intravenously administered glucose. The incremental response to ingested glucose is caused by the effects of which of the following hormones?

    a. Gastric inhibitory peptide
    b. Somatostatin
    c. Pancreatic polypeptide
    d. Secretin

COMMENT: Orally administered glucose stimulates a greater insulin response than does an equivalent amount of intravenous glucose through the release of enteric hormones that potentiate insulin secretion. This effect is known as the *enteroinsular axis.* Gastric inhibitory polypeptide appears to be an important regulator of this effect, although other gastrointestinal peptides, such as glucagon-like peptide I, also may contribute to this effect. Nutrients that regulate insulin secretion include amino acids, such as arginine, lysine, and leucine, and free fatty acids. Hormones that stimulate insulin secretion include glucagon, gastric inhibitory polypeptide, and cholecystokinin, whereas somatostatin, amylin, and pancreastatin are inhibitory. Insulin also is stimulated by sulfonylurea compounds, which act independently of glucose concentration and form the basis of management of type 2, or insulin-independent, diabetes.

ANSWER: a

REFERENCE: *Chapter 29—Pancreatic Anatomy and Physiology: Insulin Synthesis, Secretion, and Action*

CHAPTER 30

ACUTE PANCREATITIS

1. Which of the following statements describing acute pancreatitis is not true?

    a. As many as two-thirds of cases of "idiopathic" pancreatitis are associated with microlithiasis and biliary "sludge"
    b. Post-ERCP pancreatitis, which may develop in up to 4% of patients following the endoscopic procedure, may be avoided by limiting the pressure used during contrast injection of the pancreatic duct
    c. The majority of patients with pancreas divisum require dorsal duct sphincterotomy to address recurrent episodes of acute pancreatitis
    d. The majority of cases of acute pancreatitis in the United States may be attributed to gallstones or alcohol consumption

COMMENT: Large series of patients with acute pancreatitis from the United States and Great Britain reveal several important factors associated with the development of acute pancreatitis. The majority of cases, more than 80%, occur in patients with gallstones or a history of alcohol use. No identifiable cause may be identified in approximately 15% of cases, though recent studies show abnormalities in the bile of the majority of these patients. Transient biliary obstruction due to microlithiasis or biliary "sludge" may in fact be the cause of pancreatitis in these patients with "idiopathic" disease. Other important but less common causes of acute pancreatitis include hypercalcemia, hyperlipidemia, trauma, tumor obstruction of the pancreatic duct, infection, pregnancy, and a number of drugs (including thiazides, azathioprine, glucocorticoids, and pentamidine, among others). Many surgical procedures are associated with a risk of acute pancreatitis. ERCP carries a well-defined risk of post-procedure pancreatitis, which may be minimized by carefully limiting the pressure of pancreatic duct injections. Pancreas divisum is a normal variant of pancreatic anatomy that has been associated with acute pancreatitis. However, pancreatitis occurs in a small minority of these patients.

ANSWER: c

REFERENCE: *Chapter 30—Acute Pancreatitis: Etiology*

2. Choose the correct statement describing the appropriate use of ERCP in the management of acute pancreatitis.

a. The majority of patients with acute pancreatitis secondary to gallstones may be found to have a stone impacted at the ampulla that may be extracted during ERCP

b. ERCP performed routinely during the first 24 hours of an attack of is safe and may improve survival in patients with acute biliary pancreatitis

c. Choledocholithiasis may be demonstrated in the majority of patients with acute biliary pancreatitis, thus justifying the role of ERCP in patient management

d. ERCP should be used selectively to relieve biliary obstruction in appropriate patients, with best results achieved when performed in the first 24 hours after presentation

COMMENT: While gallstones appear to be the cause in a large number of cases of acute pancreatitis, choledocholithiasis may only be identified in 20% of these patients. Furthermore, an impacted stone located at the ampulla may be found in as few as 2% of cases. The transient nature of the biliary obstruction associated with gallstone pancreatitis limits the role of ERCP in the acute management of the disease. ERCP appears to be of little use as a diagnostic procedure for acute pancreatitis. Therefore it is only indicated in select patients with demonstrated biliary obstruction. Two randomized trials suggest that early ERCP in these patients may improve patient outcome. However, routine early ERCP has not been shown to be beneficial in all patients with acute pancreatitis.

ANSWER: d

REFERENCE: *Chapter 30—Acute Pancreatitis: Diagnosis; Management*

3. A 53-year-old man who was admitted six weeks previously with severe acute pancreatitis and associated acute fluid collections is seen in follow-up. He feels well, has abstained from alcohol use, and has a normal physical exam. CT scan of the abdomen is performed to follow-up his previous fluid collections. The scan reveals a 7.0-cm well-circumscribed cyst located behind the stomach adjacent to the body and tail of the pancreas. Appropriate initial management of this lesion is:

a. Percutaneous aspiration
b. Observation
c. Pseudocystgastrostomy
d. Placement of percutaneous drainage catheter

COMMENT: Recent series describing the selective management of pancreatic pseudocysts have confirmed the role of observation in asymptomatic patients. Reports from both the Mayo Clinic and the Johns Hopkins Hospital describe resolution of pseudocysts in 50%–60% of asymptomatic patients who were managed without intervention. Resolution was somewhat more likely in smaller pseudocysts, but even large (> 6 cm) pseudocysts were shown to resolve in many patients. Observation is appropriate initial management in patients with pseudocysts, as long as the patient is asymptomatic.

ANSWER: b

REFERENCE: *Chapter 30—Acute Pancreatitis: Pancreatic Pseudocysts*

4. The patient described in question 3 requires admission two weeks later with fever, leukocytosis and mild abdominal pain. CT scan reveals the same pseudocyst, slightly enlarged with some surrounding inflammatory changes. The pancreas itself appears unchanged from the previous CT. No other source of infection is identified. Aspiration of the pseudocyst reveals frank pus. The most appropriate initial management at this time is:

a. Placement of a percutaneous drainage catheter
b. Observation and intravenous imipenem
c. Exploratory laparotomy, necrosectomy, and placement of drains
d. Pseudocystgastrostomy

COMMENT: Pancreatic abscesses, previously called infected pancreatic pseudocysts, require external drainage. This may be accomplished initially with placement of a percutaneous drainage catheter. This procedure carries a low morbidity and several series have shown it to be effective in the management of patients with pancreatic abscess. However, some patients may not be drained adequately with this procedure and require operative placement of large external drainage catheters. Enteric drainage is appropriate for persistent, symptomatic pseudocysts with sterile fluid. Necrosectomy refers to the débridement of necrotic pancreatic tissue and surrounding retroperitoneal fat that may be necessary in the management of patients with infected pancreatic necrosis. This is a distinct entity from pancreatic abscess, which is not associated with pancreatic necrosis.

ANSWER: a

REFERENCE: *Chapter 30—Acute Pancreatitis: Pancreatic Pseudocysts*

5. A 42-year-old woman is admitted to the hospital with upper abdominal pain, leukocytosis, and an elevated serum amylase. Ultrasound examination reveals cholelithiasis and a normal size common bile duct. The patient is treated with analgesics and intravenous hydration, with rapid resolution of her symptoms. After three days of hospitalization, all of her laboratory values have returned to normal and her exam is notable for a significant decrease in abdominal tenderness. What is the next appropriate step in the management of this patient?

a. Discharge, with return for elective cholecystectomy in 6 to 8 weeks.
b. Laparoscopic cholecystectomy and intraoperative cholangiography prior to hospital discharge.
c. Endoscopic sphincterotomy, followed by discharge and return in 6 to 8 weeks for elective cholecystectomy.
d. Observation

COMMENT: Acute biliary pancreatitis may initially be treated with supportive care alone until resolution of symptoms. There is no acute indication for ERCP, sphincterotomy, or other biliary ductal procedure in the absence of evidence for ongoing biliary obstruction. The recurrence rate for biliary pancreatitis may be as high as 50% within 6 weeks; therefore, it is recommended that cholecystectomy be performed prior to hospital discharge. The biliary tree may be imaged either with intraoperative cholangiography or pre-operative magnetic resonance cholangiopancreatography (MRCP).

ANSWER: b

REFERENCE: *Chapter 30—Acute Pancreatitis: Management*

6. A 49-year-old female is admitted to the intensive care unit with severe acute pancreatitis that developed following ERCP. Her initial condition is notable for fever, leukocytosis, elevated serum amylase, hyperglycemia, and respiratory failure. She is aggressively managed with intravenous hydration, mechanical ventilation, and analgesia. Other appropriate steps in her initial management include:

a. Exploratory laparotomy, peritoneal lavage, and drain placement
b. Percutaneous drainage of any areas of pancreatic necrosis
c. Placement of a transhepatic biliary drain to stent open the ampulla
d. Intravenous imipenem and parenteral nutrition

COMMENT: The initial management of severe acute pancreatitis consists of supportive care and aggressive resuscitation. Important elements include sufficient analgesia, aggressive support of organ system failure, aggressive intravenous volume resuscitation, early initiation of nutritional support, deep venous thrombosis and stress ulcer prophylaxis, and careful surveillance for infection. Intravenous antibiotics do not appear to be of benefit in mild acute pancreatitis, but may improve outcome in severe cases. Operative intervention is not indicated in the absence of demonstration of infected pancreatic necrosis.

ANSWER: d

REFERENCE: *Chapter 30—Acute Pancreatitis: Management*

7. The patient described above makes some initial improvement but develops persistent fever and leukocytosis 5 to 7 days after admission. Which of the following is the next step in appropriate management?

a. Laparotomy with pancreatic débridement
b. CT scan of the abdomen with aspiration of peripancreatic fluid collections.
c. Repeat ERCP with placement of a biliary stent
d. Cholecystectomy

COMMENT: Persistent fever and leukocytosis, particularly after initial improvement of patients with severe acute pancreatitis, may suggest the diagnosis of pancreatic abscess or infected pancreatic necrosis. CT scan should be performed, and either CT or ultrasound may be used to aspirate identified peripancreatic fluid collections. All fluid should be cultured, with mandatory drainage indicated by positive culture results. The best surgical treatment in cases of infected pancreatic necrosis is wide surgical débridement of necrotic material, with placement of either large external drains or open packing of the abdomen.

ANSWER: b

REFERENCE: *Chapter 30—Acute Pancreatitis: Management*

CHAPTER 31

CHRONIC PANCREATITIS

1. Which of the following statements describing chronic pancreatitis is false?

    a. Hereditary pancreatitis is an autosomal dominant disorder associated with an abnormality in the mechanism of trypsin deactivation
    b. Chronic pancreatitis secondary to alcohol use may be correlated with type of alcohol consumed and will regress after cessation of alcohol abuse
    c. Idiopathic pancreatitis appears to have a bimodal age distribution, with older patients often presenting with a painless form of the disease characterized by exocrine insufficiency
    d. Obstructive-type chronic pancreatitis is characterized by diffuse ductal dilatation and glandular atrophy

COMMENT: The most common identified cause for chronic pancreatitis is alcohol abuse, which is responsible for 70%–80% of cases in developed countries. Alcoholic pancreatitis occurs through unknown mechanisms, and the type of alcohol consumed does not appear to correlate with disease severity. Duration of alcohol abuse may increase the severity of chronic pancreatitis, but the disease does not always regress after cessation of alcohol consumption. The majority of remaining cases of chronic pancreatitis are idiopathic, and these cases occur in a peculiar bimodal age distribution. Younger, teenage patients often present with a more aggressive and painful form of the disease, while older patients (commonly > 60 years) have a more indolent disease that often does not present until significant exocrine insufficiency develops. Other less common causes for chronic pancreatitis include tropical pancreatitis, trauma, hyperparathyroidism, and pancreatic ductal obstruction. Patients with obstructive type disease develop a characteristic diffuse dilatation of the pancreatic duct proximal to the obstruction, rather than the segmental disease seen in other forms of chronic pancreatitis. Hereditary pancreatitis is an interesting form of the disease for which a point mutation in the trypsinogen gene has been identified; this mutation is autosomal dominant with a penetrance of 80%.

ANSWER: b

REFERENCE: *Chapter 31—Chronic Pancreatitis: Etiology*

2. Which of the following is the most common clinical manifestation of chronic pancreatitis?

    a. Diabetes mellitus
    b. Steatorrhea
    c. Epigastric pain radiating to the upper lumbar vertebrae
    d. Early satiety and post-prandial emesis

COMMENT: Pain is the most common symptom of chronic pancreatitis, and it is often the most difficult symptom to manage in these patients. Patients with chronic pancreatitis often complain of epigastric pain that radiates to the back. Patients often report that leaning forward or lying prone may relieve that pain, which may be exacerbated in the supine position. Exocrine pancreatic insufficiency, which usually initially presents with fat malabsorption and steatorrhea, is a late symptom of chronic pancreatitis that occurs only after destruction of greater than 90% of the exocrine pancreas. Most patients with chronic pancreatitis may be shown to have some degree of glucose intolerance, but diabetes mellitus develops in less than 60% of patients and is often a late symptom.

ANSWER: c

REFERENCE: *Chapter 31—Chronic Pancreatitis: Clinical Presentation*

3. Which of the following is the most appropriate test to establish the diagnosis of chronic pancreatitis?

   a. Bentiromide test (para-aminobenzoic acid excretion)
   b. Serum lipase
   c. Measurement of duodenal lipase
   d. Endoscopic retrograde pancreatography

COMMENT: The diagnosis of chronic pancreatitis is suggested by clinical history, and unfortunately there are few available confirmatory tests. Serum amylase and lipase may be elevated during an acute exacerbation of pancreatitis, but are often normal between episodes and may rise only slightly as the disease progresses and exocrine function declines. Measurement of pancreatic secretions in the pancreatic duct or duodenum is possible, but no single diagnostic marker exists that confirms the diagnosis of chronic pancreatitis in distinction from other important diseases in the differential diagnosis, such as pancreatic cancer. The bentiromide test measures the excretion of para-aminobenzoic acid after administration of a precursor compound that requires chymotrypsin cleavage. This test appears only to be most sensitive in patients with severe chronic pancreatitis. ERCP is the current gold standard for diagnosis, with high sensitivity and specificity. Importantly, ERCP allows the opportunity to distinguish chronic pancreatitis from periampullary cancer, provides important anatomy of the pancreatic duct that may aid in planning surgical treatment, and may include placement of pancreatic or biliary duct stents for treatment in specific cases.

ANSWER: d

REFERENCE: *Chapter 31—Chronic Pancreatitis: Clinical Presentation*

4. Which of the following is/are appropriate indications for pancreaticoduodenectomy in the treatment of chronic pancreatitis?

   a. Chronic inflammation associated with duodenal stenosis
   b. Presence of an inflammatory mass in the head of the pancreas that cannot be distinguished from pancreatic cancer
   c. Inflammatory disease in the head of the pancreas associated with biliary obstruction
   d. Multiple pseudocysts in the head of the gland
   e. All of the above

COMMENT: Pancreatic resection is most effective in the treatment of chronic pancreatitis when disease is confined to one region of the gland. Pancreaticoduodenectomy may be used to treat disease confined to the head of the pancreas that is not amenable to a drainage procedure. In addition, pancreaticoduodenectomy plays an important role in the management of chronic pancreatitis associated with biliary obstruction, duodenal obstruction, pseudocysts located in the pancreatic head, and poorly drained head and uncinate process after a longitudinal pancreaticojejunostomy. Furthermore, pancreaticoduodenectomy should be considered in all patients with disease in the head of the pancreas when malignancy cannot be definitively ruled out. Of note, chronic pancreatitis carries a 4% risk of pancreatic cancer over 20 years.

ANSWER: e

REFERENCE: *Chapter 31—Chronic Pancreatitis: Treatment*

5. Choose the true statement describing the prognosis of chronic pancreatitis:

   a. Patients with chronic pancreatitis have an equal survival to the general population
   b. Patients with chronic pancreatitis have a decreased survival compared to the general population; complications of their disease including biliary sepsis, malnutrition, and pancreatic cancer contribute to their poor survival
   c. Patients with chronic pancreatitis have a decreased survival compared to the general population; the majority of patients die of cirrhosis, diabetic complications, or aerodigestive cancers
   d. Patients with chronic pancreatitis have a decreased survival compared to the general population; infectious complications account for the majority of excess mortalities

COMMENT: Patients with chronic pancreatitis have an excess mortality of 36% over 20 years compared to the general population. A minority of patients with chronic pancreatitis die secondary to their disease. The primary causes of death in this population may be attributed to associated tobacco and alcohol use and their sequelae, including aerodigestive cancers and cirrhosis.

ANSWER: c

REFERENCE: *Chapter 31—Chronic Pancreatitis: Prognosis*

6. Choose the correct statement describing pseudocysts in chronic pancreatitis:

   a. Pseudocysts, while common following an episode of acute pancreatitis, rarely occur in patients with chronic pancreatitis
   b. Recurrence of a pancreatic pseudocyst after aspiration implies an ongoing communication with the pancreatic duct
   c. In patients with chronic pancreatitis and a pseudocyst, adequate drainage of the pseudocyst will usually result in significant pain relief and decreased narcotic requirements
   d. Percutaneous drainage successfully treats pancreatic pseudocysts in nearly all cases

COMMENT: Pancreatic pseudocysts are the most common complication of chronic pancreatitis. The underlying ductal abnormalities in patients with chronic pancreatitis make pseudocysts less likely to regress spontaneously in these patients. Pseudocysts can be an important additional cause of pain in patients with chronic pancreatitis, but treatment of the pseudocyst rarely leads to complete pain relief. An initial attempt at percutaneous aspiration may be reasonable in these patients, but any pseudocyst that recurs has by definition and ongoing communication with the pancreatic ductal system and is best treated by operative internal drainage. This procedure can be combined with a ductal drainage procedure if indicated to address the patient's chronic pancreatitis.

ANSWER: b

REFERENCE: *Chapter 31—Chronic Pancreatitis: Treatment*

7. A 50-year-old alcoholic man is evaluated for chronic epigastric pain. Clinical history and exam are consistent with a diagnosis of chronic pancreatitis. ERCP confirms the presence of pancreatic ductal ectasia with alternating areas of stricture and dilatation. After cessation of alcohol and an appropriate trial of medical management the patient is deemed an appropriate surgical candidate. What would be the most appropriate operative procedure in this patient to treat his intractable pain?

a. 95% distal pancreatectomy
b. Distal pancreatectomy with end pancreaticojejunostomy
c. Pancreaticoduodenectomy
d. Longitudinal pancreaticojejunostomy

COMMENT: Patients with chronic pancreatitis and significant ductal dilatation are candidates for ductal drainage procedures, with longitudinal pancreaticojejunostomy being the procedure of choice. This operation provides drainage for the entire length of the pancreatic duct and preserves pancreatic parenchyma. Immediate pain relief can be achieved in more than 80% of patients, but pain may recur in 25%–50% of patients over 5 years.

ANSWER: d

REFERENCE: *Chapter 31—Chronic Pancreatitis: Treatment*

CHAPTER 32

NEOPLASMS OF THE EXOCRINE PANCREAS

1. Which of the following are risk factors strongly associated with the development of pancreatic cancer?

a. Black race
b. Caffeine consumption
c. Alcohol use
d. Smoking
e. Increasing age

COMMENT: The risk for the development of pancreatic cancer is related to age, race, sex, tobacco use, diet, and specific genetic syndromes. Incidence increases with advancing age. More than 80% of cases occur in persons between the ages of 60 and 80 years, and pancreatic cancer is rare in people under 40 years of age. The incidence and mortality rates for pancreatic cancer in African-Americans of both sexes are higher than those in whites. The gender differences in pancreatic cancer have been equalizing during recent years. Pancreatic cancer is still more common in men than in women, but the incidence and mortality rates have increased in women while they have stabilized or slightly decreased for men. The most consistently observed environmental risk for the development of pancreatic cancer is cigarette smoking. It is estimated that cigarette smoking can increase the risk of pancreatic cancer between one and one-half and five times. Alcohol consumption does not seem to be a risk factor for pancreatic cancer despite conflicting past reports. Recent studies suggest that past studies linking pancreatic cancer to alcohol use may have been confounded by tobacco use. Similarly, coffee consumption and exposure to ionized radiation have been shown not to be associated with an increased pancreatic cancer risk.

ANSWER: a, d, e

REFERENCE: *Chapter 32—Neoplasms of the Exocrine Pancreas: Epidemiology and Risk Factors*

2. Which of the following genetic alterations are found in high frequency (50% or greater) in patients with pancreatic cancer?

a. Inactivation of p53
b. Absence of DPC4
c. Point mutation in K-ras
d. Disorders of DNA mismatch-repair genes

COMMENT: The genes involved in the pathogenesis of pancreatic cancer can be divided into three categories: a) tumor-suppressor genes, b) oncogenes, and c) DNA mismatch- repair genes. Tumor suppressor genes normally function to control cellular proliferation. When these genes are inactivated by genetic events such as mutation, deletion, chromosome rearrangements, or mitotic recombination, their function as growth suppressors can be lost, and abnormal growth regulation is the result. The function of p53 appears to be inactivated in up to 75% of all pancreatic cancers. The p53 gene product is the DNA-binding protein that acts as a cell cycle checkpoint and an inducer of apoptosis. Inactivation of the p53 gene in pancreatic cancer leads to loss of two important controls of cell growth: regulation instead of the proliferation and induction of cell death. The DPC4 is a tumor-suppressor gene that has been identified on chromosome 18q. This chromosome has been shown to be missing in nearly 90% of pancreatic cancers. The DPC4 gene is inactive in almost 50% of pancreatic carcinomas. The mutation appears to be a homogeneous deletion in 30% of pancreatic cancers, and a point mutation in the other 20% of tumors. DPC4 mutations are more specific than p53 or p16 mutations for pancreatic cancer. Oncogenes are derived from normal cellular genes called protoonocogenes. When overexpressed or activated by mutation, oncogenes encode proteins with transforming properties. Activating point mutations in the K-ras oncogene is the most common genetic alteration in pancreatic carcinoma. Mutations of K-ras have been found in 80% to 100% of pancreatic cancers and therefore may be useful in the development of a molecular screening test for pancreatic cancer. Mismatch-repair genes function to insure accuracy of DNA replication, and when these genes are mutated, errors in DNA replication are not repaired. The enzymes encoded by these genes typically repair single base pair changes and small insertions and deletions that occur during DNA replication. Approximately 4% of pancreatic cancers can be characterized by disorders of DNA mismatch-repair genes.

ANSWER: a, b, c

REFERENCE: *Chapter 32—Neoplasms of the Exocrine Pancreas: Molecular Genetics*

3. Which of the following statements is/are correct regarding the pathologic findings of neoplasms of the exocrine pancreas?

a. Approximately 65% of pancreatic ductal carcinomas arise in the head, neck, or uncinate process of the pancreas; 15% originate in the body or tail of the gland, and 20% diffusely involve the whole gland.
b. Serous cystic neoplasms of the pancreas should be considered premalignant, therefore warrant aggressive surgical management.
c. Mucinous cystadenocarcinoma tends to have a better prognosis than ductal adenocarcinoma.
d. Intraductal papillary-mucinous neoplasms may be either histologically malignant or benign and warrant aggressive surgical management.

COMMENT: The most common neoplasms of the exocrine pancreas are ductal adenocarcinomas. Approximately 65% of pancreatic ductal cancers arise in the head, neck, or uncinate process of the pancreas; 15% originate in the body or tail of the gland; and 20% diffusely involve the whole gland. Cystic neoplasms also arise from the exocrine pancreas. Cystic neoplasms are much less common than ductal adenocarcinomas, tend to occur in women, and are evenly distributed throughout the gland. Serous cyst adenomas or microcystic adenomas are more common in women than in men. Most serous cystic neoplasms are benign, although malignant behavior has been reported rarely. Mucinous cystic neoplasms are also more common in women than in men. They can be divided into three types: a) mucinous cystadenoma, b) the intermediate or borderline tumor, and c) mucinous cystadenocarcinoma. Benign-appearing neoplasms may contain small foci of carcinoma. Therefore, it appears that all mucinous cystic neoplasms should be completely resected. The prognosis for patients with resected, benign or borderline tumors is excellent. Patients with mucinous cystadenocarcinoma tend to do better than patients with ductal adenocarcinoma, with a 5-year survival of approximately 50%. Intraductal papillary-mucinous neoplasms are soft villous tumors that are often found within mucous-filled, dilated pancreatic ducts. They show varying degrees of cellular atypia. Intraductal papillary-mucinous neoplasms (IPMN) appear to be more common in the head, neck, and uncinate process of the pancreas but can be found diffusely throughout the whole gland. These tumors may contain areas of invasive carcinoma and should also be considered premalignant. Aggressive surgical resection is recommended if possible.

ANSWER: a, c, d

REFERENCE: *Chapter 32—Neoplasms of the Exocrine Pancreas: Pathology*

4. A 67-year old man has itching, dark urine, and epigastric pain. Physical examination reveals jaundice. Initial laboratory tests show a total bilirubin level of 6.5 mg/dL, alkaline phosphatase is elevated at three times the upper limit of normal, and mild elevations of serum transaminase levels are seen. Which of the following is the single most useful diagnostic test?

a. Abdominal ultrasonography
b. Computed tomography of the abdomen
c. Magnetic resonance imaging of the abdomen
d. Endoscopic retrograde cholangeography

COMMENT: The early diagnosis of pancreatic cancer requires a low index of suspicion and appropriate aggressiveness in pursuing the diagnosis. Ultrasonography, CT, and magnetic resonance imaging (MRI) are all useful, non-invasive tests in the patient suspected of having a pancreatic cancer. Abdominal ultrasonography is most sensitive for detecting gallstones, an ever-present issue in the elderly patient who is jaundiced. Ultrasonography, although operator-dependent, can also demonstrate dilated intrahepatic and extrahepatic bile ducts, liver metastases, and pancreatic masses, ascites, and enlarged pancreatic lymph nodes. Ultrasonography will reveal a pancreatic mass in 60% to 70% of patients with cancer. Because helical CT is just as sensitive as ultrasonography and provides more complete information about surrounding structures and the local and distant extent of the disease, ultrasonography has largely been replaced by CT. Helical or spiral CT is currently the preferred non-invasive imaging test for the diagnosis of pancreatic cancer. Pancreatic cancer usually appears as an area of pancreatic enlargement with a localized hypodense lesion. A dual-phase intravenous contrast study is ideal not only in identifying the tumor but also in evaluating the invasion of local structures such as major visceral vessels as well as metastatic disease. MRI offers no significant advantage over CT because of a low signal-to noise-ratio, motion artifacts, lack of bowel opacification, and low spatial resolution. More recently, however, the introduction of magnetic resonance cholangiopancreatography (MRCP) has offered a promising non-invasive technique that can visualize both the bile duct and the pancreatic duct; images which are similar to those obtained with the MRCP. Traditionally, the next step in the evaluation of the jaundiced patient has been cholangeography, either by the endoscopic or percutaneous route. If the endoscopic approach is used, the duodenum and ampulla can be visualized and biopsy specimens obtained if necessary. In addition, ERCP allows direct imaging of the pancreatic duct. The sensitivity of ERCP for the diagnosis of pancreatic cancer approaches 90%. Although ERCP is reliable and confirming the presence of a clinically suspected pancreatic cancer, it should not be used routinely. Diagnostic ERCP should be reserved for patients with presumed pancreatic cancer and obstructive jaundice in whom no mass is demonstrated on a CT scan, symptomatic but non-jaundiced patients without an obvious pancreatic mass, and patients with chronic pancreatitis in whom the development of pancreatic mass is suspected based on clinical evidence or the development of jaundice.

ANSWER: b

REFERENCE: *Chapter 32—Neoplasms of the Exocrine Pancreas: Diagnosis*

5. Which of the following statements is/are true concerning the surgical technique for resection of a carcinoma of the head of the pancreas?

   a. Direct involvement or encasement of the superior mesenteric artery, superior mesenteric vein, or portal vein generally precludes resection.
   b. A histologic diagnosis of carcinoma should be obtained prior to proceeding with resection.
   c. A classic Whipple procedure with antrectomy is associated with an improvement in survival.
   d. The pancreatic-enteric anastomosis is the cause of much of the postoperative morbidity associated with the operation.

COMMENT: Once distant metastasis has been excluded, the primary tumor is assessed in regard to resectability. Local factors that preclude pancreaticoduodenal resection include retroperitoneal extension of the tumor to involve the inferior vena cava or aorta, direct involvement or encasement of the superior mesenteric artery, superior mesenteric vein, or portal vein. Although isolated focal involvement of the portal vein/SMV can be managed with venous resection, most patients with venous involvement have extension to involve the superior mesenteric artery making isolated vein resection inappropriate. If there is no evidence of other metastatic disease or local invasion, most experienced pancreatic surgeons proceed to a pancreatic resection without obtaining a tissue diagnosis. The clinical presentation, results of preoperative CT and cholangiography, and operative findings of a palpable mass in the head of the pancreas, surpass the ability of an intraoperative biopsy to define the diagnosis of malignancy. A number of techniques are used to restore gastrointestinal continuity after a pancreaticoduodenal resection. The pancreaticojejunostomy is the most problematic anastomosis in the reconstruction. Traditionally, much of the morbidity and mortality associated with this operation are related to problems with this anastomosis. The pylorus-preserving modification spares the antrum and pylorus and may reduce the incidence of troublesome post-gastroectomy problems, including marginal ulceration. A comparison of patients treated with pylorus-sparing Whipple procedure and those managed by the traditional Whipple resection including antrectomy for pancreatic cancer shows no difference in survival.

ANSWER: d

REFERENCE: *Chapter 32—Neoplasms of the Exocrine Pancreas: Resection of Pancreatic Carcinoma*

6. Which of the following statements is/are true concerning the results following pancreaticoduodenectomy for carcinoma of the pancreas?

   a. Perioperative mortality following pancreaticoduodenectomy has been consistently reported in the range of 2% to 3%.
   b. Pancreatic fistula following a pancreatic resection is associated with a mortality as high as 25%.
   c. The most frequent complication following pylorus-preserving pancreatic resection is delayed gastric emptying.
   d. The actuarial 5-year survival for patients with resected pancreatic cancer is approximately 20%.
   e. Survival following pancreatic carcinoma is independent of margin and node status.

COMMENT: During the 1960s and 1970s, many centers reported operative mortality following pancreaticoduodenectomy in the range of 20% to 40% with postoperative morbidity rates as high as 40% to 60%. During the last decade, a decline in operative morbidity and mortality following pancreaticoduodenectomy has been reported at a number of centers with operative mortality rates in the range of 2% to 3% reported. Although the operative mortality rates for pancreatic cancer have reduced significantly, the complication rates remained high (approximately 40%). Pancreatic fistula appears to remain the most frequent serious complication following pancreaticoduodenectomy, with an incidence range from 5% to 20%. In the past, the development of pancreatic fistula after a pancreaticoduodenectomy was associated with mortality rates of 10% to 40%. Although the incidence of pancreatic fistula following a pancreaticoduodenectomy remains stable, the overall associated mortality rate has diminished owing to improved management. The most frequent complications following pylorus-preserving pancreatic resection is delayed gastric emptying with an incidence in the range of 20% to 40%.

Historically, 5-year survival rates for patients undergoing resection for adenocarcinoma of the head of the pancreas were reported to be in the range of 5%. A recent report from Johns Hopkins has demonstrated an actuarial 5-year survival for all patients following pancreatic resection of 21%, with a median survival of 15.5 months. Factors found to be important predictors of survival included tumor diameter less than 3 centimeters, lymph node status, and resection margin status. The outcome is particularly favorable in the subgroup of patients who underwent pancreaticoduodenectomy with both negative lymph nodes and negative margin status with negative resection margins; the median survival was 32 months and a 5-year survival was 40%.

ANSWER: a, c, d

REFERENCE: *Chapter 32, Neoplasms of the Exocrine Pancreas: Resection of Pancreatic Carcinoma*

7. A 52-year old otherwise healthy male presents with obstructive jaundice and back pain. At laparotomy he is found to have an unresectable pancreatic cancer due to local invasion. Appropriate procedures to be performed at the time of laparotomy include:

a. A chemical splanchnicectomy
b. Hepaticojejunostomy
c. Pancreaticojejunostomy
d. Gastrojejunostomy

COMMENT: Obstructive jaundice is present in most patients who have pancreatic cancer. If left untreated, it can result in progressive liver dysfunction, hepatic failure, and early death. Nonoperative palliation with endoscopic stenting is an appropriate alternative for palliation in patients who do not undergo operation. If, however, at the time of operation the patient is found to be unresectable, the performance of a hepaticojejunostomy can provide excellent long-term palliation with minimal associated morbidity and mortality. Although true mechanical obstruction of the duodenum as seen by radiologic or endoscopic examination is infrequent at the time of presentation, duodenal obstruction develops in almost 20% of patients before they die as disease progresses. In a recent prospective, randomized trial, prophylactic gastrojejunostomy in patients with unresectable pancreatic cancer significantly decreased the rate of late gastric outlet obstruction requiring treatment without an associated increase in postoperative complication rate or length of stay. Tumor-associated pain can be incapacitating in patients with unresectable pancreatic cancer. The postulated causes of tumor-associated pain are many and include tumor infiltration into the celiac plexus, increased parenchymal pressure associated with pancreatic duct obstruction, pancreatic inflammation, gallbladder distention resulting from biliary obstruction, and gastroduodenal obstruction. Although the pancreatic duct may be obstructed and dilated, there is no indication to perform a Puestow procedure (pancreaticojejunostomy) in patients with unresectable pancreatic cancer. Patients with unresectable cancer at the time of surgical exploration should receive a chemical splanchnicectomy, with alcohol. This simple procedure has been shown to reduce the incidence of pain in patients with unresectable pancreatic cancer both with and without pain at the time of laparotomy.

ANSWER: a, b, d

REFERENCE: *Chapter 32—Neoplasms of the Exocrine Pancreas: Palliation*

CHAPTER 33

NEOPLASMS OF THE ENDOCRINE PANCREAS

1. A 35-year-old woman is evaluated for seizure disorder, mental obtundation, and personality change. The findings at physical examination are normal. The fasting serum glucose level is 44 mg/dL. Other serum values are normal. Subsequent investigations should include which of the following?
   a. Oral glucose tolerance test
   b. Determination of fasting insulin to glucose (I:G) ratios
   c. Assay of serum C peptide level
   d. Determination of serum prolactin level

COMMENT: A common mistake in evaluation for insulinoma is to begin with an oral glucose tolerance test. Instead, insulinoma is most reliably diagnosed with the technique of a monitored fast. During a monitored fast, blood for glucose and insulin determinations is sampled every 4 to 6 hours and at the time of symptom occurrence. Symptoms of hypoglycemia typically occur when glucose levels are less than 50 mg/dL. Concurrent serum insulin levels often are greater than 25 μU/mL. Additional support for the diagnosis of insulinoma comes from the calculation of the I:G ratio at different time points during the monitored fast. Healthy persons have I:G ratios less than 0.3. Patients with insulinoma typically have I:G ratios greater than 0.4 after a prolonged fast. Other measurable beta cell products synthesized in excess in patients with insulinoma include C peptide and proinsulin. Elevated levels of C peptide and proinsulin are typically found in the peripheral blood of patients with insulinoma. The possibility of surreptitious administration of insulin or oral hypoglycemic agents should be considered for all patients with suspected insulinoma. Levels of C peptide and proinsulin are not elevated if a patient is self-administering insulin. Patients self-administering either bovine or porcine insulin may have anti-insulin antibodies in circulating blood.

ANSWER: b, c

REFERENCE: *Chapter 33—Neoplasms of the Endocrine Pancreas: Insulinoma*

2. For the patient in question 1, an I:G ratio of 0.5 was documented after 28 hours of fasting. Symptoms of mental obtundation developed concurrently and were reversed by means of oral administration of glucose. Endoscopic ultrasonography showed a 1.2-cm mass in the head of the pancreas. Appropriate management consists of which of the following?
   a. Surgical enucleation of the tumor
   b. Total pancreatectomy
   c. Long-term administration of octreotide
   d. Primary radiation therapy

COMMENT: Management of insulinoma is surgical in nearly all cases. Insulinoma is evenly distributed in the pancreas, approximately one third are located in the head and uncinate process, one third in the body of the gland, and one third in the tail of the gland. Ninety percent of patients have benign solitary adenoma amenable to surgical cure. Small benign insulinomas not close to the main pancreatic duct can be removed by means of enucleation, independent of location within the gland. In the body and tail of the pancreas, insulinomas larger than 2 cm in diameter and those close to the pancreatic duct are most commonly excised by means of distal pancreatectomy. Large insulinomas deep in the head or uncinate process of the pancreas may not be amenable to local excision and may necessitate pancreatoduodenectomy.

ANSWER: a

REFERENCE: *Chapter 33—Neoplasms of the Endocrine Pancreas: Insulinoma*

3. A 45-year-old woman has upper gastrointestinal hemorrhage. Evaluation by means of upper endoscopy reveals three ulcers in the second portion of the duodenum. Bleeding is controlled with an endoscopic heat probe. Further investigation reveals a serum gastrin value of 240 pg/mL. Which of the following would support the presumptive diagnosis of gastrinoma?

a. An increase of 320 pg/mL in serum gastrin level on intravenous infusion of secretin
b. Gastric acid analysis that shows fasting acid secretion of 3 mEq/h
c. Enlarged gastric rugae on upper gastrointestinal radiographic contrast studies
d. An increase of 150 pg/mL in serum gastrin level on intravenous infusion of cholecystokinin

COMMENT: The indications for measurement of gastrin include the presence of peptic ulcer disease, prolonged undiagnosed diarrhea, being a member of a family with multiple endocrine neoplasia type 1, and prominent gastric rugal folds on upper gastrointestinal radiographic series. In most patients with gastrinoma, the fasting serum gastrin level is elevated to more than 200 pg/mL. Gastrin values greater than 1,000 pg/mL are almost enough to confirm the diagnosis of gastrinoma. Fasting hypergastrinemia alone is not sufficient for the diagnosis of gastrinoma. Gastric acid analysis is an important test in evaluation for suspected gastrinoma. It allows differentiation between ulcerogenic and nonulcerogenic causes of hypergastrinemia. The diagnosis of gastrinoma is supported by a basal acid output greater than 15 mEq/h among patients who have not undergone surgical treatment.

After documentation that hypergastrinemia is associated with excessive acid secretion, provocative testing with secretin should be performed to differentiate gastrinoma, antral G-cell hyperplasia or hyperfunction, and the other causes of ulcerogenic hypergastrinemia. The secretin stimulation test is performed while the patient is fasting. Peripheral serum samples are obtained for measurement of gastrin in the basal period, secretin (2 U/kg body weight) is administered as an intravenous bolus, and serum samples for gastrin measurement are obtained every 5 minutes for 30 minutes. An increase in gastrin level more than 200 pg/mL above the basal level supports the diagnosis of gastrinoma.

ANSWER: a, c

REFERENCE: *Chapter 33—Neoplasms of the Endocrine Pancreas: Gastrinoma*

4. The most common location(s) for development of gastrinoma is/are which of the following?

a. Pancreas to the right of the superior mesenteric vein
b. Pancreatic body and tail
c. Gastric antrum
d. Duodenum

COMMENT: Most gastrinomas have been identified to the right of the superior mesenteric vessels within the head of the pancreas or duodenum. Intraoperative ultrasonography should be performed to assist in tumor localization. Intraoperative upper gastrointestinal endoscopy may be helpful because it allows transillumination of the duodenal wall and identification of small duodenal gastrinomas. At exploration, any suspicious peripancreatic lymph nodes are excised and submitted for frozen section. Primary tumors within the substance of the pancreas that are small (less than 2 cm) and well encapsulated may be carefully enucleated. Pancreatic tumors without defined capsules or situated deep in the pancreatic parenchyma may necessitate partial pancreatic resection. In the absence of an identifiable pancreatic or duodenal tumor, longitudinal duodenotomy can be performed at the level of the second portion of the duodenum to allow eversion of the duodenum in a search of duodenal microgastrinoma. Primary gastrinoma identified within the duodenal wall is resected locally with primary closure of the duodenal defect.

ANSWER: a, d

REFERENCE: *Chapter 33—Neoplasms of the Endocrine Pancreas: Gastrinoma*

5. A patient with biochemically confirmed gastrinoma undergoes CT for tumor localization. The scans show a 2-cm mass in the head of the pancreas and numerous nodules within the right and left lobes of the liver. Appropriate management includes which of the following?

   a. Omeprazole administration
   b. Radiation therapy
   c. Pancreatoduodenectomy
   d. Proximal gastric vagotomy

COMMENT: Patients with gastrinoma who undergo localization and staging studies that suggest the presence of unresectable hepatic metastatic lesions should undergo percutaneous or laparoscopically directed liver biopsy for histologic verification. If the presence of unresectable gastrinoma is confirmed, open surgical exploration is not performed, and the patient undergoes long-term maintenance omeprazole therapy. Almost all patients can be rendered achlorhydric with appropriate dose adjustment of omeprazole. Noncompliant patients who refuse to take appropriate doses of omeprazole and who have complications related to the ulcer diathesis may need total gastrectomy. Total gastrectomy removes the end organ (parietal cell mass) and was once the procedure of choice for gastrinoma. Its use to treat patients with gastrinoma has declined markedly.

ANSWER: a

REFERENCE: *Chapter 33—Neoplasms of the Endocrine Pancreas: Gastrinoma*

6. Neoplastic hypersecretion of the hormone vasoactive intestinal peptide (VIP) is associated with which of the following features?

   a. Hypokalemia, hypochlorhydria, diarrhea
   b. Hyperglycemia, necrolytic rash, hypoaminoacidemia
   c. Constipation, gallstones, hyperglycemia
   d. Hyperkalemia, necrolytic rash, diarrhea

COMMENT: Patients characteristically have intermittent, severe diarrhea, typically of a watery nature, averaging 5 L/d. Malabsorption and steatorrhea are not common. Hypokalemia is caused by fecal loss of large amounts of potassium (as much as 400 mEq/d). Low serum potassium levels can be associated with muscular weakness, lethargy, and nausea. Most patients have hypochlorhydria or achlorhydria. One half of the patients have hyperglycemia and hypercalcemia, and cutaneous flushing occurs among a small number of patients. The diagnosis of VIPoma typically is made after other, more common causes of diarrhea are excluded. The active agent in VIPoma syndrome usually is VIP. A small number of patients have elevations in levels of other candidate mediators, such as peptide histidine-isoleucine or prostaglandins.

ANSWER: a

REFERENCE: *Chapter 33—Neoplasms of the Endocrine Pancreas: VIPoma*

Section F

LIVER AND PORTAL VENOUS SYSTEM

CHAPTER 34

HEPATOBILIARY ANATOMY

---

1. Which of the following statements is/are true concerning hepatic anatomic nomenclature?
   a. In the traditional English system, the right lobe is divided into anterior and posterior segments by an intersegmental line with no topographic landmarks or intraparenchymal septa
   b. The caudate lobe in the French, or Couinaud's, nomenclature is referred to as *segment I*
   c. The right lobe of the liver in English nomenclature is subdivided in the French system into segments V through VIII
   d. In the English system, the left lobe of the liver is divided into the medial segment and the lateral segment by the falciform ligament

COMMENT: Until recently, anatomic descriptions in the English literature began with the major divisions of liver into a right and left lobe separated by a vertical line drawn from the gallbladder fossa to the inferior vena cava. The left lobe is further divided by the falciform ligament into a medial segment and lateral segment. The right lobe is further divided into an anterior and posterior segment by an intersegmental line that has no reliable topographic landmarks and no intraparenchymal septa to allow easy identification. The French nomenclature, also known as *Couinaud's nomenclature,* enumerates the segments of the liver beginning with segment I, or the caudate lobe. Segments II, III, and IV make up most of the "English" left lobe, and segments V through VIII represent the English nomenclature right lobe.

ANSWER: a, b, c, d

REFERENCE: *Chapter 34—Hepatobiliary Anatomy: Morphologic and Functional Anatomy*

2. Which of the following statements is/are true concerning the widely accepted French, or Couinaud's, nomenclature for liver anatomy?
   a. The liver is divided into eight discrete segments based on portal pedicle branches and hepatic venous drainage
   b. This anatomic system is particularly useful in allowing less than lobar segmental anatomic resections that minimize blood loss and loss of hepatic reserve
   c. Enumeration proceeds from right to left
   d. Segments II and III are synonymous with the left lateral segment in English nomenclature

COMMENT: In the now widely accepted French (Couinaud's) nomenclature, the liver can be divided into eight discrete segments based on portal pedicle branches and hepatic venous drainage. Enumeration of the segments proceeds from left to right, beginning with segment I, the caudate lobe. The left lateral sector consists of a superior segment II and an inferior segment III and is synonymous with the left lateral segment in older terminology. The advantages of this detailed segmental anatomy, which is based on discrete portal pedicle branches, are to accurately locate individual lesions in the hepatic substance by means of preoperative imaging and intraoperative ultrasonography and to allow the possibility of less than lobar segmental anatomic resection that minimizes blood loss and functional loss of hepatic reserve.

ANSWER: a, b, d

REFERENCE: *Chapter 34—Hepatobiliary Anatomy: Morphologic and Functional Anatomy*

3. Which of the following statements is/are true concerning the arteriovenous anatomy of the liver?

   a. Most commonly, the right, left, and middle hepatic veins join the inferior vena cava as a separate trunk
   b. Most frequently, the entire length of each hepatic vein is within the parenchyma of the liver
   c. A replaced right hepatic artery may be placed in jeopardy during pancreatoduodenectomy
   d. There is little collateral arterial circulation between the right and left hepatic lobes

COMMENT: Three major hepatic veins carry blood from the central veins of the hepatic substance to the inferior vena cava (IVC). In two thirds of patients, a single large right hepatic vein joins the right anterior wall of the IVC and a middle and a left hepatic vein. These vessels converge 1 to 2 cm from the IVC and enter the left anterior wall of the IVC as a single vessel. In one third of persons, each major hepatic vein joins at the same horizontal level of the IVC as a separate trunk. Some persons have a short but definable extraparenchymal segment of one or more of the hepatic veins at the confluence with the IVC. More frequently, the entire length of the hepatic veins is intraparenchymal, which can preclude early, safe isolation of the hepatic vein during hepatic resection.

There is considerable variability in the origin and course of the right and left hepatic arteries. The most common finding (55% of persons) is a transverse common hepatic artery from the celiac trunk. This artery gives off the gastroduodenal, right gastric, and supraduodenal arteries and courses obliquely in the left anterior aspect of the hepatoduodenal ligament as a proper hepatic artery. Beyond the point at which the cystic artery branches to the gallbladder, there is a fairly low trifurcation into single right, middle, and left hepatic arteries. Knowledge of the most common variations is extremely important because unintentional division can occur during gastric, pancreatic, and hepatobiliary procedures. A replaced or accessory left hepatic artery can arise from the left gastric artery and course transversely in the lesser omentum. With nearly equal frequency, a replaced or accessory right hepatic artery arises from the superior mesenteric artery near its origin and courses posteriorly or through the head of the pancreas obliquely along the right posterior border of the hepatoduodenal ligament. Although original anatomic descriptions deny the existence of collateral vessels to the opposite hepatic lobe, image perfusion studies after ligation of main or replaced hepatic arteries clearly show the presence of collateral flow to the deprived lobe.

ANSWER: b, c

REFERENCE: *Chapter 34—Hepatobiliary Anatomy: Hepatic Veins and Arteries*

4. Intraoperative ultrasonography is commonly used by hepatic surgeons. Which of the following statements is/are true concerning intraoperative ultrasonography and hepatic surgery?

   a. Intraoperative ultrasonography offers no advantage over conventional transcorporeal ultrasound in the detection of hepatic lesions
   b. Portal structures can be differentiated from hepatic veins by the extension of Glisson's capsule surrounding these structures
   c. It is difficult to differentiate a vascular structure from a mass on ultrasound images
   d. The short hepatic veins are difficult to detect with intraoperative ultrasonography

COMMENT: Detailed anatomic description of the hepatic veins, portal pedicles, and the inferior vena cava is possible through the use of intraoperative ultrasonography. Cooperation between radiologist and hepatic surgeon with the use of intraoperative ultrasonography allows identification of lesions during surgery that are not visible with conventional transcorporeal ultrasonography or computed tomography (CT). Beginning superiorly at the inferior vena cava, the confluence and course of each hepatic vein can easily be determined. More inferiorly, the main right and left portal pedicles can be seen coursing transversely in the transverse incisura. Portal structures can easily be differentiated from hepatic veins by the hyperechoic extensions of Glisson's capsule that surround these structures. When a circular structure is encountered, a mass or metastasis can be suspected. Scanning away from the mass may reveal a tubulovascular shape that has been imaged and cross-sectioned. Flattening of the circular mass by means of external compression with the ultrasound probe also differentiates a vascular structure from a solid mass.

ANSWER: b

REFERENCE: *Chapter 34—Hepatobiliary Anatomy: Ultrasonography of the Liver*

5. A 57-year-old man with a history of Duke's C colon cancer is undergoing evaluation because of an increasing level of carcinoembryonic antigen. Which of the following statements is/are correct concerning the use of CT for this indication?

a. Conventional CT depicts lesions much smaller than 1 cm in diameter
b. Computed tomographic arterioportography involves immediate CT scanning after direct injection into both the common hepatic artery and superior mesenteric artery
c. Double helical (spiral) CT can eliminate the need for invasive angiography
d. Magnetic resonance imaging of the liver add little to the evaluation in this case

COMMENT: Computed tomography has been used increasingly to screen for hepatic and other intraabdominal or retroperitoneal lesions. Conventional CT includes 0.5 to 1.0 cm axial images of the liver after oral administration of barium and intravenous bolus injection of contrast material. Although resolution has improved, hepatic lesions smaller than 1 cm in diameter or lesions isodense with hepatic parenchyma can be missed. Resolution of hepatic lesions has been greatly enhanced by the combination of visceral angiography and CT, known as *CT arterioportography* (CTAP). Immediate CT after injection of contrast material directly into the common hepatic artery can help identify small hepatic lesions that usually show increased density relative to the surrounding hepatic parenchyma. Computed tomographic arterioportography also includes direct injection of contrast material into the splenic or superior mesenteric artery with CT imaging during the portal venous phase of this injection. Hepatic lesions supplied by the hepatic artery thus appear as discrete, hypodense lesions surrounded by normal hepatic parenchyma enhanced by portal venous contrast material.

Double helical (spiral) CT has considerable promise in complementing or replacing CTAP for preoperative imaging. This technique allows total hepatic imaging in both the arterial and the arterial and venous phases after a single, rapid, intravenous bolus injection of contrast material during a single breath hold. It is possible to visualize the portal structures and hepatic veins on a single scan and give high resolution of small hepatic lesions. In addition, three-dimensional reconstructions can be made to further delineate hepatic parenchyma and show a CT-constructed hepatic arteriogram. This technique may completely replace invasive arteriography for characterizing the blood supply to the liver before hepatic resection or after hepatic transplantation. Magnetic resonance imaging of the liver has results similar to those of CT but has not shown improvements sufficient to justify the increased cost associated with the technique.

ANSWER: b, c, d

REFERENCE: *Chapter 34—Hepatobiliary Anatomy: CT Imaging of the Liver*

6. A solitary, 6-cm lesion is identified in the right hepatic lobe in the patient described in question 5. Which of the following statements is/are true concerning initial operative management?

    a. To facilitate mobilization and assessment with intraoperative ultrasonography, complete mobilization including dividing the left and right triangular ligaments is necessary
    b. In dividing the right triangular ligament, care must be taken to avoid injury to accessory right hepatic veins draining directly into the vena cava
    c. Unless a considerable length of hepatic vein is found outside the hepatic parenchyma, early hepatic vein ligation is avoided
    d. Ligation of the portal arterial structures always is necessary before proceeding with hepatic lobectomy

COMMENT: For major hepatic resection and for complete intraoperative ultrasonography, complete mobilization of the liver is required. After detachment of the hepatic flexure of the colon and division of the falciform ligament, both the left and right triangular ligaments must be sharply taken down to fully mobilize the liver. During division of the right triangular ligament, care must be taken to avoid injury to the right diaphragm, the right adrenal gland and adrenal vein, the right phrenic vein, and several moderately sized accessory right hepatic veins draining directly into the vena cava. After mobilization, digital and bimanual palpation is performed, and intraoperative ultrasonography can be performed. Many hepatic surgeons dissect the porta hepatis to identify the main bifurcations of the hepatic artery, bile duct, and portal vein. This allows individual ligation of unilateral branches of each of these structures during hepatic lobectomy but before parenchymal dissection. In an alternative approach the main portal structures are left undisturbed and branches to a given lobe are ligated during parenchymal transection. Hemorrhage can be minimized with intermittent portal inflow occlusion by means of clamping or compression of the portal triad (Pringle maneuver). There has been considerable debate over early versus late isolation and ligation of a given hepatic vein during lobectomy because the extraparenchymal component of the hepatic vein can be quite short or absent. Because hemorrhage in this location can be difficult to control, a safe strategy is always to avoid early isolation of a given hepatic vein or to attempt isolation only when a considerable length of vein is found on mobilization of the respective triangular ligament.

ANSWER: a, b, c

REFERENCE: *Chapter 34—Hepatobiliary Anatomy: Intraoperative Assessment*

7. In the patient described in questions 5 and 6, which of the following is/are important in the performance of a right hepatic lobectomy?

    a. The use of an ultrasonic dissector is essential for division of the hepatic parenchyma
    b. If temporary portal inflow occlusion is used (Pringle maneuver), it is not necessary to reestablish blood flow during parenchymal division
    c. The greater omentum can be used to buttress the transected liver edge
    d. Control of the main right hepatic vein should eliminate all forms of venous drainage

COMMENT: The steps of right hepatic lobectomy involve adherence to the tenet of optimal operative exposure and control of vascular inflow and outflow. In select circumstances, control of the vena cava may be desired. Either the individual portal structures can be identified and ligated early in the course of the procedure or the entire portal triad can be circled with an umbilical tape tourniquet in preparation for a Pringle maneuver. If temporary portal inflow occlusion is used, intermittent 10- to 20-minute periods of clamping with 3 to 5 minutes to reestablish blood flow are recommended. Division of the hepatic parenchyma begins with scoring of Glisson's capsule with cautery or knife and proceeds with division of the hepatic surface with blunt dissection by means of finger fracture, the blunt edge of an instrument or suction tip, or an ultrasonic dissector. Individual vessels and bile ducts are cauterized, sutured, or clipped in rapid succession from anterior to posterior. The hepatic veins are encountered in the hepatic substance near the vena cava and are carefully clamped and suture ligated to complete the resection. As many as 10 posterior accessory veins drain the medial aspect of the right lobe and empty directly into the right anterior surface of the IVC.

ANSWER: c

REFERENCE: *Chapter 34—Hepatobiliary Anatomy: Major Lobectomy*

CHAPTER 35

HEPATIC PHYSIOLOGY

1. Which of the following statements is/are true concerning hepatic blood flow?

    a. Although constituting only 2.5% of total body weight, the liver receives 25% of the cardiac output

    b. Hepatic blood flow is equally derived from the portal vein and hepatic artery

    c. The liver serves as a physiologic blood reservoir either releasing blood back into the systemic circulation at times of acute blood loss or in situations of volume overload serving as a site of extra blood storage

    d. An important function of the liver, to filter particulate debris, is performed by phagocytic Kupffer cells that line the hepatic sinusoidal endothelium

COMMENT: The liver constitutes approximately 2.5% of total body weight but receives 25% of cardiac output. Total hepatic blood flow is 100 to 130 mL/min per kilogram. Approximately two thirds of total hepatic blood flow is derived from the portal vein and one third from the hepatic artery. The liver also serves as a physiologic blood reservoir. Approximately 25% to 30% of liver volume is blood. In cases of acute blood loss, as much as 30%, or 300 mL, of hepatic blood volume can be released into the systemic circulation without adverse effects on liver function. In the case of right-heart failure, however, or other causes of systemic volume overload, as much as 1 L of extra blood can be stored in the liver before passive congestion and liver injury occur. The hepatic sinusoids are lined by endothelium punctuated with pores that allow proteins and other particles to diffuse out of the vascular tree and into proximity with hepatocytes. This extreme permeability of the liver allows rapid exchange of nutrients, hormones, and environmental agents between the blood and the hepatocytes. The liver also acts as a filter for particulate debris, which enters the portal circulation through intestinal capillaries. Particles such as bacteria are ingested by Kupffer cells by the process of phagocytosis. Kupffer cells line the hepatic sinusoidal endothelium, where formed blood elements and matter may be in direct contact with these phagocytic cells.

ANSWER: a, c, d

REFERENCE: *Chapter 35—Hepatic Physiology: Hepatic Blood Flow*

2. The liver has a vital role in carbohydrate metabolism and regulation of blood glucose. Which of the following statements is/are true concerning carbohydrate metabolism by the liver?

    a. Glycogen, a complex polymer of glucose, is synthesized by hepatocytes in a remarkably energy efficient process

    b. Glucagon stimulates glycogenesis

    c. Glycolysis, the process by which glucose is converted to two molecules of pyruvate, occurs in the liver mitochondria

    d. If glycogen stores become depleted, the liver can synthesize new glucose by the process of gluconeogenesis, which is stimulated by insulin

COMMENT: Serum glucose is tightly regulated by the liver despite wide fluctuations in dietary ingestion. The liver can take up as much as 100 g/d of glucose and convert it to glycogen by the process of glycogenesis. The liver can also release glucose into the blood by means of glycogenolysis, the breakdown of glycogen, or by gluconeogenesis, the formation of new glucose from substrates such as alanine, lactate, glycerol, or dietary amino acids. Hormones are important in hepatic regulation of glucose metabolism. Insulin, for example, stimulates glycogenesis, and glucagon stimulates glycogenolysis and gluconeogenesis. Gluconeogenesis is enhanced by fasting, critical illness, and periods of anaerobic metabolism.

Glycogen is a complex polymer of glucose. Liver cells can store up to 8% of their weight as glycogen. The first step in glycogen storage is transport of glucose through the hepatocyte plasma membrane. Approximately 90% of portal venous glucose is removed from the blood by liver cells through carrier-facilitated diffusion. The rate of glucose transport is enhanced by insulin. Once in the hepatocyte, glucose and adenosine triphosphate (ATP) are converted by the enzyme glucokinase to glucose-6-phosphate (G6P), the first intermediate in the synthesis of glycogen. Because complete oxidation of one molecule of G6P generates 37 molecules of ATP, and storage uses only one molecule of ATP, the overall efficiency of glucose storage in glycogen is a remarkable 97%. Glycolysis is the pathway by which glucose is converted to two molecules of pyruvate and occurs in the cytoplasm. The citric acid cycle occurs in the mitochondria.

ANSWER: a

REFERENCE: *Chapter 35—Hepatic Physiology*

3. Which of the following statements is/are true concerning lipid metabolism in the liver?

   a. Hepatic mitochondrial hydrolysis of fatty acids is an important source of ATP
   b. Hepatic storage of triglyceride or fatty infiltration can cause hepatic fibrosis or necrosis
   c. Approximately 90% of cholesterol synthesis occurs in the liver
   d. Most cells in the body are capable of phospholipid synthesis; therefore the liver plays a minimal role in this process

COMMENT: The liver has a number of important functions in the metabolism of lipids: (a) synthesis of apolipoproteins, (b) degradation of fatty acids into energy substrates, (b) synthesis of triglycerides from carbohydrates and proteins, and (d) synthesis of cholesterol and phospholipids from fatty acids. The mitochondrial hydrolysis of fatty acids is a source of large quantities of ATP. The conversion of stearic acid to carbon dioxide and water, for example, generates 135 ATP molecules and demonstrates highly efficient storage of energy in fat. In times of unrestrained lipolysis, such as starvation, uncontrolled diabetes, or other conditions of triglyceride mobilization from adipose tissue, the ability of the liver to perform β-oxidation can be inadequate. Under these circumstances, hepatic storage of triglycerides or fatty infiltration of the liver can occur. Triglyceride storage by itself does not appear to be a cause of hepatic fibrosis or necrosis, but fatty infiltration can be a marker for derangement of normal processes by alcohol or drug toxicity, diabetes, chronic parenteral nutrition, or morbid obesity.

Cholesterol is an important regulator of membrane fluidity and is a substrate for bile acid and steroid hormone synthesis. Cholesterol may be available through dietary intake or de novo synthesis. In mammals, approximately 90% of new cholesterol is synthesized by the liver from its precursor, acetyl coenzyme A. Dietary cholesterol intake suppresses endogenous synthesis by means of inhibiting the rate-limiting enzyme in cholesterol by a synthetic pathway, 3-hydroxy-3-methylglutaryl coenzyme A (HMG-CoA) reductase. Three major classes of phospholipids are synthesized by the liver—the lecithins, the cephalins, and the sphingomyelins. Although most cells in the body are capable of some phospholipid synthesis, the liver produces 90%.

ANSWER: a, c

REFERENCE: *Chapter 35—Hepatic Physiology: Lipid Metabolism*

4. The liver is an important site of protein metabolism. Which of the following statements is/are true concerning protein metabolism by the liver?

   a. Amino acids are taken up by hepatocytes by active transport mechanisms and are generally stored long term for later synthetic activity
   b. Under certain conditions, the amine group is removed from the amino acids in the liver and the carbon chain used for carbohydrate, lipid, or nonessential amino acid synthesis
   c. The most important route of detoxification of ammonia formed as the result of deamination of amino acids is excretion of ammonia into the urine
   d. Proteins synthesized by the liver include albumin, transferrin, fibrinogen, and apolipoproteins
   e. Albumin is a sensitive indicator of hepatic synthetic function

COMMENT: Essentially all of the end products of dietary protein digestion are amino acids, which are absorbed by the enterocytes into the portal circulation in ionized states. Amino acids are taken up by hepatocytes by one of several active transport mechanisms. Amino acids are not stored in the liver but are rapidly used in the production of plasma proteins, purines, heme proteins, and hormones. Under certain conditions, the amine group is removed from the amino acids, and the carbon chain is used for synthesis of carbohydrate, lipid, or nonessential amino acids. The ammonia formed as the result of deamination of amino acids is detoxified by one of two routes. The most important pathway involves conversion of ammonia to urea by enzymes of the Krebs-Henseleit cycle, which are present only in the liver. A second route of ammonia metabolism involves deamination of l-glutamine by the kidney with excretion of ammonia into the urine.

Essentially all albumin, fibrinogen, and apolipoproteins are derived from the liver, which can total 50 g protein delivered to the plasma per day. Of the total hepatic protein synthesis, 75% is destined for export in plasma. Albumin, an important plasma protein synthesized in the liver, has a long half-life in plasma of approximately 19 days. This long half-life makes albumin an insensitive indicator of hepatic synthetic function.

ANSWER: b, d

REFERENCE: *Chapter 35—Hepatic Physiology*

5. The liver synthesizes metabolites essential for production of fuel substrates for other organs. These metabolites include:

   a. G6P
   b. Acetyl CoA
   c. Pyruvate
   d. Oxaloacetate

COMMENT: Hepatic processes in the liver are essential for production of fuel substrates for other organs. The liver, because of its terminal position in the portal system, must regulate intestinally absorbed nutrients for tissue consumption or storage. The liver accomplishes its task by synthesizing three essential metabolites—G6P, pyruvate, and acetyl CoA. Glucose-6-phosphate can be stored as glycogen or converted into glucose, pyruvate, or ribose-5-phosphate (a nucleotide precursor). Pyruvate can be converted into lactate, alanine and other amino acids, and acetyl CoA, or it can enter the tricarboxylic acid cycle. Acetyl CoA is converted to HMG-CoA (a cholesterol and ketone body precursor) or citrate (for fatty acid and triglyceride synthesis), or it is degraded to carbon dioxide and water for energy.

ANSWER: a, b, c

REFERENCE: *Chapter 35—Hepatic Physiology: Hepatic Metabolism*

6. Which of the following statements is/are true concerning formation and secretion of hepatic bile?

   a. The adult human liver secretes less than 1000 mL bile daily
   b. Most bile is secreted by hepatocytes (canalicular bile)
   c. Primary bile acids include cholic acid, chenodeoxycholic acid, and deoxycholic acid
   d. The enterohepatic circulation is extremely efficient in reabsorption of intestinal bile acids
   e. Bile acids are the primary determinant of bile flow

COMMENT: The adult human liver secretes approximately 1.5 L bile daily. Eighty percent of this volume is secreted by the hepatocytes (canalicular bile), and 20% is secreted by the bile duct epithelial cells (ductular bile). Solutes constitute approximately 3% of bile. The major solutes are conjugated bile acids, phosphatidyl choline, cholesterol, protein, and bilirubin. Bile acids are the main determinant of bile production, and canalicular bile flow is traditionally divided into bile acid-dependent and bile acid-independent components. Primary bile acids are synthesized from cholesterol in the liver; in humans they are cholic acid and chenodeoxycholic acid. Secondary bile acids are formed in the intestinal lumen by means of bacterial dehydroxylation and consist of deoxycholic acid and lithocholic acid derived from cholic acid and chenodeoxycholic acid, respectively. Essentially all primary and secondary bile acids are conjugated with the amino acids glycine and taurine. The human liver synthesizes 300 to 400 mg/d of bile acids from cholesterol, approximately 10% of the total bile salt pool. Intestinal bile acids normally are efficiently (approximately 95%) taken up by the enterohepatic circulation. Luminal bile acids are transported by carrier proteins in the distal ileum and appear in the portal venous effluent. The hepatocyte extracts more than 95% of portal venous bile acids for resecretion into the bile.

ANSWER: b, d, e

REFERENCE: *Chapter 35—Hepatic Physiology: Bile Formation*

7. Hepatic biotransformation is defined as the intracellular metabolism of endogenous and exogenous organic compounds. Which of the following enzyme families is/are responsible for hepatic bile transformation?

a. Cytochrome P-450
b. Uridine diphosphate (UDP)-glucuronyl transferase
c. Glutathione transferase
d. Sulfotransferase

COMMENT: Liver contains enzyme systems that can expose functional groups such as hydroxyl ions and alter the size and solubility of a variety of organic and inorganic compounds by means of conjugation with small polar molecules. The general strategy of the liver is to convert hydrophobic, potentially toxic compounds into hydrophilic conjugates that can be excreted into bile or urine. Four general enzyme families are responsible for hepatic bile transformation. The cytochrome P-450 enzymes catalyze reactions such as oxidation, hydroxylation, sulfoxide formation, oxidative deamination, dealcoholization, and dehalogenation. Such reactions allow further phase II conjugation with polar groups such as glucuronate, glutathione, and sulfate. Glucuronidation is the conjugation of UDP-glucuronic acid to a variety of xenobiotics by means of ester or ether linkages. The glutathione transferases and sulfotransferases play a role in conjugation of P-450 derivatives. However, the glucuronyl transferase system is the predominant mechanism.

ANSWER: a, b, c, d

REFERENCE: *Chapter 35—Hepatic Physiology: Hepatic Biotransformation*

8. Transport of substances from the blood into hepatocytes occurs through the sinusoidal membrane. Which of the following statements is/are true concerning this plasma membrane?

a. The high lipid content of this phospholipid bilayer allows lipid-soluble molecules to enter the cell by means of simple diffusion
b. Carrier proteins within the phospholipid bilayer bind to a solute in blood and by conformational change allow it to be transported into the cell
c. Large glycoprotein molecules of the sinusoidal membrane known as *receptors* always transport the binding ligand into the cell
d. Transmission of a signal to the interior of the cell by means of receptor-ligand binding, which generates intracellular second messengers, is known as *signal transduction*

COMMENT: The hepatocyte plasma membrane consists of a phospholipid bilayer in which hydrophobic fatty acid tails are oriented to the interior membrane and hydrophilic phospholipid head groups are oriented to the exterior (sinusoidal or cytoplasmic) membrane. Within this phospholipid bilayer, proteins have either structural functions or metabolic functions. The hepatocyte sinusoidal plasma membrane is heavily studded with microvilli to increase the absorptive area in contact with sinusoidal blood. The cell membrane, because of its high lipid content, allows lipid-soluble molecules to enter the cell by means of simple diffusion. Polar molecules must enter cells through membrane transport proteins. Channel proteins allow molecules to diffuse simply into cells without binding, whereas carrier proteins first bind the solute and by means of conformational change allow it to be transported into the cell. The glucose carrier in hepatocytes is an example of carrier-facilitated diffusion. The sinusoidal membrane is studded with receptors, which are large glycoprotein molecules that span the plasma membrane lipid bilayer. A ligand-binding site of this receptor molecule projects into the space of Disse. When appropriate ligand-receptor binding occurs, the entire ligand can be internalized for intracellular degradation or biliary transport. The ligand also can transmit a signal to the interior of the hepatocyte by means of a number of intracellular second-messenger systems, a process known as *signal transduction*. Such second messengers include cyclic adenosine monophosphate, inositol triphosphate, and diacylglycerol. Each of these structurally simple chemicals can amplify cell membrane events and change cellular physiologic processes.

ANSWER: a, b, d

REFERENCE: *Chapter 35—Hepatic Physiology*

CHAPTER 36

HEPATIC INFECTION AND ACUTE HEPATIC FAILURE

1. Which of the following statements is/are true concerning management of pyogenic liver abscess?

   a. Antibiotic therapy alone may be advisable in the care of patients with multiple small abscesses

   b. Percutaneous drainage provides comparable results to surgical drainage in the care of patients with unilocular large abscesses

   c. Sufficient antibiotic coverage for most hepatic abscesses includes coverage for gram-positive aerobic bacteria only

   d. Treatment of patients with a primary biliary origin of hepatic abscess must address underlying biliary pathologic conditions, such as choledocholithiasis or biliary ductal obstruction

COMMENT: The preferred treatment of most patients with hepatic abscess is broad-spectrum antibiotic coverage and drainage. A number of studies have shown for most patients with a large unilocular abscess that percutaneous catheter drainage is as effective as surgical drainage. Bacteria that predominate in pyogenic liver abscesses are gram-negative aerobes, streptococcal species, and anaerobes. Therefore, broad-spectrum antibiotic coverage is necessary. Antibiotic coverage alone may be advisable for occasional patients who have multiple small abscesses not accessible to percutaneous or surgical drainage. Because many of these patients have underlying biliary disease as the source of the hepatic abscess, correcting the underlying condition is important, such as establishing biliary drainage surgically or nonoperatively.

ANSWER: a, b, d

REFERENCE: *Chapter 36—Hepatic Infection and Acute Hepatic Failure: Pyogenic Hepatic Abscess*

2. Which of the following statements is/are true concerning the differential diagnosis of amebic and pyogenic liver abscess?

   a. The clinical presentations often can be clearly differentiated

   b. A history of travel or origin from a high-risk area suggests amebic liver abscess

   c. Results of routine hepatic chemical analysis frequently differentiate pyogenic from amebic liver abscess

   d. Serologic testing for the presence of antibody to *Entamoeba histolytica* is the only specific and sensitive way to confirm the diagnosis of amebic liver abscess

   e. Preoperative differentiation of pyogenic and hepatic abscesses is not important because surgical drainage is imperative for both

COMMENT: Differentiating amebic from pyogenic liver abscess can be a diagnostic challenge. It is important, however, because effective medical therapy with metronidazole can obviate percutaneous or surgical drainage in most cases of amebic abscess. The clinical presentations of the two conditions—acute onset of fever, abdominal pain, and results of liver function tests that show alterations—are almost identical. Important features such as travel to or origin in a high-risk area is particularly important for amebic liver abscess. Routine hepatic chemical analysis and radiographic studies rarely allow differentiation of amebic and pyogenic liver abscesses. Specific serologic tests for the presence of antibody to *E. histolytica* are specific and sensitive for amebic hepatic abscess. The results are positive in 95% of cases and therefore are essential in differentiating the two infections.

ANSWER: b, d

REFERENCE: *Chapter 36—Hepatic Infection and Acute Hepatic Failure: Amebic Hepatic Abscess*

3. Which of the following statements is/are true concerning the diagnosis and management of hydatid cysts?

   a. Percutaneous aspiration is an important aspect of diagnosis and management of hydatid cyst
   b. Computed tomography (CT) often shows the classic findings of a cystic liver lesion with a calcific rim
   c. At operation, care must be taken to protect the operative field from spillage of the cyst fluid
   d. The use of a scolecide has become obsolete with current surgical techniques

COMMENT: Hydatid cysts are most commonly the result of infection with the tapeworm *Echinococcus granulosus*. Results of routine laboratory tests in the care of patients with hydatid cysts are normal or nonspecifically abnormal. Although routine chest or abdominal radiographs may show a mass with a calcific rim, sonography and CT are the favored means of imaging hydatid cysts. The presence of calcifications and daughter cysts within the parent cyst suggests the presence of *Echinococcus* worms. Percutaneous needling of a hydatid cyst is unwise unless precautions against anaphylaxis are undertaken. Cystic fluid often is under pressure, and needling can precipitate rupture with the risk of anaphylaxis or intraperitoneal seating. The classic management of hydatid cysts is operative. The surgical aim is to remove the cyst or cysts without dissemination of the organism. At operation, the cyst is drained of fluid through a cannula after the operative field is carefully protected from fluid leakage. If the aspirate is clear, parasiticidal fluid (ethyl alcohol or 20% sterile saline solution) is injected into the cyst to kill adherent scoleces. The cyst contents and the pericystic wall are removed with careful surgical dissection.

ANSWER: b, c

REFERENCE: *Chapter 36—Hepatic Infection and Acute Hepatic Failure: Hydatid Disease of the Liver*

4. A surgeon is believed to have been exposed to hepatitis B virus by means of needle stick. Which of the following statements is/are true concerning diagnosis and outcome in this case?

   a. Incubation of hepatitis B virus takes approximately 2 weeks
   b. Jaundice is the first serologic indicator of hepatitis B infection
   c. The patient has about a 10% risk of development of a chronic carrier state
   d. All susceptible household or sexual contacts of the surgeon should receive hepatitis B virus vaccine
   e. The surgeon should receive hepatitis B immunoglobulin as soon as possible after the accidental needle stick

COMMENT: Hepatitis B infection is insidious. The incubation period is approximately 8 weeks. The first serum indicator of infection by hepatitis B virus is detection of serum hepatitis B surface antigen (HBsAg), which can precede the onset of jaundice. In most cases, hepatitis B infection is self-limited and does not progress to chronic hepatitis. However, approximately 10% of patients with acute hepatitis B infection, whether it is clinical or subclinical, eventually enter the chronic carrier state. The carrier state is defined by the presence of HBsAg in the serum for longer than 6 months. The best method of management of hepatitis B infection is primary prevention by means of vaccination. All susceptible household or sexual contacts of a person with a positive result of a serum test for HBsAg should be advised to receive a full course of hepatitis B virus vaccine. Passive prophylaxis with hepatitis B immunoglobulin should be provided to any susceptible contact who might have had recent parenteral exposure, such as an accidental needle stick.

ANSWER: c, d, e

REFERENCE: *Chapter 36—Hepatic Infection and Acute Hepatic Failure: Viral Hepatitis*

5. A patient has evidence of hepatitis approximately 8 weeks after receiving blood transfusions during a surgical procedure. Which of the following statements is/are true?

   a. The virus responsible is most likely hepatitis C
   b. Most patients enter the chronic carrier state
   c. There is no role for interferon in the management of chronic hepatitis C infection
   d. Chronic infection with hepatitis C is not associated with increased risk of development of hepatocellular carcinoma

COMMENT: Hepatitis C virus causes more than 90% of cases of posttransfusion hepatitis and most cases of sporadic non-A, non-B hepatitis worldwide. The most common identifiable sources of acquisition of hepatitis C virus are transfusion of blood or blood-derived products or a history of intravenous use of illicit drugs. The usual incubation period of posttransfusion hepatitis C infection is 5 to 10 weeks. Initial elevation of liver enzyme levels can be associated with little or no clinical disturbance. In some patients, acute hepatitis C infection does not progress to chronic infection; however, chronic hepatitis C viral infection develops among as many as 70% of patients with posttransfusion hepatitis C infection; many cases progress to cirrhosis. Hepatitis C does not appear to alter life expectancy, at least in the first 15 years of infection. However, once cirrhosis and end-stage liver disease develop, the clinical syndrome is cannot be differentiated from other forms of chronic liver disease with a predisposition to development of hepatoma. Interferon-α is the only therapy for chronic hepatitis C approved by the U.S. Food and Drug Administration. There is evidence that early administration of interferon in the management of acute hepatitis C infection can reduce the risk of progression to the chronic state. There is no evidence that interferon alters the course of chronic hepatitis C infection or changes the incidence.

ANSWER: a, b

REFERENCE: *Chapter 36—Hepatic Infection and Acute Hepatic Failure*

CHAPTER 37

CIRRHOSIS AND PORTAL HYPERTENSION

1. The most common cause of cirrhosis worldwide is:

   a. Alcoholism
   b. Wilson's disease
   c. Viral hepatitis
   d. Drug toxicity

COMMENT: Viral hepatitis is the most common cause of cirrhosis worldwide, accounting for at least 50% of cases. Hepatitis A, B, C, D, and E have all been proved to cause acute hepatitis characterized histologically by lymphocytic parenchymal and portal inflammation, focal necrosis, ballooning degeneration, cholestasis, Kupffer cell and macrophage hypertrophy and hyperplasia, and lobular disarray. Only hepatitis B, C, and D have been shown to progress to chronic hepatitis defined by persistent liver cell necrosis and inflammation for longer than 6 months.

ANSWER: c

REFERENCE: *Chapter 37—Cirrhosis and Portal Hypertension: Classification Systems*

2. Hemochromatosis is a well-characterized cause of cirrhosis. Appropriate management of liver failure caused by hemochromatosis can include:

   a. Liver transplantation
   b. Phlebotomy
   c. Iron chelation
   d. Restriction of copper intake

COMMENT: Hemochromatosis of the liver is caused by an inborn error of metabolism that causes increased absorption of iron from the gastrointestinal tract. The pathophysiologic mechanism of iron-induced hepatotoxicity is related to lipid peroxidation induced by iron in periportal regions of the liver. Activation of stellate cells by cytokines released by Kupffer cells that have phagocytosed necrotic hepatocytes injured by iron toxicity also contributes. The reaction progresses to bridging fibrosis and eventually to mixed micromacronodular cirrhosis. Treatment includes reduction of iron intake, repeated phlebotomy, and orthotopic liver transplantation.

ANSWER: a, b, c

REFERENCE: *Chapter 37—Cirrhosis and Portal Hypertension: Classification Systems*

3. A previously healthy 30-year-old woman has rapid-onset ascites, abdominal pain, fatigue, and easy bruising. Physical examination reveals ascites and hepatomegaly. Paracentesis shows bloody ascitic fluid. An appropriate next step in management is:

   a. Transjugular intrahepatic portosystemic shunting (TIPS)
   b. Duplex Doppler ultrasonography
   c. Exploratory laparotomy
   d. Intravenous pyelography

COMMENT: Budd-Chiari syndrome is a rare disease caused by mechanical obstruction of the hepatic veins. Obstruction can occur at the level of the terminal hepatic veins, major hepatic veins, or vena cava. It can be caused by obstructing webs or membranes (most commonly in Africa and Asia) or thrombosis due to hypercoagulable states and neoplasms (most common in Western countries). There is a wide range of presentations. Some patients have no symptoms, and others have acute hepatic failure or cirrhosis. This spectrum of symptoms is related to the degree and rate of progression of hepatic outflow obstruction. Classic symptoms include abdominal pain, hepatomegaly, and ascites. The diagnosis can be made with duplex Doppler ultrasonography with a sensitivity of 85% to 95%. Computed tomography is another diagnostic option.

ANSWER: b

REFERENCE: *Chapter 37—Cirrhosis and Portal Hypertension: Classification Systems*

4. A 55-year-old man with a known history of alcoholic cirrhosis falls and sustains a sprained ankle. For pain relief, he self-administers 600 mg ibuprofen 4 times a day. Five days later he has fatigue and notices a marked reduction in urine production. Initial laboratory examination reveals the following: serum creatinine, 2.5 mg/dL; urine sodium, 8 mEq/L; and urine osmolarity, 112 mOsm. The results of urinalysis were otherwise normal. The differential diagnosis should include:

   a. Nephrotic syndrome
   b. Renal calculus
   c. Hepatorenal syndrome
   d. Acute renal failure

COMMENT: Hepatorenal syndrome is a complication of cirrhosis, most often with ascites, characterized by progressive renal failure in the absence of intrinsic renal disease. This syndrome occurs among 10% of hospitalized patients with cirrhosis and ascites. Manifestations of the disease include progressive oliguria with urine outputs of 400 to 800 mL/d, an increasing serum level of creatinine, increased cardiac output, and decreased arterial pressure. The process is highly variable and is associated with marked renal cortical vasoconstriction induced by activity of the renin-angiotensin-aldosterone and sympathetic nervous systems. Hepatorenal syndrome can develop among previously well-compensated patients as a result of infection, use of nonsteroidal inflammatory drugs, variceal hemorrhage, or excessive diuretic use. Differentiation of hepatorenal syndrome from acute renal failure is possible by means of laboratory evaluation of urine and serum samples. However, at laboratory testing, hepatorenal syndrome is almost indistinguishable from prerenal azotemia. Both prerenal azotemia and hepatorenal syndrome are characterized by extremely low sodium concentrations in the urine, high urine osmolality, high urine to plasma creatinine ratios, and normal urinary sediment.

ANSWER: c

REFERENCE: *Chapter 37—Cirrhosis and Portal Hypertension: Manifestations of Cirrhosis*

5. Neurologic signs associated with liver failure include:

    a. Memory loss
    b. Parkinsonian gait disturbances
    c. Asterixis
    d. Convulsions

COMMENT: A range of neurologic symptoms occur among patients with hepatic dysfunction. Subtle deficits include changes in personality, memory loss, alterations in sleep patterns, and minor decreases in intellectual function. Defects may be detectable only with detailed psychometric testing. With progression of disease, asterixis—rapid, repetitive flexion and extension of the wrist in response to sustained extension of the forearm and fingers—can occur. The signs of liver disease usually are evident; they include fetor hepaticus and spider angioma. The combination of asterixis, elevated ammonia levels, and altered mental status in a patient with known liver disease strongly suggests the diagnosis. Electroencephalographic changes are nonspecific and can occur among patients with a variety of other conditions. Common precipitating factors that lead to hepatic encephalopathy include impairment in renal function, variceal hemorrhage, constipation, infection, excessive intake of dietary protein, and drug use, especially of benzodiazepines, and barbiturates.

ANSWER: a, c

REFERENCE: *Chapter 37—Cirrhosis and Portal Hypertension: Hepatic Encephalopathy*

6. A 37-year-old man with a history of chronic pancreatitis has acute upper gastrointestinal hemorrhage. After initial stabilization, he undergoes upper gastrointestinal endoscopy, which reveals esophageal and gastric varices. Two of the gastric varices have signs of recent hemorrhage. Angiographic evaluation reveals a patent portal vein with antegrade flow. Thrombosis is present in the splenic vein. Appropriate treatment includes:

    a. TIPS
    b. End-to-side portacaval shunt
    c. Splenectomy
    d. Side-to-side portosystemic shunt

COMMENT: Splenic venous thrombosis is most often caused by disorders of the pancreas, including acute and chronic pancreatitis, trauma, malignant tumor of the pancreas, and pseudocysts. This association is related to the location of the splenic vein behind and in close association with the pancreas. Other causes include retroperitoneal mass, abscess, inflammatory bowel disease, and idiopathic factors. Gastric varices are present in approximately 80% of patients, and esophageal varices are present in 30% to 40%. Isolated "sinistral," or left-sided, portal hypertension occurs in the setting of normal liver function. Patients are readily cured with splenectomy, although observation is acceptable if the patient does not have symptoms. The main indication for splenectomy is variceal hemorrhage.

ANSWER: c

REFERENCE: *Chapter 37—Cirrhosis and Portal Hypertension: Portal Hypertension*

7. Complications of TIPS include:

    a. Accelerated liver failure
    b. Hepatic encephalopathy
    c. Stenosis
    d. Duodenal ulceration

COMMENT: The therapeutic goal of TIPS is to reduce the hepatic vein-portal pressure gradient to less than 12 mm Hg. Transjugular intrahepatic portosystemic shunting decreases the portosystemic pressure gradient to a mean of approximately 9 to 15 mm Hg (average, 10 mm Hg) or 40% to 62% from baseline. Mortality rates are high (40% to 60% at 6 to 7 weeks) despite the relative lack of invasiveness of the procedure. The high mortality reflects the gravity of the clinical condition of most patients who need this intervention. One cause of high mortality is delay in instituting TIPS as a form of therapy after numerous unsuccessful attempts at sclerotherapy or banding. This delay allows deterioration of hepatic function and overall stability. As with all portosystemic shunts, a complication of TIPS is development of hepatic encephalopathy. After placement of a shunt, the incidence of hepatic encephalopathy increases from 10% before treatment to 25%, and there is an approximately 3% to 5% incidence of progression to accelerated liver failure. As many as 50% to 60% of patients later have stenosis or occlusion of the stent.

ANSWER: a, b, c

REFERENCE: *Chapter 37—Cirrhosis and Portal Hypertension: Surgical Intervention*

8. A 25-year-old woman who is currently on the waiting list for a liver transplant develops fever, abdominal pain, and confusion. Physical examination reveals a temperature of 101.4°F (38.6°C), diffuse abdominal pain, and increased ascites. Appropriate management includes which of the following as the next step?

    a. Paracentesis
    b. Exploratory laparotomy
    c. Barium enema
    d. Esophagogastroduodenoscopy

COMMENT: Spontaneous bacterial peritonitis is a possibly lethal complication of portal hypertension with ascites that occurs among as many as 10% of patients. The cause of spontaneous bacterial peritonitis is unknown. Antecedent gastrointestinal hemorrhage is common, and spontaneous bacterial peritonitis in this setting may be related to bacterial translocation from the intestine. Patients often have abdominal pain and fever, but 10% to 20% of cases of spontaneous bacterial peritonitis are discovered at routine paracentesis. Patients can have other signs not clearly related to spontaneous bacterial peritonitis, such as worsening encephalopathy and renal function. The diagnosis is easily made by means of examination of ascitic fluid obtained at paracentesis. An elevation in the number of white blood cells (more than 250 cells/μL) confirms the diagnosis. Most cases of spontaneous bacterial peritonitis are caused by a single organism, most commonly gram-negative enteric bacteria. Hematogenous spread can cause infection with *Streptococcus pneumoniae*. If more than one organism is present, the diagnosis of spontaneous bacterial peritonitis must be questioned, and a search for intraabdominal disease (secondary peritonitis), such as a perforated viscus or diverticulitis, should be performed.

ANSWER: a

REFERENCE: *Chapter 37—Cirrhosis and Portal Hypertension: Prevention of Recurrent Variceal Bleeding*

CHAPTER 38

HEPATIC NEOPLASMS

1. Hepatic hemangioma often is detected incidentally during investigations of upper abdominal symptoms. The finding(s) at helical contrast computed tomography (CT) most consistent with hemangioma include(s):

   a. Peripheral contrast enhancement
   b. Association with biliary ductal dilatation
   c. Water-density cyst formation
   d. Hypovascular mass

COMMENT: In the diagnosis of hemangioma, CT is useful if intravenous (IV) contrast material is administered. On noncontrast CT scans, a hypodense well-demarcated lesion is seen most often. After administration of contrast material, there is a peripheral zone of enhancement with a corrugated inner margin. The center of the lesion is hypodense, and the size remains constant throughout the study. These are classic findings of hemangioma on CT scans. At CT, however, hemangioma is consistently misinterpreted as another histologic feature if the lesion fills in during administration of contrast material, and peripheral enhancement is missed. Hemangioma also can be misinterpreted if adequate images are not obtained before and after administration of contrast material. After administration of contrast medium, the characteristic vascular pattern often is obscured if the lesion is smaller than 2 cm in diameter. Hyalinized lesions do not become enhanced and are misinterpreted at CT. Hemangioma also can be confused with other lesions, such as hypervascular metastasis or even focal fatty infiltration.

Dynamic or spiral CT is the preferred examination because it is the most accurate screening test available. The sensitivity is 75% to 80%, and the specificity is 80% to 88%. Magnetic resonance imaging (MRI) also can be used in the diagnosis of hemangioma. On T1 images, a clear-cut mass typically is present. On T2 images that are isodense to hyperintense, use of gadolinium (FLASH sequence) improves detection of lesions. There usually is peripheral rim enhancement with or without lesion enhancement. The accuracy of MRI (approximately 90%) is equal to or better than that of CT, but MRI is more expensive. The overall sensitivity of MRI is 80%, and the specificity is 99%.

ANSWER: a

REFERENCE: *Chapter 38—Hepatic Neoplasms*

2. A 35-year-old woman undergoes upper abdominal ultrasonography for evaluation of biliary colic. The ultrasound scans depict cholelithiasis and a 4-cm lesion in the left lobe of the liver. Findings at upper abdominal CT performed to evaluate the liver lesion suggest hemangioma. Appropriate management of the liver lesion includes:

   a. Left hepatic lobectomy
   b. Selective embolization of the left hepatic artery
   c. Cryoablation of the lesion
   d. No treatment

COMMENT: The clinical course of hemangioma is benign. Several large studies have shown that the size of most lesions does not change over 5 to 10 years. One study showed that approximately 10% of lesions followed for 3 years enlarged, and 12% of patients had new lesions. Most surgeons agree that patients with asymptomatic lesions less than 4 cm in diameter and fewer than three lesions should be discharged from follow-up care. Patients with asymptomatic lesions 4 to 7 cm in diameter or more than three lesions need periodic imaging studies. Resection is indicated only for patients with no symptoms, as in cases of intratumoral bleeding, or when diagnosis is uncertain. Few surgeons would recommend resection based solely on the size of lesions.

ANSWER: d

REFERENCE: *Chapter 38—Hepatic Neoplasms: Hepatic Hemangioma*

3. A 45-year-old man has a 1-year history of right upper abdominal pressure and mild early satiety. Upper abdominal CT shows a single 8- by 10-cm cystic lesion confined to the right lobe of the liver. Ultrasound examination of the cyst shows no internal echoes. Appropriate management includes:

   a. Percutaneous aspiration of the cyst
   b. Laparoscopic unroofing of the cyst
   c. Right hepatic lobectomy
   d. Cryoablation of the cyst

COMMENT: The management of hepatic cysts is straightforward. Cysts should be followed without intervention if they are asymptomatic. If hepatic cysts are symptomatic because of mass effects, they should be operatively marsupialized by means of open or laparoscopic techniques. Needle aspiration of hepatic cysts should not be performed because the cyst inevitably recurs. Needle aspiration is associated with serious complications, including infection of the cyst or perforation of a small vessel or bile duct, which causes hemorrhage or conversion of the cyst to biloma.

ANSWER: b

REFERENCE: *Chapter 38—Hepatic Neoplasms: Simple Cysts*

4. Risk factors for development of hepatocellular carcinoma include:

   a. Hepatitis C infection
   b. Hepatitis B infection
   c. Alcoholic cirrhosis
   d. Hemochromatosis

COMMENT: Hepatocellular carcinoma typically arises in livers that have been subjected to chronic stimulation and regeneration, usually because of exposure to environmental or biologic toxins that cause hepatocellular death, chronic regeneration, and cirrhosis. The most common causes are exposure to hepatitis B virus, hepatitis C virus, or hepatotoxins, notably aflatoxin B_1 (the mycotoxin of the fungus *Aspergillus flavus*), and ethanol ingestion. Hepatocellular carcinoma worldwide disproportionately affects Asians and Africans because of the high prevalence of hepatitis B and hepatitis C infection. Other diseases that cause cirrhosis can predispose to the development of hepatocellular carcinoma. These include hemochromatosis, type I glycogen storage disease, α_1-antitrypsin deficiency, tyrosinemia, use of androgenic steroids, and primary biliary cirrhosis. Dietary carcinogens include cycasin from the cycad nut.

ANSWER: a, b, c, d

REFERENCE: *Chapter 38—Hepatic Neoplasms: Angiosarcoma*

5. A 62-year-old man with known posthepatitic cirrhosis has ascites and anorexia. Investigation includes measurement of serum α-fetoprotein level; serum levels are 7 times the upper limit of normal. The most likely diagnosis and most appropriate diagnostic modality are:

a. Metastatic colon cancer and colonoscopy
b. Hepatocellular carcinoma and abdominal CT
c. Budd Chiari syndrome and hepatic venogram
d. Alcoholic hepatitis and liver biopsy

COMMENT: Diagnostic tests for hepatocellular carcinoma include spiral CT, MRI, or both. It is difficult with either of these modalities to completely differentiate hepatocellular carcinoma from adenoma and other malignant tumors of the liver. At contrast CT, lesions can appear hypointense, isointense, or mildly intense. The lesions can have calcification with thrombus in the portal or hepatic veins. After administration of gadolinium contrast material, the lesions also appear hypointense, isointense, or hyperintense. Elevation in the level of the tumor marker α-fetoprotein is highly specific and occurs among approximately 50% of patients.

ANSWER: b

REFERENCE: *Chapter 38—Hepatic Neoplasms: Angiosarcoma*

6. Patients with colorectal cancer metastatic to the liver and without evidence of extrahepatic disease are candidates for resection of the metastatic lesion. For patients undergoing such therapy, the expected 5-year survival rate approximates:

a. 10%
b. 20%
c. 50%
d. 75%

COMMENT: The most widely accepted use of hepatic metastasectomy is in the treatment of patients with colorectal cancer. In one of the largest early series of hepatic resection for metastatic cancer, investigators found a close relation between the number of lesions and the timing and relation of diagnosis of metastatic disease to the management of the primary tumor and prognosis. Patients with synchronous lesions did less well than did patients with metachronous lesions. Patients with multiple tumors had poorer survival rates than those with single lesions. This work indicated the need for a 1-cm margin around the tumor to achieve 20% to 30% long-term, disease-free survival. The results of this study, confirmed by many other investigators, also indicated that approximately 20% of patients would have only hepatic disease and no systemic disease remaining. Hepatic resection in the treatment of these patients can represent curative therapy. Approximately 150,000 cases of colon cancer occur each year in the United States; 60,000 patients eventually have hepatic metastasis. These patients are the group to be evaluated for resectional therapy.

ANSWER: b

REFERENCE: *Chapter 38—Hepatic Neoplasms: Metastatic Disease*

Section G

GALLBLADDER AND BILIARY TRACT

CHAPTER 39

BILIARY ANATOMY AND PHYSIOLOGY

1. Which of the following statements is/are true concerning the embryology of the biliary tree?
   a. The primordial anlagen of the liver and biliary tract arises from the entoderm
   b. Superior and inferior caudal buds form as the hepatic diverticulum develops
   c. The development of the liver is a separate process from that of the gallbladder and distal biliary tree
   d. The biliary tree develops in association with the dorsal pancreas

COMMENT: The primordial anlagen of the liver, extrahepatic bile ducts, gallbladder, and ventral part of the pancreas develop as a thickened area of entoderm on the ventral surface of the caudal portion of the foregut where it joins the midgut. Superior and inferior caudal buds form as the hepatic diverticulum grows out into the ventral mesogastrium. The solid mass of endodermal cells spreading with this cephalic bud forms the right and left lobes of the liver. The superior growth of the cranial portion of the hepatic diverticulum, which extends from the duodenum to the liver, results in the formation of the hepatic, common hepatic, and common bile ducts. The caudal portion of the hepatic diverticulum develops into the gallbladder and cystic duct. The common bile duct is attached to the ventral aspects of the duodenum and is in close contact with the ventral pancreatic bud.

ANSWER: a, b

REFERENCE: *Chapter 39—Biliary Anatomy and Physiology: Embryology*

2. Which of the following statements is/are true concerning the anatomy of the gallbladder?
   a. The gallbladder lies among the right, left, and quadrate hepatic lobes or hepatic segments IV and V
   b. The cystic duct contains the spiral valve of Heister, which serves an important valvular function for the gallbladder
   c. The cystic artery arises from the right hepatic artery in 95% of persons
   d. The cystic artery crosses anterior to the hepatic duct in most instances

COMMENT: The gallbladder is a pear-shaped organ bound to a fossa on the right inferior surface of the liver located among the right, left, and quadrate hepatic lobes, or hepatic segments IV and V. The gallbladder can be divided into four areas—the fundus, body, infundibulum, and neck. The body of the gallbladder extends from the fundus into the tapered portion, or neck, which curves backward and upward toward the transverse fissure of the liver and terminates in the cystic duct. The cystic duct lumen contains a thin mucosal septum, the spiral valve of Heister. The valve can make catheterization to the cystic duct difficult but does not have true valvular function. The arteries of the gallbladder are derived from the cystic branch of the hepatic artery, which in 95% of cases originates from the right hepatic artery. From its origin, the cystic artery usually crosses behind the hepatic duct (84% of cases) but is sometimes anterior to that structure. The cystic artery proceeds to the neck of the gallbladder, where it splits into anterior and posterior divisions that supply the corresponding areas of the gallbladder. The cystic veins empty into the right branch of the portal vein indirectly into the liver.

ANSWER: a, c

REFERENCE: *Chapter 39—Biliary Anatomy and Physiology: Anatomy*

3. Understanding the anatomy of the extrahepatic biliary tree is essential in performing biliary tract surgery. Which of the following statements is/are true concerning biliary ductal anatomy?

a. Most patients have the "classic" anatomic description
b. The common hepatic duct unites with the cystic duct to form the common bile duct
c. An accessory right hepatic duct is present in 5% of patients
d. A common channel or "Y" configuration of the distal bile duct and pancreatic ducts occurs in approximately 70% of persons

COMMENT: The classic anatomic description of the extrahepatic bile ducts and their arteries is present in only one third of persons. The left hepatic duct usually has a longer extrahepatic course than does the right hepatic duct. The common hepatic duct is formed by the union of the right and left hepatic ducts close to the emergence from the liver. The duct passes downward in the superior portion of the hepatoduodenal ligament and lies in front of the portal vein and to the right of the hepatic artery. The common hepatic duct unites with the cystic duct to form the common bile duct. An accessory right hepatic duct is present in 5% of cases. The cystic duct passes downward, backward, and to the left in the hepatoduodenal ligament and usually unites with the main hepatic duct at an acute angle. Its course and mode of insertion into the common duct are highly variable. The common bile duct is formed by the union of the common hepatic and cystic ducts and usually is approximately 7 to 9 cm long. The junction of the distal common bile duct and pancreatic duct at the ampulla can take one of three configurations. In approximately 70% of patients, there is a common channel of the bile and pancreatic ducts, thus a "Y" configuration. In approximately 20%, the common channel is nonexistent, and in another 10%, the two ducts enter the duodenum through separate openings.

ANSWER: b, c, d

REFERENCE: *Chapter 39—Biliary Anatomy and Physiology: Anatomy*

4. Which of the following statements is/are true concerning the relation between the biliary tree and the hepatic artery and portal vein.

a. The common hepatic and common bile duct lie immediately anterior to the portal vein
b. The cystic artery, which usually arises from the right hepatic artery, crosses behind the hepatic duct in most cases
c. A replaced right hepatic artery arising from the superior mesenteric artery system runs to the right of the common bile duct
d. The arterial supply of the extrahepatic biliary ducts is derived from major trunks running along the medial and lateral walls of the common duct at the 3 o'clock and 9 o'clock positions

COMMENT: The common hepatic duct passes downward in the superior and lateral portions of the hepatoduodenal ligament and lies in front of the portal vein and to the right of the hepatic artery. The cystic artery, which in most cases arises from the right hepatic artery, usually crosses behind the hepatic duct (84% of cases) but is sometimes anterior to that structure (16% of cases). The arterial supply of the liver has a number of anatomic variations. In patients in whom the right hepatic artery arises from the superior mesenteric artery system, the "replaced" right hepatic artery usually runs to the right of the bile duct and portal vein. The arteries to the extrahepatic biliary ducts anastomose freely within the duct walls. The ductal arterial supply is derived primarily from the gastroduodenal and right hepatic arteries. Major trunks run along the medial and lateral walls of the common duct at the 3 o'clock and 9 o'clock positions.

ANSWER: a, b, c, d

REFERENCE: *Chapter 39—Biliary Anatomy and Physiology: Anatomy*

5. Which of the following statements is/are true concerning biliary motor function?

   a. The contracted sphincter of Oddi impairs bile flow into the duodenum and directs it into the gallbladder
   b. In the postprandial state, approximately 70% of hepatic bile flows into the gallbladder before reaching the duodenum
   c. During the interdigestive period, only a small fraction of gallbladder bile enters the duodenum
   d. Gallbladder emptying during fasting is associated with phase III of the interdigestive migrating motor complex
   e. After a meal, the gallbladder empties by means of steady tonic contraction thought to be due to release of endogenous motilin from the mucosa of the small intestine

COMMENT: As bile is secreted from the liver, it flows through the hepatic ducts into the common hepatic duct and continues through the common bile duct into the duodenum. With an intact and contracted sphincter of Oddi, bile flows directly into the gallbladder, where it is concentrated and stored. In the postprandial state, approximately 70% of hepatic bile flows into the gallbladder before reaching the duodenum and entering the enterohepatic cycle. During the interdigestive phase, 90% of bile from the liver enters the gallbladder, whereas only a small fraction of gallbladder bile enters the duodenum. Gallbladder emptying during fasting is associated with phase II of the interdigestive migrating motor complex. Motilin may account for this stimulatory effect because plasma elevations of motilin seem to correlate with the onset of phase II waves. After a meal, the gallbladder empties by means of steady tonic contraction thought to be caused by release of endogenous cholecystokinin (CCK) from the mucosa of the small intestine.

ANSWER: a, b, c

REFERENCE: *Chapter 39—Biliary Anatomy and Physiology: Physiology*

6. Abnormalities of the sphincter of Oddi have been recently recognized to cause symptoms referable to the biliary tree or pancreas. Which of the following statements is/are true concerning sphincter of Oddi motor function?

   a. The basal resting pressure of the sphincter is 10 to 15 mm Hg greater than duodenal pressure
   b. Contraction of the sphincter occurs with CCK stimulation
   c. Vagal stimulation relaxes the sphincter
   d. Manometry of the sphincter of Oddi can be performed at endoscopic retrograde cholangiopancreatography to characterize basal pressure, amplitude, frequency of contraction, and direction of propagation of contractile waves
   e. Stenosis of the sphincter of Oddi is characterized by abnormally elevated basal pressure during sphincter of Oddi manometric evaluation

COMMENT: The sphincter of Oddi is approximately 4 to 6 mm long. The basal resting pressure is approximately 13 mm Hg greater than duodenal pressure. The sphincter exhibits phasic contractions at a frequency of four per minute and a duration of 8 seconds. Regulation of bile flow is controlled primarily by the sphincter and not by the surrounding smooth muscle of the duodenum. Relaxation of the sphincter occurs with CCK stimulation. The result is diminished amplitude of phasic contractions and reduced basal pressure. This allows increased passive flow of bile into the duodenum. Parasympathetic stimulation also causes intermittent relaxation of the sphincter, and sympathetic splanchnic stimulation increases pressure. Abnormalities of the sphincter of Oddi can cause symptoms referable to the biliary tree or pancreas. Manometry of the sphincter of Oddi may be performed at endoscopic retrograde cholangiopancreatography to characterize the basal pressure of the sphincter, the amplitude and frequency of contractions, and the direction of propagation of contractile waves. Stenosis of the sphincter of Oddi is characterized by abnormally elevated basal pressure (more than 39 mm Hg), whereas dyskinesia is characterized by abnormalities of other manometric values.

ANSWER: a, c, d, e

REFERENCE: *Chapter 39—Biliary Anatomy and Physiology: Physiology*

7. A 35-year-old woman has typical symptoms of biliary colic; however, sonography shows no gallstones. Which of the following statements is/are true concerning her diagnosis?

a. Chronic acalculous cholecystitis or gallbladder dyskinesia is seldom associated with classic symptoms of biliary colic

b. The most specific test for diagnosing gallbladder dyskinesia is CCK-enhanced cholescintigraphy with assessment of gallbladder ejection fraction

c. An ejection fraction greater than 75% is considered abnormal and indicative of gallbladder dyskinesia

d. Cholecystectomy is not indicated for chronic acalculous cholecystitis

COMMENT: Motility abnormalities of the gallbladder and cystic duct manifest as symptoms of gallstones. The most common presentation among patients with gallbladder motility disorders such as chronic acalculous cholecystitis or gallbladder dyskinesia is recurrent biliary type pain. The most specific test for diagnosing gallbladder dyskinesia is CCK-enhanced cholescintigraphy with assessment of gallbladder ejection fraction. Cholecystokinin is infused intravenously 15 to 30 minutes after ejection of an analogue of ^{99m}Tc-imminodiacetic acid and calculating the ejection fraction of the isotope by the contracting gallbladder. An ejection fraction less than 35% is considered abnormal, and cholecystectomy may be indicated. Most patients have relief of symptoms after cholecystectomy.

ANSWER: b

REFERENCE: *Chapter 39—Biliary Anatomy and Physiology: Physiology*

8. The gallbladder plays an important role in altering bile composition by means of absorption and secretion. Which of the following statements is/are true concerning this mucosal function?

a. Absorption of water by the gallbladder can result in twofold to tenfold concentration of the solute components of bile

b. Gallbladder mucosal absorption can occur by both active and passive mechanisms

c. Cyclic adenosine monophosphate stimulates sodium chloride-coupled transport and can influence tight junction permeability

d. Secretory products of the gallbladder include bicarbonate and glycoproteins

COMMENT: The gallbladder rapidly absorbs water and solutes from bile and concentrates the solute components twofold to tenfold. The gallbladder has an active mucosa and can absorb water and solutes against considerable concentration gradients. Water absorption is linked to the transport of ions. The two major mechanisms of absorption are active and passive. In passive absorption, sodium and chloride enter the gallbladder epithelial cells because of electrochemical gradients. This results in an osmotic gradient, and water flows into the cell. Intracellular sodium is extruded across the basolateral membrane into the lateral intercellular spaces by means of active transport. The active transport of sodium against an electrochemical gradient is associated with a Na$^+$-K$^+$-ATPase pump. Cyclic adenosine monophosphate may inhibit sodium chloride-coupled transport and may influence tight junction permeability. Other peptides, such as secretin, glucagon, and gastric inhibitory peptide, have been shown to inhibit absorption. Secretion by the gallbladder occurs by means of inhibition of net ion and fluid absorption or by means of stimulation of bicarbonate secretory mechanisms. Gallbladder epithelium also may secrete mucin and nonmucin glycoproteins, which may play a role in gallstone formation.

ANSWER: a, b, d

REFERENCE: *Chapter 39—Biliary Anatomy and Physiology: Physiology*

9. Which of the following statements is/are true with regard to biliary anatomy?

    a. The gallbladder is on the inferior surface of the liver at the junction of the right and left lobes
    b. The cystic artery most commonly arises from the proper hepatic artery
    c. The cystic artery is in the hepatocystic triangle
    d. The common bile duct is formed by the junction of the right and left hepatic ducts

COMMENT: The gallbladder lies in the anatomic plain that divides the right and left lobes of the liver. The cystic artery arises from the right hepatic artery and travels through the hepatocystic triangle. The common bile duct is formed by the junction of the common hepatic duct and cystic duct. The junction of the right and left ducts is the common hepatic duct.

ANSWER: a, c

REFERENCE: *Chapter 39—Biliary Anatomy and Physiology: Anatomy*

10. Which of the following statements correctly describe(s) the anatomy of the hepatoduodenal ligament?

    a. The hepatic artery is medial to the common bile duct
    b. The portal vein is lateral to the common bile duct
    c. The anatomic relation of the hepatic artery and common bile duct is constant
    d. The common bile duct receives its blood supply from the biliary branch of the hepatic artery

COMMENT: The hepatic artery is medial to the common bile duct and anterior to the portal vein. Hepatic artery anatomy is highly variable, as is the relation of the artery to the common bile duct. The blood supply to the common bile duct is a plexus derived from multiple sources, including the hepatic artery, gastroduodenal artery, and cystic artery, but there is no named biliary artery.

ANSWER: a

REFERENCE: *Chapter 39—Biliary Anatomy and Physiology: Anatomy*

11. Bile is composed of which of the following?

    a. Bile acids
    b. Bilirubin
    c. Cholesterol
    d. Protein
    e. Inorganic electrolytes

COMMENT: All of these substances are components of bile.

ANSWER: a, b, c, d, e

REFERENCE: *Chapter 39—Biliary Anatomy and Physiology: Physiology*

12. Which of the following statements is/are true regarding bile secretion?

    a. Bilirubin is the principal component of bile
    b. Bile acids are conjugated in the small intestine
    c. 75% of bile is secreted by the bile ducts
    d. Vasoactive intestinal peptide and secretin act on the bile ducts to increase bile secretion

COMMENT: Bile acids are the principal organic solute in bile and are conjugated in hepatocytes. Hepatocytes are responsible for 75% of bile secretion. Vasoactive intestinal peptide and secretin regulate bile duct secretion.

ANSWER: d

REFERENCE: *Chapter 39—Biliary Anatomy and Physiology: Physiology*

13. Which of the following statements is/are true regarding the sphincter of Oddi?

    a. The sphincter of Oddi relaxes during phase III of the interdigestive state
    b. Function of the sphincter of Oddi depends on duodenal contractions
    c. The sphincter of Oddi exhibits reflex relaxation with gallbladder distention
    d. The sphincter of Oddi is inhibited by CCK

COMMENT: The sphincter of Oddi exhibits basal and phasic contractions during phase III of the interdigestive state and is independent of duodenal contractions. The sphincter of Oddi is inhibited by gallbladder distention and CCK.

ANSWER: c, d

REFERENCE: *Chapter 39—Biliary Anatomy and Physiology: Dysmotility Syndromes*

14. Which of the following statements is/are correct regarding gallbladder dyskinesia?
    a. 25% of patients with biliary colic do not have gallstones on ultrasound examinations
    b. Normal gallbladder ejection fraction in response to CCK is 75%
    c. Cholecystectomy relieves biliary symptoms for all patients without gallstones
    d. Provocative CCK infusion is a quantitative test to evaluate gallbladder motility

COMMENT: Only 5% of patients with classic biliary symptoms do not have gallstones at examination. Some of these patients have symptoms related to gallbladder dysmotility. Cholecystokinin-HIDA is a quantitative test to measure gallbladder ejection fraction in response to CCK. A normal ejection fraction is 75%, and patients with a low ejection fraction (less than 39%) may respond to cholecystectomy.

ANSWER: b

REFERENCE: *Chapter 39—Biliary Anatomy and Physiology: Dysmotility Syndromes*

CHAPTER 40

CALCULOUS BILIARY DISEASE

1. Which of the following statements is/are true concerning types of gallstones and their risk factors?
    a. Cholesterol gallstones are seen in higher frequency in Asian countries.
    b. Black pigment stones are associated with bile stasis such as seen in conditions such as biliary strictures.
    c. Brown pigment stones frequently are seen in patients with hemolytic disorders.
    d. Cholesterol gallstones are more common in women, especially those who have had multiple pregnancies.

COMMENT: Cholesterol gallstones account for 85% of all stones in Western Industrialized countries. Their prevalence increases with age. In certain populations, such as American Indians, the incidence is extremely high especially in women. In Chileans and Bolvarians of Indian ancestry, the incidence of gallstones is also very high. Cholesterol gallstones are more common in women, especially those who have had multiple pregnancies, in the woman who is taking birth control pills, in the obese, in patients undergoing rapid weight loss, and in some persons with hypolipidemia. Cholesterol gallstones are common in populations consuming a Western diet, which is relatively high in animal fat. Black pigment stones account for 10% to 15% of stones in Western industrialized countries but are at a much higher percentage of stones in Asian countries, such as Japan. Black stones are common in hemolytic disorders such as hereditary spherocytosis and sickle cell anemia. Brown stones are uncommon in Western Industrialized countries and account for only a small percentage of stones. In these countries, the bile stasis that causes brown stones to form is usually secondary to biliary strictures or to the passage of cholesterol or black stones into the bile ducts. Brown stones are more common in geographic regions, such as Southeast Asia, where biliary parasites are endemic.

ANSWER: d

REFERENCE: *Chapter 40—Calculous Biliary Disease: Incidence and Risk Factors*

2. Which of the following statement is/are true concerning solubilization and transport of cholesterol in bile?

a. Cholesterol is secreted into bile as cholesterol-phospholipid vesicles.

b. A concentration of cholesterol in excess of its solubility results in formation of solid cholesterol monohydrate crystals.

c. The combination of phospholipid and cholesterol monomers incorporated with a bile salt leads to formation of a mixed micelle.

d. A cholesterol saturation index above 1.0 is considered supersaturated and cholesterol crystals will form.

COMMENT: Hepatic cholesterol is derived either from preformed cholesterol taken up from the serum by hepatocytes or is synthesized by hepatocytes. Cholesterol is secreted into bile as cholesterol-phospholipid vesicles. Cholesterol exists in bile in various phases. The phases of cholesterol are the monomeric phase, the micellar phase, the vesicular phase and solid cholesterol crystals. The vesicular and crystalline phases are referred to as solid phases, the monomers and micelles being the soluble phases. Movement of cholesterol occurs between phases as governed by energetics. Phospholipid and cholesterol monomers are incorporated into simple bile salt micelles to create mixed micelles. The presence of phospholipid in mixed micelles greatly increases their capacity to incorporate cholesterol. If micelles or vesicles become supersaturated with cholesterol, cholesterol may move out to form cholesterol crystals. This process continues until a state of equilibrium is reached. Equilibrium is the final state of a physical-chemical system, a condition in which all acting influences are cancelled by others so that a stable, unchanging system results. Whether bile is supersaturated with cholesterol can be determined by measuring the concentration of lipids in bile and plotting its relative composition on the phase diagram. A cumbersome mathematical index has been described, the cholesterol saturation index. If bile has a cholesterol saturation index above 1.0, it is supersaturated with cholesterol and will contain cholesterol crystals when it reaches it reaches equilibrium. Bile not in a state of equilibrium may be supersaturated with cholesterol yet not contain cholesterol crystals.

ANSWER: a, b, c

REFERENCE: *Chapter 40—Calculous Biliary Disease: Pathogenesis*

3. A number of risk factors for gallstone disease affect cholesterol saturation. Which of the following statements is/are true concerning the relationship of cholesterol super-saturation and risk factors?

a. During the last two trimesters of pregnancy, cholesterol secretion into bile decreases relative to bile salt and phospholipids secretion.

b. Cholesterol gallstones are common in vegetarians.

c. During rapid weight loss, cholesterol secretion of the bile is decreased.

d. Supersaturation of bile increases with age because cholesterol secretion increases.

COMMENT: Supersaturation of bile is almost always caused by cholesterol hypersecretion rather than by a reduced secretion of phospholipid or bile salts. Multiple mechanisms produce cholesterol hypersecretion, and many of these are related to known risk factors for cholesterol gallstone formation. Supersaturation of bile increases with age because cholesterol secretion increases. Cholesterol synthesis increases with increasing weight. In addition, rapid weight loss in the obese patient also contributes to gallstone formation because during rapid weight loss, the secretion of cholesterol in the bile is sharply increased. Altered gallbladder motility and accelerated crystalization rates may also contribute to gallstone formation during rapid weight loss. Estrogen promotes the secretion of cholesterol into bile. During the last two trimesters of pregnancy, cholesterol secretion to bile increases relative to bile salt and phospholipid secretion, with the result that cholesterol saturation index rises. In pregnant women and in those taking contraceptive steroids, the rate of gallbladder emptying is also reduced and the gastrointestinal transit time is prolonged. The relationship between diet and gallstones is complex. Cholesterol gallstones do not form in vegetarians. Cholesterol gallstones are common in populations that consume a Western diet, which is relatively high in animal fat.

ANSWER: d

REFERENCE: *Chapter 40—Calculous Biliary Disease: Pathogenesis*

4. Which of the following statements is/are true concerning the pathogenesis of pigment gallstones?

    a. Black pigment stones contain three calcium salts, calcium bilirubinate, calcium carbonate, and calcium phosphate.

    b. Stasis of bile contributes to the formation of brown but not black pigment stones.

    c. The bacterial enzyme, beta-glucuronidase contributes to the formation of brown pigment stones.

    d. Foreign bodies in bile may contribute to the formation of brown pigment stones.

COMMENT: Black pigment stones contain three calcium salts—calcium bilirubinate as a polymer, calcium carbonate, and calcium phosphate. The factors governing the solubility of calcium salts in bile are complex. Congenital or acquired hemolytic states result in excessive levels of conjugated bilirubin in bile, which increases the rate of production of unconjugated bilirubin. Stasis of bile within the gallbladder has also been implicated as an important etiologic factor in the pathogenesis of black pigment stones. This is underscored by the finding that calcium bilirubin stones tend to form in patients on total parental nutrition, a clinical setting characterized by gallbladder stasis. When a foreign body such as a parasite or stone lodges in the bile duct, bile stasis and bacterial contamination follow. The same happens in the presence of a biliary stricture. Bile is normally sterile and it is maintained in this state by the mechanical action of bile flow in addition to some of the constituents of bile, such as immunoglobulin A and perhaps bile salts. Once bacterial contamination occurs, organisms such as Escherichia coli secrete a beta-glucuronidase that enzymatically cleaves bilirubin glucuronide to produce insoluble, unconjugated bilirubin. This substance precipitates and, along with dead bacterial cell bodies, produces a thick sludge that forms soft brown stones throughout the biliary tree and gallbladder.

ANSWER: a, c, d

REFERENCE: *Chapter 40—Calculous Biliary Disease: Pathogenesis*

5. Which of the following statements is/are true concerning the natural history of gallstones?

    a. Most patients with gallstones are symptomatic.

    b. About 10% of asymptomatic patients annually become symptomatic per year.

    c. Complicated gallstone disease develops in about 5% of symptomatic patients per year.

    d. About 25% of patients with complicated gallstone disease have had no prior symptoms.

COMMENT: When gallstones first form, they are asymptomatic, and most patients remain in this clinical stage throughout life. The pool of asymptomatic patients is huge, about 20 million in the United States, because the disease is so common. Annually, about 3% of asymptomatic patients or about 600,000 people, become symptomatic (i.e., biliary colic develops). Symptomatic patients tend to have recurring bouts of biliary colic. Complicated gallstone disease develops in 3% to 5% of symptomatic patients per year. It is unusual (less than 0.5% annually) for complicated gallstone disease to develop in an asymptomatic person who has not previously had an interval of symptomatic disease without complications.

ANSWER: c

REFERENCE: *Chapter 40—Calculous Biliary Disease: Natural History of Gallstones*

6. Which of the following statements is/are true concerning asymptomatic gallstones?

a. Gallbladder cancer forms only in association with gallstones, therefore prophylactic cholecystectomy should be performed routinely.

b. Between 20% and 30% of patients with asymptomatic gallstones will become symptomatic within 20 years.

c. Diabetic patients have an aggressive natural history for gallstones and therefore cholecystectomy should be performed routinely when gallstones are detected.

d. A porcelain gallbladder is an absolute indication for cholecystectomy.

COMMENT: The diagnosis of asymptomatic gallstones is incidental, as screening is not performed or indicated for this disease. Several studies have followed asymptomatic patients for many years. Between 20% and 30% of patients become symptomatic within 20 years. In very few patients do complications develop prior without symptoms, so prophylactic cholecystectomy is not indicated to prevent sudden, unexpected complications in persons with asymptomatic stones. Gallbladder cancer occurs only in association with gallstones, but it is so uncommon in the United States that the screening programs and prophylactic cholecystectomy are not indicated. Diabetic patients with asymptomatic gallstones have the same natural history as other persons in that symptoms appear, presenting a window of opportunity for treatment, before complications develop. Cholecystectomy during the asymptomatic stage is indicated in a few uncommon situations. Porcelain gallbladder, a rare pre-malignant condition in which the wall of the gallbladder becomes calcified, is an absolute indication for cholecystectomy. Malignant transformation occurs in about 25% of untreated patients. The calcification of gallstones is not associated with cancer risk.

ANSWER: b, d

REFERENCE: *Chapter 40—Calculous Biliary Disease: Asymptomatic Gallstones*

7. The chief symptom of gallstones is biliary colic, which develops when the pressure in the gallbladder is increased by contraction of the gallbladder against an obstructing stone. Which of the following traits are characteristic of typical biliary colic?

a. Constant

b. Mild

c. Located in the epigastrium or right upper quadrant

d. Tends to occur after a meal

COMMENT: Four traits are characteristic of typical biliary colic. It is episodic; patients suffer discreet attacks of pain, between which they feel well. It is severe, bringing the patients to care quickly; the pain is often so severe that patients cry or compare the pain to labor. It is located in the epigastrium or right upper quadrant, and it comes on in the middle of the night or after a meal, often after a fatty or heavy meal. Patients whose attacks of pain have the characteristic location, severity, and timing and who have gallstones demonstrated on ultrasonography may be confidently advised that they have symptomatic gallstones. Other common features of the pain are that it is steady, increases in severity during 30 minutes and lasts two to four hours, often radiates to the back, and is associated with nausea and vomiting, and may be followed by episodes of diarrhea.

ANSWER: c, d

REFERENCE: *Chapter 40—Calculous Biliary Disease: Symptomatic Gallstones*

8. A 48-year-old woman has acute right upper quadrant pain, which is consistent with biliary colic. Which of the following statements is/are true concerning her diagnosis?

    a. Gallstones are the only biliary tract condition that can result in these symptoms.

    b. Ultrasonography is the most sensitive test available for diagnosis.

    c. Nonvisualization of the gallbladder on oral cholecystogram may represent the presence of gallstones.

    d. A quantitative gallbladder ejection fraction of less than 40% may represent gallbladder dismotility and might cause such symptoms.

COMMENT: Diagnostic imaging is used to confirm the presence of gallstones. Abdominal sonography is the standard diagnostic test. Oral cholecystography is an older test. A radioopaque dye, administered orally, is absorbed by the intestines, secreted by the liver, and concentrated in the gallbladder. When the gallbladder is imaged 12 hours later, the stones appear as filling defects. Another sign indicative of stones is nonvisualization of the gallbladder, provided the pills were taken and intestinal hepatic function is normal. This indicates that the cystic duct is obstructed or that the gallbladder wall inflammation has progressed to the point where the gallbladder cannot concentrate the dye. Cholecystography is slightly less sensitive than ultrasonography (95% versus 98%). Occasionally, patients with typical attacks of biliary pain have no evidence of stones on ultrasonography. This pain may be caused by sludge or by very small stones not detectable by ultrasonography. Sludge and gallstones are not the only conditions capable of inducing biliary colic. Cholesterolosis is a condition in which cholesterol accumulates within macrophages in the gallbladder mucosa, either diffusely or locally as polyps. It may sometimes cause biliary colic. The polypoid form is often detected by ultrasonography. Adenomyomatosis is a non-neoplastic condition characterized by the ingrowth of gallbladder mucosal glands into the muscle layer, either diffusely or focally in the fundus. It may cause biliary colic. Functional abnormalities of the gallbladder contraction may lead to pain. Hypomotility is detectable by measuring the gallbladder ejection fraction with the cholecystokinin/biliary scintigraphy test. The test is considered positive when the ejection fraction is reduced (<40%) on repeat exam.

ANSWER: b, c, d

REFERENCE: *Chapter 40—Calculous Biliary Disease: Symptomatic Gallstones*

9. Which of the following statements is/are true concerning the nonoperative treatment of gallstones?

    a. Oral dissolution of gallstones using the bile acid ursodeoxycholic acid is highly successful with good long-term results.

    b. Extracorporeal shock wave biliary lithotripsy is a technique that is widely applicable in patients with symptomatic gallstones.

    c. Contact dissolution using a cholesterol solvent is an effective though invasive technique that is not widely practiced.

    d. Oral dissolution of bile salts works best in patients with small cholesterol gallstones.

COMMENT: A number of nonoperative methods for treating symptomatic gallstones exist. Contact dissolution of stones with the cholesterol solvent methyl tert butyl ether and percutaneous cholecystolithotripsy with extraction are invasive techniques that involve percutaneous intubation of the gallbladder. In the former procedure, stones are bathed in a cholesterol solvent for several hours until they dissolve; the technique is not widely used today. In the latter technique, the tract is enlarged and the stones are destroyed by direct lithotripsy and mechanically extracted. Nonoperative treatment also includes dissolution of gallstones with the bile acid ursodeoxycholic acid and extracorporeal shock wave lithotripsy (ESWL). These treatments are rarely used today. Bile salt dissolution works consistently well only in patients who are not obese and who have small cholesterol gallstones (5% to 10% of patients presenting with stones), and stones eventually reform in more than 50% of these patients. ESWL is a reasonable therapy for patients with single stones 0.5 to 2 cm in diameter since single stones have a lower recurrence rate of about 20%. Again, only a small percentage of patients with stones fit in these categories.

ANSWER: c, d

REFERENCE: *Chapter 40—Calculous Biliary Disease: Symptomatic Gallstones*

10. Laparoscopic cholecystectomy has become the standard management of symptomatic gallstone disease. Which of the following statements is/are true concerning this technique?

   a. Correct traction of the gallbladder aligns the cystic duct with the common bile duct.
   b. Operative cholangiography prevents biliary tract injury during laparoscopic cholecystectomy.
   c. The incidence of major bile duct injury during laparoscopic cholecystectomy is between 0.3% and 0.6%.
   d. Spillage of stones into the peritoneal cavity during laparoscopic cholecystectomy is a totally innocuous event.

COMMENT: The goal of dissection in laparoscopic cholecystectomy is the conclusive identification of the cystic artery and cystic duct, as these are the structures to be divided. During the dissection leading up to the conclusive identification, normal structures must not be injured. These surgical principles govern the conduct of the operation. Retraction on the gallbladder fundus should be upward and to the right and traction on the pouch of Hartmann laterally to the right. This combination "disaligns" the common duct and cystic duct so that they appear as distinct structures. Incorrect traction aligns the ducts so that they appear as a continuous structure, and as a consequence the chance of biliary injury is increased. The single greatest problem in laparoscopic cholecystectomy is biliary injury. The reliable data available places the rate of major bile duct injury between 0.3% and 0.6%, but if all biliary injuries are considered, the injury rate in these reports ranges from 0.6% to 1.5% which is three to four times the injury rate at open surgery. The use of routine operative cholangiography is controversial. Biliary injuries appear to be less frequent in the hands of surgeons who perform operative cholangiography routinely. In about 50% of ductal injuries, a cholangiogram fails to prevent the injury although abnormal anatomy is present.

ANSWER: c

REFERENCE: Chapter 40—Calculous Biliary Disease: Laparoscopic Cholecystectomy and Open Cholecystectomy

11. A 48-year-old woman has acute right upper quadrant pain, low grade fever, and nausea and vomiting for 12 hours. Which of the following statements is/are true concerning the diagnosis management of this patient?

   a. Mild elevation of bilirubin level (less than 3 mg/dL) strongly suggests a common bile duct stone.
   b. A positive bile culture almost always can be expected in this setting.
   c. Laparoscopic cholecystectomy is clearly contraindicated.
   d. Appropriate antibiotics includes coverage for gram negative anaerobes.

COMMENT: The diagnosis of acute cholecystitis depends on the constellation of symptoms, signs, and characteristic findings on diagnostic imaging modalities. The pain of acute cholecystitis is similar to, but more severe than, the pain of biliary colic. The pain is typically in the right upper quadrant or epigastrium and is unremitting in comparison to time-limited pain of biliary colic. Local inflammatory signs, including tenderness and guarding, and peritoneal signs are usually present in the right upper quadrant or more diffusely. Severe jaundice is rare, but mild jaundice may be present: up to 6mg/dL. Severe jaundice suggests the presence of common bile duct stones, cholangitis, or obstruction of the common hepatic duct by severe pericholecystic inflammation resulting from impaction of a large stone in Hartmann's pouch. Acute calculous cholecystitis is an inflammatory complication of cholelithiasis. It is usually a sterile chemical inflammation, but secondary bacterial inflammation may occur. The initial management of patients with acute cholecystitis includes hospitalization, intravenous fluid resuscitation, and systemic antibiotics. The antibiotic regimen should be appropriate for typical bowel flora (gram-negative rods and anaerobes). The definitive treatment of acute cholecystitis is cholecystectomy. Laparoscopic cholecystectomy is the preferred approach particularly early in the course of the disease, when inflammation around the gallbladder is still minimal. Although associated with a higher rate of conversion and perhaps higher morbidity, it remains the procedure of choice.

ANSWER: d

REFERENCE: Chapter 40—Calculous Biliary Disease: Complicated Gallstone Disease

12. Appropriate options for management of common bile duct stones identified at laparoscopic cholecystectomy include:

a. Conversion to open cholecystectomy and common duct exploration.
b. Transcystic ductal dilatation and exploration.
c. Laparoscopic choledochotomy.
d. Completion of laparoscopic cholecystectomy with postoperative endoscopic retrograde cholangiography and stone removal.

COMMENT: Laparoscopic bile duct exploration can be performed by means of flouroscopic cholangiography, biliary balloon catheters, stone baskets, and direct laparoscopic common bile duct exploration. All requires an institutional commitment to equipment and expertise that is not available at every site. Transcystic ductal dilatation exploration with stone removal is being performed at increasing numbers and appears to be safe and effective. Although limited experience with laparoscopic choledochotomy and common bile duct exploration has been reported, this technique is probably not appropriate for the average surgeon. Many surgeons, depending on the clinical situation, may choose to convert the patient to an open procedure, to perform a traditional open choledochotomy and common duct exploration. Finally, depending on the clinical situation, an option is to complete the procedure and plan a postoperative ERCP with sphincterotomy and clearance of the bile duct.

ANSWER: a, b, d

REFERENCE: *Chapter 40—Calculous Biliary Disease: Complicated Gallstone Disease*

13. A 65-year-old woman presents with shaking, chills, and a fever to 102 degrees. There is evidence of jaundice. She also complains of right upper quadrant pain and has some slight tenderness to palpation in that area. Which of the following statements is/are true concerning her diagnosis and management?

a. Initial management should consist of intravenous antibiotics appropriate for gram-negative rods.
b. Nonoperative biliary drainage is indicated in patients who do not respond to initial antibiotic therapy.
c. If acute operative intervention is necessary, common duct exploration, choledochoscopy, and cholecystectomy should be performed.
d. The condition requires the presence of both bacteria and biliary obstruction.

COMMENT: In acute cholangitis, infection develops behind a partially obstructing stone. It is likely that bacteria intermittently enter the biliary tree through the ampulla, bloodstream, or lymphatics. Normally, bacteria are cleared mechanically by bile flow and by the presence of anti-bacterial substances in bile. In the presence of a stone, mechanical clearance is interrupted, bile formation is inhibited and contamination may become infection. Infection spreads rapidly through the biliary tree, a huge surface area, and bacteria readily enter the systemic circulation to cause septicemia. These factors explain why acute cholangitis is a much more serious inflammation than acute cholecystitis. Acute cholangitis should always be considered potentially life-threatening, although cholangitis encompasses a spectrum of diseases, ranging from a subclinical illness to acute toxic cholangitis. Patients presenting with gallstone induced cholangitis are often older and female. They often present with a combination of systemic and local symptoms. Commonly the illness commences with a sudden shaking chill (rigor) followed by a high fever of septicemia. The patient may become disoriented secondary to septic shock. Jaundice and right upper quadrant pain are frequent symptoms. The initial management of cholangitis includes intravenous antibiotics appropriate for coverage of the most commonly cultured organisms (gram-negative rods, *Streptococcus faecalis*, and less commonly *Bacteroides fragilis*). For patients with acute toxicalangitis or who fail to respond to antibiotic therapy, emergency decompression of the biliary tree is required. This is typically accomplished by endoscopic sphincterotomy and trans-biliary drainage or temporary stenting. Percutaneous transhepatic drainage is used when ERCP fails or is unavailable. If decompression by less invasive means is not available or possible, then operative intervention to decompress a biliary tree is indicated. In such an unstable patient, operative intervention should be restricted to insertion of a T-tube in the common bile duct. Stone extraction should be limited to those stones that can be extracted easily within a short period of time.

ANSWER: a, b, d

REFERENCE: *Chapter 40—Calculous Biliary Disease: Complicated Gallstone Disease*

14. A 46-year-old man who suffered pelvic and extremity fractures, pulmonary contusions, and required a laparotomy for a fractured spleen remains intubated in the intensive care unit. On the eighth postoperative day, the patient develops a fever and elevation of white blood cell count. His level of bilirubin rises significantly. He grimaces with tenderness in the right upper quadrant. Which of the following statements is/are true concerning the diagnosis?

a. An abdominal ultrasound should be performed at the bedside.
b. Percutaneous cholecystomy is the treatment of choice.
c. If improvement is not seen in 24 hours, laparotomy may be indicated.
d. The process is usually sterile, therefore antibiotics play no role in management.

COMMENT: Acalculous cholecystitis typically occurs in a patient with other acute systemic illness (e.g., after major burns, major trauma, or significant abdominal or thoracic operation). Symptoms and signs depend largely on the patient's concurrent medical conditions. In patients with severe systemic illness, the symptoms and signs may not be evident because of sedation or alteration of consciousness because of illness. In such patients, elevated alkaline phosphatase or bilirubin levels are indications for further investigation. Further laboratory evaluation may demonstrate an elevated white blood cell count. Diagnostic imaging is the key to establishing the diagnosis of acalculus and cholecystitis. Ultrasonography is inexpensive, can be performed at the bedside of a critically ill patient, and can demonstrate the typical findings of acalculous or calculus cholecystitis, including gallbladder wall thickening, pericholecystic fluid, and abscess formation in the right upper quadrant. An abdominal CT scan is as sensitive as ultrasonography for this condition and allows imaging of the remainder of the abdominal cavity. The management of acalculous cholecystitis must be tailored to the individual patient. Definitive management includes urgent cholecystectomy. However, most affected patients are unfit to tolerate a major abdominal operation. In these cases, percutaneous cholecystostomy is the procedure of choice. It resolves the cholecystitis in more than 90% of patients and generally is well tolerated. Concomitant management must include systemic antibiotics, maintenance of NPO status, and treatment of the concomitant illnesses that have placed the patient at risk for the disease. The response to treatment must be monitored, and if improvement is not apparent within 24 hours, then other steps including cholecystectomy must be taken. Failure is usually caused by gangrene with perforation or a mistaken diagnosis.

ANSWER: a, b, c

REFERENCE: *Chapter 40—Calculus Biliary Tract Disease: Acalculous Cholecystitis*

CHAPTER 41

BILIARY NEOPLASMS

1. Gallbladder cancer is a rare malignancy with a dismal outlook because of its insidious onset, propensity for local invasion, and rapid disease progression. Which of the following statements is/are true concerning incidence of and risk factors for this disease?

   a. Up to 90% of patients with carcinoma of the gallbladder have gallstones
   b. Gallbladder cancer is found incidentally after elective cholecystectomy for gallstones in 1% of patients
   c. Routine cholecystectomy for asymptomatic gallstones is indicated because of the risk of gallbladder cancer
   d. A porcelain gallbladder is at no higher risk for gallbladder cancer than is a patient with calcified gallstones
   e. Larger gallstones are associated with an increased risk of gallbladder cancer when compared to smaller stones

COMMENT: The increased risk of gallbladder cancer with cholelithiasis is well established; 70%–90% of all patients with carcinoma also have gallstones. However, less than 0.5% of patients with gallstones are found to have gallbladder cancer. After elective cholecystectomy for gallstones, gallbladder cancer is found incidentally in 1% of patients. The association of gallstones with carcinoma is probably related to chronic inflammation. Larger stones (> 3 cm) are associated with a tenfold increased risk of cancer. Epidemiologic studies have found the 20-year risk for development of cancer in patients with gallstones is less than 0.5% for the overall population, and 1.5% for high-risk groups. Therefore, routine cholecystectomy for symptomatic gallstones because of concern about gallbladder cancer does not appear to be warranted. However, because of the 25%–60% incidence of cancer in those with "porcelain gallbladder" or calcification of the gallbladder wall, all patients with this finding should undergo cholecystectomy even if asymptomatic.

ANSWER: a, b, e

REFERENCE: *Chapter 41—Biliary Neoplasms: Gallbladder Carcinoma*

2. The surgical treatment of gallbladder cancer is highly dependent on the clinical presentation and stage of the cancer. Which of the following statements is/are true concerning surgical management of gallbladder cancer:

a. For tumors limited to the muscular layer of the gallbladder (T1) simple cholecystectomy is adequate treatment

b. For T2 gallbladder cancers, cholecystectomy plus portal lymph node dissection represents appropriate treatment

c. A T2 gallbladder cancer identified postoperatively after laparoscoptic cholecystectomy should undergo clinical observation only

d. A patient with bile duct obstruction due to gallbladder cancer should be considered unresectable due to the extent of the disease

e. Most patients presented with gallbladder cancer are candidates for surgical resection

COMMENT: Gallbladder cancer, if not completely surgically removed, results in rapid local progression and death. Although surgical resection represents the treatment of choice and the only potentially curative treatment, resection is possible in only 25% of patients because of the advanced stage of the disease at the time of presentation. For tumors limited to the muscular wall of the gallbladder (T1) there is near-universal agreement that simple cholecystectomy is adequate. T1 tumors have not yet invaded the subscrosal layer, which contains lymphatics, and therefore lymphadenectomy is not required. Attesting to the fact that early gallbladder carcinoma is completely curable, simple cholecystectomy has resulted in nearly 100% survival rates when early cancer is an incidental finding after elective cholecystectomy. The extent of surgical resection for T2 or greater tumors is controversial. For tumors with full-thickness invasion into the perimuscular connective tissue but not to the serosa (T2), radical cholecystectomy, with resection of segments for 4b and 5 of the liver is required. Because the gallbladder is not surrounded by serosa where it is attached to the liver, even T2 tumors may invade into the plane of dissection on the hepatic side of the gallbladder for a simple cholecystectomy. Therefore, T2 tumors cannot be completely removed with cholecystectomy alone. Complete excision of tumors is more likely with a procedure involving resection of segments 4b and 5, the segments immediately surrounding the gallbladder bed where tumor direct extension into the liver occurs. Regional lymphadenectomy is an important part of this procedure. Since half the patients with T2 tumors are found to have nodal spread after resection. Dissection of lymph nodes should include all tissue from the bifurcation of the hepatic duct to the distal common bile duct D and include nodes along the hepatic artery to the celiac axis. If a tumor rises in the gallbladder infundibulum, the CBD is often involved with the tumor, either by direct extension or external invasion of the hepato-duodenal ligament. In this case, an extended liver resection with removal of the portion of the CBD should be performed. Reconstruction is then performed by Roux-en-Y hepatico jejunostomy.

Gallbladder cancer is often discovered during pathologic examination after cholecystectomy for presumed benign gallbladder disease. Patients with T2 or greater tumors and no signs of distaut metastasis should be offered radical resection to eradicate all disease. Even if they are normal, excision laparoscopic port sites should also be performed because of the well-documented history of port site seeding.

ANSWER: a, e

REFERENCE: *Chapter 41—Biliary Neoplasms: Gallbladder Carcinoma*

3. Which of the following statements is/are true concerning the survival for patients with gallbladder carcinoma?

a. Overall survival is approximately 20%

b. Survival for T1 disease (limited to the muscular level) is nearly 100% after simple cholecystectomy

c. T2 and T3 tumors without nodal disease have 5-year survival rates greater than 50%

d. The most common site of recurrence after resection of gallbladder cancer is intraabdominal

COMMENT: The five-year survival rate for all patients with gallbladder cancer is less than 5% in most series, with median survival of six months. This is primarily because most patients present with unresectable disease. Of the patients undergoing resection, survival depends on the depth of penetration and nodal status. Nearly 100% survival rates are reported after simple cholecystectomy for T1 disease, whereas T2 and T3 tumors without nodal disease have a five-year survival rate greater than 50%. Node positivity is an ominous finding, with few series reporting five-year survivors. The most common site of recurrence after resection of gallbladder cancer is intraabdominal, specifically in the liver or the celiac or retro-pancreatic nodal basins.

ANSWER: b, c, d

REFERENCE: *Chapter 41—Biliary Neoplasms: Gallbladder Carcinoma*

4. Which of the following are risk factors for the development of bile duct carcinoma?

    a. Primary sclerosing cholangitis
    b. Choledochal cyst
    c. Crohn's disease
    d. Biliary infection with clonorchis

COMMENT: Cholangiocarcinoma is a rare cancer that arises from the biliary epithelium and occurs in less than 4,500 patients in the United States each year. Cholangiocarcinoma has a relatively even distribution between men and women with a male:female ratio of 1.3:1. The average age of patients presented with bile duct cancer is between 50 and 70 years. Risk factors for this disease include primary sclerosing cholangitis, ulcerative colitis, choledochal cyst, biliary tract infection, either with clonorchis or in chronic typhoid carriers.

ANSWER: a, b, d

REFERENCE: *Chapter 41—Biliary Neoplasms: Bile Duct Carcinoma*

5. Which of the following statements is/are true concerning the pathology and clinical findings of bile duct carcinoma?

    a. Most bile duct carcinomas are located in the perihilar area
    b. Cholangitis is a common presentation for patients with bile duct carcinoma
    c. Mid-bile duct obstruction is most commonly due to gallbladder carcinoma rather than bile duct carcinoma
    d. Klatskin's tumors refer to cholangiocarcinoma at the hepatic duct bifurcation

COMMENT: Cholangiocarcinomas have been classified according to their location in the upper (60%), middle (15%–20%) or lower third (15%–20%) of the bile duct. Middle-third lesions arise between the cystic duct and the superior border of the duodenum. Lower-third lesions are found below the superior border of the duodenum but above the ampula. Most mid-bile duct malignant obstructions are due to gallbladder cancers. Cholangiocarcinoma occurring at the hepatic hilus is commonly referred to as a hilar cholangiocarcinoma or Klatskin's tumor. Most patients with cholangiocarcinoma present with painless jaundice, although mild right upper quadrant pain, pruritis, anorexia, malaise, and weight-loss may also be reported. Cholangitis is the presenting symptom in only 10%–30% of patients.

ANSWER: c, d

REFERENCE: *Chapter 41—Biliary Neoplasms: Bile Duct Carcinoma*

6. Which of the following statements is/are true concerning surgical treatment of cholangiocarcinoma?

    a. The greatest risk for recurrence following resection of a hilar cholangiocarcinoma is the presence of positive margins and no-positive tumors
    b. Pancreaticoduodenectomy is required for the treatment of most distal bile duct carcinomas
    c. Patients with resectable distal bile duct cancer have a five-year survival rate in excess of 75%
    d. The performance of hepatic resection has resulted in improved survival in the resection of Klatskin's tumors

COMMENT: Results of major studies of hilar cholangiocarcinoma have shown five-year survival rates ranging from 10%–30%. In recent years, more aggressive surgical approaches with an increasing number of hepatic resections have resulted in a higher incidence of negative margins and improved survival. The greatest risk factors for recurrence of disease include the presence of positive margins and node-positive tumors. Patients with distal cholangiocarcinoma generally require pancreaticoduodenectomy to obtain clearance of the tumor because of the intrapancreatic location of the distal CBD. Patients with cholangiocarcinoma arising in the distal bile duct have both an increased resectability rate and an improved prognosis over those with hilar cholangiocarcinoma. Patients with resectable distal bile duct cancer have a five-year survival rate of 30%–50% with decreased survival if nodes are positive with the tumor.

ANSWER: a, b, d

REFERENCE: *Chapter 41—Biliary Neoplasms: Bile Duct Carcinoma*

7. Which of the following statements is/are true concerning benign gallbladder neoplasms?

    a. Cholesterol polyps (cholesterolosis) account for half of all gallbladder polyploid lesions
    b. Gallbladder adenomas should be considered pre-malignant
    c. Adenomyomatosis is a benign condition with no evidence of malignant transformation
    d. Large polyps greater than 10 mm should be treated with cholecystectomy
    e. Benign gallbladder tumors are usually symptomatic with symptoms consistent with cholelithiasis

COMMENT: Benign gallbladder tumors are rare with a reported incidence of 0.5%–3.0%. Benign gallbladder tumors are most frequently polyps or polyploid lesions. The incidence of polyps in asymptomatic patients is approximately 5%. Cholesterol polyps (cholesterolosis) account for half of all gallbladder polyploid lesions, and arise from epithelium-covered cholesterol-laden macrophages in the lamina propria. This lesion is not considered pre-malignant. Gallbladder adenomas may be tubular or papillary, both arising from the epithelial layer of the gallbladder. The direct association between benign adenomas, adenomas containing carcinoma in situ, and invasive carcinoma has been demonstrated and therefore these lesions are considered pre-malignant. In general, adenomas less than 12 mm in size are typically all benign whereas adenomas with cancerous foci are usually greater than 12 mm. Adenomyomatosis of the gallbladders is characterized by localized or diffuse hyperplastic extension of the mucosa into, and often beyond, a hypertrophic gallbladder muscular layer. The etiology is unknown. This lesion may be pre-malignant because cases of adenocarcinoma arising in or near adenomyomatosis have been reported. Patients with benign gall bladder tumors typically present with symptoms consistent with cholelithiasis, including right-upper quadrant pain, fatty food intolerance, and nausea. Many benign gallbladder lesions are also discovered incidentally after elective cholecystectomy, therefore symptoms due to benign lesions are difficult to separate from those due to gallstones. Most lesions are, however, asymptomatic and are discovered incidentally during imaging for other abdominal conditions. Large polyps, greater than 10 mm, have the greatest malignant potential. Therefore if a large polyp is present, even in asymptomatic patients without stones, cholecystectomy is warranted. Smaller pedunculated lesions with gross characteristics of a benign cholesterol polyp may be observed and resected only if symptomatic.

ANSWER: a, b, d

REFERENCE: *Chapter 41—Biliary Neoplasms: Benign Gallbladder Neoplasms*

CHAPTER 42

BILIARY STRICTURES AND SCLEROSING CHOLANGITIS

1. Most benign bile duct strictures occur after operations in or near the right upper quadrant. Other causes of benign bile duct strictures include:

    a. Chronic pancreatitis
    b. Ulcerative colitis
    c. Primary sclerosing cholangitis
    d. Intrahepatic arterial infusion of 5-fluorouracil

COMMENT: Most bile duct strictures are postoperative; more than 80% occur after injury to the bile duct during cholecystectomy. A number of inflammatory conditions also can cause strictures of the biliary tree. The chronic inflammation and fibrosis associated with chronic pancreatitis can cause stricture of the intrapancreatic bile duct. Primary sclerosing cholangitis is an idiopathic disease believed to be autoimmune; it is characterized by intrahepatic and extrahepatic inflammatory strictures of the biliary tree. Although primary sclerosing cholangitis frequently is associated with ulcerative colitis, this colonic disease has no direct causal relation to benign bile duct strictures. A rare cause of benign bile duct strictures in both the intrahepatic and extrahepatic biliary tree has been the use of intrahepatic arterial infusion of 5-fluorouracil to manage hepatic metastasis from colorectal carcinoma.

ANSWER: a, c, d

REFERENCE: *Chapter 42—Biliary Strictures and Sclerosing Cholangitis: Postoperative Bile Duct Strictures*

2. Which of the following statements is/are true concerning the incidence of bile duct injury after cholecystectomy?

   a. Data from the era before laparoscopic cholecystectomy suggest the incidence of bile duct injury during open cholecystectomy is 0.1% to 0.2%

   b. The current incidence of bile duct injury during laparoscopic cholecystectomy is greater than 1%

   c. The experience of the surgeon performing laparoscopic cholecystectomy can be correlated with the incidence of bile duct injury

   d. Intraoperative cholangiography during laparoscopic cholecystectomy prevents bile duct injury in almost all cases

COMMENT: Results of a number of surveys encompassing thousands of patients undergoing open cholecystectomy suggest the incidence of bile duct injury is 0.1% to 0.2%. In a number of early individual series of laparoscopic cholecystectomy, bile duct injuries occurred among 1% of patients. As larger series have been reported and surveys including thousands of patients have appeared, the true incidence appears to be 0.3% to 0.6%. A number of factors are associated with bile duct injury during laparoscopic cholecystectomy, including the experience of the surgeon. This reflects the steep learning curve with this procedure. Although strongly debated, there is no evidence that intraoperative cholangiography prevents bile duct injury during laparoscopic cholecystectomy. The use of intraoperative cholangiography, however, may allow detection of the injury early in the procedure and thus minimize the extent of injury.

ANSWER: a, c

REFERENCE: *Chapter 42—Biliary Strictures and Sclerosing Cholangitis: Postoperative Bile Duct Strictures*

3. Most postoperative bile duct strictures after cholecystectomy manifest soon after the operation. Which of the following is a manifestation of bile duct strictures after cholecystectomy?

   a. Obstructive jaundice

   b. External biliary fistula

   c. Progressive accumulation of bile in the peritoneal cavity (bile ascites)

   d. Biliary cirrhosis

COMMENT: Most benign postoperative bile duct strictures present soon after the operation. Patients believed to have postoperative bile duct strictures within days to 1 week of an initial operation usually have one of two presentations. One is progressive elevation of levels of markers of liver function, particularly serum bilirubin and alkaline phosphatase. These changes can occur as early as the second or third postoperative day. The second mode of early presentation is leakage of bile from the injured bile duct. Bilious drainage from the operatively placed drains or through the wound after cholecystectomy is abnormal and represents biliary injury. Among patients without drains, or in patients from whom drains have been removed, bile can leak into the peritoneal cavity as bile ascites or accumulate in loculations. Patients with markedly delayed diagnosis of bile duct stricture may have advanced biliary cirrhosis and other evidence of liver dysfunction when they come to medical attention.

ANSWER a, b, c

REFERENCE: *Chapter 42—Benign Biliary Strictures and Sclerosing Cholangitis: Postoperative Bile Duct Strictures*

4. The standard for evaluation of bile duct strictures is cholangiography. The two routes for cholangiography are percutaneous transhepatic cholangiography (PTC) or endoscopic retrograde cholangiography (ERC). Which of the following statements is/are true?

    a. Percutaneous transhepatic cholangiography is generally more valuable than ERC in defining the proximal biliary tree to be used in reconstruction
    b. Endoscopic retrograde cholangiography is technically easier in the care of patients with bile leaks because the biliary tree usually is not dilated
    c. Parenteral antibiotics should be administered before either procedure to prevent cholangitis
    d. Biliary stents can be placed by means of either technique to control biliary leaks

COMMENT: The standard for evaluation of bile duct stricture is cholangiography. Percutaneous transhepatic cholangiography is generally more valuable than ERC in that it defines the anatomy of the proximal biliary tree used in the surgical reconstruction. Endoscopic retrograde cholangiography is often less useful than PTC because the discontinuity of the extrahepatic biliary tree usually prevents adequate filling of the proximal biliary tree. However, in patients with biliary fistulas, the proximal biliary tree often is not dilated, making PTC somewhat technically more challenging. Parenteral antibiotics should be administered before either procedure to decrease the risk of cholangitis. Biliary stents used to temporarily control biliary leaks or to stent a stricture after nonsurgical dilation can be placed by the percutaneous or the endoscopic route.

ANSWER: a, b, c, d

REFERENCE: *Chapter 42—Biliary Strictures and Sclerosing Cholangitis: Postoperative Bile Duct Strictures*

5. Management of a suspected bile duct injury depends on a number of factors; most important are the mode and timing of presentation. Which of the following statements is/are true concerning a patient with suspected bile leak after laparoscopic cholecystectomy?

    a. Laparotomy should be performed immediately
    b. Cholangiography should be performed to determine the nature of the injury
    c. Surgically placed drains should be removed to allow the fistula to close
    d. The patient should be discharged to home to allow the leak to close spontaneously

COMMENT: Patients with a biliary leak in the early postoperative period may have sepsis with either cholangitis or intraabdominal bile collections. Sepsis must be controlled first with broad-spectrum parenteral antibiotics, cholangiography with percutaneous biliary drainage, and percutaneous or operative drainage of biliary leaks. Once sepsis is controlled, there is no hurry in proceeding with surgical reconstruction of the bile duct stricture. The combination of proximal biliary decompression and external drainage allows most biliary fistulas to be controlled or even closed. At that time, the external drains can be removed. The patient can then be discharged to home to allow several months to lapse for resolution of the inflammation in the periportal region and recovery of overall health status.

ANSWER: b

REFERENCE: *Chapter 42—Biliary Strictures and Sclerosing Cholangitis: Postoperative Bile Duct Strictures*

6. If a bile duct injury is suspected at laparoscopic cholecystectomy, appropriate management includes which of the following?

   a. Conversion to open cholecystectomy and intraoperative cholangiography
   b. Small ducts (less than 3 mm in diameter) seen at cholangiography to drain a single liver segment can be ligated
   c. If the injured segment is longer than 1 cm, end-to-end ductal anastomosis is the procedure of choice
   d. Postoperative external drainage should be avoided

COMMENT: In many cases, proper initial management of a bile duct injury recognized at cholecystectomy can avoid development of a bile duct stricture. Recognition of a bile duct injury is uncommon, however, during either open or laparoscopic cholecystectomy. If bile leakage is found or if "atypical" anatomy is encountered during laparoscopic cholecystectomy, early conversion to an open technique and prompt cholangiography are imperative. If a segment of accessory duct narrower than 3 mm has been injured and cholangiography shows segmental or subsegmental drainage of the injured ductal system, simple ligation of the injured duct is indicated. If the injured duct is 4 mm or larger, however, it is likely to drain several hepatic segments or the entire right or left lobe and requires operative repair. If the injured segment of bile duct is short (less than 1 cm) and the two ends can be opposed without tension, end-to-end anastomosis can be performed with placement of a T tube through a separate choledochotomy either above or below the anastomosis. For proximal injuries, or if the injured segment of bile duct is longer than 1 cm, an end-to-end bile duct anastomosis should be avoided because of the excessive tension that usually exists in these situations. The use of a Roux-en-Y jejunal limb is preferable for anastomosis. Regardless of the type of anastomosis, all repairs at the initial operation should involve external drainage with either a T tube or an intraoperatively placed transanastomotic stent.

ANSWER: a, b

REFERENCE: *Chapter 42—Biliary Strictures and Sclerosing Cholangitis: Postoperative Bile Duct Strictures*

7. Which of the following statements regarding elective repair of a bile duct stricture is/are true?

   a. A transanastomotic stent is necessary for a successful result
   b. Stenting for approximately 1 year is necessary for an anastomosis performed at the distal common hepatic duct
   c. A Roux-en-Y hepatojejunostomy provides the best route for restoring biliary-enteric continuity
   d. Preoperatively placed biliary catheters facilitate dissection and identification of the stricture and are useful in placement of transanastomotic stents if necessary

COMMENT: Several principles are associated with successful repair of a biliary stricture. Although many surgeons favor the use of transanastomotic stents, a number of series have had successful results without the use of such stents. The length of stenting depends on the location of the stricture. If the injury involves the common bile duct or common hepatic duct at least 2 cm distal to the hepatic duct bifurcation, and adequate proximal bile duct mucosa can be defined, the use of long-term biliary stenting is not necessary. In these situations, transanastomotic stenting for 4 to 6 weeks after the operation is adequate. When adequate proximal bile duct is not available for a good mucosa-to-mucosa anastomosis, long-term stenting of the biliary-enteric anastomosis with polymeric silicone transanastomotic stents for at least 1 year is recommended. For established strictures, simple excision and end-to-end anastomosis or repair of the damaged duct can rarely be accomplished because of the invariable loss of duct length as a result of fibrosis associated with injury. In almost all cases, hepatojejunostomy constructed to a Roux-en-Y limb of jejunum is the preferred procedure. The use of preoperatively placed transhepatic biliary catheters can aid in dissection and identification of the biliary tree, especially in operations on patients with previous attempts at repair, in which scarring and fibrosis can be severe. The biliary catheters also can assist in placement of long-term transanastomotic stents.

ANSWER: c, d

REFERENCE: *Chapter 42—Biliary Strictures and Sclerosing Cholangitis: Postoperative Bile Duct Strictures*

8. A 37-year-old woman has obstructive jaundice caused by a mid-bile duct stricture 4 months after laparoscopic cholecystectomy. Which of the following statements is/are true?

a. Surgical reconstruction is the only option for treatment of this patient
b. Excellent long-term results can be expected among approximately 80% of patients who undergo surgical biliary reconstruction
c. One year follow-up results after successful repair are satisfactory regardless of the method of management
d. Surgical reconstruction offers a better chance of long-term success than either percutaneous or endoscopic dilation

COMMENT: Excellent long-term results can be achieved among 70% to 90% of patients who undergo surgical repair of bile duct strictures. The definition of satisfactory results in most series requires no symptoms of jaundice or cholangitis. Length of the follow-up period is important in analyzing results, however, because recurrent strictures can occur as late as 20 years after the initial procedure. Approximately two thirds of recurrent strictures are evident within 2 years and 90% within 7 years. Although operative management of bile duct strictures in most cases gives excellent results, the nonoperative approaches of percutaneous or endoscopic dilation are suitable alternatives for many patients. Although comparisons of techniques are difficult, results of two retrospective comparative studies from single institutions suggested surgical reconstruction offers a better chance of long-term success than does either percutaneous or endoscopic management.

ANSWER: b, d

REFERENCE: *Chapter 42—Biliary Strictures and Sclerosing Cholangitis: Postoperative Bile Duct Strictures*

9. Nonoperative dilation, performed either endoscopically or percutaneously, can be used successfully to manage which of the following causes of bile duct strictures?

a. Postoperative bile duct strictures following hepatojejunostomy for reconstruction during a Whipple procedure
b. Complete transection of the bile duct during laparoscopic cholecystectomy (the so-called "classic laparoscopic cholecystectomy injury")
c. Primary sclerosing cholangitis
d. Oriental cholangiohepatitis

COMMENT: Nonoperative management of bile duct strictures can be provided at most institutions; however, it has technical limitations due to the anatomic situation. In so-called "classic laparoscopic bile duct injury" however, complete bile duct transection and discontinuity of the biliary tree eliminate the possibility of nonoperative management. Percutaneous dilation of a biliary-enteric anastomosis has been shown in a number of series to have a success rate approaching that of surgical reconstruction. Although limited experience with percutaneous or endoscopic dilation to manage primary sclerosing cholangitis has been reported, this alternative may provide at least temporary improvement in symptoms and radiologic appearance. Oriental cholangiohepatitis is an unusual infection of the biliary tree frequently associated with infection by *Clonorchis sinensis* and other parasites. Cholangiography shows numerous strictures of both the intrahepatic and extrahepatic biliary tree and bile ducts filled with sludge and stones. Surgical management consisting of cholecystectomy and improving biliary drainage by means of Roux-en-Y choledochojejunostomy or choledochoduodenostomy is necessary for almost all patients. Access to the biliary tree for postoperative management of intrahepatic stones or sludge should be maintained, however, with transhepatic biliary stents.

ANSWER: a, c

REFERENCE: *Chapter 42—Biliary Strictures and Sclerosing Cholangitis*

10. Primary sclerosing cholangitis has a number of treatment options—both medical and surgical. Which of the following statements is/are true?

a. A number of immunosuppressive oral agents can provide specific effective therapy for primary sclerosing cholangitis
b. Biliary reconstruction with long-term transanastomotic stents can be useful in the care of selected patients with focal strictures at the bifurcation of the hepatic duct
c. Biliary reconstruction should be reserved for patients with established biliary cirrhosis
d. Hepatic transplantation for primary sclerosing cholangitis can be associated with survival rates similar to those of other indications for transplantation

COMMENT: There is no known specific, effective medical therapy for primary sclerosing cholangitis. Encouraging results from a prospective, randomized, placebo-controlled trial, however, suggest that ursodeoxycholic acid greatly improves results of serum liver function tests and clinical symptoms. Because of the lack of effective medical therapy, an aggressive surgical approach is indicated for most instances of symptomatic primary sclerosing cholangitis. One surgical approach to the treatment of patients with a predominant stricture at the hepatic duct bifurcation is resection of the bifurcation and long-term transhepatic stenting with polymeric silicone stents. Results among patients without established cirrhosis are excellent. However, among patients with secondary biliary cirrhosis present before surgery, perioperative morbidity and mortality have been high and long-term results poor. Patients with established secondary biliary cirrhosis should be referred for hepatic transplantation. Reviews of experience with hepatic transplantation for primary sclerosing cholangitis suggest survival is similar to that reported for hepatic transplantation for any diagnosis.

ANSWER: b, d

REFERENCE: *Chapter 42—Biliary Strictures and Sclerosing Cholangitis: Primary Sclerosing Cholangitis*

11. Which of the following statements is/are true concerning bile duct strictures due to chronic pancreatitis?

a. Most patients have progressive jaundice
b. Strictures are classically long and tapered and involve the entire intrapancreatic bile duct
c. Patients may have no symptoms, and the condition is diagnosed only because of persistent elevation of serum alkaline phosphatase level
d. An excellent option for surgical management is choledochoduodenostomy

COMMENT: The clinical presentation of common bile duct strictures secondary to chronic pancreatitis is variable. A large number of patients have no symptoms, and the diagnosis of bile duct strictures is suggested only by abnormal results of liver function tests. Measurement of serum alkaline phosphatase appears to be the most sensitive laboratory finding; the level is elevated in more than 80% of patients. Although transient jaundice can occur in most cases, progressive jaundice is rare. Cholangiography shows classic long, smooth gradual tapering of the common bile duct throughout the intrapancreatic segment. Biliary reconstruction is the appropriate treatment of most patients. Many surgeons prefer choledochoduodenostomy because it does not divert bile from the duodenum, is technically easier to perform, and leaves the jejunum intact for any associated procedures needed for decompression of the obstructed gastrointestinal tract or pancreatic duct.

ANSWER: b, c, d

REFERENCE: *Chapter 42—Biliary Strictures and Sclerosing Cholangitis: Bile Duct Strictures Secondary to Chronic Pancreatitis*

Section H

COLON, RECTUM, AND ANUS

COLONIC ANATOMY AND PHYSIOLOGY

1. Which of the following statements is/are true regarding colonic anatomy?

   a. The transverse colon is suspended by its own mesocolon and is extremely mobile
   b. The columnar epithelium of the colon is made up of regularly arranged crypts, goblet cells. and microvilli
   c. The cecum is the widest portion of the colon
   d. Haustra coli are sacculations between the taeniae
   e. There is one antimesenteric and two mesenteric taeniae

COMMENT: The mucosal surface of the colon consists of columnar epithelium made up of regularly arranged crypts and numerous goblet cells. Unlike that of the small intestine, the columnar epithelium of the colon does not possess villi. The muscularis propria of the colon consists of an inner circular layer and an outer longitudinal layer. The thick circular muscle forms a continuous layer around the entire circumference of the colon. The outer longitudinal muscle layer is grouped into three bands known as *taeniae.* These bands are positioned approximately 120 degrees apart around the circumference of the colon with one taenia along the mesenteric border and the other two on the antimesenteric border of the colon. The sacculations seen between the taeniae are called *haustra coli.* The transverse colon is suspended by the transverse mesocolon and is considered completely intraperitoneal. It is the most mobile portion of the colon and can be present anywhere from the upper abdomen down into the pelvis. The greater omentum descends from the greater curvature of the stomach in front of the transverse colon and ascends to attach to the transverse colon on its anterosuperior edge.

ANSWER: a, c, d

REFERENCE: *Chapter 43—Colonic Anatomy and Physiology: Anatomy of the Colon; General Considerations*

2. Which of the following statements is/are true regarding colonic physiology?

   a. The colon can absorb as much as 5 to 6 L of water during a 24-hour period
   b. Water absorption in the colon is an energy-dependent process that depends on the breakdown of short-chain fatty acids by the colonic microflora
   c. Salt and water absorption is greatest in the right colon
   d. Sodium absorption is an energy-dependent process controlled by the Na^+-K^+-ATPase pump at the apical membrane of the colonic epithelium
   e. Short-chain fatty acids are the primary intraluminal colonic anion

COMMENT: Approximately 1500 mL of ileal effluent reaches the cecum over a 24-hour period, of which 90% is water. Of this amount, only 100 to 150 mL of water appears in the stool. The colon has a tremendous reserve capacity that allows it to absorb as much as 5 to 6 L of water over a 24-hour period. Water absorption in the colon is a passive process that depends primarily on the osmotic gradient established by the active transport of sodium across the colonic epithelium. Salt and water absorption is greater in the right colon than in the left colon and sigmoid colon. Patients undergoing a right hemicolectomy should be counseled preoperatively that they might experience loose bowel movements or frank diarrhea in the early postoperative period. Sodium absorption involves the passive movement of sodium across the apical membrane into the mucosal cell down an electrochemical gradient. To maintain an adequate electrochemical gradient, intracellular sodium is removed from the cell into the interstitial space in exchange for potassium. This is an energy-dependent process controlled by a Na^+-K^+-ATPase pump at the basolateral membrane of the colonic epithelium. Short-chain fatty acids, which include acetate, butyrate, and propionate, are absorbed in a concentration-dependent manner. They are an important energy substrate for the colonic epithelial cells and are the major fecal anions.

ANSWER: a, c, e

REFERENCE: *Chapter 43—Colonic Anatomy and Physiology: Physiology; Absorption*

3. A 72-year-old woman patient in a nursing home falls out of bed and sustains a fracture of the right hip. The patient undergoes uncomplicated open reduction and internal fixation of the right hip. On postoperative day 3 she reports abdominal pain and bloating. Abdominal radiographs are obtained (Fig. 43. 1). The following is/are true about the treatment of this patient:

a. Treatment involves exploratory laparotomy with decompressive transverse loop colostomy

b. Initial therapy consists of nasogastric decompression, correction of fluid and electrolyte imbalances, gentle enemas, and avoidance of narcotics and anticholinergics

c. Cecostomy is warranted if conservative measures fail to decompress the colon

d. Neostigmine 2.5 mg intravenously over 2 to 3 minutes decompresses the colon

COMMENT: Colonic pseudoobstruction is a clinical entity in which signs and symptoms of bowel obstruction are present without actual mechanical obstruction. Pseudoobstruction usually is found among patients with serious underlying medical conditions who have undergone a major, usually extraabdominal, surgical procedure. The most frequent symptoms include abdominal pain and distention. Constipation and obstipation, diarrhea, and nausea and vomiting also can occur. Physical examination usually shows tympani to percussion and mild tenderness with palpation. Abdominal radiographs show marked colonic distention typically localized to the right colon. The management of colonic pseudoobstruction is nonoperative initially and consists of nasogastric decompression, correction of fluid and electrolyte imbalances, gentle enemas, rectal tube placement, and avoidance of narcotics and anticholinergics. With these conservative measures, colonic pseudoobstruction usually resolves in more than 75% of cases. If conservative measures fail or when the luminal diameter of the cecum reaches 10 to 12 cm, a more aggressive approach is warranted because of the risk of cecal perforation. Decompressive colonoscopy has historically been the method of choice in this setting. Intravenous administration of 2.5 mg neostigmine over 2 to 3 minutes has been found to promptly decompress the colon for nearly all patients. Surgery is reserved for patients with obvious peritoneal signs or instances in which all forms of nonoperative therapy fail. In the latter setting, in which the possibility of cecal perforation is high, cecostomy is warranted.

ANSWER: b, c, d

REFERENCE: *Chapter 43—Colonic Anatomy and Physiology: Colonic Pseudoobstruction*

4. Which of the following statements is/are true regarding the arterial and venous systems of the colon?

a. The right colic artery always arises from the superior mesenteric artery

b. The inferior mesenteric vein joins the superior mesenteric vein to form the portal vein

c. The superior hemorrhoidal veins drain into the portal system through the inferior mesenteric vein, whereas the middle and inferior hemorrhoidal veins drain blood into the systemic venous circulation through the internal iliac veins

d. The marginal artery of Drummond is made up of a series of arterial arcades along the mesenteric border of the colon

e. The superior mesenteric artery arises from the infrarenal aorta, passes posteriorly to the pancreas, and passes anteriorly to the third portion of the duodenum

COMMENT: The superior mesenteric artery arises from the suprarenal aorta, runs posteriorly to the pancreas, and passes anteriorly to the third portion of the duodenum. The superior mesenteric artery gives rise to the ileocolic and middle colic branches that supply the cecum, ascending colon, and proximal transverse colon. The right colic artery, which also supplies the ascending colon, can originate as a branch of the ileocolic artery or it can arise directly from the superior mesenteric artery. The inferior mesenteric artery arises from the infrarenal aorta and supplies the distal transverse colon, descending colon, sigmoid colon, and upper rectum through its left colic, sigmoidal, and superior hemorrhoidal branches. The middle and inferior hemorrhoidal arteries arise from the hypogastric arteries and supply the distal two thirds of the rectum. A series of arterial arcades along the mesenteric border of the entire colon, known as the *marginal artery of Drummond*, connect the superior mesenteric and inferior mesenteric arterial systems.

The veins that drain the large intestine bear the same terminology and follow a similar course to the corresponding arteries. The veins from the right colon and transverse colon, along with the veins draining the small intestine, drain into the superior mesenteric vein. The superior mesenteric vein runs slightly anterior and to the right of the superior mesenteric artery. The superior mesenteric vein courses beneath the neck of the pancreas, where it joins the splenic vein to form the portal vein. The inferior mesenteric vein drains blood from the left colon, sigmoid colon, rectum, and superior anal canal. The inferior mesenteric vein ascends over the psoas muscle in a retroperitoneal plane. The vein courses under the body of the pancreas to drain into the splenic vein. The superior hemorrhoidal veins drain blood from the rectum into the portal system through the inferior mesenteric vein. The middle and inferior hemorrhoidal veins drain blood from the lower rectum and anal canal into the systemic venous circulation through the internal iliac veins.

ANSWER: c, d

REFERENCE: *Chapter 43—Colonic Anatomy and Physiology: Anatomy of the Colon; Arterial Blood Supply*

5. Which if the following statements is/are true about the neural components of the colon?
   a. Meissner's plexus is located in the submucosa between the muscularis mucosa and the circular muscle of the muscularis propria
   b. Auerbach's plexus is located between the circular and longitudinal muscles of the colon
   c. Input from sympathetic nerves generally stimulates colonic motility
   d. Input from parasympathetic nerves generally stimulates colonic motility

COMMENT: The colon possesses extrinsic and intrinsic (enteric) neuronal systems. The extrinsic system consists of sympathetic nerves that generally inhibit and parasympathetic nerves that stimulate colonic peristalsis. The intrinsic or enteric nervous system consists of two groups of plexuses in the wall of the colon. These plexuses are identified by their location within the wall of the colon. Meissner's plexus is located in the submucosa between the muscularis mucosae and the circular muscle of the muscularis propria. The myenteric plexus, also known as Auerbach's plexus, is located between the inner circular muscle and outer longitudinal muscle layers of the colon.

ANSWER: a, b, d

REFERENCE: *Chapter 43—Colonic Anatomy and Physiology: Anatomy of the Colon; Neural Components*

CHAPTER 44

ULCERATIVE COLITIS

1. Which of the following statements is/are correct regarding ulcerative colitis?

   a. The most common age at onset for ulcerative colitis is early adulthood
   b. Approximately 25% of cases of ulcerative colitis occur after the age of 60 years
   c. The frequency is the same for both sexes
   d. Approximately 10% to 25% of patients with ulcerative colitis have first-degree relatives with the disease

COMMENT: Most cases of ulcerative colitis have an onset between the ages of 15 and 40 years. Although the age at onset can extend to old age, only 3% to 5% of cases have an onset after 60 years of age. The sexes are affected equally frequently. Clear-cut familial patterns of ulcerative colitis have been observed. Ten percent to 25% of patients with this disease have first-degree relatives with ulcerative colitis. Monozygotic twins have higher concordance for inflammatory bowel disease than do dizygotic twins. Geographic and racial differences influence the occurrence of the disease. There is no definitive evidence regarding the role of genetic and environmental influences in the determination of familial patterns.

ANSWER: a, d

REFERENCE: *Chapter 44—Ulcerative Colitis: Epidemiology*

2. Which of the following features would be more consistent with Crohn's disease than with ulcerative colitis?

   a. Transmural inflammation
   b. Microscopic evidence of granuloma within mucosal biopsy specimens
   c. Microscopic evidence of submucosal thickening and fibrosis
   d. Microscopic evidence of submucosal inflammation

COMMENT: Transmural changes are found in Crohn's disease of the colon, in which all layers of the colonic wall can be involved in a granulomatous inflammatory process. In the earliest stages, the lesions consist of infiltration of round cells and polymorphonuclear leukocytes into the crypts of Lieberkühn at the base of the mucosa. Crypt abscesses are common. Microscopic examination shows vacuolization of overlying epithelial cells, swelling of mitochondria, and widening of intercellular spaces. Submucosal thickening and fibrosis associated with recurrent submucosal inflammation are more common in Crohn's disease than in ulcerative colitis.

ANSWER: a, b, c, d

REFERENCE: *Chapter 44—Ulcerative Colitis: Pathology*

3. Which of the following ocular manifestations of ulcerative colitis respond(s) to therapy with steroids or immunosuppressive agents?

   a. Iritis
   b. Uveitis
   c. Retrobulbar neuritis
   d. Ulcerative panophthalmitis

COMMENT: A number of ocular manifestations of ulcerative colitis exist. Included in this group are iritis, uveitis, conjunctivitis, episcleritis, retinitis, and retrobulbar neuritis. With the exception of ulcerative panophthalmitis, ocular symptoms are closely related to disease activity and respond to therapy with steroids or immunosuppressive agents.

ANSWER: a, b, c

REFERENCE: *Chapter 44—Ulcerative Colitis: Clinical Features*

4. A 19-year-old man has bloody diarrhea (10 bowel movements per day) and weight loss (10 pounds [4.5 kg]). Physical examination reveals two circular, 4-cm erythematous lesions on the trunk. Each lesion has an area of necrosis in the center. The abdominal examination reveals mild hypogastric tenderness. The stool is guaiac positive. The most appropriate next diagnostic step is which of the following?

   a. Barium enema
   b. Flexible sigmoidoscopy
   c. Liver biopsy
   d. Chest radiograph

COMMENT: The diagnosis of ulcerative colitis is one of exclusion. There are no definitive, laboratory, radiologic, or histologic features. All patients with bloody diarrhea should have an infectious cause excluded. Stool samples and biopsy specimens should be evaluated for *Campylobacter, Salmonella,* pathogenic *Escherichia coli,* and *Clostridium difficile* organisms and amebic colitis. Flexible sigmoidoscopy is the first step in diagnosis, because ulcerative colitis involves the distal colon and rectum in 90% to 95% of cases. Mild cases may show only a loss of normal vascular pattern, a granular texture, and microhemorrhages when the friable mucosa is touched with the endoscope. Advanced cases are characterized by spontaneous bleeding, ulceration, and purulent exudate. Mucosal biopsy is essential in establishing the diagnosis. Lesions of the skin and oral cavity are frequently found among patients with ulcerative colitis. Pyoderma gangrenosum occurs among approximately 1% of patients.

ANSWER: b

REFERENCE: *Chapter 44—Ulcerative Colitis: Diagnosis*

5. Which of the following statements is/are correct regarding the risk of cancer in the context of ulcerative colitis?

   a. After 10 years of active disease, the risk of cancer approximates 20% to 30%
   b. After 10 years of active disease, the risk of cancer approximates 2% to 3%
   c. The risk of colon cancer among persons with ulcerative colitis is identical to than among healthy controls
   d. After 20 years of disease activity, the risk of colon cancer approximates 80%

COMMENT: Marked dysplasia or suspected colon cancer is a clear indication for colectomy in the care of patients with ulcerative colitis. Earlier studies have suggested that the risk of cancer is relatively low for the first 10 years after the onset of disease activity (approximately 2% to 3%). The incidence of colon cancer then begins to climb at a rate of 1% to 2% per year. By the time the patient has had ulcerative colitis for 20 years, the risk of colon cancer approximates 20%. Many epidemiologists believe that earlier studies overestimated the risk of malignant disease because of referral bias and the imperfection of retrospective surveys performed in tertiary referral hospitals.

ANSWER: b

REFERENCE: *Chapter 44—Ulcerative Colitis: Indications for Surgery; Cancer Prophylaxis*

6. A 25-year-old woman with known ulcerative colitis arrives in the emergency department with a 24-hour history of abdominal pain, distention, and obstipation. Physical examination reveals a temperature of 38.6°C, abdominal distention, and diffuse abdominal tenderness. Abdominal radiographs show marked colonic dilatation, most pronounced in the transverse colon. Laboratory examination reveals a white blood cell count of 19,000/µL. Over the first 24 hours of hospitalization, symptoms are progressive despite intravenous fluid resuscitation, nasogastric suctioning, and intravenous administration of antibiotics. The most appropriate treatment of this patient includes which of the following?

a. Decompressive colonoscopy
b. Proctocolectomy with formation of end ileostomy
c. Total abdominal colectomy with formation of Hartmann pouch and end ileostomy
d. Cecostomy

COMMENT: Acute toxic megacolon occurs among 6% to 13% of patients with ulcerative colitis. Initial management of toxic megacolon includes intravenous fluid and electrolyte resuscitation, nasogastric suctioning, administration of broad-spectrum antibiotics, and total parenteral nutrition. The therapeutic role of intravenous steroids in toxic megacolon is controversial. Most patients with a severe attack of ulcerative colitis are already receiving steroid therapy and need stress doses of glucocorticoids to prevent adrenal crisis. When symptoms are progressive or when there is evidence of colonic perforation, emergency surgery is indicated.

Postoperative complications, including sepsis, wound infection, intraperitoneal abscess, fistula formation, and delayed wound healing, are common and have been reported among as many as 50% of patients. The presence of colonic perforation doubles operative risk. In the presence of toxic megacolon or colonic perforation, the operation should be definitive without being overly aggressive. Abdominal colectomy with ileostomy and Hartmann closure of the rectum is the best procedure. After recovery, a delayed operation for restoration of continence can be performed. Leaving the rectum intact allows it to be used for subsequent mucosal proctectomy and ileoanal anastomosis.

ANSWER: c

REFERENCE: *Chapter 44—Ulcerative Colitis: Indications for Surgery; Surgical Emergencies*

7. The most common postoperative complication after formation of a continent ileostomy (Kock pouch) is which of the following?

a. Failure of the nipple valve
b. Small-bowel obstruction
c. Pancreatitis
d. Ischemic necrosis of the pouch

COMMENT: Continent ileostomy has been associated with a high postoperative complication rate. Most complications are related to displacement of the nipple valve, which produces fecal incontinence and difficulty inserting the tube and emptying the pouch. Valve failure has been reported to occur among as many as 40% of patients. Ten percent to 20% of patients have postoperative bowel obstruction. Several syndromes of ileostomy dysfunction related to the Kock pouch have been reported. These are variably described as stagnant loop syndrome, pouchitis, and nonspecific ileitis. Clinical features include diarrhea, malabsorption of fat and vitamin B_{12}, proliferation of anaerobic bacteria, inflammation of the pouch, and incontinence. Crohn's disease is a clear contraindication for this operation, because the rate of postoperative complication is much higher in this group.

ANSWER: a

REFERENCE: *Chapter 44—Ulcerative Colitis: Indications for Surgery; Continent Ileostomy*

8. Many patients with ulcerative colitis undergo elective total abdominal colectomy, rectal mucosectomy, formation of a small-intestinal reservoir, and ileoanal anastomosis. The most common postoperative complication after this operation is which of the following?

a. Enterocutaneous fistula
b. Small-bowel obstruction
c. Pulmonary embolism
d. Urinary retention

COMMENT: The most common complication of restorative proctocolectomy is small-bowel obstruction. The rate of bowel obstruction necessitating reoperation has been reported to be 10% to 20% in most series of patients undergoing ileal pouch–anal anastomosis. Pelvic and wound infections have been reported to occur among 10% of patients undergoing ileoanal anastomosis, although the overall infection rate has been approximately 5% in several series. Conversion to permanent ileostomy because of postoperative complications is necessary for fewer than 5% of patients.

ANSWER: b

REFERENCE: *Chapter 44—Ulcerative Colitis: Indications for Surgery; Ileoanal Anastomosis*

9. A 30-year-old man who had undergone total abdominal colectomy with ileoanal anastomosis 2 years previously reports a sudden increase in stool frequency, nocturnal leakage, and low-grade fevers. The findings at physical examination are unremarkable. Flexible endoscopic examination of the small-intestinal pouch reveals friable erythematous mucosa. Biopsy specimens of the mucosa are obtained. While awaiting biopsy results, which of the following is the most appropriate empiric therapy?

a. Oral glucocorticoids
b. Oral vancomycin
c. Oral metronidazole
d. Glucocorticoid enema

COMMENT: Nonspecific enteritis or pouchitis is the most common late complication of ileal pouch–anal anastomosis, occurring among as many as 15% of patients. The clinical symptoms include high stool frequency, watery stools, fat malabsorption, urgency, nocturnal leakage, and rectal bleeding. Patients may have fever, malaise, and arthralgia. The cause of this condition is unknown. Most patients respond to treatment with metronidazole.

ANSWER: c

REFERENCE: *Chapter 44—Ulcerative Colitis: Indications for Surgery; Ileoanal Anastomosis*

10. One year after ileal pouch–anal anastomosis, mean 24-hour stool frequency is which of the following?

a. Two to three
b. Five to six
c. Eight to nine
d. Eleven to twelve

COMMENT: Overall mean 24-hour stool frequency is five or six bowel movements in the late follow-up period after ileal pouch–anal anastomosis.

ANSWER: b

REFERENCE: *Chapter 44—Ulcerative Colitis: Indications for Surgery; Ileoanal Anastomosis*

CHAPTER 45

COLONIC POLYPS AND POLYPOSIS SYNDROMES

1. A 52-year-old man undergoes screening colonoscopy. A 3-cm sessile polyp is found in the mid transverse colon. Biopsy reveals that the lesion is an adenomatous polyp. The risk that the lesion harbors carcinoma approximates:

a. 10%
b. 20%
c. 40%
d. 80%

COMMENT: Although all adenocarcinoma of the colon and rectum arises in adenomatous polyps, not all polyps evolve into carcinoma. The malignant potential of adenomatous polyps is related to polyp size and histologic characteristics. Large polyps and those with a higher proportion of villous architecture are more likely to contain coincident carcinoma. These features are interdependent, however, because large polyps are more likely to be villous and to contain higher degrees of dysplasia. Adenomas 0.5 cm or less in diameter are most often tubular adenoma and rarely contain severe dysplasia or carcinoma (less than 0.5% in autopsy series). Likewise, only 1% to 2% of adenomatous polyps smaller than 1 cm contain carcinoma, but autopsy studies suggest that 40% of adenomas larger than 2 cm contain cancer. Data derived from examination of colonoscopic polypectomy specimens indicate similar trends but suggest a lower incidence of cancer-containing polyps.

ANSWER: c

REFERENCE: *Chapter 45—Colonic Polyps and Polyposis Syndromes: Neoplastic Mucosal Polyps; Histopathology and Malignant Potential*

2. For adults without symptoms, the recommended program for screening for colorectal carcinoma is:

 a. Yearly colonoscopy and semiannual fecal occult blood testing beginning at 40 years of age
 b. Colonoscopy every 5 years and yearly fecal occult blood testing beginning at 50 years of age
 c. Yearly colonoscopy and yearly fecal occult blood testing beginning at 50 years of age
 d. Yearly barium enema beginning at 60 years of age

COMMENT: The National Cancer Institute, the American Cancer Society, the American College of Physicians, the American Gastroenterological Association, and the World Health Organization Collaborating Center for Prevention of Colorectal Cancer advocate screening sigmoidoscopy every 5 years in conjunction with yearly fecal occult blood tests beginning at 50 years of age. The benefit of sigmoidoscopy in interrupting the adenoma to carcinoma sequence is suggested by results of a number of studies. Investigators compared the use of rigid sigmoidoscopy to examine 261 members of the Kaiser Permanente Medical Care Program who died of cancer of the rectum or distal colon with use of the procedure to examine 868 matched controls. Only 8.8% of those with cancer had undergone screening sigmoidoscopy; 24.2% of controls had done so. The helpfulness of sigmoidoscopy was limited to development of fatal colon cancer within reach of the sigmoidoscope and was long standing, at least 10 years.

ANSWER: b

REFERENCE: *Chapter 45—Colonic Polyps and Polyposis Syndromes; Neoplastic Mucosal Polyps, Pathogenesis*

3. During colonoscopy for investigation of occult fecal blood loss, an ulcerated lesion is identified in the sigmoid colon that suggests carcinoma. In the cecum, a second 3-mm lesion is found. Appropriate treatment includes:

 a. Electrical ablation of the cecal lesion with biopsy forceps
 b. Subtotal colectomy
 c. Segmental ascending and sigmoid colectomy
 d. Observation only for the cecal lesion

COMMENT: Once detected, adenoma should be completely removed, preferably by means of endoscopic snare polypectomy. Polypectomy is relatively safe and easily performed when adenomas are small or pedunculated but is more difficult when polyps are large or sessile. Potential complications include bleeding and perforation of the polypectomy site. Large sessile villous adenoma (more than 2 cm in diameter) have great potential for malignant degeneration. If such lesions cannot be completely removed by means of snare polypectomy, segmental surgical resection may be necessary. Diminutive polyps have little malignant potential. If they are too small for snare polypectomy, ablation with a hot biopsy forceps is a reasonable approach. Because 30% to 50% of patients with one adenoma have synchronous adenoma elsewhere in the colon, the entire colon should be "cleared" by means of colonoscopy if a patient has a polyp.

ANSWER: a

REFERENCE: *Chapter 45—Colonic Polyps and Polyposis Syndromes: Neoplastic Mucosal Polyps; Management of Adenomas*

4. A pedunculated polyp is found during colonoscopy of the ascending colon and is removed by means of snare technique. Histologic examination reveals carcinoma in the head of the polyp. The stalk margin does not contain neoplasia. Lymphatic invasion is not found. Appropriate therapy includes:

a. Colonoscopy in 1 year
b. Right hemicolectomy
c. Subtotal colectomy
d. Radiation therapy

COMMENT: Endoscopic polypectomy is adequate therapy for an adenomatous polyp that contains cancer if the polyp is known to be confined to the head of the polyp (carcinoma in situ or intramucosal carcinoma). The adequacy of simple polypectomy has been controversial in cases in which malignant cells have invaded the polyp stalk, but most studies indicate that polypectomy is adequate treatment provided a margin greater than 2 mm is present, the cancer is not poorly differentiated, and there is no vascular or lymphatic invasion. The presence of cancer at or near the margin is associated with adverse outcome, even in the absence of other unfavorable factors. In the absence of unfavorable histologic findings and with a negative margin, the incidence of residual cancer is low (less than 1%). These criteria are more difficult to assess for sessile polyps. If an adequate margin cannot be assured or histologic findings are abnormal, surgery is recommended to control the risk of regional lymph node metastasis.

ANSWER: a

REFERENCE: *Chapter 45—Colonic Polyps and Polyposis Syndromes: Neoplastic Mucosal Polyps; Management of Adenomas*

5. A 24-year-old has rectal bleeding. Sigmoidoscopic evaluation reveals approximately 30 polyps in the rectum and sigmoid colon. The likely diagnosis and appropriate therapy are:

a. Familial adenomatous polyposis (FAP) and colectomy
b. Familial adenomatous polyposis and colonoscopic polypectomy
c. Ulcerative colitis and colectomy
d. Ulcerative colitis and steroid enemas

COMMENT: Surgery is the only reasonable management option for FAP. The clinical decision involves selection of the operation and its timing. The diagnosis of FAP often is made in adolescence, but there is typically a delay of 20 years or more from the appearance of the first adenoma until cancer develops. It usually is prudent to wait until the patient has reached full physical maturity before surgery is planned. The safest surgical approach is total proctocolectomy with ileoanal anastomosis. Any residual rectal mucosa left behind is at risk of neoplasia. Even with careful endoscopic surveillance of the rectal segment, invasive carcinomas can develop.

ANSWER: a

REFERENCE: *Chapter 45—Colonic Polyps and Polyposis Syndromes: Gastrointestinal Polyposis Syndromes; Management*

CHAPTER 46

COLORECTAL CANCER

1. Dietary risk factors thought to play a causative role in development of colorectal cancer include which of the following?
   a. High fat intake
   b. Low fiber intake
   c. High intake of smoked food
   d. High vegetable intake

COMMENT: Evidence from epidemiologic studies suggests that dietary factors play important causative roles in the development of large bowel cancer. Fat intake has had the most consistently positive association and fiber intake the most consistently inverse association with incidence of colorectal cancer. In comparisons between countries, the rates of colon cancer are strongly associated with the intake of animal fat and meat. The associations between per capita consumption of total fat, saturated fat, and cholesterol and national incidences of colon cancer are strongly positive. The proposed mechanism by which dietary fat increases the risk of colonic cancer is interaction with bile acids.

The relation between fiber intake and colon cancer was initially described by Burkitt, who reported low rates of colon cancer in areas of Africa where fiber consumption and stool bulk were high. In general, epidemiologic studies have shown that fiber intake is higher in non-western countries with lower incidences of colon cancer. The role of fiber was originally seen simply as providing bulk to dilute potential carcinogens and speed their transit through the colon. This appears to be an oversimplification—the relation between fiber intake and colon cancer is more complex. Results of additional studies suggest that certain fibers may bind mutagens, which may reduce their contact with colonic epithelium, favorably change fecal pH, and participate in other complex interactions.

ANSWER: a, b

REFERENCE: *Chapter 46—Colorectal Cancer: Etiology; Dietary Factors*

2. The most common oncogene abnormality observed in association with colorectal cancer is which of the following?
   a. Overexpression of the N-*myc* oncogene
   b. Amplification of the K-*ras* oncogene
   c. Suppression of the *erb*-B oncogene
   d. Amplification of the L-*myc* oncogene

COMMENT: In colon cancer, an important genetic alteration is mutation of the K-*ras* protooncogene. The *ras* protooncogenes are a family of normal genes (N-*ras*, H-*ras,* and K-*ras*) highly conserved in nature that encode for the production of guanosine triphosphate binding proteins (G proteins), which are important for signal transduction. G proteins are involved in transduction of proliferative signals induced by growth factors or factors involved in cell differentiation. The product of a mutated *ras* gene is an abnormal G protein that has lost its ability to become inactivated and thus causes continuous growth stimulation and autonomous cell growth or differentiation. In experiments, transfection of normal fibroblasts by mutated *ras* genes confers neoplastic properties to those cells.

Approximately one half of cases of colorectal carcinoma and a similar percentage of cases of adenoma larger than 1 cm in diameter have been found to have the *ras* gene mutations. In contrast, fewer than 10% of patients with adenoma smaller than 1 cm have this mutation. It has been postulated that the *ras* gene mutation may be the initiating event in some types of colorectal carcinoma or may promote clonal expansion of a mutated cell population. It appears that the *ras* gene mutation alone is not responsible for tumorigenesis. Additional molecular events appear to be necessary.

ANSWER: b

REFERENCE: *Chapter 46—Colorectal Cancer: Etiology; Molecular Genetics*

3. Which of the following tumor suppressor genes has/have been associated with the development of colorectal cancer?

   a. The *DCC* gene
   b. The *APC* gene
   c. The *p53* gene
   d. The *Rb* gene

COMMENT: Loss of specific chromosomal regions represents genetic alteration associated with the development of colorectal neoplasms in a high percentage of cases. These chromosomal regions have been hypothesized to contain tumor suppressor genes the products of which normally regulate growth and differentiation in a negative manner. One such gene linked to familial adenomatous polyposis was mapped to the long arm of chromosome 5q and referred to as the APC (adenomatosis polyposis coli) gene. The gene codes for a 300-kd protein that binds to β-catenin, implying an important role in cell adhesion and possibly cytoskeleton function. It is hypothesized that disruption of cell adhesion and cytoskeleton function can lead to loss of contact inhibition, which may promote neoplastic transformation and invasiveness of cancer cells.

Another tumor suppressor gene thought to be important in colorectal tumorigenesis is the p53 gene located on chromosome 17p. Alteration in p53 is one of the most common genetic events in malignant disease among humans. The p53 gene produces a DNA-binding phosphoprotein important in cell proliferation, differentiation, and cell survival. Allelic loss of p53 has been found in more than 75% of persons with colorectal carcinoma.

Another common genetic alteration associated with colorectal tumors is allelic loss of chromosome 18q. This is where the "deleted in colorectal carcinoma" gene, also called *DCC,* is located. Mutations in DCC are present in 47% of persons with late adenoma and 73% of those with carcinoma. The DCC protein shares homology with the neural cell adhesion molecule family that regulates cell adhesion and recognition.

ANSWER: a, b, c

REFERENCE: *Chapter 46—Colorectal Cancer: Etiology; Molecular Genetics*

4. Which of the following types of colonic polyps is/are associated with the highest incidence of malignant degeneration?

   a. Tubular adenoma
   b. Tubulovillous adenoma
   c. Villous adenoma
   d. Hamartomatous polyp

COMMENT: Adenoma can be tubular (75% to 100% tubular component), tubulovillous (25% to 75% villous component), or villous (75% to 100% villous). The most common type is tubular adenoma, or adenomatous polyp, which constitutes approximately 75% of neoplastic polyps. Tubulovillous adenoma represents 15% and pure villous adenoma 10% of neoplastic polyps. All adenomas contain some degree of dysplasia or cellular atypia. This dysplasia can be graded from mild to severe. Carcinoma in situ and severe dysplasia have been grouped together under the classification high-grade dysplasia. In carcinoma in situ, there is no invasion into the muscularis mucosa as there is in invasive carcinoma. The incidence of invasive malignant growth differs markedly for the three types of adenomas and increases with the size of the lesion. In general, malignant growth occurs in 5% of adenomatous polyps, 22% of tubulovillous adenomas, and in 40% of villous lesions. Although villous lesions are much less common, they are more likely to harbor a malignant tumor.

ANSWER: c

REFERENCE: *Chapter 46—Colorectal Cancer: Clinical Risk Factors; Polyps*

5. A 52-year-old man undergoes right hemicolectomy for carcinoma of the ascending colon. Pathologic examination of the resected specimen reveals invasion of the tumor to the level of the muscularis propria. Three of 17 lymph nodes contain microscopic tumor. What are the correct Dukes classification (Astler-Coller modification) and associated 5-year survival rate for this lesion?

a. Dukes C2, 45% 5-year survival rate
b. Dukes B1, 75% 5-year survival rate
c. Dukes C1, 45% 5-year survival rate
d. Dukes B3, 65% 5-year survival rate

COMMENT: One of the more commonly used staging systems is the modified Astler-Coller system. According to this system, stage A represents tumors that invade into the mucosa only. Stage B1 tumors invade into but not through the muscularis propria. Stage B2 lesions invade through the bowel wall without adjacent organ involvement, whereas stage B3 tumors involve adjacent organs. Stage C tumors involve regional lymph nodes and are subgrouped into stages C1, C2, and C3, according to depth of bowel-wall penetration. Stage D represents evidence of distant organ involvement. In general, the 5-year survival rate among patients with stage D disease is less than 10%. Overall, the 5-year survival rates for stages A, B, and C are 90%, 77%, and 47%, respectively. Additional studies have revealed that among patients with Dukes stage C disease, the number of positive nodes is an important predictor of survival.

ANSWER: c

REFERENCE: *Chapter 46—Colorectal Cancer: Staging; Modified Astler-Coller Staging System*

6. A pedunculated polyp, found incidentally at colonoscopy, is removed by means of snare polypectomy from the ascending colon. Invasive cancer to the level of the submucosa is identified histologically within the polyp. The lesion is well differentiated. No lymphatic or vascular invasion is found. The cauterized margin does not contain neoplasia. Appropriate subsequent management includes which of the following?

a. Endoscopy in 6 months
b. Right hemicolectomy
c. Subtotal colectomy
d. Repeat endoscopy with fulguration of the polypectomy site

COMMENT: With the availability of colonoscopy, endoscopic polypectomy has become the standard approach to the management of neoplastic polyps. The risk of this procedure is extremely low; the complication rate is less than 1%. Almost all pedunculated polyps can be removed endoscopically with a snare. A dilemma in the management of colonic polyps occurs when a resected lesion contains a malignant focus. A decision must be made about the need for colectomy. If the lesion does not penetrate the muscularis mucosae, it should be considered an in situ malignant tumor that does not have the propensity to metastasize and therefore does not necessitate further surgery. If the lesion penetrates the muscularis mucosae, it is invasive cancer and may necessitate surgery. In selected cases of pedunculated polyps, conservative management without colectomy can be undertaken if the lesion does not contain poorly differentiated tumor cells or evidence of vascular invasion and if a negative resection margin has been obtained at the level of the stalk. Lesions that are poorly differentiated or have evidence of vascular invasion, regardless of a negative surgical margin, should be managed by means of colectomy.

ANSWER: a

REFERENCE: *Chapter 46—Colorectal Cancer: Treatment of Primary Colorectal Tumors; Neoplastic Polyps*

7. Which of the following statements is/are true with regard to resection of rectal cancer?

a. A distal margin of 5 cm should be obtained because 42% of patients have microscopic evidence of intramural spread beyond 3 cm from the palpable tumor
b. A distal margin of 3 cm should be obtained because only 3% of patients have microscopic evidence of intramural spread beyond 2 cm from the palpable tumor
c. Local recurrence rates correlate strongly with distal margins less than 4 cm
d. There is no correlation between local recurrence and distal margins beyond 2 cm

COMMENT: One of the controversies surrounding sphincter-saving procedures for rectal tumors is the length of adequate distal mucosal margin. The traditional dictum of 5 cm for a margin is not substantiated by any studies. Only 2.5% of patients have intramural spread beyond 2 cm from the palpable tumor, and these patients generally have dissemination of tumor despite aggressive local therapy. There is no correlation between local recurrence and the extent of distal margin when it is greater than 2 cm. A surgical margin of 3 cm, measured on the fresh specimen, ideally should be achieved.

ANSWER: b, d

REFERENCE: *Chapter 46—Colorectal Cancer: Treatment of Primary Colorectal Tumors; Intraperitoneal Colon and Upper Third of the Rectum*

8. A 72-year-old woman undergoes anterior resection of a rectal tumor located 7 cm proximal to the anal verge. Pathologic examination of the resected specimen reveals invasion of the tumor into the muscularis propria. Five of eight lymph nodes contain microscopic tumor. There is no evidence of disseminated disease. Appropriate subsequent management includes which of the following?

a. Postoperative radiation plus intravenous 5-fluorouracil
b. Postoperative radiation alone
c. Observation
d. Postoperative radiation plus intravenous doxorubicin hydrochloride (Adriamycin)

COMMENT: In the management of rectal cancer, it is almost as important to prevent local failure and ensuing symptoms as it is to prevent death of distant failure. Radiation therapy is recommended for patients with stage II or III rectal cancers. In a randomized, prospective study, 204 patients with stage II or III rectal cancer were randomized to receive postoperative radiation alone or radiation therapy plus 5-fluorouracil and semustine chemotherapy. The group who received chemotherapy had improved local tumor control and a higher overall survival rate. In another prospective study, semustine was found not to be an essential component of effective adjuvant therapy. Because of these results and those of other clinical studies, the National Institutes of Health has recommended that patients with stage II or III rectal cancer receive postoperative chemotherapy and radiation therapy as standard care.

ANSWER: a

REFERENCE: *Chapter 46—Colorectal Cancer: Treatment of Primary Colorectal Tumors; Adjuvant Chemotherapy*

9. Which of the following statements is/are correct with regard to the use of carcinoembryonic antigen (CEA) determinations in the management of colorectal cancer?

   a. Carcinoembryonic antigen determination has 95% specificity when used for screening for development of colon cancer among patients with ulcerative colitis
   b. Carcinoembryonic antigen levels are increased among 20% of patients with local recurrence after resection
   c. Carcinoembryonic antigen measurements are increased among 90% of patients with disseminated disease
   d. Carcinoembryonic antigen levels are increased among 90% of patients with local recurrence after resection

COMMENT: Carcinoembryonic antigen is a glycoprotein originally described to be a tumor-specific antigen derived from neoplasms of the gastrointestinal tract. Carcinoembryonic antigen is an oncofetal antigen because it also is expressed by early embryonic or fetal cells. It is now known that CEA is not tumor specific because it can be elevated by a variety of malignant tumors from different sites and by some benign conditions. Measurement of CEA is not useful as a screening or diagnostic test but is useful as a tumor marker. The level of CEA is elevated among more than 90% of patients with disseminated colorectal cancer and approximately 20% of patients with localized disease. Serum levels generally are elevated in proportion to the mass of the tumor and often correlate with response to therapy. Levels of CEA are useful when elevated levels decrease to normal after curative resection. Among approximately two thirds of patients with recurrent disease, increased CEA level is the first indicator of the tumor, and serial CEA measurement, combined with regular physical examinations, is one of the most useful tests for detecting recurrent colorectal cancer.

ANSWER: b, c

REFERENCE: *Chapter 46—Colorectal Cancer: Treatment of Recurrent Colorectal Cancer*

10. A 58-year-old man undergoes resection of Dukes C2 carcinoma of the colon by means of right hemicolectomy. Three years postoperatively, increasing CEA levels prompt evaluation, including abdominal computed tomography. Two lesions, each measuring 2 cm, are found in the right hepatic lobe. No other abnormalities are found. Right hepatic lobectomy is performed without complication. Which of the following most closely approximates the anticipated 5-year survival rate?

   a. 85% to 90%
   b. 65% to 70%
   c. 45% to 50%
   d. 25% to 30%

COMMENT: The liver is the most frequent site of blood-borne metastasis from primary colorectal cancer. In a subgroup of patients, the liver may be the only site of recurrent disease, and surgical excision of the metastatic lesions is the only curative option for these patients. Overall, surgical resection is associated with a 25% to 30% 5-year survival rate. Patients eligible for hepatic resection of metastatic disease are those who have no evidence of extrahepatic tumor, no medical contraindications to surgery, and fewer than four lesions amenable to resection with negative surgical margins.

ANSWER: d

REFERENCE: *Chapter 46—Colorectal Cancer: Treatment of Colorectal Cancer; Hepatic Metastases*

11. A 52-year-old man without symptoms is undergoing screening sigmoidoscopy. A 2-cm, yellow, submucosal nodule is found in the rectum 6 cm from the anal verge. Findings at deep endoscopic biopsy suggest carcinoid. Appropriate management includes which of the following?

    a. Observation
    b. Transanal excision
    c. Low anterior resection
    d. Abdominoperineal resection

COMMENT: Most carcinoids in the gastrointestinal tract occur in the ileum and the appendix. The rectum is the next most common site, and occasional carcinoid tumors occur in the colon. Tumor size is an extremely important prognostic factor. Approximately 60% of rectal carcinoids manifest as asymptomatic submucosal nodules less than 2 cm in diameter. Transanal local excision suffices for definitive therapy because small tumors rarely metastasize. Malignant potential is seen almost exclusively among patients with tumors larger than 2 cm. More radical excision of larger rectal lesions may be needed for local control; however, the results of radical excision of large rectal carcinoids are poor because the lesions are likely to metastasize.

ANSWER: b

REFERENCE: *Chapter 46—Colorectal Cancer: Other Colorectal Tumors; Carcinoid Tumors*

CHAPTER 47

ANAL CANCER

1. A 43-year-old woman has anal pain and spotting of blood with defecation. Physical examination reveals a 2 by 3 cm area of ulceration within the anal canal. The other findings at physical examination are normal. Incisional biopsy shows squamous cell carcinoma. Appropriate management includes which of the following?

    a. Abdominoperineal resection
    b. Wide local excision, skin grafting, proximal diverting colostomy
    c. Primary radiation therapy
    d. Local excision and primary closure

COMMENT: For localized squamous cell cancer of the anal canal, the most effective protocol consists of primary radiation therapy and chemotherapy. The treatment regimen includes the following:

1. External irradiation—3,000 rad (30 Gy) to the primary tumor and pelvic and inguinal nodes from day 1 to day 21 (200 rad/d, 5 days a week)
2. Systemic chemotherapy—1,000 mg 5-fluorouracil per square meter per 24 hours as a continuous infusion for 4 days, starting on day 1 of radiation therapy and repeated on days 28 through 31
3. Mitomycin C—15 mg/m^2 intravenous bolus on day 1

If the lesion cannot be seen at gross inspection and its microscopic absence is confirmed by means of biopsy, no further treatment is necessary.

ANSWER: c

REFERENCE: *Chapter 47—Anal Cancer: Neoplasms of the Anal Canal; Squamous Cell Carcinoma*

2. A 72-year-old woman has anal itching and burning. Physical examination reveals an erythematous, scaly lesion, 3 cm in circumference, within the anal canal. The intersphincteric groove can not be appreciated in the area of the lesion. The other findings at physical examination are normal. Appropriate initial management includes which of the following?

a. Acyclovir 200 mg four times a day for 10 days
b. Hydrocortisone cream 0.1% topically for 14 days
c. Incisional biopsy
d. Metronidazole 250 mg by mouth four times a day for 14 days

COMMENT: Extramammary Paget's disease can be found in the axilla and in the anogenital region, including the labia majora, penis, scrotum, groin, pubic area, perineum, perianal region, thigh, and buttock. Paget's disease of the perianal area is a malignant neoplasm of the intraepidermal portion of apocrine glands with or without associated dermal involvement. Paget's disease has a long preinvasive phase, but if the patient is not treated, invasive adenocarcinoma of the apocrine gland type develops. The disease is more common among women than among men, with the highest incidence in the seventh decade of life.

Macroscopically the lesion appears as an erythematous scaly or eczematoid plaque-like lesion similar to other benign perianal lesions, making clinical diagnosis difficult. A definite diagnosis is made by means of biopsy, which shows a characteristic histologic appearance—large, pale, vacuolated cells with hyperchromatic eccentric nuclei. The cells invariably contain acid mucosubstances, an important feature in differentiating this lesion from melanoma and Bowen's disease.

ANSWER: c

REFERENCE: *Chapter 47—Anal Cancer: Perianal Neoplasms; Perianal Paget Disease*

3. For the patient in question 2, biopsy revealed an invasive apocrine gland neoplasm. The deep margins include striated muscle infiltrated by neoplastic cells. Appropriate management includes which of the following?

a. Primary radiation
b. Abdominoperineal resection with bilateral inguinal lymph node dissection
c. Abdominoperineal resection only
d. Carbon dioxide laser fulguration

COMMENT: Wide local excision is the best treatment in the absence of invasive carcinoma. Because of the high incidence of local recurrence and residual tumor, it is vital to obtain an adequate margin of resection. At gross inspection, the extent of involvement is ill defined, and multiple punch biopsies may be needed to determine the extent of involvement. For more advanced lesions with underlying carcinoma, abdominoperineal resection is indicated. Inguinal lymph node dissection is performed only if groin lymph nodes are clinically positive for metastasis. Because of the commonly delayed diagnosis (average, 4 years), approximately 25% of patients with perianal Paget's disease have metastasis when they seek treatment. The sites of metastasis, in order of frequency, are inguinal and pelvic lymph nodes, liver, bone, lung, brain, bladder, prostate, and adrenal gland. The prognosis is poor once metastasis has occurred.

ANSWER: c

REFERENCE: *Chapter 47—Anal Cancer: Perianal Neoplasms; Perianal Paget Disease*

4. Human papillomavirus (HPV) infection has been shown to increase the risk of anal carcinoma in a manner that clinically parallels the role of HPV infection in the genesis of cervical carcinoma. Which of the following statements is/are true?

   a. Human papillomavirus types 6 and 11 are generally associated with benign lesions such as warts
   b. Human papillomavirus virus is associated with melanoma
   c. Human papillomavirus types 16 and 18 are most commonly associated with invasive carcinoma of the anus
   d. Human papillomavirus infection can be prevented by means of vaccination

COMMENT: Human papillomavirus types 6 and 11 are associated with lesions such as warts and anal intraepithelial neoplasia or low-grade dysplasia that rarely progresses to invasive carcinoma. In contrast, HPV types 16, 18, 31, 33, 34, and 35 are most commonly associated with high-grade dysplasia, anal intraepithelial neoplasia, and carcinoma of the anus and cervix. Human papillomavirus types 6 and 11 are maintained as extrachromosomal episomes, whereas HPV types 16 and 18 are integrated into host DNA. This explains the differing propensities to initiate development of carcinoma. Immunosuppressed patients, such as recipients of renal transplants or cardiac allografts and in patients who have recently completed chemotherapy, are at increased risk of anal carcinoma. Approximately 50% of patients with HIV infection have detectable HPV DNA.

ANSWER: a, c

REFERENCE: *Chapter 47—Anal Cancer: Etiology and Pathogenesis*

5. Which of the following statements is/are true regarding Paget's disease of the perianal area?

   a. It originates from the anal mucosa
   b. It is an invasive squamous cell carcinoma
   c. The lesion is characterized by an exophytic mass with rolled, everted edges with central ulceration
   d. The likelihood of coexistence of visceral carcinoma, such as carcinoma of the rectum, is high

COMMENT: Most authors agree with the concept that Paget cells are glandular and probably of apocrine origin. Unlike Paget's disease of the nipple, which is invariably associated with an underlying invasive or in situ ductal adenocarcinoma, perianal Paget's disease starts out as a benign neoplasm. It can eventually become invasive and give rise to an adenocarcinoma. The lesions appear as a slowly enlarging erythematous, eczematous, and often sharply demarcated anal rash that can ooze or scale and usually is accompanied by pruritus. The coexistence of visceral carcinoma is well known, with an incidence of 50% in some series. Total colonoscopy is indicated.

ANSWER: d

REFERENCE: *Chapter 47—Anal Cancer: Perianal Neoplasms; Perianal Paget Disease*

6. 65-year-old woman has dull aching pain in the anorectum for 6 months associated with intermittent bleeding mixed with stool. Examination shows a 3-cm, indurated polypoid mass in the anal canal with the lower margin at the dentate line and the upper margin 3 cm above the dentate line. There is no groin lymphadenopathy. Computed tomography of the abdomen shows no metastasis to the liver and no enlargement of pelvic lymph nodes. Which of the following statements is/are true?

a. The lesion is classified as T3N0
b. The treatment of choice is abdominoperineal resection followed by chemoradiation
c. The lesion is a Dukes B
d. Prophylactic chemoradiation to the groin is advisable to reduce the risk of late metastasis

COMMENT: The TNM system has now become the standard staging for carcinoma of the anus. It is important to note that the most recent addition of World Health Organization standards and the unified American Joint Committee on Cancer introduced major changes in the staging of primary carcinoma. The T category is now determined by the largest diameter of the primary carcinoma measured in centimeters. It formerly was necessary to estimate clinically the circumferential extent of the anal carcinoma and whether the external sphincter was invaded: T1, 2 cm; T2, 2 to 5 cm; T3, more than 5 cm. Although it is important in carcinoma of the colon and rectum, the Dukes staging system is irrelevant in carcinoma of the anus because part of the lymphatic drainage is in the inguinal region and outside the extent of resection. Abdominoperineal resection is no longer the primary management of invasive squamous cell carcinoma of the anal canal. It has a high recurrence rate, and local recurrence after abdominoperineal resection has a less favorable prognosis. Abdominoperineal resection is reserved for local failure of chemoradiation therapy, for anorectal complications of treatment, especially fecal incontinence, and for treatment of patients who cannot tolerate chemoradiation therapy. The combination of 5-fluorouracil, mitomycin C, and pelvic radiation therapy has become standard treatment. Elective radiation to clinically normal inguinal nodes reduces the risk of lymph node failure and carries little morbidity. Only 1 of 38 such patients had a late recurrence in the inguinal area after undergoing combination chemotherapy and radiation therapy. In a series in which inguinal nodes were not treated electively, the late nodal recurrence rate was 15% to 25%.

ANSWER: d

REFERENCE: *Chapter 47—Anal Cancer: Etiology and Pathogenesis*

7. Which of the following statements is/are true, regarding verrucous carcinoma of perianal skin?

a. It is a malignant lesion of the perianal skin
b. The mode of metastasis is to the inguinal nodes
c. The lesion can invade adjacent organs, such as anal sphincter, vagina, uterus
d. The basic treatment is wide local excision

COMMENT: Giant condyloma acuminatum or Buschke-Löwenstein tumor represents verrucous carcinoma. The lesion typically manifests as a large (8 by 8 cm) slow-growing, painful, wartlike growth that is relatively soft and has a cauliflower-like appearance. Although the lesion is histologically benign, its behavior is clinically malignant. The clinical course of this lesion is relentless progression and expansion of the tumor by means of extensive erosion and pressure necrosis of surrounding tissues, which can cause numerous sinuses and fistulous tracts. Metastasis from this tumor has not been reported. The basic treatment is wide local excision. If, however, the lesion involves the adjacent organs, abdominoperineal resection is performed.

ANSWER: c, d

REFERENCE: *Chapter 47—Anal Cancer: Perianal Neoplasms; Verrucous Carcinoma*

8. A 55-year-old woman is referred by a general practitioner because of bleeding hemorrhoids. Proctoscopic examination reveals a brownish, nonulcerated, polypoid lesion, 1.5 cm in diameter in the anal canal 2 cm above the dentate line. Intrarectal ultrasound examination shows the depth of invasion into the submucosa and no enlargement of perirectal lymph nodes. Neither side of the groin has lymphadenopathy. The patient has good anal continence. Biopsy shows melanoma. Which of the following statements is/are true?

a. The treatment of choice is wide full-thickness local excision
b. Preoperative chemoradiation therapy followed by wide local excision is the best treatment
c. The anal canal is the most common site of melanoma
d. Another option for treatment is immunotherapy

COMMENT: Melanoma is a rare malignant tumor of the anal canal. The anal canal nevertheless represents the third most common site of melanomas, exceeded only by the skin and eyes. Melanoma of the anal canal is radioresistant and does not respond to chemotherapy or immunotherapy. It has a marked tendency to spread submucosally into the rectum but rarely invades adjacent organs, probably because most patients die before this occurs. Lymphatic spread to the mesenteric nodes has occurred among approximately one third of the patients by the time of diagnosis. Spread to the inguinal nodes occurs less often. Hematogenous spread to the liver and lung is early and rapid, accounting for most deaths. The surgical approach to this malignant neoplasm is controversial. There is no statistical difference in survival rates when patients treated by means of abdominoperineal resection are compared with those treated by means of local excision. Both 5-year survival rates are approximately 15% to 17%. It appears that local control of the disease after the operation is not as much a problem as distant metastasis, which is the main cause of death. For small lesions, wide local excision is the best procedure.

ANSWER: a

REFERENCE: *Chapter 47—Anal Cancer: Melanoma*

CHAPTER 48

DIVERTICULAR DISEASE

1. A 65-year-old woman has obstipation, lower abdominal pain, and fever. Physical examination reveals a temperature of 38.5°C, left lower quadrant tenderness, and an ill-defined lower abdominal mass. The white blood cell count is 17,500/μL. Intravenous hydration, broad-spectrum antibiotics, and analgesics are ordered. After 48 hours, the symptoms are not alleviated. Appropriate management includes which of the following?

a. Barium enema
b. Computed tomography (CT) of the abdomen
c. Immediate laparotomy
d. Intravenous pyelography

COMMENT: Signs and symptoms of diverticulitis include fever, tachycardia, leukocytosis with left shift of the differential count, abdominal pain, and a tender lower abdominal mass. Most patients with an acute episode of diverticulitis can be treated with intravenous fluids, bowel rest, broad-spectrum antibiotics, and analgesics. If the patient's condition does not improve within 48 hours, complications of diverticulitis may exist, and further investigation is necessary. Only approximately 20% of patients have complications of diverticulitis with their first episode. This percentage increases to 60% with recurrent episodes. Although water-soluble contrast enema radiography can provide the diagnosis of diverticulitis, CT has become the preferred diagnostic test for patients who do not improve within 48 hours. Computed tomography is especially useful in delineating the complications of diverticulitis, including perforation and abscess formation. At CT, percutaneous drainage catheters can be placed if an abscess is identified. After CT drainage of an abscess, 50% to 90% of patients can undergo successful one-stage segmented colectomy and primary anastomosis. If percutaneous drainage is not feasible or an abscess is not identified, surgical intervention is recommended.

ANSWER: b

REFERENCE: *Chapter 48—Diverticular Disease: Peridiverticulitis*

2. Recurrent episodes of sigmoid colonic diverticulitis prompt operative therapy. Which of the following describe(s) the appropriate margins for resection?

    a. Proximal margin, splenic flexure; distal margin, rectosigmoid junction
    b. Proximal margin, descending colon; distal margin, rectosigmoid junction
    c. Proximal margin, descending colon; distal margin, mid-rectum
    d. Proximal margin, transverse colon; distal margin, mid-rectum

COMMENT: At exploratory laparotomy, if the disease is localized, segmental colectomy should be performed. Distal resection always should extend to the proximal rectum to decrease the chance of recurrence. The proximal extent of resection should include the segment involved with the acute disease and any colon with signs of chronic disease or large numbers of diverticula. With this approach, the recurrence rate after surgical resection is less than 10%. The only absolute contraindications to primary anastomosis are free perforation with generalized peritonitis, obstruction with unprepared bowel, and intraoperative conditions that do not warrant primary anastomosis, such as septic shock, ureteral injury, or other medical conditions that make a prolonged operation inadvisable. If resection is thought to be unsafe in the presence of a massive phlegmon or if the patient's condition is too unstable for resection, diverting end colostomy with mucous fistula may be appropriate. Colonic resection is planned for a later date, after inflammation subsides.

ANSWER: b

REFERENCE: *Chapter 48—Diverticular Disease: Peridiverticulitis*

3. An elderly man reports he is passing gas with urination. The medical history includes one episode of diverticulitis for which the patient was treated medically, transurethral resection of the prostate for benign prostatic hypertrophy, and diabetes. Which of the following diagnostic tests is most appropriate initially?

    a. Computed tomography of the abdomen and pelvis
    b. Cystoscopy
    c. Barium enema
    d. Intravenous pyelography

COMMENT: Colovesical fistulas account for approximately one half of fistulas due to diverticulitis. Most patients with colovesical fistula have urinary tract symptoms, including urgency, dysuria, pneumaturia, and fecaluria. In spite of obvious symptoms, the diagnosis of colovesical fistula can be difficult to establish conclusively. Recurrent urinary tract infections in an elderly man should increase suspicion. Barium enema radiographic examination usually shows diverticula or occasionally sigmoid narrowing. Only rarely is the fistulous tract actually filled. Cystoscopy shows hyperemia and inflammation consistent with chronic cystitis. Although these findings can be localized to some extent, indicating the presence of fistulous communication, the fistulous opening is seldom seen. Computed tomography with intraluminal contrast material has emerged as the most sensitive test for the presence of a colovesical fistula. The presence of barium in the urine confirms the diagnosis of colovesical fistula. In more than 90% of patients, air is seen in the urinary bladder, and an indurated segment of sigmoid colon is found adjacent to a locally thickened bladder wall.

ANSWER: a

REFERENCE: *Chapter 48—Diverticular Disease: Fistula Formation*

4. For the patient in question 3, a colovesical fistula originating from the sigmoid colon is found. Colonoscopy reveals diverticula and excludes carcinoma. During laparotomy, thickened sigmoid colon is found adherent to the dome of the bladder. A definite fistula is not found. Appropriate operative management includes which of the following?

   a. Sigmoid resection, primary colonic anastomosis, catheter drainage of bladder
   b. En bloc resection of sigmoid colon and adjacent bladder wall, primary colonic anastomosis, suprapubic cystostomy
   c. En bloc resection of sigmoid colon and adjacent bladder wall, formation of descending colostomy and Hartmann's pouch, suprapubic cystostomy
   d. Sigmoid resection, primary colonic anastomosis, bilateral percutaneous nephrostomy

COMMENT: Most patients with colovesical fistulas are treated effectively with a one-stage procedure consisting of segmental colectomy and closure of the fistulous opening in the bladder. The proximal margin of resection should include the entire segment of thickened, contracted colon and any additional colon involved in the acute inflammation. If the fistulous opening cannot be identified, implying that it is small in diameter, nothing needs to be done to identify the bladder fistula. Urinary catheter drainage for 7 to 10 days followed by cystographic verification of closure of the fistula is sufficient therapy. Depending on the severity of the related complications of diverticulitis (obstruction, inflammation, abscess, sepsis, other fistula), it may occasionally be necessary to perform a two-stage procedure, the first stage being segmental colectomy and colostomy formation and the second stage closure of the colostomy. Either the one- or two-stage procedure can be performed with low morbidity and mortality and with a recurrence rate less than 5%.

ANSWER: a

REFERENCE: *Chapter 48—Diverticular Disease: Fistula Formation*

CHAPTER 49

ACUTE GASTROINTESTINAL HEMORRHAGE

1. A 45-year-old man with a history of alcohol abuse arrives in the emergency department with hematemesis. He has tachycardia but not hypotension. Intravenous infusion of 1,000 mL lactated Ringer's solution normalizes the pulse rate. Placement of a nasogastric tube produces bloody drainage, which rapidly clears with warmed saline lavage. Appropriate management includes which of the following?

   a. Immediate esophagogastroduodenoscopy
   b. Observation in an intensive care unit followed by esophagogastroduodenoscopy in 24 hours
   c. Immediate upper gastrointestinal contrast examination
   d. Immediate intravenous infusion of vasopressin followed by endoscopy in 24 hours

COMMENT: Numerous studies have documented the unequivocal diagnostic superiority of endoscopy over contrast radiography in showing sites of upper gastrointestinal hemorrhage with a diagnostic sensitivity of 70% to 85% and a high specificity (approximately 90%) for endoscopy among bleeding patients. The timing of endoscopy is crucial. Early endoscopy (within 12 hours of admission) increases the likelihood of finding the suspect lesion. Fewer than 20% of lesions found 24 hours or more after hemorrhage have endoscopic signs of active or recent bleeding. This assumes importance in the care of patients with more than one disease process identified at endoscopy. When performed early, endoscopy is more than 90% sensitive in showing the site of hemorrhage.

Performance of emergency or urgent esophagogastroduodenoscopy for an actively bleeding or recently bleeding patient is associated with an increased incidence of complications. Complications include aspiration, recurrent or increased hemorrhage, respiratory depression from sedatives, and perforation of the esophagus, stomach, or duodenum. The risks of endoscopy can be minimized when the procedure is performed in an intensive care unit with adequate monitoring of the patient's respiratory and hemodynamic values. Endoscopy should be performed when the patient is in hemodynamically stable condition after volume resuscitation.

ANSWER: a

REFERENCE: *Chapter 49—Acute Gastrointestinal Hemorrhage*

2. Which of the following statements is/are correct with regard to use of visceral angiography for diagnosis in gastrointestinal hemorrhage?

a. Identification of visceral bleeding sites with angiography requires a bleeding rate of 0.5 to 1.0 mL/min at the time of the study
b. Identification of visceral bleeding sites with angiography requires a bleeding rate of 5 to 10 mL/min at the time of the study
c. With selective catheterization of visceral vessels, the site of hemorrhage is identified for approximately one half of patients
d. With selective catheterization of visceral vessels, the site of hemorrhage is identified for approximately four fifths of patients

COMMENT: Diagnostic angiography is used to examine patients who cannot undergo endoscopy or when endoscopy has been unsuccessful in finding the source of hemorrhage. Successful angiographic identification of the source of hemorrhage depends on the presence of active arterial bleeding at the time of the study. Extravasation of contrast material occurs if the patient is bleeding at a rate greater than 0.5 to 1 mL/min. This figure, derived from animal studies, correlates with the loss of four to five units of blood per day by humans. Patients are likely to be bleeding at a rate angiographically detectable if they need continuous volume infusion to maintain hemodynamic stability. Selective visceral angiography and endoscopy are complementary in the evaluation of active bleeding. In examinations of massively bleeding patients, endoscopic visualization often is severely limited, and selective mesenteric arteriography often shows the site of bleeding. With selective catheterization and injection of the celiac axis and superior mesenteric artery, the site of hemorrhage is identified in 40% to 60% of patients.

ANSWER: a, c

REFERENCE: *Chapter 49—Acute Gastrointestinal Hemorrhage: Selective Visceral Angiography*

3. Comorbidities that represent risk factors for upper gastrointestinal hemorrhage include which of the following?

a. Congestive heart failure
b. Cirrhosis
c. Pneumonia
d. Chronic obstructive pulmonary disease
e. Cardiac arrhythmia

COMMENT: The mortality rate reported for acute gastrointestinal hemorrhage is 10%; a large number of deaths are directly related to exsanguination. Age is a significant prognostic factor; it is found to influence outcome in nearly every report. Concurrent chronic illness also markedly affects morbidity and mortality rates. Congestive heart failure, cardiac arrhythmia, central nervous system disease, cirrhosis, cancer, pneumonia, chronic obstructive pulmonary disease, and renal disease have been associated with increased death rates among patients bleeding from upper gastrointestinal sources. Patients who bleed while in the hospital for other medical conditions have a particularly high risk of dying. In one survey, the mortality rate among patients who bled while hospitalized for other conditions was 33%. Those arriving at the hospital with hemorrhage had an 8% mortality rate.

ANSWER: a, b, c, d, e

REFERENCE: *Chapter 49—Acute Gastrointestinal Hemorrhage: Common Causes of GI Hemorrhage and Treatment; Upper GI Hemorrhage*

4. The endoscopic appearance of duodenal ulcers can be used to predict the likelihood of rebleeding. Which of the following are signs of increased risk of recurrent hemorrhage?

a. Ulcer size greater than 1.5 cm in diameter
b. Ulcer located in the pyloric channel
c. Visible vessel within the ulcer base
d. Oozing beneath an adherent clot
e. Ulcer located in the second portion of the duodenum

COMMENT: The appearance of duodenal ulcers during endoscopy has been correlated with the likelihood of persistent or recurrent hemorrhage and the necessity for operative intervention. A visible vessel in the base of an ulcer has been associated with a 49% to 70% risk of rebleeding and increased mortality. Endoscopic signs of active bleeding include spurting or oozing of blood from under a clot and suggest that the patient is at increased risk of needing numerous units of blood, of operative treatment, and of death.

ANSWER: c, d

REFERENCE: *Chapter 49—Acute Gastrointestinal Hemorrhage: Common Causes of GI Hemorrhage and Treatment; Upper GI Hemorrhage*

5. Which of the following statements is/are correct with regard to Mallory-Weiss tears?
   a. Mallory-Weiss tears represent 49% of cases of upper gastrointestinal hemorrhage
   b. The tear, which is full-thickness at the esophagogastric junction, is associated with severe mediastinitis
   c. When bleeding is associated with a Mallory-Weiss tear, balloon tamponade usually results in prompt cessation of hemorrhage
   d. Mallory-Weiss tears represent 5% to 15% of cases of upper gastrointestinal hemorrhage

COMMENT: Mallory-Weiss syndrome involves acute upper gastrointestinal hemorrhage that occurs after retching or vomiting. These lesions account for approximately 5% to 15% of cases of patients with upper gastrointestinal bleeding. Mallory and Weiss described the presence of a laceration of the gastric cardia and postulated that violent emesis against an unrelaxed cardia was the mechanism of injury. Although the syndrome initially was associated with alcohol abuse, endoscopy has shown large numbers of patients with Mallory-Weiss syndrome without a history of alcohol abuse.

Initial management includes volume resuscitation, gastric lavage, and nasogastric decompression. Most patients with Mallory-Weiss tears stop bleeding spontaneously either before treatment or after these early measures. Once bleeding has stopped, rebleeding is rare. Nonoperative management consisting of endoscopic electrocoagulation or injection therapy has been successfully applied to these lesions. Esophageal balloon tamponade is contraindicated, because it can convert a partial thickness tear into a full-thickness esophageal laceration. In cases not amenable to endoscopic therapy, operative management consists of oversewing the laceration through an anterior longitudinal gastrotomy in the middle third of the stomach. The mortality rate in recent series has been between 5% and 10%; deaths were related to associated disease, most notably cirrhosis.

ANSWER: d

REFERENCE: *Chapter 49—Acute Gastrointestinal Hemorrhage: Common Causes of GI Hemorrhage and Treatment; Upper GI Hemorrhage, Mallory-Weiss Tears*

6. Which of the following statements is/are correct regarding vascular ectasia of the colon?
   a. Approximately 90% of patients with hemorrhage stop bleeding spontaneously
   b. One half of affected patients have associated cardiac disease, most commonly coronary atherosclerosis
   c. Colonic vascular ectasia occurs most commonly in the cecum and ascending colon
   d. Endoscopic ablation is the preferred therapy for colonic ectasia

COMMENT: Vascular ectasia occurs most frequently in the cecum and ascending colon, although it is found in the transverse and left colon or rectum in as many as 20% to 30% of cases. At endoscopic examination, these lesions are flat or slightly raised, red, and 2 to 10 mm in diameter. At microscopic examination, vascular ectasia consists of dilated, thin-walled vessels that appear to be ectatic veins, venules, and capillaries localized to the submucosa and mucosa. Advanced lesions, histologically characterized as arteriovenous communications, manifest as massive hemorrhage and hematochezia. More than 90% of patients stop bleeding spontaneously, allowing time for adequate evaluation before definitive treatment. Approximately one half of patients with vascular ectasia have cardiac disease, most commonly atherosclerotic coronary disease. One fourth of patients have aortic stenosis.

Vascular ectasia can be diagnosed with colonoscopy or selective mesenteric angiography. Colonoscopy has been reported to have a sensitivity of 80% in the detection of vascular ectasia. Patients bleeding from colonic vascular ectasia can be treated by means of endoscopic modalities with a procedure-related morbidity of 2% to 10%. Patients bleeding from vascular ectasia for whom endoscopic hemostatic modalities are unsuccessful or unavailable can be treated with resection of the colon after preoperative localization of the bleeding site. For the usual patient, right colectomy with ileotransverse colostomy is the best treatment.

ANSWER: a, b, c, d

REFERENCE: *Chapter 49—Acute Gastrointestinal Hemorrhage: Lower Gastrointestinal Hemorrhage*

7. The most common site of Dieulafoy vascular malformation is which of the following?

    a. Stomach
    b. Duodenum
    c. Ileum
    d. Cecum

COMMENT: Dieulafoy vascular malformation is an unusual cause of recurrent hematemesis in which bleeding originates from an unusually large (1 to 3 mm in diameter) artery running through the gastric submucosa for variable distances. Erosion of the gastric mucosa overlying the vessel results in necrosis of the arterial wall and brisk hemorrhage. The mucosal defect usually is small, 2 to 5 mm, and without evidence of chronic inflammation. The diagnosis is most frequently made at endoscopy with the detection of an arterial bleeding from a pinpoint mucosal defect. In some instances, a small arterial vessel can be seen protruding from the gastric mucosa. The lesions characteristically are located within 6 cm of the esophagogastric junction along the lesser curvature. Management consists of excision of the gastric wall bearing the lesion by means of wedge resection of the proximal lesser curvature.

ANSWER: a

REFERENCE: *Chapter 49—Acute Gastrointestinal Hemorrhage: Unusual Causes of Acute Gastrointestinal Hemorrhage; Dieulafoy Vascular Malformation*

8. A 60-year-old man has orthostatic symptoms and maroon blood per anus. During the initial evaluation, he tells you he underwent a barium enema examination last year that showed diverticulitis. The most appropriate next step is:

    a. Placement of a nasogastric tube
    b. Colonoscopy
    c. Visceral angiography
    d. Tagged red blood cell scanning

COMMENT: The history of diverticulosis is noncontributory because most patients in this age group have diverticula. Maroon stool suggests that blood has been present in the gastrointestinal tract for some time, but it is not a sufficiently accurate finding to pinpoint the location of the bleeding. The best initial step is placement of a nasogastric tube to determine whether blood is present in the stomach. An aspirate that does not show blood does not exclude an upper gastrointestinal source. However, the presence of bile in the nasogastric aspirate without blood usually suggests the source of bleeding is distal to the ligament of Treitz.

ANSWER: a

REFERENCE: *Chapter 49—Acute Gastrointestinal Hemorrhage: Lower GI Hemorrhage*

9. A 32-year-old otherwise healthy man has massive upper gastrointestinal bleeding. Upper endoscopic examination reveals a posterior duodenal ulcer with a visible, nonbleeding vessel. The patient responds to initial volume resuscitation and shows no evidence of active bleeding after 12 hours. Optimal care of this patient should include:

    a. Management of *Helicobacter pylori* infection
    b. Antacids
    c. Histamine H_2 blocker
    d. Initiation of a proton pump inhibitor
    e. Urgent vagotomy, oversewing of the vessel, and pyloroplasty

COMMENT: Proton pump inhibitors and management of *H. pylori* infection both have been shown to decrease the recurrence rate of hemorrhage. Antacids and histamine H_2 blockers have largely been supplanted by the more efficacious proton pump inhibitors. Operation can be considered at this point in some cases because of the substantial risk of rebleeding associated with this lesion. This would be especially true in the care of older, debilitated patients. In this young, otherwise healthy person, most surgeons would not recommend operation at this point. If bleeding reoccurs, the decision to operate or to perform a second endoscopic examination must be individualized. Either alternative would be appropriate in most cases.

ANSWER: a, d

REFERENCE: *Chapter 49—Acute Gastrointestinal Hemorrhage: Common Causes of GI Hemorrhage and Treatment; Upper GI Hemorrhage*

10. A 45-year-old woman with a history of chronic, active hepatitis is being considered for hepatic transplantation. She has a life-threatening variceal hemorrhage that is controlled after some difficulty with endoscopic ligation. The best treatment option(s) while the patient awaits transplantation is/are:

   a. Open portacaval shunt
   b. Repeated, elective sclerotherapy
   c. Transjugular intrahepatic portacaval shunt
   d. Octreotide

COMMENT: The ideal treatment of this patient will control the variceal hemorrhage while not making transplantation more difficult or dangerous. Repetition of sclerotherapy is effective management of the varices and will not interfere with transplantation. Transjugular intrahepatic portacaval shunting also is highly effective at decompressing the portal vein. This procedure carries added risk of hepatic encephalopathy. The most durable management of portal hypertension is surgical portacaval shunting. Octreotide is useful during acute bleeding episodes but is not good long-term therapy for esophageal varices.

ANSWER: b, c

REFERENCE: *Chapter 49—Acute Gastrointestinal Hemorrhage: Common Causes of GI Hemorrhage and Treatment; Upper GI Hemorrhage*

11. Gastrointestinal hemorrhage usually stops spontaneously when caused by which of the following:

   a. Mallory-Weiss tear
   b. Colonic diverticulum
   c. Colonic angiodysplasia
   d. Peptic gastric ulcer

COMMENT: Gastrointestinal hemorrhage stops spontaneously in most patients, regardless of the cause. The exact fraction varies from cause to cause, as does the risk of rebleeding.

ANSWER: a, b, c, d

REFERENCE: *Chapter 49—Acute Gastrointestinal Hemorrhage: Common Causes of GI Hemorrhage and Treatment; Upper GI Hemorrhage*

12. A 75-year-old man has a single episode of hematemesis. History reveals aortofemoral bypass 10 years earlier. Upper endoscopy shows blood but no etiologic factor is found. The appropriate next step(s) is/are:

   a. Follow-up endoscopy under ideal elective conditions the following week
   b. Colonoscopy
   c. Computed tomography
   d. Laparotomy
   e. Meckel's scan

COMMENTS: The history of aortofemoral bypass should raise the possibility of an aortoenteric fistula. These patients commonly have a herald bleed that can be followed by rapidly exsanguinating hemorrhage. Computed tomography may be useful to confirm the diagnosis by showing evidence of graft infection or pseudoaneurysm at the proximal anastomosis. However, normal findings at computed tomography do not exclude the presence of an aortoenteric fistula. Many patients need laparotomy to confirm or refute the diagnosis. Endoscopy in the evaluation of gastrointestinal hemorrhage is most accurate immediately, and repetition of the procedure the following week is unlikely to be helpful. Meckel's diverticulum that causes bleeding is exceedingly unlikely in this age group and does not cause hematemesis in any case.

ANSWER: c, d

REFERENCE: *Chapter 49—Acute Gastrointestinal Hemorrhage: Lower GI Hemorrhage*

13. A 55-year-old woman has several episodes of gastrointestinal hemorrhage over the course of a year. Upper endoscopy, tagged red blood cell scanning, and colonoscopy repeatedly show normal findings except for the presence of diverticula in the sigmoid colon. The next option for this patient is:

    a. Left hemicolectomy
    b. Total abdominal colectomy
    c. Intraoperative enteroscopy
    d. Enteroclysis
    e. Observation only

COMMENT: The presence of diverticula is not sufficient to implicate them as the source of bleeding without another localizing study. Blind left hemicolectomy or total abdominal colectomy carries substantial risk of rebleeding and should be considered only under unusual circumstances. Enteroclysis can help detect a small-bowel lesion that could cause repeated hemorrhage. Intraoperative enteroscopy may be necessary if findings at enteroclysis are normal and should be more sensitive to detection of mucosal lesions such as angiodysplasia of the small bowel.

ANSWER: e

REFERENCE: *Chapter 49—Acute Gastrointestinal Hemorrhage: Lower GI Hemorrhage*

CHAPTER 50

ANORECTAL DISORDERS

1. Which of the following statements is/are correct relating to anal sphincteric function?

    a. When the rectum is distended, the internal anal sphincter relaxes and the external anal sphincter contracts
    b. When the rectum is distended, the internal anal sphincter contracts and the external anal sphincter relaxes
    c. The external anal sphincter is responsible for resting anal pressure
    d. The internal anal sphincter is responsible for resting anal pressure

COMMENT: The internal sphincter, because it is innervated by the autonomic nervous system, is not subject to voluntary control. This powerful muscle exists in a continuously tonic state and is responsible for maintaining closure of the resting anal canal. The high-pressure zone of the anal canal at rest is the result of actions of the internal sphincter. The external sphincter contributes to anal pressure only when a bolus of stool is present within the anal canal. The increase in pressure during voluntary contraction (squeeze pressure) is exclusively caused by the activity of the external sphincter. The high resting pressure in the anal canal acts as a barrier to prevent leakage of mucus and gas.

When the rectum is distended, the internal sphincter relaxes. This relaxation allows the rectal content to move down to the anal canal. When the rectum is distended, the external sphincter contracts. Reflex contraction of the external sphincter prevents rectal content from leaking through the anus. Although volitional contraction of the external sphincter can only be sustained for short periods, it is the most important mechanism of voluntary continence.

ANSWER: a, d

REFERENCE: *Chapter 50—Anorectal Disorders: Mechanisms of Anal Continence*

2. The most common complication after hemorrhoidectomy is which of the following?

a. Urinary retention
b. Rectal bleeding
c. Incontinence
d. Wound infection

COMMENT: Hemorrhoidectomy should be considered when the hemorrhoids are severely prolapsed through the anus, necessitating manual replacement, or are complicated by associated pathologic conditions, such as ulceration, fissure, fistula, large hypertrophied anal papilla, or extensive skin tags. An elliptical excision starts at the perianal skin, includes external and internal hemorrhoids, and ends at the anorectal ring. The mucosa and submucosa are dissected from the underlying internal sphincter muscle. Unless there is an associated anal stenosis or chronic anal fissure, internal sphincterotomy is not performed. The entire wound is closed with running absorbable suture. The largest and the most redundant hemorrhoid should be excised first. No packing is placed in the anal canal. Urinary retention is the most common complication of hemorrhoidectomy. It can be avoided if intravenous fluids are restricted during the procedure and minimized for the next 6 to 8 hours.

ANSWER: a

REFERENCE: *Chapter 50—Anorectal Disorders: Hemorrhoidectomy*

3. A 65-year-old man has mucous discharge and perianal discomfort. Physical examination reveals a fistulous opening lateral to the anus. Anoscopic examination allows passage of a probe through the fistula track. The fistula traverses the internal anal sphincter, the intersphincteric plane, and a portion of the external anal sphincter. The fistula is categorized as which type?

a. Intersphincteric
b. Transsphincteric
c. Suprasphincteric
d. Extrasphincteric

COMMENT: The four main forms of fistula-in-ano are based on the relation of the fistula to the sphincter muscles. An intersphincteric fistula track is in the intersphincteric plane. The external opening usually is in the perianal skin close to the anal verge. A transsphincteric fistula starts in the intersphincteric plane or in the deep postanal space. The fistula track traverses the external sphincter, and the external opening is at the ischioanal fossa. Horseshoe fistulas are in this category. Suprasphincteric fistulas start in the intersphincteric plane in the mid anal canal and pass upward to a point above the puborectalis muscle. The fistula passes laterally over this muscle and downward between the puborectalis and levator ani muscles into the ischioanal fossa. An extrasphincteric fistula passes from the perineal skin through the ischioanal fossa and the levator ani muscle and penetrates the rectal wall. Extrasphincteric fistulas can arise from cryptoglandular origin, trauma, foreign body, or pelvic abscess.

ANSWER: b

REFERENCE: *Chapter 50—Anorectal Disorders: Fistula-in-Ano*

4. For the patient in question 3, appropriate management includes which of the following?

a. Division of the tissues over the probe with an electrocautery and leaving the wound open to heal by means of secondary intention

b. Division of the tissues over the probe with an electrocautery and closing the wound with a pedicled skin flap

c. Division of the internal anal sphincter with an electrocautery and encircling the external sphincter with a seton

d. Proximal diverting colostomy and antibiotics

COMMENT: For young patients, transection of internal and external sphincter muscles in the posterior half in the course of fistulotomy does not always jeopardize anal continence. Among older patients and women, however, transection of the external sphincter muscle, particularly in the anterior half, risks incontinence. When transection of the external sphincter appears likely, some surgeons recommend use of a seton. A seton is a suture drawn through a fistula. The rationale for use of a seton is to produce fibrosis. The seton is threaded through the fistula track and tied over the muscles. In the second stage (average interval, 6 to 8 weeks), fistulotomy is performed. Incontinence after the proper use of a seton is uncommon, even when the fistula is deep.

ANSWER: c

REFERENCE: *Chapter 50—Anorectal Disorders: Fistula-in-Ano*

5. Appropriate management of chlamydial proctitis includes which of the following?

a. Tetracycline 500 mg four times a day

b. Metronidazole 250 mg four times a day

c. Acyclovir 200 mg four times a day

d. Erythromycin 500 mg four times a day

COMMENT: *Chlamydia trachomatis* is the most common cause of sexually transmitted disease in the United States, affecting 4 million Americans each year. Proctoscopy reveals nonspecific proctitis with friable, granular, and edematous mucosa. Immunofluorescent microscopic examination provides an accurate and a rapid diagnosis. Treatment includes tetracycline hydrochloride, 500 mg by mouth four times a day for 7 days, or doxycycline, 100 mg by mouth twice a day for 7 days. For patients with contraindications to tetracycline, erythromycin base or stearate, 500 mg by mouth four times a day for 7 days, or erythromycin ethylsuccinate, 800 mg by mouth four times a day for 7 days, can be used. Two new drugs have been approved by the U.S. Food and Drug Administration (FDA) for the management of chlamydia—azithromycin, 1 gm orally in a single dose, and ofloxacin, 300 mg orally two times a day for 7 days. A substantial advantage of azithromycin, in comparison with all other therapies, is that a single dose is effective. This antimicrobial agent may prove most useful in situations in which compliance with a 7-day regimen of another antimicrobial agent cannot be ensured. In view of the high efficacy of tetracycline and doxycycline, cost also should be considered in the selection of a treatment regimen.

ANSWER: a, d

REFERENCE: *Chapter 50—Anorectal Disorders: Sexually Transmitted Diseases*

6. A 30-year-old healthy man is concerned about a 6-month history of fresh blood dripping in the toilet bowel at completion of a bowel movement. He also has noticed occasional protrusion of "hemorrhoids" but has never needed to push them back. Proctoscopy reveals a red, soft mass on the anterior anal cushion with some metaplastic changes. There is no anal stenosis or other abnormality. The following statement(s) is/are true:
   a. The patient has a first-degree hemorrhoid
   b. Because of bleeding, hemorrhoidectomy is indicated
   c. Hemorrhoids are varicose veins of the anal canal
   d. Rubber band ligation is the best treatment

COMMENT: In first-degree hemorrhoids, the anal cushions slide down beyond the dentate line on straining. In second-degree hemorrhoids, the anal cushions prolapse through the anus on straining but reduce spontaneously, as in this case. In third-degree hemorrhoids, the anal cushions prolapse through the anus on straining or exertion and require manual replacement into the anal canal. In fourth-degree hemorrhoids, the prolapse is not manually reducible. The best management of second-degree hemorrhoids is rubber band ligation. Hemorrhoids are not varicose veins, as was previously understood. *Hemorrhoid* is the pathologic term to describe downward displacement of prolapse of the anal cushions causing dilatation of the contained venules. A hemorrhoid develops when the supporting tissues of the anal cushion deteriorate. This patient has a second-degree hemorrhoid. Rubber band ligation is the best treatment. Hemorrhoidectomy is indicated mostly for severe third-degree and fourth-degree hemorrhoids.

ANSWER: d

REFERENCE: *Chapter 50—Anorectal Disorders: Hemorrhoids*

7. Rectal prolapse is an uncommon condition of unknown causation. The following statement(s) is/are true:
   a. Rectal prolapse is intussusception of the rectum
   b. Prolonged protrusion of the rectum that stretches the anus eventually leads to anal incontinence
   c. In spite of high recurrence rates, perineal rectosigmoidectomy is a lesser procedure with low morbidity and mortality and acceptable results
   d. Abdominal rectopexy corrects the prolapse and constipation

COMMENT: Although the cause of rectal prolapse is poorly understood, the disorder is considered a form of intussusception. It usually starts in the anterior aspect of the lower rectum, approximately 8 cm from the anal verge. By the time rectal prolapse is diagnosed, one half of patients already have anal incontinence. Loss of continence is not caused by prolonged protrusion that causes mechanical stretching of the sphincter. Incontinence in rectal prolapse is caused by damage to the pudendal nerve, which supplies the sphincter muscles, from prolonged stretching. Approximately 50% of patients with fecal incontinence from rectal prolapse improve after repair of the prolapse. Because the return of incontinence takes as long as 6 to 12 months, operative management of incontinence should be postponed for 1 year. Perineal rectosigmoidectomy has appeal as a lesser procedure, particularly for elderly patients or patients in a high surgical risk category. Most patients have little postoperative pain and stay in the hospital only a few days. The short-term recurrence rate is approximately 10%. Abdominal rectopexy with or without resection is a major operation with high risk of morbidity and mortality, but it has a low recurrence rate. Patients should be cautioned that despite successful transabdominal repair, almost one half of the patients continue to have defecation problems.

ANSWER: a, c

REFERENCE: *Chapter 50—Anorectal Disorders: Rectal Prolapse*

8. A 20-year-old man visits the office because he has had anal pain during and after bowel movements for more than 2 months. There is also bright red blood on wiping. There is no problem with diarrhea or abdominal cramps. Examination of the anal canal reveals a 5 mm by 5 mm deep anal fissure in the posterior midline of the anus. The following statement(s) is/are true:

a. The unhealed fissure is caused by repeated trauma from bowel movements
b. Lateral sphincterotomy is the best treatment
c. The triad of anal fissure consists of fissure, sentinel skin tag, and internal hemorrhoid
d. Nitroglycerin paste decreases anal resting pressure

COMMENT: Chronic anal fissure usually is deep, exposing the internal anal sphincter. Chronic anal fissure occasionally has a triad of fissure, sentinel skin tag, and hypertrophied anal papilla. Conservative management of chronic anal fissure is application of 0.2% to 0.3% nitroglycerin paste directly to the anal fissure. Nitroglycerin decreases anal resting pressure and increases anodermal blood flow. Doppler flowmetry shows lower anodermal blood flow at the fissure site, suggesting that unhealed fissure is caused by ischemia. Reduction of anal pressure by means of sphincterotomy improves anodermal blood flow, resulting in fissure healing. Lateral internal sphincterotomy is the best operation. Fissurectomy should be avoided because a midline wound, particularly posterior, may not heal.

ANSWER: b, d

REFERENCE: *Chapter 50—Anorectal Disorders: Anal Fissure*

9. A 25-year-old man has a 3-cm perianal abscess that has lasted approximately 4 days. The patient otherwise has been in good health. There was no history of diabetes. The following statement(s) is/are true:

a. Antibiotic therapy for 7 days is needed
b. A subsequent anal fistula, if deep, should be managed with a seton as a first stage
c. Unroofing the fistula or fistulotomy is the basic management of anal fistula
d. Fistulectomy is the best management of fistula, to avoid recurrence

COMMENT: Like an abscess in any part of the body, an anorectal abscess must be drained as soon as possible. In general, antibiotics are not necessary after the abscess is adequately drained and should not be used as the primary treatment. Fistula-in-ano is a chronic form of perianal abscess that is spontaneously or surgically drained but in which the abscess cavity does not heal completely. Instead it becomes an inflammatory track with a primary opening (internal opening) in the anal crypt at the dentate line and a secondary opening (external opening) in the perianal skin. The principles of fistula surgery include unroofing the fistula, eliminating the primary opening (infective source), and establishing adequate drainage. Failure to open the entire track can lead to recurrence. Fistulectomy, excision of the fistula track, has no advantages over fistulotomy and is more likely to cause anal incontinence. Transection of a large amount of the external sphincter muscle, particularly in the anterior half and to treat women, risks incontinence. A seton should be applied. A seton is a suture, usually silk, rubber band, or a strip of Penrose drain, drawn through a fistula. It is used to tie the muscles covering the fistula to cause fibrosis or to cut the muscles. In the second stage (average interval, 6 to 8 weeks), fistulotomy is performed. Incontinence after proper use of a seton is uncommon, even when the fistula is deep.

ANSWER: b, c

REFERENCE: *Chapter 50—Anorectal Disorders: Anorectal Abscesses*

10. A 25-year-old woman gave birth 1 month ago. A midline episiotomy became infected. The wound has now completely healed with no residual infection, but the patient passes gas and stool into the vagina. Examination reveals a 2-mm rectovaginal fistula at the level of the dentate line anteriorly. The following statement(s) is/are true:

a. Start antibiotics and continue for 2 weeks
b. Endorectal advancement anorectal flap repair gives satisfactory results
c. Wait 3 to 6 months before repair of the fistula
d. The patient needs a permanent colostomy

COMMENT: Obstetric injury accounts for most rectovaginal fistulas. Spontaneous or nonoperative healing of a rectovaginal fistula depends primarily on the cause and to a lesser extent on the size. Approximately one half of small rectovaginal fistulas caused by obstetric trauma heal spontaneously. For a low, simple fistula endorectal advancement of an anorectal flap gives the best results. It is important to wait, usually 3 to 6 months, until the inflammation has subsided before considering a surgical repair; otherwise the wound will not heal and the risk of recurrent fistula is high. An alternative repair is to lay open the rectovaginal fistula and convert it to a fourth-degree perineal tear. Layered closure of the anal and vaginal defect is performed with synthetic absorbable sutures.

ANSWER: b, c

REFERENCE: *Chapter 50—Anorectal Disorders: Rectovaginal Fistula*

11. Which of the following statements is/are true regarding anal incontinence?

a. Anal ultrasonography is useful to detect defects of the external sphincter
b. Biofeedback helps and should be used in selected cases
c. Gracilis muscle transposition has fallen out of favor
d. Artificial anal sphincter is a new operation with a promising future

COMMENT: Ultrasonographic examination of the anal canal provides a clear image of the internal and external sphincter all around. It has decreased the need for other examinations, such as electromyography, because the ultrasonographic image can help accurately localize defects and asymmetry. Ultrasonographic examination of the anal canal is reliable for mapping defects of the external sphincter and is more comfortable for patients than is electromyographic mapping. Biofeedback is used in the management of anal incontinence to retrain the anus and rectum, to be aware of the sensation of rectal fullness, and to retrain contraction of the sphincteric muscles. Biofeedback training helps 85% of patients with various causes of anal incontinence.

Gracilis muscle transposition, once a popular operative technique, has fallen out of favor because of an unsatisfactory short-term success rate of approximately 50%. This striate muscle is capable of producing voluntary contraction to occlude the anal canal. It is, however, unable to preserve a closed lumen at all times because of lack of an inherent tone within the muscles, unlike the resting anal tone generated by the internal sphincter muscle. Use of an electrostimulating device has a better short-term success rate of 75%. Long-term, low-frequency electrical stimulation of skeletal muscle converts fast-twitch muscle into slow-twitch muscle capable of sustained activity. This operation is expensive and is experimental.

There has been enthusiasm for use of an artificial anal sphincter. The sphincter consists of an inflatable cuff of silicone rubber placed around the upper anal canal. The pressure-regulating balloon is placed to the left or right of the bladder, and the pump with which the patient can inflate and deflate the cuff is placed in the labia majora or in the scrotum. This operation has been received with enthusiasm in Europe but is not approved for clinical application by the FDA. For patients who are incapacitated by complete fecal incontinence and whose chances of success from anal sphincter repair are slim, permanent end-sigmoid colostomy is the best choice.

ANSWER: a, b, c, d

REFERENCE: *Chapter 50—Anorectal Disorders: Anal Incontinence*

Section I
HERNIA, ACUTE ABDOMEN, AND SPLEEN

CHAPTER 51

ABDOMINAL WALL HERNIAS

1. Direct inguinal hernias involve Hesselbach's triangle, the border of which are composed of:
   a. Inguinal ligament
   b. Border of rectus abdominis muscle
   c. Inferior epigastric vessels
   d. Transversus abdominis muscle

COMMENT: The inguinal triangle is the site of direct inguinal hernias. This triangle is most often described from the anterior aspect, in which case the inguinal ligament forms the base of the triangle, the rectus abdominis muscle the medial border, and the inferior epigastric vessels the superolateral border. The triangle as originally described by Hesselbach had the pectineal ligament as the base. The latter description is useful to surgeons viewing the abdomen from within, because the inguinal ligament cannot be seen from this viewpoint. When the inguinal triangle is transilluminated, the thin translucent abdominal wall within the triangle emphasizes its importance in hernia development and repair. The most translucent area indicates that little or no muscle is present. Only the peritoneum and the transversalis fascia cover the triangle in this area. The aponeurotic arch of the transversus abdominis muscle crosses the triangle just below the apex in most persons. A high aponeurotic arch affords less reinforcement to the triangle and can be a predisposing factor for formation of a direct inguinal hernia.

ANSWER: a, b, c

REFERENCE: *Chapter 51—Abdominal Wall Hernias: Anatomy of the Abdominal Wall and Groin; The Inguinal (Hesselbach's) Triangle*

2. A 45-year-old man arrives in the emergency department with a 12-hour history of abdominal distention, vomiting, and lower abdominal pain. Physical examination reveals abdominal tympany and an exquisitely tender mass in the right inguinal canal. The mass cannot be reduced. The skin overlying the mass is red and edematous. The diagnosis this presentation suggests is inguinal hernia with:
   a. Incarceration
   b. Hydrocele
   c. Testicular torsion
   d. Strangulation

COMMENT: In addition to an irreducible hernia and intestinal obstruction, the patient is toxic, dehydrated, and febrile. Examination of the abdomen reveals the signs of intestinal obstruction with distention and increased bowel sounds. The patient also has had absolute constipation and vomiting. The hernia itself is tense, irreducible, and tender, and the overlying skin may be discolored with a reddish or bluish tinge. No bowel sounds are present within the hernia itself. The patient commonly has leukocytosis with a predominance of polymorphonuclear leukocytes. Blood gas measurements may reveal metabolic acidosis.

Treatment of these patients requires urgent attention to detail. No attempt should be made to reduce the hernia. Rapid resuscitation should begin immediately with nasogastric suction and fluid and electrolyte replacement. The patient should be given antibiotics. Once the patient is resuscitated, urgent surgery is performed to expose the hernia, open the sac, and assess the viability of the bowel. More bowel can be pulled into the hernia so that viable bowel can be transected and the gangrenous portion removed. End-to-end anastomosis should be performed and the bowel reduced into the abdominal cavity. The hernia is repaired.

ANSWER: d

REFERENCE: *Chapter 51—Abdominal Wall Hernias: Clinical Features of Hernia; Complications of Hernia*

3. The most common form of abdominal herniation is:
   a. Femoral
   b. Umbilical
   c. Epigastric
   d. Inguinal

COMMENT: Spontaneous abdominal hernias occur among approximately 5% of the world population over a lifetime. The prevalence may be as high as 10%. Inguinal hernias are the most common abdominal wall hernias and constitute about 80% of cases. Femoral hernias occur in approximately 5% of instances. Incisional, umbilical, epigastric, and a host of miscellaneous types of hernia make up the other 15%. Most inguinal hernias occur among men and boys with a male to female ratio of 7:1. Femoral hernia has a female dominance of approximately 1.8:1.

ANSWER: d

REFERENCE: *Chapter 51—Abdominal Wall Hernias: Etiology, Epidemiology, and Natural History*

4. The processus vaginalis is the result of migration of the testis from its abdominal location to
   the scrotum, which is completed by about 28
   weeks of gestation. The processus normally is
   obliterated in the first few months of life. Failure
   of the processus vaginalis to become obliterated
   is the cause of:
   a. Indirect inguinal hernia
   b. Scrotal hydrocele .
   c. Testicular torsion
   d. Direct inguinal hernia

COMMENT: The prime cause of indirect inguinal hernia is a patent processus vaginalis. If all or part of the processus remains patent, the defect can give rise to indirect inguinal hernia, scrotal hydrocele, and encysted hydrocele of the cord or hydrocele of the canal of Nuck in women and girls. In a 38-year follow-up study of 1,944 patients, investigators found a contralateral lesion in 15.8% of the patients. In a large series of hernias occurring in childhood, other authors reported that the patent processus vaginalis closed in most patients. In premature infants, both sides were patent. In the neonatal period, in 60% of cases, the contralateral side was patent, but by the time the child reached 2 years of age, only 40% of processes were patent. This 40% rate persists into adult life, but only 20% of these produce a symptomatic hernia. The other 20% of patients have lifelong patent processus, which does not produce any symptoms.

ANSWER: a, b

REFERENCE: *Chapter 51—Abdominal Wall Hernias: Etiology, Epidemiology, and Natural History*

5. For a 25-year-old man, the lifetime risk of strangulation if an inguinal hernia is untreated approximates:
   a. 1%
   b. 5%
   c. 20%
   d. 50%

COMMENT: The course of untreated inguinal hernia is poorly understood; almost no modern data are available. This lack of information has occurred because of the commonly held opinion that all inguinal hernias should be repaired when diagnosed to prevent complications. In fact, the risk of a major complication such as incarceration, obstruction, and strangulation is low. It has been estimated that an 18-year-old man has a 0.272 lifetime risk of strangulation; the risk for a 75-year-old man is 0.034. This extremely low incidence of major complications may offset the ninefold to tenfold higher mortality risk among patients with intestinal obstruction than among patients without obstruction. Other investigators have reported the annual risk of a major complication to be 0.002 to 0.0037.

ANSWER: a

REFERENCE: *Chapter 51—Abdominal Wall Hernias: Etiology, Epidemiology, and Natural History*

6. Repair of inguinal hernia with the Lichtenstein
   technique is associated with a recurrence rate
   approximating:
   a. 1%
   b. 5%
   c. 20%
   d. 50%

COMMENT: The recurrence rate has been reduced with modern hernioplasty techniques. Although the Shouldice clinic has a recurrence rate of less than 1% for hernia repair, other centers using this technique have had a slightly higher recurrence rate. Tension-free repair with synthetic mesh has a uniformly reported recurrence rate less than 1%. A 0.1% recurrence rate was reported in one study with 4,000 patients. Published studies of the Lichtenstein repair consistently show a recurrence rate of less then 1%. Investigators have reported a 9-year experience in treatment of almost 3,300 patients with mesh plug repair. The recurrence rate with this method was 0.2%, and the morbidity was minimal. The recurrence rate for laparoscopic repair performed by experienced surgeons is equally low.

ANSWER: a

REFERENCE: *Chapter 51—Abdominal Wall Hernias: Treatment; Periumbilical Hernias*

7. During a routine infant examination, a pediatrician finds an asymptomatic umbilical hernia. The physician reassures the mother that the hernia has a possibility of spontaneous closure. By 2 years of age, the likelihood that an umbilical hernia will close approximates:

a. 10%
b. 20%
c. 50%
d. 80%

COMMENT: Umbilical and paraumbilical hernias are caused by improper healing of the umbilical scar. The result is a defect in the fascia covered by skin. Among infants the fascial defect varies in size but is most commonly 1 to 2 cm in diameter. A large proportion of pediatric umbilical hernias heal spontaneously. By 2 years of age, 80% of have closed. Persistent umbilical hernias necessitate surgery. Among older patients, the onset usually is sudden, and the defect is relatively small. An underlying cause of increased intraabdominal pressure, such as ascites or intraabdominal tumor, should be sought.

ANSWER: d

REFERENCE: *Chapter 51—Abdominal Wall Hernias: Periumbilical Hernias*

8. Spigelian hernias are located:

a. In the upper one third of the linea alba
b. Medial to the femoral vein
c. Within Hesselbach's triangle
d. Lateral to the rectus abdominis muscle

COMMENT: The Flemish anatomist Adriaan van der Spieghel first described the semilunar line, which is the lower limit of the posterior rectus sheath. A spigelian hernia protrudes through an area of weakness just lateral to the rectus sheath and just below this line. The hernia usually is interparietal, rarely penetrating the external oblique fascia, and therefore can be difficult to appreciate. The usual presentation is lower abdominal swelling just lateral to the border of the rectus muscle. Spigelian hernia often occurs among elderly women. These hernias usually are small, approximately 1 to 2 cm in diameter, although large examples up to 14 cm in diameter have been described. Omentum or small or large bowel may enter the sac. Incarceration and strangulation are common complications of this hernia. Because the hernia is deep to the external oblique fascia, the clinical presentation may not be obvious. Pain and tenderness may be the only signs. Plain radiographs may show a bowel shadow in this area. Computed tomography can show the defect well. Treatment is operative repair. Recurrence is uncommon.

ANSWER: d

REFERENCE: *Chapter 51—Abdominal Wall Hernias: Unusual Hernias; Spigelian Hernias*

CHAPTER 52

ACUTE ABDOMEN AND APPENDIX

1. Which of the following are not covered by visceral peritoneum?

   a. Spleen
   b. Pancreas
   c. Gallbladder
   d. Rectum

COMMENT: Peritoneum is made up of a continuous visceral and parietal layer. The intestinal tract from stomach to distal sigmoid colon is lined by visceral peritoneum. Likewise, the liver, spleen, and gallbladder are almost entirely covered by visceral peritoneum. The pancreas and duodenum are largely located within a retroperitoneum. The rectum is entirely extraperitoneal.

ANSWER: b, d

REFERENCE: *Chapter 52—Acute Abdomen and Appendix: Embryologic and Physiologic Considerations*

2. Pelvic appendicitis is frequently associated with which of the following physical signs?

   a. Tenderness at McBurney's point
   b. Psoas sign
   c. Obturator sign
   d. Cervical motion tenderness

COMMENT: Acute appendicitis typically begins with poorly localized central abdominal pain associated with anorexia and nausea. This reflects pain of visceral origin. As the inflammatory process becomes transmural, a transition to somatic-type pain develops. This is associated with rigidity and tenderness of overlying muscle groups and organs in direct continuity with the inflammatory process. In typical cases of appendicitis, when the organ is located within the right lower quadrant of the abdomen, patients will display tenderness over McBurney's point and often an associated psoas sign (pain on thigh extension). However, when the location of the appendix is deep within the pelvis, there may be little or no abdominal findings. Proximity of the inflamed appendix to the obturator internus muscle may be associated with a positive obturator test (suprapubic pain on internal and external rotation of the thigh). Tenderness on rectal examination may be present. Additionally, a peri-appendiceal inflammatory process and abscess in continuity with the right adnexa may be associated with cervical motion tenderness. In cases of pelvic appendicitis, a psoas sign is not present because the psoas muscle does not lie in direct continuity with the inflamed organ.

ANSWER: c, d

REFERENCE: *Chapter 52—Acute Abdomen and Appendix: Embryologic and Physiologic Considerations*

3. Abdominal examination in patients with abdominal pain is unreliable in which of the following conditions?

   a. Pregnancy
   b. Spinal cord injury
   c. Children
   d. Immunosuppression

COMMENT: In a number of special circumstances, the evaluation of the patient with acute abdominal pain is particularly challenging. Abdominal pain during pregnancy may be difficult due to a variety of non-surgical causes associated with this condition. Moreover, interpretation of blood work must recognize physiologic alterations such as leukocytosis. Radiologic testing may be limited due to concerns over fetal exposure. The gravid uterus causes marked distortion of anatomical relationships that may confuse the examining physician. However, physical findings such as peritonitis are not known to be altered by this condition. The diagnosis of acute abdominal pain in the pediatric population is difficult due to difficulties in obtaining a proper history. However, findings on physical exam are generally reliable. Acute abdominal pain in immunosuppressed patients (e.g., organ transplantation, immunosuppressive therapy, chemotherapy, AIDS) represents a particular diagnostic challenge. Unusual infectious causes are frequently seen. Physical findings may be subtle. The physical findings may be absent despite the presence of serious intraabdominal pathology. Patients with spinal cord injury have notoriously unreliable physical examinations. Classic signs such as tenderness, guarding, and fever are unreliable. The presence of shoulder pain, abdominal distension, nausea, vomiting, and autonomic dysreflexia are particularly important to document in this setting.

ANSWER: b, d

REFERENCE: *Chapter 52—Acute Abdomen and Appendix: Abdominal Pain in Special Circumstances*

4. Referred pain to the genitalia may be caused by:

   a. Ruptured iliac artery aneurysm
   b. Ureteral stone
   c. Cystitis
   d. Pelvic inflammatory disease

COMMENT: In addition to pain of somatic and visceral categories a third form of pain related to acute abdominal disorders is referred pain. Referred pain is perceived as at a site removed from the anatomic location of the pathology but in a region that shares a common embryonic origin. The most common example is radiation of biliary pain origin to the right subscapular region. Pain due to ureteral stones commonly radiates to the groin or genitalia. Additionally, pain of kidney origin or pathology associated with the iliac artery may also radiate to the genitalia. Uterine and rectal pain typically radiate posteriorly to the coccyx.

ANSWER: a, b

REFERENCE: *Chapter 52—Acute Abdomen and Appendix: Embryologic and Physiologic Considerations*

5. The typical patient with acute appendicitis will describe the onset of symptoms in the following order:

   a. Nausea/vomiting, fever, right lower quadrant pain and tenderness
   b. Periumbilical pain, nausea/vomiting, right lower quadrant pain and tenderness, fever
   c. Nausea/vomiting, periumbilical pain, right lower quadrant pain and tenderness, fever
   d. Fever, periumbilical pain, nausea/vomiting, right lower quadrant pain and tenderness

COMMENT: Most patients with acute appendicitis will describe a characteristic set of symptoms and these symptoms almost always follow a precise temporal pattern. The initial symptom is the periumbilical pain which is visceral in nature. This is followed by nausea and/or vomiting. The pain then shifts to the right lower quadrant as the inflammatory process involves the overlying parietal peritoneum. At this point, the patient may describe pain in the right lower quadrant that is exacerbated by various movements. Physical exam will reveal tenderness in the right lower quadrant with signs of peritoneal irritation. Fever then ensues, and is usually of a low-grade nature, especially early on in the course. Eventually, laboratory tests will reveal a leukocytosis, usually mild in nature. In those patients where the symptoms do not follow this temporal pattern, one must be suspicious of a diagnosis other than acute appendicitis.

ANSWER: b

REFERENCE: *Chapter 52—Acute Abdomen and Appendix: Appendix, Diagnosis*

6. A 35-year-old male presents with a ten-day history of abdominal pain. The symptoms were fairly mild but have increased somewhat over the past couple of days with localized pain in the right lower quadrant. On exam, the temperature is 101.2 degrees Fahrenheit and the patient has a tender mass in the right lower quadrant. There is no tenderness that can be elicited elsewhere within the abdomen. Appropriate management of this patient would be:

   a. IV hydration and antibiotics, urgent appendectomy through a McBirney incision
   b. IV hydration and antibiotics, CT-guided drainage, interval appendectomy at approximately 10 weeks
   c. IV hydration and antibiotics, ileocecectomy via midline laparotomy
   d. IV hydration and antibiotics, operative drainage of abscess through a McBirney incision, interval appendectomy at approximately 10 weeks
   e. IV hydration and antibiotics, interval appendectomy at approximately 10 weeks

COMMENT: In patients who present with a prolonged history (greater than 5 days) and have localized tenderness in the right lower quadrant, perhaps with a palpable mass, the likely diagnosis is a periappendiceal abscess/phlegmon. Such patients have already "walled-off" the appendiceal inflammation and are best treated initially with nonoperative therapy, including intravenous hydration and antibiotics. A CT scan may be performed and if a large collection/abscess is identified, then a CT-guided catheter can be placed. In many patients, antibiotics alone will be sufficient. Urgent operation in these patients is associated with increased morbidity, including the possible injury of surrounding structures such as the small intestine, and the possible need for an ileocecectomy or cecostomy tube placement. Initial nonoperative management is therefore recommended, and an interval appendectomy can be performed once the inflammatory process has completely resolved, usually at approximately 10 weeks following the initial presentation. Whether or not an interval appendectomy is required remains a controversial issue, since the incidence of recurrent appendicitis is probably quite low (approximately 10%).

ANSWER: b, e

REFERENCE: *Chapter 52—Acute Abdomen and Appendix: Appendiceal Mass*

7. The following statements are true regarding carcinoid tumors of the appendix:

   a. For tumors greater than 2 cm in diameter, a formal right hemicolectomy is indicated
   b. Regardless of tumor size, if the surgical margins are clear, then simple appendectomy is the proper surgical therapy
   c. Approximately 10% of appendectomy specimens will contain microscopic evidence of carcinoid tumor
   d. Carcinoids are thought to derive from the endocrine cells within the appendiceal wall

COMMENT: Approximately one percent of all appendectomy specimens contain a neoplasm, two thirds of which are carcinoids. These tumors are of neural crest origin and are thought to be derived from entro-endocrine cells in the appendiceal wall. The prognosis of patients with appendiceal carcinoid tumors is directly related to size. For tumors greater than or equal to two centimeters, formal right hemicolectomy is indicated in order to ensure adequate lymphatic clearance. Smaller tumors can be safely treated by appendectomy alone, assuming the surgical margins are clear.

ANSWER: a, d

REFERENCE: *Chapter 52—Acute Abdomen and Appendix: Appendiceal Neoplasms*

8. Regarding physical signs suggestive of acute appendicitis, the following are true:

   a. Rovsing's sign refers to pain on internal rotation of the right hip
   b. Iliopsoas sign refers to pain on extension of the right hip
   c. Dumphy's sign refers to pain on internal rotation of the right hip
   d. Rovsing's sign refers to right lower quadrant pain induced by palpation in the left lower quadrant

COMMENT: A variety of classical physical signs have been described and are suggestive of the presence of acute appendicitis. Dumphy's sign refers to increased pain with any coughing or movement and is related to inflammation that involves the parietal peritoneum. Rovsing's sign is right lower quadrant pain that is induced by palpation of the left lower quadrant and is highly suggestive of a right lower quadrant inflammatory process. The obturator sign is seen with inflammation of a pelvic appendix and refers to pain on internal rotation of the right hip. Finally, the iliopsoas sign is most often seen with a retrocecal appendix and refers to pain on extension of the right hip.

ANSWER: b, d

REFERENCE: *Chapter 52—Acute Appendicitis and Appendix: Appendix, Diagnosis*

CHAPTER 53

SPLEEN

1. Choose the correct statement describing normal splenic anatomy:
   a. Normal arterial inflow to the spleen includes the splenic artery and short gastric branches of the left gastric artery
   b. The majority of the splenic artery extends into the posterior surface of the pancreas
   c. The splenoomental attachments are associated with the splenic capsule along the superior pole and can lead to inadvertent injury to the spleen from traction on the omentum
   d. The majority of the splenic parenchyma is made up of the red pulp, which is made up of splenic cords with intervening sinuses

COMMENT: The spleen receives its arterial inflow from the splenic artery, a branch of the celiac trunk, and short gastric branches of the left gastroepiploic artery that travel in the splenogastric ligament. The splenic artery travels in its characteristic tortuous course through the lesser sac, with some of its most inferior loops projecting into the posterior surface of the pancreas. The splenic parenchyma is divided into red and white pulp. The white pulp is primarily located surrounding the arterioles, while the majority of the parenchyma is made up of the cord-like red pulp, divided by the splenic sinuses. The spleen is suspended by the splenogastric, splenorenal, and splenocolic ligaments. The splenoomental ligament is not always present, but is important to recognize because the attachments to the lower pole of the spleen can be avulsed , tearing the splenic capsule, when downward traction is applied to the omentum.

ANSWER: d

REFERENCE: *Chapter 53—Spleen: Embryology and Anatomy*

2. Which of the following statements is/are true regarding the normal immune function of the spleen?
   a. The red pulp plays the primary role in immune surveillance, as antigens are processed and presented by macrophages lining the splenic sinuses
   b. The periarteriolar lymphatic sheath, which is composed of both T cells and B cell follicles, can expand greatly in response to antigen stimulation
   c. The spleen is a site of synthesis for the opsonins tuftsin and properdin, which play an important role in phagocyte and complement activation
   d. The spleen plays an important role in the opsonization and clearance of encapsulated bacteria

COMMENT: The red pulp is primarily involved in erythrocyte maintenance and removal, while the white pulp and the marginal zones that surround the small arterioles are the site of the spleen's immune functions. The periarteriolar zone contains both B and T cells involved in generation of humoral and cellular responses, and it can expand greatly in response to antigen stimulation. The spleen plays an important role in the production of opsonins, small molecules that play critical roles in the activation of phagocytosis and the complement cascade. These opsonins contribute to the important role that the spleen plays in clearing encapsulated bacteria from the blood stream. It is the loss of this function that creates the need for vaccination against S. pneumoniae, N. meningitides, *and* H. influenzae *in all patients who have undergone splenectomy.*

ANSWER: b, c, d

REFERENCE: *Chapter 53—Spleen: Physiology*

3. Choose the correct statement(s) describing splenic artery aneurysms:

a. The splenic artery is the second most common abdominal artery to be affect by aneurysmal changes

b. Splenic artery aneurysms are typically asymptomatic and may be detected by a rim of calcifications in the left upper quadrant visible on plain film

c. While symptomatic splenic artery aneurysms are best treated with splenectomy, the majority of patients with asymptomatic aneurysms require no therapy

d. Splenic artery aneurysms occur more commonly in women by a 2:1 ratio

e. All of the above

COMMENT: Splenic artery aneurysms are rare, but are the second most common site of abdominal artery aneurysms. They occur in women twice as often as in men and are most often asymptomatic. They may be discovered by the appearance of calcifications in the left upper quadrant noted on plain film or by CT scan. Symptomatic splenic artery aneurysms are best treated with splenectomy. Asymptomatic calcified atherosclerotic aneurysms in elderly patients require no intervention, but an aneurysm found in a younger patient should be treated with elective splenectomy. This is particularly true in young women of childbearing age, as the risk of rupture increases substantially during pregnancy.

ANSWER: a, b, d

REFERENCE: *Chapter 53—Spleen: Indications for Splenectomy not Related to Hypersplenism*

4. A 23-year-old man presents to the emergency room after being thrown over the handlebars of his mountain bike, landing on his left side. He complains only of left sided abdominal pain. Initial vital signs are P = 100, BP = 110/70, RR = 18. Abdominal exam is notable for focal left upper quadrant tenderness. CT scan of the abdomen reveals a 3 cm laceration through the inferior pole of the spleen with small hematoma and modest amount of free fluid in the left upper quadrant and paracolic gutter. No other injuries are identified. Appropriate initial management of this patient is:

a. Selective embolization of the splenic artery branches to the inferior pole

b. Diagnostic laparoscopy including evaluation of the left hemi-diaphragm

c. Observation, with serial examinations and hemoglobins in a monitored unit

d. Splenectomy

e. Exploratory laparotomy with attempted splenic salvage

COMMENT: Recent series have confirmed the safety of nonoperative management of blunt splenic injury. Eligible patients should be hemodynamically stable and have no other injuries that require either operative management or that could interfere with obtaining a reliable exam (i.e., head injury). Patients should be admitted to a monitored unit where they can be closely monitored with serial examinations and hemoglobins. Between 3% and 15% of patients will ultimately require laparotomy for ongoing or recurrent bleeding. Embolization and laparoscopy do not play a role in the initial management of patients with splenic injury secondary to blunt trauma.

ANSWER: c

REFERENCE: *Chapter 53—Spleen: Indications for Splenectomy not Related to Hypersplenism*

5. A 55-year-old man is undergoing a left hemi-colectomy when upon exploration of the abdomen, three small (2 cm) cystic lesions are discovered arising from the superior pole of the spleen. The spleen is otherwise normal in size and appearance. The most appropriate management of these lesions is:

a. Aspiration and cyst wall biopsy
b. Partial splenectomy
c. Splenectomy
d. No intervention required

COMMENT: Simple cysts of the spleen are relatively common and are often multifocal. They have co clinical significance unless they reach a large size and become symptomatic. Incidentally discovered splenic cysts require no intervention. Metastases to the spleen are very uncommon and would likely not appear cystic.

ANSWER: d

REFERENCE: *Chapter 53—Spleen: Indications for Splenectomy not Related to Hypersplenism*

6. A 47-year-old man with a history of chronic hereditary pancreatitis presents with upper gastrointestinal bleeding. Upper endoscopy reveals several large varices along the greater curvature of the stomach. What is the most likely underlying diagnosis and indicated treatment?

a. Hypersplenism; splenectomy
b. Portal hypertension; transjugular intrahepatic portocaval shunt
c. Splenic vein thrombosis; splenectomy
d. Hypersplenism; splenic artery embolization
e. Splenic vein thrombosis; portocaval shunt

COMMENT: Chronic pancreatitis is the most common cause of splenic vein thrombosis. Thrombosis of the splenic vein can lead to sinistral or "left-sided" portal hypertension, with the development of splenomegaly and gastric varices at the site of venous collaterals in the splenogastric ligament. Upper GI bleeding is the most common presentation of this disease, and is an indication for splenectomy. Traditional procedure to treat portal hypertension will not affect this disorder.

ANSWER: c

REFERENCE: *Chapter 53—Spleen: Hypersplenism*

7. Which of the following diseases often require splenectomy for long-term management?

a. Sickle cell anemia
b. Hereditary spherocytosis
c. Hodgkin's lymphoma
d. Immune thrombocytopenic purpura
e. Autoimmune hemolytic anemia

COMMENT: Hereditary spherocytosis is treated primarily with splenectomy, which eliminates the symptoms of anemia, jaundice, and splenomegaly. ITP also often requires splenectomy to achieve lasting clinical remission, which is achieved in 60%–80% of patients after splenectomy. Autoimmune hemolytic anemia is also an indication for splenectomy in patients that do not respond or who cannot be treated with splenectomy. Sickle cell anemia rarely requires splenectomy for hypersplenism and most patients with this disorder have a small atrophied spleen that results from recurrent infarctions. Hodgkin's disease does not require splenectomy, and routine splenectomy for staging has not been shown to improve patient survival when compared to clinical staging alone.

ANSWER: b, d, e

REFERENCE: *Chapter 53—Spleen: Hypersplenism*

8. Which of the following statements is/are true concerning immune thrombocytopenic purpura?

a. The central defect in patients with ITP is the development of IgG specific to a platelet antigen, most commonly the fibrinogen receptor
b. The majority of patients with ITP will have palpable spleens, with spleens greater than 1,000 g in mass
c. Standard medical therapy for ITP includes corticosteroids, platelet transfusions, and Rho(D) immunoglobulin
d. Recurrence of ITP after laparoscopic splenectomy should prompt investigation into an alternative diagnosis

COMMENT: ITP is an autoimmune disease characterized by the production of IgG antibodies against a platelt antigen, most commonly the fibrinogen receptor. The spleen has been implicated as both a site of antibody production and platelet destruction in this disorder. Patients are initially managed with medical therapies aimed at increasing the platelet count including corticosteroids, platelet transfusions, and infusion therapy with gamma-immunoglobulin and Rho(D) immunoglobulin (which specifically targets Fc receptors). Sustained remission is rarely achieved by medical therapy alone and most patients are treated with splenectomy. As these patients have relatively normal to slightly-enlarged spleens, they are good candidates for laparoscopic splenectomy. Complete remission is achieved in 60%–80% of patients after splenectomy. Patients who fail treatment with splenectomy should be evaluated for accessory spleens, which may be detected through the use of indium-labeled platelets and single-photon emission computed tomography (SPECT).

ANSWER: a, c

REFERENCE: *Chapter 53—Spleen: Embryology and Anatomy*

CHAPTER 54

THYROID GLAND

1. A nonrecurrent right "recurrent laryngeal nerve" is most likely mistaken for which of the following structures?

   a. Superior thyroid artery
   b. Middle thyroid vein
   c. External branch of the superior laryngeal nerve
   d. Inferior thyroid artery

COMMENT: A nonrecurrent laryngeal nerve is present on the right in approximately 1% of persons (see Fig. 54.4). The nonrecurrent laryngeal nerve runs parallel to the inferior thyroid artery and can be mistaken for an arterial branch and is therefore subject to injury.

ANSWER: d

REFERENCE: *Chapter 54—Thyroid Gland: Surgical Anatomy*

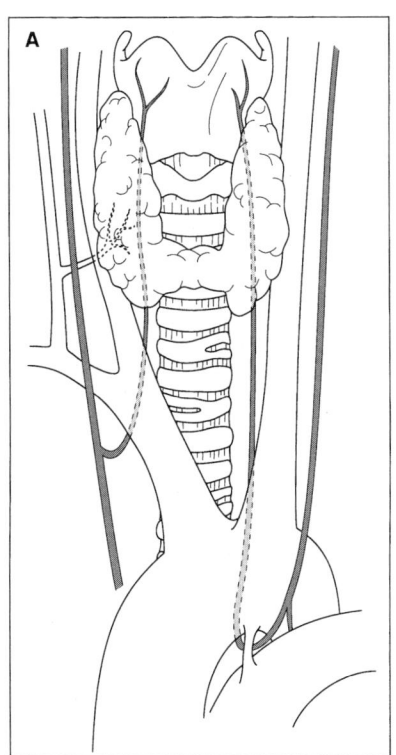
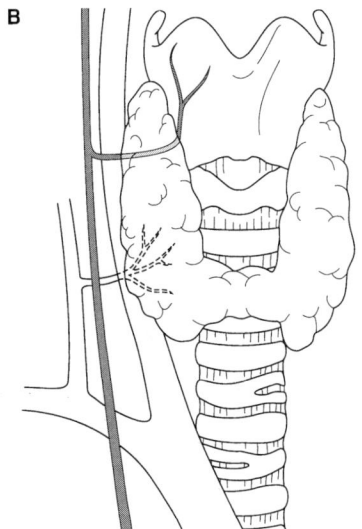
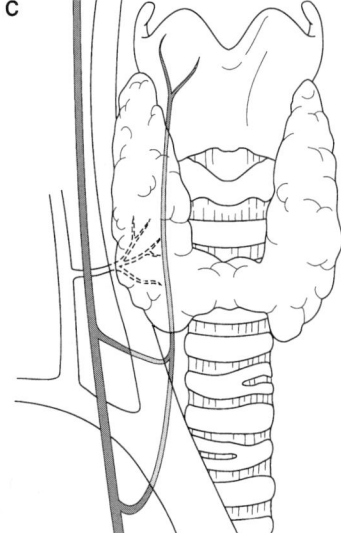

Figure 54.4

2. Patients with Graves' disease often present with:
   a. Thyrotoxicosis
   b. Exophthalmos
   c. Elevated serum thyroxine (T_4) level
   d. Suppressed thyroid-stimulating hormone (TSH)

COMMENT: Graves' disease is an autoimmune disorder with a genetic predisposition, a higher incidence among women, and the presence of thyroid-stimulating immunoglobulins. In addition to classic symptoms and signs of thyrotoxicosis, patients also have exophthalmos.

ANSWER: a, b, c, d

REFERENCE: *Chapter 54—Thyroid Gland: Functional Disorders*

3. The most important diagnostic study for a patient with normal thyroid function and a dominant thyroid nodule is:
   a. Ultrasonography of the thyroid
   b. Technetium 99m pertechnetate scan
   c. Fine needle aspiration (FNA)
   d. Thyroid lobectomy

COMMENT: After a careful history interview and physical examination, FNA is the single most important diagnostic procedure for patients with normal thyroid function and dominant thyroid nodules. Patients with hyperthyroidism due to toxic adenoma do not benefit from FNA.

ANSWER: c

REFERENCE: *Chapter 54—Thyroid Gland: Solitary or Dominant Thyroid Nodule*

4. A 57-year-old man has a 3-cm left thyroid nodule. Fine-needle aspiration shows a follicular neoplasm. The most appropriate procedure for this patient is:
   a. Suppression of thyroid hormone
   b. Core biopsy
   c. Left thyroid lobectomy
   d. Total thyroidectomy

COMMENT: Approximately 20% of follicular neoplasms of the thyroid prove malignant on histologic review of permanent resected specimens. Neither FNA cytologic examination nor intraoperative frozen section analysis can help reliably differentiate follicular adenoma from follicular carcinoma.

ANSWER: c

REFERENCE: *Chapter 54—Thyroid Gland: Fine Needle Aspiration (FNA)*

5. A 26-year-old woman with a thyroid nodule undergoes FNA, the results of which confirm the diagnosis of medullary carcinoma of the thyroid. Additional preoperative studies likely to be useful to this patient include:
   a. Measurement of serum level of carcinoembryonic antigen
   b. Measurement of serum level of calcitonin
   c. Measurement of serum level of parathyroid hormone
   d. Urinary metanephrine screen

COMMENT: This patient may have an index case of multiple endocrine neoplasia type 2A. All of these preoperative studies are appropriate.

ANSWER: a, b, c, d

REFERENCE: *Chapter 54—Thyroid Gland: Medullary Carcinoma*

CHAPTER 55

PARATHYROID GLANDS

1. A 30-year-old man has severe peptic ulcer disease and hypergastrinemia. His father and one sibling have had pancreatic islet cell tumor. Which of the following tests is/are appropriate?

   a. Measurement of serum level of calcium
   b. Twenty-four-hour urine collection to measure catecholamines and metanephrine
   c. Somatostatin receptor scintigraphy
   d. Measurement of serum level of prolactin
   e. Calcium pentagastrin stimulation test for calcitonin

COMMENT: Pancreatic islet cell tumor associated with Zollinger-Ellison syndrome (gastrinoma), especially with a family history, may be a feature of multiple endocrine neoplasia type 1. This syndrome includes primary hyperparathyroidism, duodenal pancreatic islet cell tumor, and adenoma of the anterior pituitary gland. Appropriate tests include screening for primary hyperparathyroidism with a serum level of calcium and screening for pituitary adenoma with prolactin level, because this is the most frequent functional pituitary tumor in the syndrome. Somatostatin receptor scintigraphy can be helpful for localizing primary tumors and metastatic lesions. Multiple endocrine neoplasia type II includes medullary carcinoma of the thyroid gland, pheochromocytoma, and primary hyperparathyroidism. Urine catecholamine testing and serum calcitonin testing may be appropriate for patients believed to have multiple endocrine neoplasia type 2.

ANSWER: a, c, d

REFERENCE: *Chapter 55—Parathyroid Glands: Hyperparathyroidism*

2. In a patient with primary hyperparathyroidism, three normal parathyroid glands are identified at exploration. Appropriate further investigation to identify the fourth, presumably abnormal, gland during the operation include(s):

   a. Intraoperative ultrasound examination of the neck
   b. Removal of the thyroid lobe on the side of the missing gland
   c. Removal of the cervically accessible thymus gland
   d. Exploration of the carotid sheath
   e. Exploration of the retropharyngeal tissues

COMMENT: The parathyroid glands can be situated in several unusual sites in the neck, such as within the thyroid and any site from the retropharyngeal area through the carotid sheath and well down into the mediastinum. Variations in parathyroid anatomy are caused primarily by differences in patterns of embryogenesis. During the fourth and fifth weeks of fetal development, the embryo develops a series of four pharyngeal pouches (see Fig. 55.2). The superior parathyroid glands arise from the fourth pharyngeal pouch in conjunction with the lateral part of the thyroid, and the inferior glands arise from the third pouch along with the thymus. The derivatives of each pouch migrate together so that the superior parathyroid glands usually remain in close association with the upper pole of the thyroid. They can, however, occasionally be loosely attached by a long vascular pedicle and migrate caudally along the esophagus into the posterior mediastinum. In some instances, a gland is totally embedded in the thyroid parenchyma. The inferior parathyroid glands descend with the thymus, but this migration may be extremely variable. Inferior glands can be found anywhere from the pharynx to the mediastinum. Regardless of their location, they usually adhere to the thymus or are within the thyrothymic ligament. Supernumerary glands can be identified in as many as 15% of patients, most often in association with the thymus. Results of autopsy studies suggest that four parathyroid glands almost always are present.

ANSWER: a, b, c, d, e

REFERENCE: *Chapter 55—Parathyroid Glands: Hyperparathyroidism; Principles of Surgical Correction*

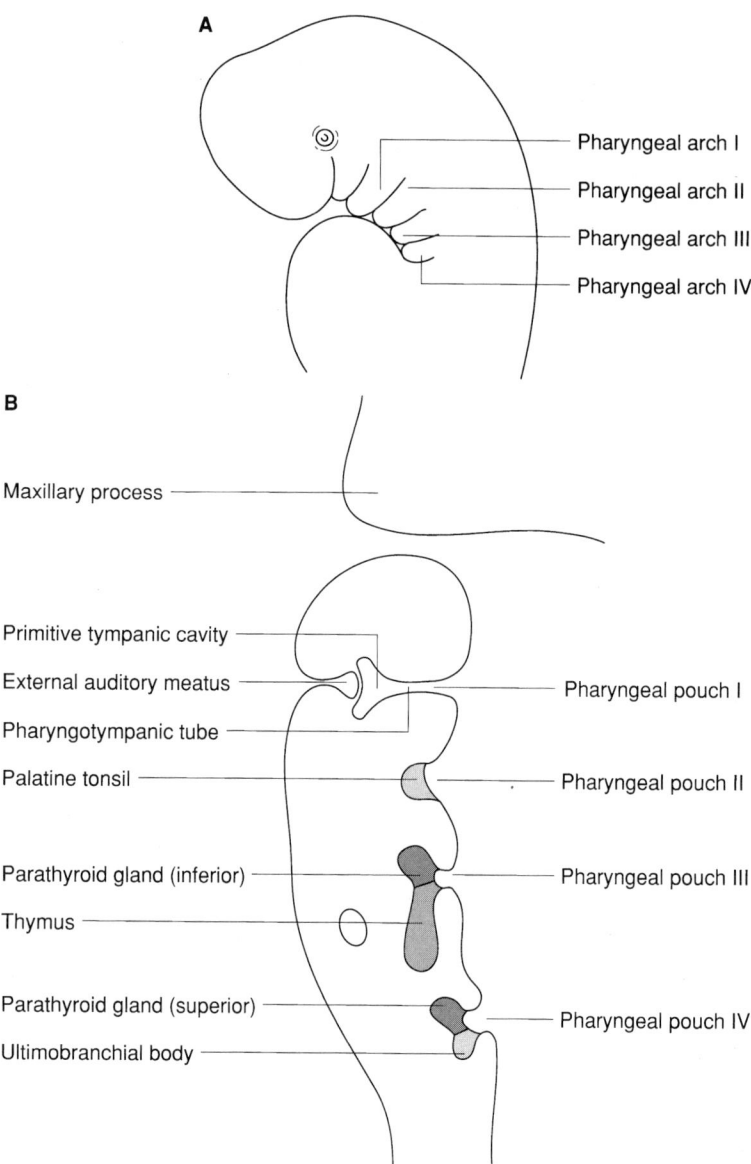

A

Pharyngeal arch I
Pharyngeal arch II
Pharyngeal arch III
Pharyngeal arch IV

B

Maxillary process

Primitive tympanic cavity
External auditory meatus — Pharyngeal pouch I
Pharyngotympanic tube
Palatine tonsil — Pharyngeal pouch II
Parathyroid gland (inferior) — Pharyngeal pouch III
Thymus
Parathyroid gland (superior) — Pharyngeal pouch IV
Ultimobranchial body

Figure 55.2

3. Parathyroid hormone level:
   a. Is most reliably measured by means of amino-terminal assay
   b. Can be a useful intraoperative adjunct as a rapid assay
   c. Is confounded by the presence of high serum levels of parathyroid hormone–related protein
   d. Is depressed among patients with renal failure because of low levels of vitamin D
   e. Generally is elevated among patients with humoral hypercalcemia of malignant disease

COMMENT: The level of parathyroid hormone in serum is most reliably measured with an intact parathyroid hormone assay, which can be performed rapidly as an intraoperative adjunct. The intact assay does not have cross reactivity with parathyroid hormone–related protein, and thus parathyroid hormone levels are typically low among patients with this humoral hypercalcemia of malignant disease. Parathyroid hormone levels are elevated among most patients with dialysis-dependent renal failure.

Parathyroid hormone is synthesized initially as a precursor, preproparathyroid hormone, that is sequentially cleaved in the parathyroid gland to proparathyroid hormone and then to parathyroid hormone (see Fig. 55.5). Secretion of this 84-amino-acid molecule is controlled by a negative feedback loop with extracellular fluid calcium. Most parathyroid hormone is secreted in this form and then cleaved in the liver into N- and C-terminal fragments. The N terminus contains most of the biologic activity and is rapidly degraded by the liver, whereas the inactive C terminus is slowly metabolized by the kidney.

ANSWER: b

REFERENCE: *Chapter 55—Parathyroid Glands: Physiology*

4. Hypocalcemia:
   a. Is most frequently a result of operative damage to the parathyroid glands
   b. Causes symptoms of neurologic and muscular excitability, including numbness, tingling, and muscle spasms
   c. If symptomatic, should be managed with intravenous administration of calcium chloride
   d. Usually occurs within 6 hours of thyroid surgery if it occurs at all
   e. Can be effectively managed over the long term with calcium and vitamin D supplementation

COMMENT: Thyroid surgery is the most common cause of hypocalcemia. The nadir of calcium levels after thyroid surgery is typically 48 to 72 hours after the operation. Hypocalcemia can generally be managed with oral calcium, vitamin D, or both. Patients with severe symptoms may need treatment with intravenous calcium; however, this should always be calcium gluconate rather than calcium chloride because of the risk of soft-tissue damage with calcium chloride infusion.

ANSWER: a, b, e

REFERENCE: *Chapter 55—Parathyroid Glands: Hypocalcemia*

5. Biochemical hyperparathyroidism among patients with minimal or no symptoms:
   a. Is an absolute indication for operative intervention
   b. Should never be approached operatively
   c. May be managed with medical monitoring with careful follow-up evaluation
   d. Necessitates individualized assessment of the situation
   e. May necessitate direct bone mass measurement to determine the best course of management

COMMENT: The treatment of patients with asymptomatic primary hyperparathyroidism is controversial. It is clear from the available data that the patient's condition does not deteriorate rapidly, so immediate operation is not necessary. However, biochemical correction can be obtained and improvement in bone mass maintained over the long term with operative cure, so operation is appropriate for some patients. Management of this condition must be individualized.

ANSWER: c, d, e

REFERENCE: *Chapter 55—Parathyroid Glands: Hyperparathyroidism*

CHAPTER 56

ADRENAL GLANDS

1. Which of the following statements is/are true regarding the function of the adrenal gland?
   a. Release of corticotropin-releasing hormone (CRH) is regulated principally by negative feedback by corticotropin
   b. Plasma 17-ketosteroid levels reflect the degree of adrenal cortisol production
   c. Renin undergoes enzymatic cleavage in the lung to angiotensin I
   d. The plasma half-life of corticotropin is relatively long (>24 hours)
   e. None of the above

COMMENT: The proximate stimulator of cortisol production is the peptide hormone, adrenocorticotropic hormone (corticotropin). It originates in the anterior pituitary gland and is regulated by CRH. Regulation of CRH is controlled by various neural influences. These include intrinsic central nervous system influences and negative feedback inhibition by cortisol. Although there is evidence of short-loop feedback of corticotropin on CRH, both slow and fast feedback by cortisol on the pituitary release mechanism are the primary sources of clinically relevant CRH regulation.

The steroidogenic pathway involves conversion of cholesterol to pregnenolone, progesterone, or 17-hydroxyprogesterone and then to either adrenal androgen or cortisol through several intermediates. The 17-ketosteroids reflect adrenal androgen synthesis, and the 17-hydroxysteroids reflect cortisol synthesis.

Renin is produced predominantly in the juxtaglomerular apparatus of the kidney, where it acts locally and is released into the systemic circulation. Renin cleaves angiotensin I, a decapeptide derived from the liver, which serves as renin substrate. Angiotensin I undergoes enzymatic cleavage in the lung to angiotensin II, which is the biologically active form of the peptide. The plasma half-life of corticotropin is short (minutes), and the hormone has a rapid onset of action. This is in contrast to a longer plasma half-life and a slower onset of action of cortisol.

ANSWER: e

REFERENCE: *Chapter 56—Adrenal Glands: Physiology*

2. Which of the following are normal systemic effects of glucocorticoids?
   a. Enhanced proteolysis
   b. Increased gluconeogenesis
   c. Diminished lipolysis
   d. Decreased rate of intestinal epithelial replication

COMMENT: The many systemic effects of glucocorticoids are related to regulation of intermediary metabolism. In this regard, perhaps the most important action is the effect of steroids on protein breakdown. A direct proteolytic effect of steroids is suggested by several lines of evidence.

Glucocorticoids enhance gluconeogenesis by both a direct effect on gluconeogenic hepatic enzymes and provision of substrate for gluconeogenesis by means of proteolysis. Glucocorticoid influence leads to the accentuation of lipolysis. The truncal obesity of steroid excess is related to the predominance of the lipogenic effect of insulin on truncal adipocytes over the lipolytic effect of glucocorticoids. The opposite relation may hold for the receptors in fat of the extremities and would explain the comparatively scant fat in these areas with steroid excess.

The most notable effect of glucocorticoids in the intestinal tract is a decrease in the rate of mucosal cell replication. Mucosal and pancreatic prostaglandin synthesis is decreased. This may have important implications for the cytoprotective mechanisms in the stomach.

ANSWER: a, b, d

REFERENCE: *Chapter 56—Adrenal Glands: Cortisol*

3. Which of the following statements is/are true regarding androgens and estrogens in the fetus?

   a. The development of normal female external genitalia requires estrogen production by the ovary
   b. A girl with congenital adrenal hyperplasia is likely to be masculinized in appearance
   c. The development of normal male external genitalia requires adrenal androgen production
   d. A boy with congenital adrenal hyperplasia is likely to be feminized in appearance

COMMENT: Adrenal androgens in the fetus stimulate wolffian duct development and elongate the genital tubercle. They promote midline migration of the labial folds and fusion of these folds to form the scrotum. To complete the male transformation, the urethral opening migrates to the tip of the phallus. All of these events are androgen dependent. Because a normal female fetus does not secrete androgens, the genital tubercle, labial folds, and urethral opening all remain in the female position in this circumstance. Thus the female phenotype is associated with the absence of production of fetal sex hormones. Excess androgen in a female fetus causes neonatal virilization, as in congenital adrenal hyperplasia. A male infant with congenital adrenal hyperplasia is likely to have normal-looking external genitalia as a neonate. Precocious puberty develops over a period of years in the latter circumstance.

ANSWER: b, c

REFERENCE: *Chapter 56—Adrenal Glands: Androgens and Estrogens*

4. A term neonate is found to have ambiguous female genitalia. This infant is at risk of which of the following life-threatening problems?

   a. Cardiomyopathy with congestive heart failure
   b. Sodium-wasting nephropathy with hypovolemia
   c. Respiratory failure from surfactant deficiency
   d. Spontaneous hemorrhage from thrombocytopenia
   e. Pulmonary embolus from a hypercoagulable state

COMMENT: Enzymatic defects in the steroidogenic pathway produce a syndrome known as *congenital adrenal hyperplasia*. This syndrome presents predominantly in the neonatal period with sexual ambiguity. These enzymatic defects decrease cortisol secretion. The specific enzyme defects present determine the clinical form of the syndromes. These include 21-hydroxylase deficiency, 11β-hydroxylase deficiency, and 17-hydroxylase-deficiency. The 21-hydroxylase deficiency and the 11β-hydroxylase deficiency result in excess androgen production in utero and result in masculinization with ambiguous genitalia of a female newborn. Masculinizing effects in a boy may not be detected until precocious puberty becomes obvious. Approximately 40% of patients with 21-hydroxylase deficiency, the most common form, have salt wasting or sodium loss by urine. Hypovolemic shock can result. Cardiomyopathy, respiratory failure, thrombocytopenia, and pulmonary emboli are not associated with this syndrome.

ANSWER: b

REFERENCE: *Chapter 56—Adrenal Glands: Excess Sex Steroids*

5. Which of the following statements is/are true regarding aldosterone?

    a. Secretion is directly related to serum potassium concentration
    b. Angiotensin II is a more potent regulatory factor than is corticotropin
    c. Primary hyperaldosteronism is characterized by hyperkalemia
    d. Secondary hyperaldosteronism occurs with renal arterial stenosis

COMMENT: Aldosterone secretion is controlled by changes in afferent arteriolar pressure in the renal cortex and by changes in sodium content in the renal tubule. These changes are sensed by the juxtaglomerular apparatus and macula densa and act through the renin angiotensin system. At least two other factors influence aldosterone secretion. Aldosterone secretion is directly related to serum potassium concentration. An increase in serum level of potassium directly stimulates aldosterone production. A decrease in serum level of potassium has the opposite effect. Because of its early point of action in the steroidogenic pathway, corticotropin increases secretion of aldosterone, although it is much less potent in this regard than in its stimulation of cortisol. The stimulatory effects of potassium and corticotropin on aldosterone secretion can be overcome by means of angiotensin II stimulation.

Primary hyperaldosteronism is characterized by mineralocorticoid hypersecretion, which promotes a positive sodium balance and hypokalemia. Approximately 80% of patients with primary hyperaldosteronism have serum potassium levels of 3.5 mEq/L or less. Causes of secondary hyperaldosteronism are related to increased renin secretion. These include renal arterial stenosis, congestive heart failure, and renal salt wasting.

ANSWER: a, b, d

REFERENCE: *Chapter 56—Adrenal Glands: Control of Aldosterone Secretion; Aldosterone Excess*

6. The causes of Cushing syndrome include which of the following?

    a. Posterior pituitary adenoma
    b. Adrenal hyperplasia
    c. Small-cell carcinoma of the lung
    d. Pheochromocytoma
    e. Adrenal carcinoma

COMMENT: The varied causes of cortisol excess produce clinical features collectively called *Cushing's syndrome.* These include administration of exogenous steroids, Cushing's disease (excessive corticotropin production by the anterior pituitary gland, usually from adenoma), ectopic corticotropin production (small-cell carcinoma of the lung), adrenal adenoma or carcinoma, micronodular pigmented hyperplasia, macronodular hyperplasia, and steroid-dependent adrenal hyperplasia. Pheochromocytoma is characterized by catecholamine rather than cortisol excess because it arises from the adrenal medulla rather than the adrenal cortex.

ANSWER: b, c, e

REFERENCE: *Chapter 56—Adrenal Glands: Cortisol Excess; Catecholamine Excess*

7. A 10-year-old child has hypertension, tachycardia, nervousness, and sweating. The best initial diagnostic evaluation is which of the following?

a. Radioimmunoassays for norepinephrine and epinephrine in serum
b. Magnetic resonance imaging (MRI) of the adrenal gland
c. Iodine 131 metaiodobenzylguanidine (MIBG) scintigraphy
d. Measurement of catecholamines and their degradation products in a 24-hour urine specimen

COMMENT: The first diagnostic step in determining the functional state of an adrenal gland or lesion is to screen the urine or plasma for secretory products. Once hypersecretion is found, the specific pathologic condition producing a syndrome must be determined with the aid of functional tests and relevant scanning and imaging. The most efficient and sensitive means of screening when a patient is believed to have pheochromocytoma, as in this case, is measurement of the catecholamines or metabolic products thereof in the urine. Although 24-hour samples can smooth out the possible episodic variations in catecholamine secretion, shorter sampling periods can be useful, especially if corrected for creatinine excretion. Timing of the collection is critical for patients who have only episodic hypertension. Urine collection should be started immediately after a suspected attack of hypertension. Fluctuations in plasma catecholamine concentration are much greater than those in urinary excretion, even among healthy persons. Plasma determinations are quite sensitive and specific with radioimmunoassays and high-performance liquid chromatographic measurement of plasma levels of catecholamines. The specificity can be low, however, because of the overlap of normal spikes in catecholamine concentration with concentration produced by minimally secreting pheochromocytoma. Magnetic resonance imaging and MIBG scintigraphy both can be useful after catecholamine excess is confirmed. Magnetic resonance imaging shows anatomic features well. Iodine 131 metaiodobenzylguanidine scintigraphy is particularly useful in looking for nonadrenal and bilateral pheochromocytoma.

ANSWER: d

REFERENCE: *Chapter 56—Adrenal Glands: Diagnostic Investigations*

8. Which of the following diagnostic tests help(s) differentiate the pituitary gland and adrenal glands as the cause of hypercortisolism?

a. High-dose dexamethasone suppression test
b. Corticotropin-releasing hormone stimulation test
c. Low-dose dexamethasone test
d. Day and night measurement of cortisol in the plasma

COMMENT: Diurnal variation of plasma cortisol levels is lost in hypercortisolism caused by adrenal tumors or pituitary lesions. Dexamethasone, by means of negative feedback, suppresses hypothalamic-pituitary secretion of corticotropin and affects consequent decreases in plasma excretion of cortisol and urinary 17-hydroxycorticosteroid. Administration of a single dose of 2 mg dexamethasone suppresses plasma cortisol and urinary 17-hydroxycorticosteroids at least one half compared with the control value for untreated healthy persons (low-dose suppression test). In Cushing's disease, in which the setpoint of corticotropin secretion is higher than normal, low-dose dexamethasone is insufficient to suppress corticotropin. High-dose dexamethasone suppression is achieved with 2 mg dexamethasone administered every 6 hours for 24 hours. A normal response is to decrease 17-hydroxycorticosteroid excretion more than one half. In the case of Cushing's disease, the hypothalamic steroid receptors that allow negative feedback are intact but at a higher setpoint. In this case, 17-hydroxycorticosteroid secretion decrease considerably after high-dose administration of dexamethasone. Adrenal tumors, other causes of ectopic production of corticotropin, and most cases of nodular hyperplasia do not respond to dexamethasone suppression with a decrease in steroid secretion. With an adrenal tumor, pituitary corticotropin is already suppressed, and dexamethasone cannot suppress it further. With ectopic corticotropin secretion, the tissue that produces corticotropin has no receptors for steroids, and negative feedback cannot be achieved. Therefore high-dose dexamethasone suppression differentiates hypercortisolism of pituitary and adrenal origin.

Possibly the most helpful new test for this purpose entails administration of recombinant CRH to release corticotropin and to stimulate cortisol secretion. Corticotropin-releasing hormone (1 mg/kg) is administered intravenously, and serial blood samples are obtained for 3 hours after administration. The normal pituitary adrenal axis responds with a moderate increase in corticotropin and cortisol. In Cushing's disease, the increases in corticotropin and cortisol are accentuated. With adrenal autonomous production of cortisol and with ectopic corticotropin production, there is almost no response to CRH.

ANSWER: a, b

REFERENCE: *Chapter 56—Adrenal Glands: Hypercortisolism; Cushing Syndrome*

9. Imaging of the adrenal glands is best achieved with which of the following techniques?
   a. Ultrasound
   b. Computed tomography (CT)
   c. Arteriography
   d. Scintigraphy with iodine 131 6-β-iodomethyl-19-norcholesterol (NP-59)
   e. Scintigraphy with MIBG

COMMENT: Although ultrasonography is the least expensive of the imaging procedures, its value is limited by the relative inaccessibility of the adrenal glands and by the small size of some adrenal lesions. Computed tomography is the technique most commonly used to examine patients with suspected adrenal abnormalities. Computed tomography reliably depicts adrenal tumors larger than 1 cm in diameter. The sensitivity of CT for tumors 1 cm in diameter is approximately 80% and reaches 100% for tumors 3 to 4 cm in diameter. Although CT is noninvasive and reasonably sensitive, it is nonspecific. It does not differentiate functioning from nonfunctioning tumors or benign from malignant tumors with any degree of reliability.

Magnetic resonance imaging has developed a certain usefulness even after retrenchment from early optimistic predictions. Magnetic resonance imaging is more expensive than CT and requires greater patient cooperation, but it has greater versatility because of the use of T1- and T2-weighted images. In some cases, T2-weighted images provide a differential diagnosis and help differentiate entities such as metastatic or primary carcinoma and pheochromocytoma from adenoma, lipoma, myelolipoma, and cysts. In a sense, MRI is complementary to CT in that the latter can better depict the lesion whereas the former can differentiate one type of lesion from the other. Magnetic resonance imaging is probably better than CT for differentiating anatomic relationships and the extent of involvement of the surrounding tissues.

Two radiopharmaceuticals have proved useful in imaging the adrenal gland. Adrenocortical lesions can be imaged with NP-59, which is taken up as cholesterol in the adrenocortical steroidogenic pathway. The other agent is MIBG, a norepinephrine analogue. It indicates norepinephrine accumulation in storage vesicles and can help detect sympathoadrenal tumors at any site in the body. Scintigraphy with NP-56 can localize the adrenal cortex and any functioning tumors. It can help differentiate adrenocortical hyperplasia from functioning adenoma or carcinoma. Scintigraphy with MIBG is useful in localizing pheochromocytoma throughout the body, especially when the tumors are multiple, extraadrenal, recurrent, or metastatic.

Arteriography, venography, and selective venous sampling have become less popular as experience with other imaging techniques has become greater. Invasive procedures with intravascular contrast agents have clear disadvantages. Arteriography is especially dangerous in examinations of patients with pheochromocytoma.

ANSWER: b

REFERENCE: *Chapter 56—Adrenal Glands: Diagnostic Investigations*

10. Which of the following adrenal lesions can be managed definitively by medical means?

   a. Benign functional adrenocortical adenoma
   b. Adrenocortical carcinoma
   c. Congenital adrenal hyperplasia
   d. Cushing's disease
   e. Pheochromocytoma

COMMENT: Management of adrenal tumors is primarily surgical removal. Although pharmaceutical agents are useful in preparing the patient for surgery or in palliative treatment of patients with recurrent adrenal carcinoma, no agent is definitive therapy for adrenal tumors. Congenital adrenal hyperplasia stands alone among the primary, hyperfunctioning adrenal syndromes amenable to medical therapy for definitive control. Functioning benign lesions of the adrenal cortex that are not corticotropin dependent, such as adenoma or macronodular hyperplasia, respond to metyrapone and aminoglutethimide, which are inhibitors of enzymes in the adrenal steroidogenic pathway. Both agents can effect a decrease in production of cortisol when there is no increase in corticotropin due to feedback stimulation. These drugs are not satisfactory long-term agents because of a high incidence of drug reactions, patient noncompliance, and continued growth of the lesions. They may be useful when surgery must be delayed. Although malignant, functioning adrenocortical lesions should be debulked whenever possible. Several chemotherapeutic agents can be used for adjunctive therapy. The most noteworthy is mitotane (*o,p,*-DDD). This cytolytic agent has a 30% to 70% response rate in terms of decreasing steroid output. Patient survival is not affected, however. Nonoperative treatment with cortisone acetate and possibly fludrocortisone is definitive therapy for congenital adrenal hyperplasia. Cushing's disease is best managed by means of transsphenoidal resection of the pituitary adenoma. Pheochromocytoma necessitates definitive surgical resection, although preoperative pharmacologic preparation with catecholamine blockade is needed.

ANSWER: c

REFERENCE: *Chapter 56—Adrenal Glands: Treatment*

11. A 45-year-old woman is found to have a 2-cm solid nodule in the right adrenal gland during abdominal CT after an automobile accident. The adrenal lesion is asymptomatic, and it is found nonfunctional on evaluation. You would recommend which of the following?

   a. Extraperitoneal right adrenalectomy through either a flank or a posterior approach
   b. Suppression with 5 mg prednisone by mouth every other day
   c. Follow-up CT in 1 to 3 months
   d. Excisional biopsy through a laparoscopic approach

COMMENT: The indication for operation in the care of a patient with a unilateral functioning adrenal tumor is clear. For a patient with a nonfunctioning adrenal tumor, the need for surgery is related to the size of the tumor and its rate of growth. There is consensus that a tumor larger than 6 cm should be removed. Some experts recommend that the acceptable size limit be 3 cm, especially when MRI findings suggest carcinoma or when results of functional studies suggest activity. When nonoperative therapy is chosen, the patient should undergo adrenal CT 1, 3, and 6 months after the initial scan and yearly thereafter to assess the growth of the lesion. If the tumor has grown, surgical removal is indicated.

ANSWER: c

REFERENCE: *Chapter 56—Adrenal Glands: Treatment*

12. A 25-year-old man has been taking 40 mg prednisone by mouth every other day for ulcerative colitis for 5 years. He undergoes an uneventful colectomy with endorectal pull-through and ileoanal anastomosis. Which of the following statements is/are correct regarding steroid management?

   a. On the day of the operation he should receive 100 mg hydrocortisone intravenously every 6 hours
   b. The postoperative steroid dose should be halved every 12 hours to reduce the risk of infectious complications and improve would healing
   c. Prophylactic treatment with a somatostatin analogue decreases the risk of postoperative pancreatitis
   d. Exogenous steroid replacement can be stopped after 3 months

COMMENT: Postoperative treatment of a patient with pituitary adrenal suppression from exogenous steroids involves tapering the exogenous steroid doses to maintenance levels after high-dose replacement at the time of operation. One simple regimen involves administering 100 mg hydrocortisone intravenously every 6 hours during the first 48 hours. Some experts prefer alternating intramuscular doses of cortisone acetate in the event that intravenous access is lost. If no intervening complications occur, the doses can be halved every 48 to 72 hours. In the care of patients who have been exposed preoperatively to glucocorticoid excess, the maintenance dose can be as high as 100 mg/d for several months. Both high doses and normal maintenance of 35 to 55 mg/d can be given in the form of oral cortisone acetate as long as reliable alimentation and absorption have been achieved. The pituitary-adrenal axis remains suppressed for 6 to 12 months after an operation. Complications in the postoperative period include wound infection, pancreatitis, and thromboembolism. There are no data to suggest that the risk of postoperative pancreatitis can be diminished with somatostatin analogue therapy.

ANSWER: a

REFERENCE: *Chapter 56—Adrenal Glands: Operative Treatment*

13. A 20-year-old man with a 10-cm left adrenal mass is found to have 10 mg norepinephrine in a 24-hour urine collection and a plasma 18-hydroxycorticosterone level of 50 mg/dL. Initial reoperative preparation includes which of the following?

   a. Treatment with spironolactone
   b. Intravenous potassium loading to prevent intraoperative hypokalemia
   c. Treatment with phenoxybenzamine
   d. Treatment with labetalol

COMMENT: This patient has a pheochromocytoma. The most efficient and sensitive means of screening for pheochromocytoma is measurement of catecholamines, or metabolic products thereof, in the urine. The catecholamines norepinephrine and epinephrine are excreted in amounts less than 100 µg/d among healthy persons. Because of overlap in values, specificity can be improved by use of a normal range of up to 250 mg/d. Measurement of plasma level 18-hydroxycorticosterone is helpful in the evaluation of patients with hyperaldosteronism, because it is an intermediate product in aldosterone synthesis. The levels of 18-hydroxycorticosterone are greater than 100 mg/dL in almost all patients with aldosterone-producing adenoma. The plasma value for this patient is normal. Perioperative treatment with spironolactone and potassium replacement is appropriate for patients with hyperaldosteronism but not for those with pheochromocytoma.

Nonoperative management of pheochromocytoma is generally unsatisfactory and entails pharmacologic blockade of the effects of catecholamines. Phenoxybenzamine and prazosin are two preferred agents that block the α-adrenergic effects of the catecholamines preoperatively with pheochromocytoma. The use of β-adrenergic blockers, such as labetalol, may be required in the care of patients with obvious β-adrenergic effects, such as resting heart rates greater than 100 beats/min.

Because of the risk of wide swings in blood pressure and other effects of chronic catecholamine secretion, careful preoperative preparation is required by patients with pheochromocytoma. It is customary to institute α-adrenergic blockade 2 to 3 weeks before anticipated surgery. This has beneficial effects of controlling blood pressure and allowing restoration of a decrease in blood volume. It is the consensus that preoperative preparation in this manner makes intraoperative care of the patient much safer. For patients who need β-adrenergic blockade, it is essential to first establish good α-adrenergic blockade. These patients are prone to cardiac failure induced by β-adrenergic blockade because of possible preexisting cardiomyopathy. β-Adrenergic blockade in the treatment of a patient with cardiomyopathy after failure to first reduce the afterload with α-adrenergic blockade can precipitate cardiac failure.

ANSWER: c

REFERENCE: *Chapter 56—Adrenal Glands: Pheochromocytoma*

14. The approximate 5-year survival rate for adrenocortical carcinoma is which of the following?
    a. Zero
    b. 20% to 25%
    c. 50% to 60%
    d. Nearly 100%

COMMENT: The prognosis for adrenocortical carcinoma is not good. The overall 5-year survival rate is 20% to 25% for these malignant tumors. When there is localized disease at surgery, the 5-year survival may be higher, in the 40% to 50% range. The true prognosis among children is not clear, but the data suggest a 2-year survival rate of approximately 20%.

ANSWER: b

REFERENCE: *Chapter 56—Adrenal Glands: Outcomes*

15. Which of the following statements is/are true with respect to pheochromocytoma?

    a. Pheochromocytoma associated with multiple endocrine neoplasia type 2a usually is unilateral and rarely is malignant; therefore, unilateral exploration through a posterior flank incision usually is sufficient

    b. Clonidine does not suppress basal plasma levels of catecholamines in patients with pheochromocytoma

    c. Iodine 131 6-β-iodomethyl-19-norcholesterol is taken up as cholesterol by the adrenal medulla

    d. The ratio of plasma 3,4-dihydroxyphenylglycol (DHPG) to norepinephrine is generally higher among patients with pheochromocytoma than among patients with essential hypertension

COMMENT: Pheochromocytoma associated with multiple endocrine neoplasia type 2a syndrome is often bilateral and malignant; therefore abdominal exploration through an anterior approach is indicated. The ability to measure catecholamines in the plasma has made possible the clonidine suppression test. In patients without pheochromocytoma, clonidine suppresses high basal plasma concentrations into the normal range, whereas concentrations in patients with pheochromocytoma are not suppressed. Another use of plasma catecholamine measurement is to examine the ratio of DHPG to norepinephrine in plasma. 3,4-Dihydroxyphenylglycol is released from the chromaffin cells and adrenergic neurons to a much greater extent than is norepinephrine in pheochromocytoma patients than in patients with essential hypertension. That is, the ratio of DHPG to norepinephrine is higher among patients with pheochromocytoma.

Iodine 131 6-β-iodomethyl-19-norcholesterol is taken up as cholesterol by the adrenal cortex and is incorporated in the adrenocortical steroidogenic pathway. It is a useful agent for imaging adrenocortical lesions. Iodine 131 metaiodobenzylguanidine is a norepinephrine analogue useful in localizing pheochromocytoma throughout the body, especially when the tumors are multiple, extraadrenal, recurrent, or metastatic.

ANSWER: b, d

REFERENCE: *Chapter 56—Adrenal Glands: Diagnostic Investigations*

CHAPTER 57

PITUITARY GLAND

1. Which of the following statements is/are true regarding the pituitary gland?

    a. Antidiuretic hormone is a product of the neurohypophysis

    b. The preferred surgical approach to the pituitary gland is through the sphenoid sinus

    c. Growth hormone (GH), corticotropin, luteinizing hormone, follicle-stimulating hormone (FSH), and serotonin are products of the adenohypophysis

    d. The adenohypophysis is regulated by neurotransmitters released by the supraoptic hypophyseal tract

COMMENT: The anterior pituitary gland is the adenohypophysis, which constitutes 80% of the gland. The posterior pituitary gland, the neurohypophysis, constitutes the remainder and should be considered almost an extension of the hypothalamus of the brain. The pituitary glands are situated within the bony confines of the sella turcica (Turkish saddle) and are bordered laterally by the cavernous sinuses (venous), inferiorly and anteriorly by the sphenoid sinus (air), posteriorly by the dorsum sella, and superiorly by the membranous diaphragma sella. Each cavernous sinus contains the siphon region of the internal carotid artery and portions of cranial nerves III, IV, V, and VI, all within the venous plexus. The optic chiasm lies immediately above the diaphragma sella. Directly below the anterior and inferior portions of the sella is the aerated sphenoid sinus. This is sufficiently large in 97% of patients to allow a transnasal, transsphenoidal surgical approach to the pituitary gland.

The adenohypophysis is regulated by a portal venous system between the median eminence of the hypothalamus and the adenohypophysis itself. This system involves transport of (a) thyrotropin-releasing hormone to stimulate secretion of the thyroid-stimulating hormone (TSH), (b) corticotropin-releasing hormone to stimulate corticotropin, (c) GH-releasing hormone to stimulate secretion of GH, (d) gonadotropin-releasing hormone to stimulate luteinizing hormone and FSH, and (e) prolactin-inhibitory factor (dopamine) to inhibit prolactin. The neurohypophysis is regulated by means of direct transport of hormones through nerve fibers from the supraoptic and paraventricular nuclei in the hypothalamus. The neurohypophysis is almost an extension of the hypothalamus. Products of the neurohypophysis are antidiuretic hormone (vasopressin) and oxytocin. The pituitary gland is not known to release serotonin.

ANSWER: a, b

REFERENCE: *Chapter 57—Pituitary Gland: Embryology, Anatomy, and Physiology*

2. Pituitary adenoma is best classified according to functional hormone output. This information may be derived from which of the following?
   a. Hematoxylin and eosin staining
   b. Immunohistochemical staining of pituitary tissue
   c. In situ hybridization studies
   d. Selective venous sampling from the inferior petrosal sinuses

COMMENT: Pituitary adenoma has been classified historically as acidophilic, basophilic, and chromophobic. Adenoma can have a variable staining pattern with conventional hematoxylin and eosin, so it is difficult to classify adenoma with these stains. Immunohistochemical analysis, ultrastructural studies, and in situ hybridization analysis for specific hormones are the most reliable methods of classifying pituitary adenoma. Immunohistochemical staining of pituitary adenoma with specific antibodies has reliably classified adenoma with highly purified polyclonal and monoclonal antibodies against prolactin, GH, corticotropin, FSH-β, luteinizing hormone β, and TSH-β. Many studies with these antibodies have revealed that some pituitary tumors are composed of several cell types, which produce various hormones. Some adenomas may not store specific hormones, so immunohistochemical staining may be weak or absent. Messenger RNA (mRNA) usually is present in the cytoplasm of adenoma. Localization of mRNA for specific protein hormones is becoming widely used in the classification of pituitary adenoma. As many as 25% of pituitary neoplasms are null-cell adenoma. Selective venous sampling from the inferior petrosal sinus by means of transfemoral catheterization is an effective method to compare venous effluent from the pituitary gland with systemic levels for a specific hormone. This technique also can show laterality. The latter issue may be important because certain small adenomas may not be discernible on the basis of gross appearance at surgery.

ANSWER: b, c, d

REFERENCE: *Chapter 57—Pituitary Gland: Methods of Cell Analysis; Clinical and Endocrine Evaluation, Cushing Disease*

3. A 30-year-old woman has amenorrhea, headache, and bitemporal hemianopsia. Appropriate diagnostic testing includes which of the following?

a. Cerebral angiography
b. Measurement of serum level of prolactin
c. Magnetic resonance imaging of the brain
d. Abdominal and pelvic computed tomography (CT)

COMMENT: Patients with pituitary lesions have symptoms and signs related to a mass effect on the pituitary gland and surrounding structures, to hypersecretion of the hormones by the lesion itself, or to a combination of both. As mass lesions in the pituitary enlarge, they encounter the contents of the cavernous sinuses, including the third, fourth, and sixth cranial nerves and the first two divisions of the fifth cranial nerve, as well as the internal carotid artery. Growth of a tumor in the relatively unrestricted upward direction is much more common than other forms of growth. It often results in compression of the optic chiasm and loss of vision, typically bitemporal hemianopsia. Prolactin-secreting pituitary adenoma often manifests as endocrine symptoms, including amenorrhea and galactorrhea among women. Among men, loss of libido, infertility, and visual loss are typical. Magnetic resonance imaging (MRI) has evolved as the first choice for diagnostic imaging and often is the only tool needed to reach a therapeutic decision with regard to pituitary adenoma. With intravenous infusion of a paramagnetic substance such as gadolinium, MRI depicts intrasellar tumors as small as 5 mm in diameter. The extent of suprasellar and sphenoid sinus extension as well as lateral extension into the cavernous sinuses also can be depicted. Cysts and hemorrhage can be differentiated, as can blood flowing within an aneurysm. Computed tomography has a place in pituitary imaging if MRI is not available. Plain radiographs of the skull usually are not needed. Cerebral angiography is performed only if an aneurysm is suspected or if a lesion is so large that occlusion or compression of the internal carotid artery is in question. For this patient, the symptoms clearly point to a central nervous system, pituitary cause rather than abdominal end-organ failure with regard to the amenorrhea.

ANSWER: b, c

REFERENCE: *Chapter 57—Pituitary Gland: Imaging of the Pituitary and Parasellar Region; Clinical and Endocrine Evaluation, Hyperprolactinemia*

4. Which of the following conditions is/are associated with hyperprolactinemia?

a. Chronic renal failure
b. Exogenous estrogen administration
c. Diabetes mellitus
d. Cirrhosis

COMMENT: Elevated serum levels of prolactin do not always indicate the presence of a pituitary tumor. Important alternative causes are chronic renal failure, hypothyroidism, and various drugs, including phenothiazines, tricyclic antidepressants, exogenous estrogen, opiates, reserpine, verapamil, and others. Hepatic disease, pregnancy, and a variety of pituitary and hypothalamic lesions also cause hyperprolactinemia. If the prolactin level is greater than 150 ng/mL, a pituitary tumor is almost invariably the cause, but often microadenoma produces prolactin levels less than 100 ng/mL. The size of pituitary tumors has been shown to relate to the degree of prolactin elevation, which may reach into the thousands of nanograms per milliliter. There are no reliable provocative tests to differentiate prolactinoma from other causes of hyperprolactinemia, so the diagnosis relies on ruling out other causes and imaging of the adenoma.

ANSWER: a, b, d

REFERENCE: *Chapter 57—Pituitary Gland: Clinical and Endocrine Evaluation; Hyperprolactinemia*

5. A 45 year-old woman seeks evaluation of hypertension, recent-onset obesity, hirsutism, and depression. Cerebral MRI does not show a pituitary lesion. Evaluation may include determination of which of the following?

a. Daytime serum cortisol level after low-dose dexamethasone suppression
b. Simultaneous serum corticotropin measurement in peripheral and inferior petrosal sinus sites
c. Chest and abdominal CT
d. Urinary free cortisol excretion

COMMENT: The findings of Cushing's syndrome often include central obesity, hypertension, hirsutism, fatigue, easy bruising, stria, moonlike facies, dorsal fat pad, and often depression or other mental changes. Less common abnormalities include headache, osteoporosis, diabetes mellitus, galactorrhea, peripheral edema, and amenorrhea. Often a patient comes to medical attention without the classic cushingoid appearance and reports only severe fatigue or depression. The cause of hypercortisolism is corticotropin-secreting pituitary adenoma (Cushing's disease) in as many as 80% of cases. The others are caused by an adrenocortical tumor or an ectopic neoplasm secreting corticotropin or corticotropin-releasing factor. Pituitary-dependent hypercortisolism is much more common among women (80%), and an ectopic cause is more common among men.

As many as 60% of patients with pituitary causes undergo imaging studies that do not provide enough information for a diagnosis. Therefore the diagnosis often relies completely on endocrine testing. Multiple measurements of cortisol and corticotropin to evaluate the diurnal pattern are important but often are misleading. They are mainly of value when the levels are clearly elevated. Measurement of urinary free cortisol excretion over 24 hours is extremely important. If the overnight dexamethasone screening test yields an 8 a.m. serum cortisol level less than 5 μg/dL, then hypercortisolism rarely is present. Most patients with a pituitary cause of hypercortisolism do not have suppression with the low-dose dexamethasone test but do with the higher-dose test. Patients with adrenal or ectopic causes do not have suppression with either dose. Chest and abdominal CT is appropriate to look for adrenal or lung tumors. The most specific test when the MRI findings are normal and evidence implicates the pituitary gland is simultaneous measurement of corticotropin levels in both inferior petrosal sinuses with concurrent measurement of peripheral corticotropin level. This approach produces specific information about the existence of corticotropin-secreting pituitary tumor and even the laterality of the tumor.

ANSWER: b, c, d

REFERENCE: *Chapter 57—Pituitary Gland: Clinical and Endocrine Evaluation; Cushing Disease*

6. Which of the following statements is/are true with respect to GH-secreting pituitary adenoma?

    a. Fewer than 50% of patients have GH levels greater than 10 ng/mL

    b. Oral glucose administration suppresses GH levels among patients with acromegaly

    c. More than 80% of cases of GH-secreting microadenoma can be cured with transphenoidal resection

    d. Preoperative therapy for macroadenoma with a somatostatin analogue may improve postoperative remission rates

COMMENT: The endocrine diagnosis of acromegaly rests largely on serum levels of insulin-like growth factor 1, also known as somatomedin-C, because both healthy patients and those with acromegaly can have GH levels less than 5 ng/mL. Even though 90% of patients with acromegaly have GH levels greater than 10 ng/mL and the normal GH level of a resting, non-stressed patient is less than 5 ng/mL, both healthy persons and patients with acromegaly may have levels less than 5 ng/mL. Insulin-like growth factor 1, which mediates the effect of GH on peripheral tissues, should be measured whenever acromegaly is suspected (see Fig. 57.7). The cause of acromegaly usually is GH-secreting pituitary adenoma, but in rare instances elevated GH levels are caused by production of GH-releasing hormone by ectopic tumor.

The goals of treatment are to decrease circulating GH or somatomedin C levels to within a normal range and to shrink the mass lesion causing compression-related symptoms. When microadenoma is removed transsphenoidally, endocrine remission can be expected in 80% to 88% of cases. When macroadenoma is resected, postoperative remission occurs in 30% to 68% of cases. The rate of remission is inversely related to preoperative GH level and tumor size. Preoperative therapy for macroadenoma with a somatostatin analogue may improve the postoperative remission rate.

ANSWER: c, d

REFERENCE: *Chapter 57—Pituitary Gland: Acromegaly*

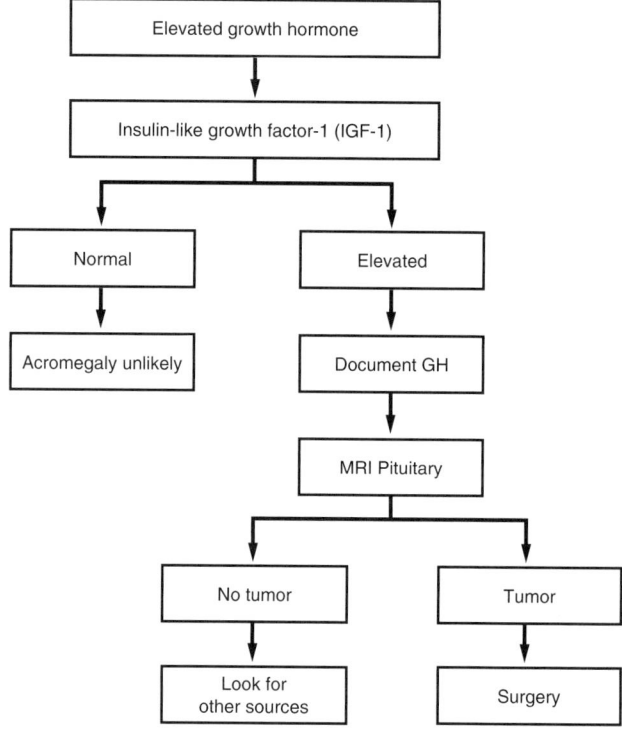

Figure 57.7

7. Which of the following statements is true with respect to Cushing's disease?

    a. Pituitary microadenoma often is small and deep within the gland itself

    b. The best therapy for hypercortisolism due to pituitary adenoma among women of child-bearing age is transsphenoidal total hypophysectomy

    c. Patients who do not have a remission after both surgery and radiation to the pituitary gland need medical or surgical adrenalectomy

    d. The long-term recurrence rate after resection of corticotropin-producing pituitary microadenoma is approximately 40%

COMMENT: Pituitary microadenoma that secretes corticotropin can be very small and often is situated deep within the gland itself. If the tumor is not evident when the dura is opened, incisions must be made into the gland and internal exploration performed. If no tumor is identified, a decision must be made whether to resect all or a portion of the gland. If the endocrine evidence is convincing of pituitary origin and the patient has no desire to have children, total hypophysectomy is warranted. If results of petrosal sinus sampling clearly indicate laterality, hemiresection of the gland can be performed.

Approximately 75% of patients have microadenoma as the source of corticotropin secretion. The postoperative remission rate among these patients is 88% to 96%, and the long-term recurrence rate appears to be no more than 5%. Ten percent to 20% of patients who undergo exploration have macroadenoma. The postoperative remission rate among these patients has been reported to be 33% to 61%. Most of these patients need postoperative radiation therapy. When both surgical and radiation therapy fail, the patient needs surgical adrenalectomy or medical suppression of adrenal function.

ANSWER: a, c

REFERENCE: *Chapter 57—Pituitary Gland: Clinical and Endocrine Evaluation; Cushing Disease, Treatment*

8. Pharmacologic management of GH excess caused by pituitary adenoma includes use of which of the following?
   a. Bromocriptine
   b. Vasopressin
   c. Octreotide
   d. Prednisone

COMMENT: Bromocriptine, a dopamine receptor agonist, was found to decrease GH levels for 71% of 126 patients with acromegaly. A clinical response was achieved by as many as 95% of patients with acromegaly, and decreased somatomedin C levels were found in some patients with persistently elevated GH levels. Bromocriptine does not appear to be effective primary management of acromegaly, but it may help to control GH and somatomedin C levels in adjuvant therapy. A somatostatin analogue, octreotide, has been used to manage acromegaly. It has been found to greatly decrease GH and somatomedin C levels for most patients and to normalize values for 50%. This treatment provides only minimal tumor shrinkage, and GH levels increase again immediately after cessation of the drug. This drug may prove useful for preoperative treatment or when surgery fails. Vasopressin and prednisone have no role in the management of acromegaly.

ANSWER: a, c

REFERENCE: *Chapter 57—Pituitary Gland: Clinical and Endocrine Evaluation; Acromegaly*

9. The most common mass lesion in the sella turcica is which of the following?
   a. Craniopharyngioma
   b. Aneurysm
   c. Benign pituitary cyst
   d. Pituitary adenoma

COMMENT: Pituitary adenoma is the most common mass lesion in the sella turcica or parasellar region. It constitutes 8% to 10% of all brain tumors. Some cases are cystic and can be confused with other lesions. Craniopharyngioma is the next most common tumor, although it is more often suprasellar in location. Tumors of the sella turcica are more common among children, but as many as one third occur among adults. The tumor usually is cystic. It is calcified in 70% of children and 40% of adults. Rarer lesions include meningioma, germinoma, metastatic lesion from primary tumor of the lung and breast, glioma, dermoid and benign epidermoid, Rathke cysts, aneurysm, and a variety of inflammatory and granulomatous processes.

ANSWER: d

REFERENCE: *Chapter 57—Pituitary Gland: Clinical and Endocrine Evaluation; Differential Diagnosis*

CHAPTER 58

BREAST

1. Which of the following statements is/are true concerning the anatomy of the breast?

   a. About 25% of the lymphatic drainage of the breast courses to the internal mammary nodes

   b. Nerves within the axillary fat pad include the intercostal brachial nerve, the long thoracic nerve, and thoracodorsal nerve

   c. Fascial bands projecting through the breast to the skin form a supporting framework known as Cooper's ligaments

   d. The ductal system of the breast from the alveoli to the skin is lined with columnar epithelium

COMMENT: The breast abuts the fascia of the pectoralis major and serratus anterior muscles. Projections of the fascia course through the breast to the skin, forming a supporting framework of the breast parenchyma. These fascial bands, called *suspensory ligaments of Cooper,* are better developed in the upper breast. The structure of the breast can be divided into lobular and ductal elements. The lobule is the functional unit of the breast. Within a lobule, the terminal elongated tubular ducts are called *alveoli.* Ten to 100 alveoli coalesce to form a larger duct, which defines a lobular unit. The lobular ducts join to form progressively larger ducts and ultimately an excretory duct. The alveolar ducts, lobular ducts, and excretory ducts are lined with either cuboidal or columnar epithelium. Eventually, 10 to 20 excretory ducts dilate into a short excretory sinus (lined with squamous epithelium) just beneath the areola. Excretory ducts then course perpendicularly to exit through the nipple.

The lymphatic anatomy of the breast is of interest to surgeons because of the tendency of breast cancer to involve the regional lymph nodes. Studies with radioactive tracers show at least 97% of lymphatic flow from the breast is into the axilla. The remainder courses into the internal mammary nodes. These studies also show that lymph flowing into the internal mammary gland chain is not restricted in origin to the medial half and subareolar region of the breast, as was thought, but can originate in any quadrant of the breast. In the axilla, lymphatic vessels terminate in the lymph nodes embedded in the axillary fat pad. Also within the axillary fat pad are the intercostal brachial nerves (sensory nerve supply in the underarm), the long thoracic nerve (a motor nerve to the serratus anterior and subscapularis muscles), and the thoracodorsal nerve (a motor nerve to the latissimus dorsi muscle adjacent to its accompanying arteries and veins).

ANSWER: b, c

REFERENCE: *Chapter 58—Breast: Anatomy and Embryology*

2. Which of the following statements is/are true concerning the effect of various hormones on breast function?

   a. Estrogen receptors are present only in breast cancer cells
   b. Mammary ductal dilatation and differentiation of alveolar epithelial cells and secretory cells are the result of increasing progesterone levels
   c. Breast changes in the early first trimester are primarily caused by increased progesterone effects of pregnancy
   d. Milk production and secretion after childbirth are maintained by continuing secretion of prolactin by the anterior pituitary gland

COMMENT: Breast growth, development, and function are orchestrated by a variety of hormones and growth factors. Estrogen plays a central role in breast development, growth, and differentiation. Lipid-soluble estrogens enter the normal and malignant breast cells by diffusing through the cell membrane. Once within the cell, estrogens bind with the estrogen receptor. Both normal and malignant breast cells contain estrogen receptors, but the low levels of receptors in normal breast tissue and in some breast cancers result in negative results of clinical assays. Cyclic changes associated with the menstrual cycle have a profound influence on breast structure and function. During the period of relative quiescence, increasing secretion of estrogen by the graafian follicle stimulates epithelial proliferation in the breast. As the luteal phase of the cycle begins, progesterone levels increase. Mammary ductal dilatation and differentiation of alveolar epithelial cells into secretory cells result. At the onset of menstruation, the rapid decrease in levels of circulating sex hormones leads to breast involution, and the cycle begins anew. During pregnancy, marked ductular, lobular, and alveolar growth occurs under the influence of estrogen, progesterone, placental lactogen, prolactin, and chorionic gonadotropin. These changes prepare the breasts for milk production at parturition. Early in the first trimester, ductal sprouting and lobular formation proceed under estrogenic influence. During the second trimester, lobular events predominate under the influence of progestins. The abrupt withdrawal of placental lactogen and sex hormones that occurs with delivery leaves the breast predominately under the influence of pituitary-derived prolactin. Milk production and secretion are maintained during lactation by continued secretion of prolactin by the anterior pituitary gland.

ANSWER: b, d

REFERENCE: *Chapter 58—Breast: Physiology*

3. Which of the following statements is/are true concerning mammography?

   a. As many as 50% of cases of cancer detected with mammography are not palpable
   b. One third of palpable breast cancers are not detected with mammography
   c. The sensitivity of mammography increases with age
   d. The American Cancer Society currently recommends routine screening mammography beginning at 40 years of age
   e. Only approximately 10% of nonpalpable lesions detected with mammography are found malignant at biopsy

COMMENT: Although mammography has been available for years, it did not become widely used until the findings of the Health Insurance Plan of New York and the Breast Cancer Detection Demonstration project studies of screening mammography were disseminated. These and other investigators found that 10% to 50% of cancers detected with mammography are not palpable. Conversely, 10% to 20% of tumors not detected with mammography are found by means of palpation. The incidence of breast cancer begins to increase sharply at 40 years of age, and the sensitivity of mammograms increases with age as the dense parenchymal tissue of young women is progressively replaced by fatty tissue. Routine screening mammography has been shown to decrease breast cancer–related mortality among women older than 50 years of age without symptoms. Controversy exists concerning the role of screening among younger women. The American Cancer Society recommends that mammographic screening begin at 40 years of age. Although sensitive, mammography is not specific. Only approximately 25% of nonpalpable lesions detected with mammography are found malignant at biopsy. A spiculated density with ill-defined margins on a mammogram is almost certainly malignant. In most instances, features are seen that suggest but do not confirm the diagnosis of cancer. These include clustered microcalcifications, asymmetric density, ductal asymmetry, distortion of normal breast architecture, or skin or nipple distortion.

ANSWER: a, c, d

REFERENCE: *Chapter 58—Breast: Breast Examination*

4. Which of the following statements is/are true concerning tissue sampling techniques for breast masses?

    a. The sensitivity of fine-needle aspiration (FNA) biopsy is such that mastectomy can be performed in the case of malignant diagnosis
    b. The accuracy of mammographically directed FNA biopsy is comparable with that for FNA biopsy of palpable lesions
    c. Core-needle biopsy showing normal breast tissue is an acceptable diagnosis
    d. The technique of core-needle biopsy is not applicable to radiographically detected lesions

COMMENT: Whatever tissue sampling method is chosen, only biopsy (examination of cells or tissue) and not physical examination or mammography can establish a definitive diagnosis and avoid delay in treatment. Fine needle aspiration biopsy allows rapid, minimally invasive diagnosis of many palpable and some nonpalpable, radiologically detected breast masses. The technique is both reliable and accurate. The incidence of false-positive findings is generally less than 0.5%. Fine needle aspiration biopsy is not, however, so highly specific that definitive surgery, particularly mastectomy, should be performed without previous intraoperative frozen-section confirmation of the presence of cancer. The reported sensitivity of FNA biopsy ranges from 7% to 99%; 85% is a good estimate of the true sensitivity in clinically relevant settings. X-ray-guided FNA biopsy has been used for minimally invasive diagnosis of nonpalpable breast lesions detected mammographically. The technique is quite effective, especially for mass lesions. The accuracy is comparable with that achieved with FNA biopsy of palpable lesions. Core-needle biopsy is a helpful tissue sampling method for palpable masses. The tissue obtained is useful for histologic analysis although inadequate for cytosol hormone receptor determination. The technique also can be used with mammographic guidance to evaluate nonpalpable lesions.

ANSWER: b

REFERENCE: *Chapter 58—Breast: Evaluation of Breast Masses*

5. Which of the following treatments is/are of proven benefit in the management of mastodynia associated with fibrocystic breast disease?

    a. Avoidance of methylxanthine compounds, particularly caffeine
    b. Cessation of smoking
    c. Vitamin E
    d. Danazol

COMMENT: The relation of methylxanthines, particularly caffeine, to mastodynia and breast nodularity is controversial. Most women do, however, experience diminution of symptoms and improvement in breast nodularity when they limit or eliminate caffeine intake. Patients with mastodynia should be advised to eliminate caffeine beverages for 2 to 3 months to determine whether there has been improvement in the symptoms. In addition to caffeine abstention, patients should be urged to stop smoking because nicotine is purported to worsen mastodynia.

A number of medications have been advocated for the management of mastodynia. Because of the subjective nature of the disease, however, and its propensity to be better tolerated by patients with reassurance, the exact method of most of these interventions is unclear. Vitamin E has been touted as beneficial, but clinical data do not support the use of this or other vitamins for this condition. The use of hormonal agents to manage mastodynia has been more extensively examined. Danazol, a weak antigen, is the most effective drug for management of mastodynia related to fibrocystic disease. The androgenic side effects of danazol, however, are troublesome enough to restrict its use to the most difficult cases of mastodynia. Other hormonal agents have been investigated for the management of mastodynia. Among young women, oral contraceptives have a variable effect on mastodynia. A trial and error search for optimal preparations may be necessary because the effect of oral contraceptives depends on the formulation of the agent.

ANSWER: a, b, d

REFERENCE: *Chapter 58—Breast: Benign Breast Disorders*

6. A 33-year-old woman is referred with nipple discharge. Which of the following statements is/are true concerning diagnosis and management in this case?
   a. Bilateral galactorrhea suggests underlying endocrinopathy
   b. Brownish discharge usually suggests old blood and is worrisome for underlying breast cancer
   c. Expressible bloody nipple discharge should be evaluated with ductography
   d. Milky breast discharge would not be expected 1 year after discontinuation of breast feeding

COMMENT: At one time or another, many women notice nipple discharge. The most common physiologic basis for nipple discharge is lactation. Milk may continue to be secreted intermittently for as long as 2 years after breast-feeding has stopped, particularly with breast stimulation. A milky, whitish discharge, usually bilateral, not related to lactation or breast stimulation, is called *galactorrhea.* The presence of bilateral galactorrhea should prompt an evaluation for underlying endocrinopathy causing increased prolactin secretion by the pituitary gland. Classically this is associated with amenorrhea, but galactorrhea may be the only sign of hypoprolactinemia. Nipple discharge associated with fibrocystic disease generally is green, yellow, or brown. Intraductal papilloma and cancer produce a bloody or blood-tinged serous discharge. The brownish discharge of fibrocystic disease can be easily confused with old blood. A guaiac test or simply dabbing the discharge with a gauze pad and examining the stain can usually differentiate the two. A bloody or blood-tinged discharge must be promptly evaluated to exclude carcinoma. If the discharge is expressible when the patient is examined, contrast ductography can be performed.

ANSWER: a, c

REFERENCE: *Chapter 58—Breast: Benign Breast Disorders*

7. A 21-year-old woman has an asymptomatic breast mass. Which of the following statements is/are true concerning diagnosis and management in this case?
   a. Mammography has an important role in diagnosis of the lesion
   b. Ultrasonography often is useful in the differential diagnosis of this lesion
   c. The mass always should be excised
   d. The lesion should be considered premalignant

COMMENT: Fibroadenoma is the most common tumor among adolescents and young women, but it also is frequently encountered among older women. It generally manifests as a palpable breast mass and must be differentiated from cancer. Fibroadenoma typically manifests as a painless, slow-growing mass found incidentally at self-examination of the breast. Palpation of a mass usually reveals a well-circumscribed, oval or round, mobile mass with a firm, rubbery texture. Because the mammographic appearance of a fibroadenoma rarely is characteristic, mammography plays little role in the diagnosis of this lesion. Ultrasonography can help differentiate a solid mass from a cyst. The ultrasonographic appearance of a well-marginated, homogenous mass may be sufficiently characteristic to allow diagnosis of fibroadenoma. Excisional biopsy is not necessary for every fibroadenoma. Women younger than 30 years with characteristic physical findings and sonographic appearance of the fibroadenoma can be given the option of observation. Most fibroadenomas are not believed to be premalignant lesions or to indicate increased risk of development of breast cancer.

ANSWER: b

REFERENCE: *Chapter 58—Breast: Benign Breast Disorders*

8. A 42-year-old woman undergoes her first mammogram. Clustered microcalcifications are seen, but no mass is palpable. Which of the following statements is/are true concerning diagnosis and management in this case?

a. Needle localization and excision of the mass are necessary to establish the diagnosis
b. Frozen-section examination is particularly useful in the diagnosis of this lesion
c. Intense interlobular fibrosis and proliferation of small ductules with loss of orientation of lobules and epithelial cells may suggest carcinoma
d. This finding is associated with increased risk of cancer

COMMENT: Sclerosing adenosis is a histologic subtype of fibrocystic change not associated with increased risk of cancer. It is, however, one of the benign breast processes most likely to be confused radiologically and histologically with cancer. It usually is detected at routine mammography as cluster microcalcifications without an associated palpable mass. In these cases, needle localization and excision are needed to establish a diagnosis. Sclerosing adenosis microscopically is characterized by interlobular fibrosis and proliferation of small ductules. If the fibrous component is particularly intense, the orientation of lobules and epithelial cells may be lost, mimicking carcinoma. Differentiating sclerosing adenosis from cancer at frozen-section examination can be particularly difficult and should not be attempted.

ANSWER: a, c

REFERENCE: *Chapter 58—Breast: Benign Breast Disorders*

9. A 35-year-old woman, who is currently breast-feeding her firstborn child, has an erythematous and inflamed fluctuant area at breast examination. Which of the following statements is/are true concerning diagnosis and management in this case?

a. The most common organism to expect on a culture is *Staphylococcus aureus*
b. Open surgical drainage likely is indicated
c. Breast-feeding absolutely should be discontinued
d. If the inflammatory process does not completely respond, biopsy may be indicated

COMMENT: Infection complicates breast-feeding for fewer than 1 in 100 women, but these lactational infections still account for 80% of all breast infections. Presumably gaining access through the skin of the irritated nipple of the nursing woman, *S. aureus* organisms are by far the most common pathogens in this setting. Many breast infections begin as cellulitis without abscess formation. When an actual abscess is suspected, percutaneous aspiration can establish the diagnosis and allow for bacterial culture and sensitivity testing. Open surgical drainage is the most prudent and effective treatment. Although women may choose to cease breast-feeding, there is no absolute indication for this. When mastitis or breast infection is suspected clinically, the possibility of inflammatory carcinoma must be entertained. Any inflammatory process that does not respond completely and promptly to antibiotics or drainage should be subjected to biopsy to rule out cancer.

ANSWER: a, b, d

REFERENCE: *Chapter 58—Breast: Benign Breast Disorders*

10. Which of the following statements is/are true concerning intraductal papilloma?

   a. This lesion is the most common cause of bloody nipple discharge
   b. Serous, nonbloody discharge is unlikely to be caused by intraductal papilloma
   c. A nonpalpable lesion often can be diagnosed with ductography
   d. An isolated lesion is considered premalignant

COMMENT: Intraductal papilloma is the most common cause of bloody nipple discharge, although in one half of cases, the discharge is serous. Because the average size of intraductal papilloma is 3 to 4 mm, the lesion rarely is palpable. Ductography can depict the lesion, or the lesion can be found after subareolar duct excision performed to control the discharge. Isolated intraductal papilloma is not considered premalignant, nor does it place the patient at increased risk of breast cancer. Unlike isolated papilloma, diffuse papillomatosis is associated with increased risk of breast cancer, perhaps as high as 40%.

ANSWER: a, c

REFERENCE: *Chapter 58—Breast: Benign Breast Disorders*

11. Which of the following is/are associated with increased risk of breast cancer?

   a. Nulliparity
   b. Oophorectomy before 35 years of age
   c. Use of oral contraceptives
   d. High-fat, high-calorie diet
   e. Postmenopausal use of conjugated estrogen

COMMENT: Women who undergo oophorectomy before 35 years of age and do not take replacement estrogen have a two-thirds reduction in breast cancer risk (see Table 58.7). Replacement estrogen therapy eliminates the beneficial effect of oophorectomy. Most studies of oral contraceptive use do not show associated increased risk of development of breast cancer. Studies of estrogen replacement therapy among postmenopausal women have yielded equivocal results. Most studies have not shown an association between breast cancer risk and postmenopausal use of conjugated estrogen.

ANSWER: a, d

REFERENCE: *Chapter 58—Breast: Breast Cancer*

12. Which of the following chromosomal or genetic abnormalities is/are associated with the development of breast cancer?

   a. Mutations in the p53 tumor suppressor gene
   b. Mutation in the short arm of chromosome 2
   c. The presence of the *BRCA1* gene on chromosome 17
   d. The presence of the *BRCA2* gene on chromosome 13

COMMENT: Four inherited syndromes are associated with the development of breast cancer. Li-Fraumeni syndrome has an autosomal dominant mode of inheritance. The syndrome is attributed to mutations in the p53 tumor suppressor gene, a gene that codes for a protein that serves as a G1-S checkpoint regulator of the cell cycle. A mutation has been characterized on the short arm of chromosome 2 in a gene associated with DNA repair. Predisposition to a wide range of malignant diseases, including breast and colon cancer, is associated with abnormalities at this locus. The most exciting development in inherited susceptibility to breast cancer relates to identification and cloning of the *BRCA1* gene, which was initially localized on the long arm of chromosome 17 by means of linkage analysis. Germline abnormalities in *BRCA1* may be responsible for as many as 5% of all cases of breast cancer in the United States. The gene is characterized by autosomal dominant inheritance with a high degree of penetrance. Almost 60% of women inheriting the gene have breast cancer by 50 years of age, and lifelong risk approaches 85%. Another breast cancer susceptibility gene, *BRCA2,* has been localized by means of linkage analysis to a small region of chromosome 13q12-13. *BRCA2* apparently confers high risk of early-onset breast cancer among women. Like those with *BRCA1,* carriers of *BRCA2* have a lifetime risk of breast cancer that approaches 90%.

ANSWER: a, b, c, d

REFERENCE: *Chapter 58—Breast: Breast Cancer*

13. Which of the following statements is/are true concerning the histologic variants of invasive carcinoma of the breast?

a. The presence of an in situ component with invasive ductal carcinoma adversely affects prognosis

b. Medullary carcinoma, although often large, is associated with a better overall prognosis than is common invasive ductal cancer

c. Mucinous or colloid carcinoma is one of the more common variants of invasive ductal cancer

d. Invasive lobular carcinoma is associated with a higher incidence of bilateral breast cancer

COMMENT: Although the breast is composed of both lobular and ductal elements, most breast cancer arises in the ductal elements. Invasive ductal carcinoma accounts for 70% to 80% of all cases of breast cancer. Although there is no single microscopic feature specific for infiltrating ductal carcinoma, the lesion can be recognized histologically as invasive adenocarcinoma involving ductal elements. The malignant ductal cells often are dispersed within the fibrous stroma, leading to the appellation *scirrhous carcinoma.* A number of less common types of breast cancer arise from the ductal epithelium and are hence classified as variants of invasive ductal carcinoma. There are distinct histologic criteria for classifying these lesions; the criteria must be met throughout the tumor. Histologically pure examples of these variant tumors are associated with better long-term survival than is ordinary invasive ductal carcinoma. When mixed histologic features are encountered, the clinical behavior parallels that of the invasive ductal element, not the other subtype. These mixed tumors are considered together with pure invasive ductal carcinoma for prognostic purposes. In many cases, when areas of in situ ductal carcinoma are seen, the presence of an in situ component does not adversely affect prognosis, although it jeopardizes attempts at breast conservation.

Medullary carcinoma is one of the more common variants, accounting for approximately 6% of all invasive breast cancers. These tumors can grow to be large within the breast (5 to 10 cm) and are characteristically well circumscribed. Mucinous carcinoma, also called *colloid carcinoma,* is encountered in 1% to 2% of cases of breast cancer. Invasive lobular carcinoma arises from the lobular component of the breast and in most series accounts for approximately 10% of breast cancers. Almost every series has a higher incidence of bilateral cancer among patients with invasive lobular carcinoma. The contralateral breast is involved either synchronously (3% of patients) or metachronously among as many as 30% of patients.

ANSWER: b, d

REFERENCE: *Chapter 58—Breast: Breast Cancer*

14. Clinical features of breast cancer associated with a particularly poor prognosis include:

a. Edema of the skin of the breast
b. Skin ulceration
c. Lateral arm edema
d. Dermal lymphatic invasion

COMMENT: The histologic hallmark of inflammatory breast cancer is dermal lymphatic invasion found at skin biopsy. The signs of this clinical syndrome include breast warmth, tenderness, erythema, and edema (see Table 58.10).

ANSWER: a, b, c, d

REFERENCE: *Chapter 58—Breast: Breast Cancer*

15. Which of the following statements is/are true concerning the surgical staging of breast cancer?

a. All biopsy specimens should be transported to the pathology laboratory in formalin within 24 hours of the procedure

b. Removal of only level I axillary lymph nodes can lead to understaging of breast cancer in as many as one fourth of cases

c. Level III axillary lymph nodes should be removed in all axillary lymph node dissections

d. A clinically negative axilla is found to have histologically positive metastasis in approximately one third of patients

COMMENT: Pathologic staging begins with the initial biopsy. Unless previously secured, fresh tumor needs to be obtained for hormone receptor analysis before placement into formalin solution. A period of warm ischemia as short as 30 minutes can cause underestimation of estrogen receptor levels. The need to remove axillary nodes must be determined preoperatively. Axillary lymph node metastasis is found in approximately one third of clinically negative axillae but only if proper axillary dissection is performed. Removal of only level I nodes or "sampling" of axillary lymph nodes in a haphazard manner increases the risk of injury to important axillary neurovascular structures and may lead to understaging in as many as 25% of cases. Proper staging of axillary lymph nodes includes en bloc removal and examination of level I and level II nodes. When conducted for staging, axillary lymph node dissection should not include removal of level III axillary nodes; in fewer than 2% of cases are metastatic lesions present in level III nodes when level I and level II nodes are negative. Removal of level III nodes, however, increases the incidence of postoperative lymphedema of the arm almost fivefold. Therapeutic axillary lymph node dissection performed for palpable disease in the axilla should include removal of all levels to clear gross disease.

ANSWER: b, d

REFERENCE: *Chapter 58—Breast: Breast Cancer*

16. Which of the following statements is/are correct concerning prognostic factors for carcinoma of the breast?
    a. Prognosis is improved with estrogen or progesterone receptor positivity
    b. Increase in the thymidine-labeling index, a measure of the proportion of cells in the DNA synthetic phase (S phase), is associated with improved survival
    c. High tumor levels of cathepsin D are associated with improved prognosis
    d. Immunohistochemical demonstration of active angiogenesis correlates with increased metastatic potential and poor prognosis

COMMENT: See Table 58.11.

ANSWER: a, d

REFERENCE: *Chapter 58—Breast: Breast Cancer*

17. Which of the following conclusion can be drawn from the results of the National Surgical Adjuvant Breast Project (NSABP) prospective, randomized trials completed in the 1970s and 1980s?
    a. Delay of axillary node dissection until there is clinical evidence of disease does not influence overall survival
    b. Removal of clinically negative nodes has no therapeutic benefit
    c. Breast irradiation reduces both local recurrence and overall survival
    d. Modified radical mastectomy offers no advantage over lumpectomy with axillary node dissection

COMMENT: The scientific basis of local-regional therapeutic strategies for stage I and stage II breast cancer was established by a series of studies conducted during the 1970s and 1980s by the NSABP. In the first of these protocols, total mastectomy with delayed node dissection only for nodes that subsequently turned positive, total mastectomy with local-regional radiation therapy, and radical mastectomy were clinically equivalent. The finding that delay of axillary node dissection until there is clinical evidence of disease does not influence survival emphasizes that the role of axillary dissection in the care of patients with clinically negative nodes is solely for staging. The removal of clinically negative nodes has no therapeutic benefit if regional recurrences are detected and managed promptly. In the second of these protocols, modified radical mastectomy, lumpectomy with axillary node dissection, and lumpectomy with axillary node dissection and irradiation were compared in the management of small breast cancers. Modified radical mastectomy offered no advantage over other treatments when analyzed according to disease-free or overall survival rates in the care of patients with node-negative or node-positive disease. Breast irradiation after lumpectomy reduced the likelihood of in-breast tumor recurrence from 39% to 10% but did not affect overall survival rate compared with lumpectomy alone.

ANSWER: a, b, d

REFERENCE: *Chapter 58—Breast: Breast Cancer*

18. Which of the following statements is/are true concerning breast reconstruction?

    a. The timing of breast reconstruction is of no oncologic significance
    b. Breast reconstruction can interfere with detection of local recurrence of breast cancer
    c. Maintenance of an effective subpectoral pocket for a breast implant requires preservation of the pectoralis fascia
    d. Because of its complexity, the transverse rectus abdominis musculocutaneous (TRAM) flap is seldom used for primary breast reconstruction

COMMENT: Breast reconstruction is suitable for any woman who has undergone mastectomy who desires reconstruction. Breast reconstruction can be performed at mastectomy (immediate) or later (delayed). Because the presence of reconstruction can interfere with accurate planning and administration of radiation therapy, reconstruction usually is delayed if the use of local or regional radiation therapy is anticipated. Otherwise, timing of breast reconstruction is of no oncologic significance. Because most local recurrences occur in the subcutaneous tissues, reconstruction does not interfere with detection. Reconstruction does not complicate administration of chemotherapy.

Breast reconstruction techniques entail autogenous tissue or synthetic prostheses to recreate a breast mound. Prosthetic reconstruction usually is accomplished by means of subpectoral placement of an implant filled with saline solution or silicone gel. Maintenance of an effective subpectoral pocket for an implant requires preservation of the pectoralis fascia and the medial pectoral nerve during mastectomy. The TRAM flap is the best autogenous reconstruction. The TRAM operation is complex and time consuming. Despite the magnitude of the procedure, it is still commonly used for immediate reconstruction.

ANSWER: a, c

REFERENCE: *Chapter 58—Breast: Breast Cancer*

19. Which of the following statements is/are true concerning radiation therapy after lumpectomy?

    a. The total dose given to the breast usually is in the range of 2,500 to 3,000 cGy
    b. Radiation to the axillary nodal bed is a normal part of the procedure for most patients
    c. Long-term complications of radiation therapy include rib fractures and arm edema
    d. Breast edema and skin erythema usually resolves within a few weeks
    e. None of the above

COMMENT: Breast conservation usually involves lumpectomy and radiation therapy to achieve local control of breast cancer. Any technique of postlumpectomy irradiation of the breast must adequately cover the volume at risk, deliver a homogenous dose throughout the target tissues, avoid overlapping or inadequate apposition of fields, and minimize the dose reaching the heart and lung. The entire breast should be treated with a total dose of 4,500 to 5,000 cGy. There is no good evidence to support a radiation boost to the site of the primary tumor. Complications from breast irradiation are uncommon if the procedure is performed correctly. Acute complications of radiation therapy include fatigue, breast edema, and skin erythema; these are almost always self-limited and resolve over weeks (fatigue) to months (erythema) or years (edema). The most common long-term problems are rib fractures and minor arm edema, each of which occurs approximately 5% of the time.

ANSWER: c

REFERENCE: *Chapter 58—Breast: Breast Cancer*

20. Which of the following statements is/are true concerning adjuvant systemic therapy?

    a. Adjuvant tamoxifen in the care of post-menopausal women with node-positive, estrogen receptor (ER)–positive disease is equivalent to cytotoxic chemotherapy
    b. Tamoxifen clearly improves survival among all patients with hormone receptor–positive disease
    c. Treatment with cyclophosphamide, methotrexate, and 5-fluorouracil (CMF) is associated with improved overall survival among both premenopausal and postmenopausal patients with node-positive disease
    d. There is no evidence to suggest a role for chemotherapy in the care of patients with node-negative disease

COMMENT: Adjuvant therapy with tamoxifen leads to a prolonged disease-free period for post-menopausal women with ER-positive disease and histologically positive nodes and for premenopausal and postmenopausal women with ER-positive disease and negative nodes. Because of similar results and because tamoxifen is generally less toxic than chemotherapy, this therapy is the best treatment of postmenopausal women with node-positive, ER-positive disease. Therapy with CMF is associated with both longer disease-free survival and overall survival among premenopausal patients with positive lymph nodes. Postmenopausal women with positive nodes have improved disease-free survival rates, but there is no significant difference in overall survival rate. Several trials of adjuvant chemotherapy with CMF or related regimens have been conducted in the treatment of patients with node-negative disease. The early results of all of these trials have been similar—disease-free survival rate is definitely improved with adjuvant chemotherapy. These studies are not mature enough to draw definitive conclusions regarding overall survival. The National Cancer Institute therefore has recommended the use of adjuvant chemotherapy in the care of all patients with tumors large enough to have hormonal receptor levels measured.

ANSWER: a

REFERENCE: *Chapter 58—Breast: Breast Cancer*

21. Which of the following statements is/are true concerning the recurrence of breast cancer?

    a. Most patients have a recurrence within 5 years of diagnosis
    b. More than 70% of recurrences of breast cancer involve distant metastasis
    c. Pulmonary metastatic lesions are the most common initial form of distant recurrence
    d. The local recurrence rate after breast-conserving procedures varies from 10% to 40% whether or not radiation is used
    e. Disease recurs among at least 35% of patients with node-negative disease undergoing appropriate primary breast therapy

COMMENT: Metastatic disease after primary therapy for breast cancer can recur at any time. Fifty percent to 70% of relapses occur within 2 years and more than 85% occur within 5 years. More than 70% of recurrences are distant, but anywhere from 10% to 30% of recurrences are local. Bone and lung are the most common initial sites of distant relapse—50% and 25%, respectively. A breast-conserving procedure can be associated with a low local tumor recurrence rate. The rate of local recurrence decreases from 40% to 10% if postoperative radiation therapy is given to the entire breast. Despite potentially curative resection, at least 20% of patients with node-negative and 60% of those with node-positive breast cancer have recurrence of the disease after surgical treatment.

ANSWER: a, b, d

REFERENCE: *Chapter 58—Breast: Breast Cancer*

22. Which of the following statements is/are true concerning local recurrence of breast cancer?

   a. The percentage of patients with chest wall recurrence as the initial site of failure after mastectomy is similar for node-negative and node-positive disease
   b. Most patients with local-regional recurrence of disease die of metastatic disease
   c. Management of local recurrence after mastectomy includes local radiation therapy and systemic chemotherapy
   d. In-breast recurrence after breast-conserving surgery is not a negative prognostic factor
   e. Regional lymph node recurrence after axillary node dissection is rare

COMMENT: Recurrence in the chest wall after mastectomy is ominous. In a large series of patients treated with mastectomy, 6.5% of women with node-negative and 8.8% of those with node-positive disease had chest wall recurrence as the initial site of failure. Ten years after local-regional recurrence, approximately 60% of patients with initially node-negative and almost all (>90%) of those with initially node-positive disease had evidence of metastatic disease. Patients with local recurrence who have not undergone chest wall radiation need radiation therapy. A full course of at least 4,500 to 5,000 cGy should be delivered to the entire chest wall, and consideration should be given to a boost dose at any sites of gross tumor. Because postmastectomy recurrence often is followed rapidly by metastatic disease, it is logical to postulate a role for adjuvant systemic therapy once local measures have achieved control of chest wall disease.

Evidence suggests that in-breast recurrence after breast conservation is a prognostic factor. Women who have in-breast recurrence are at higher risk of systemic disease than are women who do not have recurrence in the breast. Fewer than 3% of patients have recurrence of disease in the axilla after axillary node dissection.

ANSWER: a, b, c, e

REFERENCE: *Chapter 58—Breast: Breast Cancer*

23. A premenopausal woman who underwent mastectomy for breast cancer 3 years previously has pulmonary metastasis. Which of the following statements is/are true concerning management in this case?

   a. If the patient received adjuvant therapy, her response is likely to be better
   b. If the patient has ER-positive disease, hormonal therapy should be the first line of treatment
   c. The response to chemotherapy will likely be dose dependent
   d. Combination chemotherapy will likely work better for this patient than for a woman who is postmenopausal

COMMENT: Chemotherapy for metastatic breast cancer is more likely to be used to treat young women, those with ER-negative tumors, those with visceral involvement, and those with rapidly advancing or life-threatening disease. Combinations of agents usually are used to manage metastatic breast cancer, and the response rate usually is dose dependent. All regimens are slightly less active for postmenopausal women. Response rates are highest among women who have not received previous therapy for metastatic disease. Previous adjuvant therapy is not consistently associated with a poorer response to therapy, particularly if a long time has lapsed between adjuvant therapy and the development of metastasis. Endocrine therapy is appropriate for first-line treatment of nearly all women with ER-positive metastatic breast disease. Tamoxifen is the best agent for first-line hormonal therapy for metastatic breast cancer. Both premenopausal and postmenopausal patients can receive this agent. Side effects are minimal.

ANSWER: b, c, d

REFERENCE: *Chapter 58—Breast: Breast Cancer*

24. Which of the following statements is/are true concerning noninvasive carcinoma of the breast?

   a. Ductal carcinoma in situ (DCIS) is associated with a high risk of development of invasive ductal carcinoma in the same quadrant of the same breast as the initial lesion
   b. Patients with DCIS should not be treated with breast conservation therapy
   c. Lobular carcinoma in situ (LCIS) is the most common form of noninvasive breast cancer
   d. When LCIS is found, the likelihood of development of lobular carcinoma in situ of the contralateral breast is as high as 50%
   e. Approximately one third of patients with biopsy-proven LCIS eventually have invasive cancer, always of the same breast

COMMENT: Noninvasive (in situ) cancer is defined as a neoplastic entity within the epithelium of origin and without invasion to the basement membrane. Ductal carcinoma in situ arises from the ductular elements. The age distribution of DCIS does not differ greatly from that of invasive ductal carcinoma. Not every woman who undergoes complete excision of focal DCIS eventually has invasive ductal cancer. Results of several studies suggest one half or more of patients have invasive breast cancer after excisional biopsy alone. When subsequent invasive cancer does occur, it is almost always of the invasive ductal type and occurs in the same quadrant of the breast as the initial DCIS. The latent period before development of invasive cancer usually is more than 5 years. Total mastectomy usually is associated with a nearly 100% cure rate for this condition. Although total mastectomy remains the standard of therapy for DCIS, there is increasing experience with breast-conserving therapy. Breast conservation can be offered to patients with DCIS if the entire tumor can be surgically removed with negative histologic margins and if the remaining breast tissue can be reliably assessed clinically and radiographically. It appears as if the disease-free survival rate after lumpectomy and radiation therapy is worse than that after simple mastectomy. Therefore, breast conservation for DCIS commits patients to more careful long-term follow-up evaluation and likely necessitates additional treatment to control recurrences.

Lobular carcinoma in situ accounts for one third of cases of noninvasive breast cancer. Patients with LCIS are considerably younger than patients with invasive breast cancer. Three fourths of women with this disease are premenopausal. Lobular carcinoma in situ is an infrequent finding among women older than 75 years. When the opposite breast is sampled at the time of diagnosis, contralateral LCIS is found in 30% to 50% of cases. The prognosis for LCIS is solely related to subsequent development of invasive carcinoma. Approximately one third of patients with biopsy-demonstrated LCIS eventually have invasive cancer. One half of cases occur in the index breast and one half in the contralateral breast. Subsequent breast cancer can be either lobular or ductal.

ANSWER: a, d

REFERENCE: *Chapter 58—Breast: Breast Cancer*

25. Which of the following statements is/are correct concerning cystosarcoma phyllodes?
    a. The tumor occurs most commonly among postmenopausal women
    b. Total mastectomy is necessary for all patients with this diagnosis
    c. Axillary lymph node dissection is not necessary for malignant cystosarcoma phyllodes
    d. Most patients with the malignant variant of cystosarcoma phyllodes die of metastatic disease

COMMENT: Cystosarcoma phyllodes is a tumor arising in the mesenchymal tissue of the breast. The tumor usually manifests as a painless breast mass. Phyllodes tumor is most common among women 30 to 40 years of age but can occur at any age, even before puberty. Differentiation of benign from a malignant phyllodes tumor can be difficult. Approximately one fourth of all phyllodes tumors are histologically malignant, but only a fraction of these patients actually have metastatic disease. The optimum management of benign or malignant phyllodes tumor is wide excision with a margin of normal breast tissue. The margin must be histologically free of involvement because even benign lesions can recur after incomplete excision. If this can be done leaving an adequate appearance, mastectomy is not necessary. Total mastectomy is reserved for large lesions in small-breasted women or recurrences after previous local excision that is not amenable to repeat local excision. Axillary lymph node dissection is not performed in the absence of biopsy-proven nodal involvement, even for malignant phyllodes tumors, because axillary metastasis is uncommon.

ANSWER: c

REFERENCE: *Chapter 58—Breast: Breast Cancer*

26. A 45-year-old woman has a weeping eczematoid lesion of the nipple. Which of the following statements is/are true concerning diagnosis and management in this case?

   a. Treatment is with warm compresses and oral antibiotics
   b. Biopsy of the nipple revealing malignant cells within the milk ducts is invariably associated with underlying invasive carcinoma
   c. Appropriate treatment is mastectomy
   d. The lesion always carries high risk of subsequent metastatic disease

COMMENT: Paget's disease is characterized by a weeping, eczematoid lesion of the nipple. There is often accompanying edema and inflammation. Biopsy of the nipple reveals malignant cells within the milk ducts. The lesion is invariably associated with underlying invasive or in situ ductal carcinoma. The prognosis of Paget's disease is that of the underlying cancer. Standard treatment is mastectomy with axillary lymph node dissection only if invasive cancer is present.

ANSWER: c

REFERENCE: *Chapter 58—Breast: Breast Cancer*

27. Which of the following statements is/are true concerning gynecomastia?

   a. If the disease is unilateral, it is unlikely to be drug related
   b. Standard surgical treatment is subcutaneous mastectomy
   c. The presence of gynecomastia often is associated with development of breast cancer
   d. A formal endocrine evaluation is indicated for most patients with gynecomastia

COMMENT: Gynecomastia is defined as palpable enlargement of the male breast. Pathologic causes of estrogen excess or testosterone deficiency are associated with gynecomastia. In many cases, no cause is found. Clinically significant gynecomastia has been associated with the use of a number of drugs, including cimetidine, digoxin, spironolactone, and tricyclic antidepressants. The use of marijuana also has been associated with gynecomastia. Drug-related gynecomastia often is unilateral or unequal between the two breasts, and discontinuation of the offending drug does not always lead to resolution of the condition. A formal endocrine evaluation is not indicated for gynecomastia unless another sign of hormonal imbalance is found at routine evaluation. Standard surgical management of gynecomastia is subcutaneous mastectomy performed with local anesthesia. The presence of gynecomastia is not associated with subsequent development of cancer, yet protracted hyperestrogenemic states, which are associated with gynecomastia, are linked to development of breast cancer.

ANSWER: b

REFERENCE: *Chapter 58—Breast: Male Breast Diseases*

Section K
THORAX

CHAPTER 59

LUNG NEOPLASMS

1. The relation between small-cell and non-small-cell lung cancer can be described as follows:

   a. They differ in histologic features, clinical behavior, and cell of origin
   b. Of all lung cancers, approximately 80% are non-small-cell and 20% are small-cell
   c. Both cell types are predictably responsive to chemotherapy
   d. The International Staging System can be applied to both tumor types
   e. The majority of patients with non-small-cell cancer unlike the minority of patients with small-cell cancer are candidates for pulmonary resection

COMMENT: Although small-cell and non-small-cell carcinomas of the lung differ in histologic features and clinical behavior, they probably have a common origin; c-*myc* or n-*myc* amplified small-cell lung cancer lines undergo transition to non-small-cell phenotypes after insertion of an activated *ras* gene. The overall incidence of lung cancer is 80% non-small-cell and 20% small-cell. Only small-cell carcinoma is predictably responsive to chemotherapy.

The staging system for small-cell lung cancer is based on limited as opposed to extensive disease outside a tolerable radiation therapy portal. The International Staging System uses TNM descriptors for four clinical stages. Only approximately 30% of patients with non-small-cell lung cancer have potentially resectable tumors.

ANSWER: b

REFERENCE: *Chapter 59—Lung Neoplasms: Small-cell and Non-small Cell Lung Cancer*

2. A 2-cm peripheral squamous cell carcinoma of the lung of a 60-year-old man with a pleural effusion positive for malignant cells would be classified as:

   a. T1N0M1
   b. T3N0M0
   c. T3N0M1
   d. T4N0M0
   e. T4N0M1

COMMENT: The presence of a pleural effusion in association with primary lung cancer usually is an ominous sign that precludes surgical resection. If more than one sample of the effusion is negative for malignant cells and is nonbloody, the effusion can be considered unrelated to the tumor and excluded as a staging element. When the results of cytologic examination of the effusion are abnormal, the tumor is considered T4 regardless of size or nodal status.

ANSWER: d, e

REFERENCE: *Chapter 59—Lung Neoplasms: Non-small Cell Lung Cancer*

3. Which of the following is/are true regarding the evaluation and preparation of a 55-year-old smoker for resection of a 3-cm pulmonary adenocarcinoma?

   a. Preoperative cessation of smoking does not reduce the risk of postoperative pulmonary complications
   b. Resting $Paco_2$ is of more value than Pao_2
   c. Forced expiratory volume in 1 minute (FEV_1) is of more value than is measured vital capacity
   d. Diffusion capacity should be measured routinely
   e. A ventilation-perfusion (V/Q) lung scan is useful when pulmonary reserve is marginal

COMMENT: Preoperative cessation of smoking for 2 weeks can reduce the risk of pulmonary complications and should be required. In preoperative assessment for pulmonary resection, the $Paco_2$ is of more value than Pao_2 because a $Paco_2$ greater than 50 mm Hg indicates a patient with chronic lung disease is at very high risk. Hypoxemia may be secondary to the mechanical effects of the tumor and produce V/Q mismatch. The latter can be confirmed with a V/Q lung scan, which also helps identify areas of functioning lung in patients with marginal pulmonary function. The best screening test for adequacy of pulmonary reserve is FEV_1. It helps identify obstructive pulmonary disease, which is more important than the restrictive lung disease identified by means of measurement of vital capacity. Diffusion capacity measurement provides little additional information of value.

ANSWER: b, c, e

REFERENCE: *Chapter 59—Lung Neoplasms: Non-small Cell Lung Cancer; Selection of Treatment*

4. A 62-year-old male smoker has right anterior chest pain. A 3-cm mass is attached to the chest wall, and there is radiographic evidence of rib erosion and positive cytologic results for non-small-cell carcinoma. Which of the following is/are true?

   a. The patient cannot undergo surgical treatment because of the tumor size and chest wall involvement
   b. Radiation therapy is the preferred initial treatment
   c. Operative resection should be performed with en bloc removal of the tumor and adjacent chest wall as well as mediastinal lymph node resection
   d. Positive mediastinal nodes have little effect on survival
   e. The disease is classified stage IIIa

COMMENT: Survival after resection for non-small-cell lung cancer is related to the stage of the disease with a strong adverse effect of nodal involvement. This is true even for large peripheral tumors that extend into the chest wall, as in this case, in which a 40% to 50% survival rate would be expected in the absence of nodes (T3N0, stage IIIa) but only a 15% survival with nodal involvement. Radiation therapy would be a postoperative consideration to reduce the incidence of local recurrence. En bloc operative resection of the involved lobe and mediastinal nodes for staging would offer the greatest likelihood of cure.

ANSWER: c, e

REFERENCE: *Chapter 59—Lung Neoplasms: Non-small Cell Lung Cancer*

5. Which of the following statements is/are true concerning resection of T1N1 squamous cell cancer from a 47-year-old man?

   a. There is a higher risk of local recurrence than with any other histologic type of non-small-cell cancer
   b. The greatest risk to the patient is distant metastasis
   c. The liver is the most likely site of metastasis
   d. If the patient survives 5 years, there is a greater risk of new lung cancer than of recurrence
   e. To improve survival, the patient should be considered for adjuvant chemotherapy

COMMENT: The risk of local recurrence of non-small-cell carcinoma of the lung is much more common for squamous cell lesions than the others. It averages 20% to 30% overall. The greatest risk, however is of distant metastasis, which occurs among 70% to 80% of patients, regardless of stage of the tumor. Almost all recurrences take place within 5 years. The brain is the most common site of distant metastasis. For this patient with stage II disease, radiation therapy but not chemotherapy would be a consideration to reduce the incidence of local recurrence. After 5 years, the highest risk is of new lung cancer rather than recurrence.

ANSWER: a, b, d

REFERENCE: *Chapter 59—Lung Neoplasms: Non-small Cell Lung Cancer*

6. A 42-year-old woman with hemoptysis has a 2-cm mulberry-appearing polypoid lesion in the left main stem bronchus that may be bronchial adenoma. The differential diagnosis includes which of the following?

   a. Mucoepidermoid carcinoma
   b. Plasma cell granuloma
   c. Carcinoid tumor
   d. Adenoid cystic carcinoma
   e. Mucous gland adenoma

COMMENT: The term *bronchial adenoma* includes a spectrum of tumors arising from epithelial stem cells that vary from benign mucous gland adenoma to malignant adenoid cystic and mucoepidermoid carcinoma as well as the carcinoid tumor of similar varied behavior. Among these variants, carcinoids are most common, representing 80% to 90% of all bronchial adenomas.

ANSWER: a, b, c, d, e

REFERENCE: *Chapter 59—Lung Neoplasms: Bronchial Adenomas*

7. Biopsy of the lesion described in question 6 is reported as "bronchial carcinoid with no signs of atypia." Which of the following statements is/are true?

   a. Sleeve resection of the bronchus would be appropriate
   b. Lymph node biopsy at resection is unnecessary
   c. Associated carcinoid syndrome is unlikely
   d. If carcinoid syndrome were found in a tumor this size, hepatic metastasis would be likely
   e. When bronchial carcinoid syndrome occurs, right-sided cardiac valves are affected

COMMENT: In the absence of atypia, carcinoids are only locally malignant and can be managed by means of limited resection of the lung, bronchus, or both. Sleeve resection of the bronchus that preserves distal lung would be appropriate. Lymph node sampling at resection, however, is advisable to ensure that complete resection has been performed. Carcinoid syndrome is rare, except in the presence of a large primary tumor or hepatic metastasis. When carcinoid syndrome does occur, left-sided cardiac valves are affected rather than right-sided valves, which one would expect with gastrointestinal carcinoids.

ANSWER: a, c, d

REFERENCE: *Chapter 59—Lung Neoplasms: Bronchial Adenomas*

8. A 42-year-old man has a solitary "coin lesion" 2 cm in diameter in the area of the right upper lobe on a routine chest radiograph. Which of the following statements is/are true?

a. A radiograph from 5 years earlier shows the lesion to be 1.2 cm in diameter and suggests malignant growth
b. If computed tomography (CT) shows mediastinal adenopathy, mediastinoscopy is preferable to thoracotomy
c. In the absence of previous radiographs, the lesion should be followed by serial radiographs every 6 months
d. Calcification in a concentric or "popcorn" configuration denotes a benign lesion
e. Needle aspiration that yields "chronic inflammatory cells" denotes a benign lesion

COMMENT: In the evaluation of a solitary lung lesion, previous radiographs are important, particularly if the lesion is new. A coin lesion that is growing slowly does not necessarily indicate malignant growth, because the most common benign tumor, hamartoma, has a variable pattern of slow growth and typically shows popcorn calcification. Concentric calcification also is most suggestive of benign granuloma. In the absence of previous radiographs, the lesion must be assumed malignant until proved otherwise and should not be dismissed to follow-up evaluation. If CT shows mediastinal adenopathy, mediastinoscopy with biopsy is appropriate to make a diagnosis. Needle aspiration results of "chronic inflammatory cells" are not enough information for a diagnosis.

ANSWER: b, d

REFERENCE: *Chapter 59—Lung Neoplasms: Non-small Cell Lung Cancer*

9. A 53-year-old woman who underwent removal of a malignant tumor 2 years earlier has a solitary lung nodule 1.5 cm in diameter. Which of the following statements is/are true?

a. If the primary tumor originated in the breast, the lesion is most likely to represent new primary lung cancer
b. If the primary tumor was melanoma, the lesion is most likely metastatic
c. If the rest of the lung fields are clear, CT is unnecessary
d. If the primary tumor was in the gastrointestinal tract, there is little likelihood that the lesion is new primary lung cancer
e. Fine-needle aspiration always should be performed before resection of a lung lesion

COMMENT: A new pulmonary lesion in a patient who has undergone therapy for malignant disease poses a diagnostic and therapeutic challenge. Computed tomography always should be performed because plain radiographs depict only lesions 9 mm in diameter or greater. The lesion is most likely to be metastatic if the previous malignant tumor was sarcoma or melanoma and most likely to be a new primary lung cancer if the previous malignant lesion originated in the head, neck, or breast. When the original lesion was in the gastrointestinal or genitourinary tract, there is an equal chance that it is metastatic or a new primary lesion. Results of fine-needle aspiration do not usually alter the plan for excision. This procedure is performed only when the patient is not an operative candidate or wants to know the diagnosis.

ANSWER: a, b

REFERENCE: *Chapter 59—Lung Neoplasms: Surgical Resection of Pulmonary Metastases*

10. For the patient in question 9 to become an operative candidate, which of the following criteria must be met?

   a. It must be possible to control extrathoracic metastasis with another modality, such as radiation therapy
   b. The tumor doubling time must be longer than 40 days
   c. Recurrence at the primary site must be managed before therapy for metastatic disease is begun
   d. Even if effective systemic therapy is available, resection of metastatic lesions is preferred
   e. If pulmonary reserve is marginal, resection of the maximal number of metastatic foci should be performed

COMMENT: There are a number of controversies in the area of operative approaches to metastatic disease of the lung. There is general agreement, however, that extrathoracic metastasis precludes eligibility for pulmonary resection. Although tumor doubling time is a measure of aggressiveness, it is too variable to have prognostic significance and is generally disregarded as a criterion for resection. Recurrence at the primary site must be controlled before the metastatic focus is managed to prevent further seeding. If effective systemic therapy is available, as would be expected for breast or testicular cancer or osteogenic sarcoma, it is preferred over surgical resection. Pulmonary resection should not be undertaken unless the pulmonary reserve allows resection of all metastatic foci.

ANSWER: c

REFERENCE: *Chapter 59—Lung Neoplasms: Surgical Resection of Pulmonary Metastases*

CHAPTER 60

CHEST WALL, PLEURA, MEDIASTINUM, AND NONNEOPLASTIC LUNG DISEASE

1. Which of the following statements is/are true concerning the sternum?

   a. The xiphoid process is the anterior border of the thoracic outlet
   b. The gladiolus is the body of the sternum
   c. The angle of Louis is at the level of the second costal cartilage
   d. The eleventh rib is attached by the costal cartilage to the xiphoid
   e. The sternomanubrial junction is at the level of T4 posteriorly

COMMENT: The sternum consists of three segments—the upper manubrium, the body or gladiolus, and the xiphoid process, which ends in the rectus sheath and has no costal attachments. The xiphoid marks the anterior border of the thoracic outlet. The junction of the manubrium and body is the sternal angle or angle of Louis, which corresponds to the level of T4 posteriorly and attaches to the second costal cartilage anteriorly.

ANSWER: a, b, c, e

REFERENCE: *Chapter 60—Chest Wall, Pleura, Mediastinum, and Nonneoplastic Lung Disease: Anatomy of the Chest Wall*

2. After a shotgun wound of the chest wall, a 39-year-old woman wants reconstruction without a foreign-body prosthesis. Old incisions prohibit use of the rectus abdominis muscle. Which of the following statements is/are true concerning chest wall muscles for reconstruction?

   a. The pectoralis major muscle is available and innervated by the medial and lateral pectoral nerves, so named to describe their relation to the pectoralis minor muscle
   b. The serratus anterior muscle is available because its absence has no functional significance
   c. There is no serratus posterior muscle
   d. The latissimus dorsi muscle is available and supplied by the thoracodorsal artery
   e. The latissimus dorsi muscle is innervated by the thoracodorsal nerve with fibers from C6, C7, and C8

COMMENT: The pectoralis major muscle can be used for reconstruction, but the medial and lateral pectoral nerves are named for the respective cords of the brachial plexus. The serratus anterior muscle holds the scapula to the chest wall and its absence produces the functional and cosmetically disabling winged scapula. The serratus posterior muscle is attached to the seventh cervical and first three thoracic vertebrae posteriorly and functions as an accessory muscle of respiration. The constancy of the vascular pedicle to the latissimus dorsi muscle and its size allow this muscle to be used to reconstruct defects of the head, neck, chest wall, and pleural cavity. It is innervated by the thoracodorsal nerve with fibers from C6, C7, and C8.

ANSWER: d, e

REFERENCE: *Chapter 60—Chest Wall, Pleura, Mediastinum, and Nonneoplastic Lung Disease*

3. A 61-year-old man has a painful mass 3.5 cm in diameter below the clavicle and attached to the chest wall. Which of the following statements is/are true?

   a. Computed tomography (CT) is the best study to determine rib destruction
   b. The lesion should be removed en bloc without biopsy to minimize risk of local recurrence
   c. The likelihood is approximately 40% that the lesion is metastatic
   d. If the lesion is metastatic, the most likely primary tumor is in the lung or pancreas
   e. Fewer than 50% of chest wall tumors are malignant

COMMENT: Chest wall tumors are uncommon, accounting for only 1% to 2% of all tumors. Approximately 57% of chest wall tumors are primary, whereas 43% are metastatic. Solitary metastatic lesions most frequently arise from the thyroid gland, the genitourinary tract, and the colon. Overall, approximately 60% of chest wall tumors are malignant, most arising from bone or cartilage. Computed tomography is of value in showing the relation between the mass and contiguous structures but is of little value in determining the presence of bone destruction because of the oblique course of the ribs. Specific rib radiographs are most helpful. Now that multimodality therapy is available, core-needle biopsy is recommended and has not increased the incidence of local recurrence.

ANSWER: c

REFERENCE: *Chapter 60—Chest Wall, Pleura, Mediastinum, and Nonneoplastic Lung Disease: Chest Wall Tumors*

4. The lesion in Fig. 60.12 was found when a 32-year-old man needed a routine chest radiograph for employment. Which of the following statements is/are true?

   a. The stippled calcification and intact cortex of the rib are characteristic of osteochondroma
   b. The stippled calcification is characteristic of osteogenic sarcoma
   c. If the lesion is osteogenic sarcoma, the optimum treatment is resection and radiation therapy
   d. If the lesion is osteochondroma, it need not be resected in this age group
   e. The radiographic findings are typical of Ewing sarcoma

COMMENT: Osteochondroma is the most common benign rib tumor and has a 3:1 male predominance. The stippled calcification and intact rib cortex are characteristic of this lesion in contrast to the bone destruction of Ewing sarcoma and combined bone destruction and sunburst calcification of osteogenic sarcoma. For both Ewing and osteogenic sarcoma, multimodality therapy with preoperative chemotherapy followed by resection yields better results than does radiation therapy. Osteochondroma among prepubertal children can be observed unless the lesion becomes painful or enlarged. It is routinely resected for adults.

ANSWER: a

REFERENCE: *Chapter 60—Chest Wall, Pleura, Mediastinum, and Nonneoplastic Lung Disease: Chest Wall Tumors*

5. To resect a chondrosarcoma of the chest wall from a 42-year-old man, the second through fourth ribs are removed, leaving a defect 8 cm by 8 cm. Which of the following statements is/are true regarding reconstruction?

a. If this were posterior, beneath the scapula, reconstruction would not be needed
b. If the defect is anterior, the primary benefit of reconstruction is improved cosmetic results
c. Whenever chest wall reconstruction is considered, it should be delayed 6 to 12 months to allow detection of recurrent tumor
d. If polypropylene mesh (Marlex) is used for reconstruction, no wound drainage tube is necessary
e. If polytetrafluoroethylene (PTFE) is used for reconstruction, both pleural and wound tubes should be used

COMMENT: Skeletal chest wall defects that are full thickness and occur posteriorly where they can be covered by the scapula do not require reconstruction. Anterior chest wall defects do require reconstruction, primarily to stabilize the chest wall and prevent paradoxical motion. The reconstruction should be immediate for optimal physiologic benefit. Because Marlex mesh is porous, only a wound catheter is needed because pleural fluid will drain through it. Polytetrafluoroethylene, however, is a solid sheet and necessitates both pleural and wound drainage.

ANSWER: a, d, e

REFERENCE: *Chapter 60—Chest Wall, Pleura, Mediastinum, and Nonneoplastic Lung Disease: Reconstruction*

6. An upright chest radiograph of a homeless 47-year-old woman with cachexia shows blunting of the right costophrenic angle. Which of the following statements is/are true?

a. A lateral decubitus film rather than a CT scan should be obtained to confirm the presence of fluid
b. Tuberculous effusion can readily be identified by means of stain and culture of aspirated fluid
c. A pleural fluid level of glucose lower than the serum level confirms the diagnosis of empyema
d. The presence of bloody pleural effusion in this case confirms the diagnosis of underlying malignant disease
e. A report that reads lymphoma after cytologic examination of the pleural fluid should be viewed with skepticism

COMMENT: Although the CT is a very sensitive indicator of pleural effusion, a lateral decubitus radiograph is the simplest way to differentiate fluid from pleural thickening or fibrosis. Tuberculous pleuritis is difficult to diagnose with stain or culture, which have a 30% yield, but the diagnosis is facilitated by needle biopsy of the pleura. Pleural fluid level of glucose lower than the serum level is characteristic of rheumatoid arthritis, neoplasia, and tuberculosis as well as empyema. Red-tinged fluid can be caused by needle trauma, but even frankly bloody fluid in this patient may reflect trauma as well as underlying malignant disease. Pleural inflammation induces reactive changes in mesothelial cells that make the cells resemble lymphocytes, so a diagnosis of lymphoma is suspect.

ANSWER: a, e

REFERENCE: *Chapter 60—Chest Wall, Pleura, Mediastinum, and Nonneoplastic Lung Disease: Pleural Effusions*

7. A 52-year-old patient with alcoholism, a fever, and a cough productive of purulent sputum is found to have opacity on chest film consistent with a posterior, loculated fluid collection. Which of the following statements is/are true?

    a. The findings suggest parapneumonic empyema
    b. If pus is found at aspiration of the pleural space, a chest tube should be placed
    c. If pus is found at aspiration, bronchoscopy is a necessary part of the evaluation
    d. In this situation, rib resection for drainage is preferred to insertion of a large-bore chest tube
    e. Decortication of the lung should be considered if the lung does not expand within 4 weeks

COMMENT: The posterior location of the infiltrate and fluid collection is typical of a parapneumonic empyema. The most important test is pleural aspiration, which usually yields frank pus; if it does, a chest tube should be placed. Oily propyliodone (Dionosil) once was used to perform empyemography, but this substance is no longer commercially available. In the case of parapneumonic empyema, tube drainage alone may be sufficient to allow full expansion of the lung. If this is not the case, formal rib resection or early decortication should be performed. Decortication or marsupialization is indicated if the lungs do not expand after 6 to 8 weeks. Every patient with spontaneous empyema should undergo bronchoscopy to rule out endobronchial obstruction by a foreign body or tumor.

ANSWER: a, b, c

REFERENCE: *Chapter 60—Chest Wall, Pleura, Mediastinum, and Nonneoplastic Lung Disease: Empyema*

8. A 38-year-old man has facial and upper extremity edema, venous distention in the neck and arms, and a cyanotic appearance. Which of the following statements is/are true?

    a. The most likely cause of the problem is mediastinal granulomatous disease
    b. A venogram should be obtained to confirm the diagnosis
    c. Mediastinoscopy for diagnosis is contraindicated
    d. If a malignant lesion is identified, resection is indicated for palliation
    e. If the cause is benign disease, gradual improvement without operation is expected

COMMENT: Although mediastinal granulomatous disease is one cause of superior vena cava syndrome, the most common cause (75%) is malignant disease. A venogram adds little information to the typical findings and increases risk of subcutaneous extravasation of contrast medium from the venous hypertension. Mediastinoscopy can be used for tissue diagnosis to recognize increased risk of bleeding and airway problems caused by the edema associated with the endotracheal intubation needed for the procedure. If a malignant tumor is found, operative resection usually is precluded by the extent of mediastinal invasion. In the case of benign disease, the symptoms tend to improve as chest wall and mediastinal collaterals enlarge.

ANSWER: e

REFERENCE: *Chapter 60—Chest Wall, Pleura, Mediastinum, and Nonneoplastic Lung Disease: SVC Syndrome*

9. A 39-year-old woman with hypertension and radicular chest wall pain is found to have a solid posterior mediastinal mass. Which of the following statements is/are true?

    a. The location of the lesion suggests teratoma
    b. High levels of vanillylmandelic acid in the urine indicate the lesion is paraganglioma
    c. If the lesion had been seen on a radiograph 5 years earlier, resection would not be indicated
    d. A neurosurgical consultation should be obtained
    e. Elevation of the level of vasoactive intestinal polypeptide suggests ganglioneuroma

COMMENT: The posterior mediastinal location of the tumor is most indicative of a neurogenic tumor. Teratoma is characteristically found in the anterior mediastinum. Neurogenic tumors can undergo malignant degeneration and should be resected, particularly in this patient with symptoms, even if known to be present for years. The radicular pain suggests the possibility of intraspinous extension of the tumor, and therefore neurosurgical consultation is appropriate. Elevation of both urinary vanillylmandelic acid and vasoactive intestinal polypeptide can be caused by ganglioneuroma but would not be characteristic of paraganglioma.

ANSWER: d, e

REFERENCE: *Chapter 60—Chest Wall, Pleura, Mediastinum, and Nonneoplastic Lung Disease: Mediastinal Masses*

10. A 22-year-old woman recovering from traumatic head injury has bright red bleeding when the tracheostomy is suctioned. Which of the following statements is/are true?

a. Antibiotics should be administered to manage bronchitis

b. Deflation of the tracheal tube cuff is a useful diagnostic maneuver

c. If massive bleeding occurs, a finger should be used to compress the innominate artery against the sternum

d. Operative management of a tracheoinnominate fistula includes resection and prosthetic replacement of the innominate artery

e. Tracheal resection usually is needed for a tracheoinnominate fistula to prevent recurrence

COMMENT: The complication of tracheoinnominate artery fistula characteristically occurs among young women and often is heralded by bleeding during tracheostomy suctioning. Deflation of the tracheal tube cuff confirms the diagnosis if massive bleeding occurs. At that point the tracheal tube cuff should be overinflated and a finger inserted into the tracheostomy incision to tamponade the bleeding. Throughout this maneuver, the airway must be protected. Operative repair through an upper sternal split requires resection of the innominate artery and coverage of the oversewn vessels with viable tissue because the wound is contaminated. No prosthetic material should be inserted, and tracheal resection is not necessary.

ANSWER: b, c

REFERENCE: *Chapter 60—Chest Wall, Pleura, Mediastinum, and Nonneoplastic Lung Disease: Complications of Surgical Airways*

CHAPTER 61

CONGENITAL HEART DISEASE AND CARDIAC TUMORS

1. A 5-year-old girl is found at routine examination to have a pulmonic flow murmur, fixed splitting of P2, and a right ventricular lift. Which of the following statements is/are true?

a. Cardiac catheterization is indicated if the chest radiograph shows cardiomegaly

b. A radiology report of "scimitar syndrome" findings on the chest radiograph indicates the need for an arteriogram

c. If the catheterization report is "ostium secundum defect," at least one pulmonary vein drains anomalously

d. Measured pulmonary vascular resistance of 14 Wood units/m^2 with an atrial septal defect (ASD) mandates early repair

e. An ASD with a Qp/Qs ratio of 1.8 can be observed until symptoms occur

COMMENT: The findings suggest an ASD that can be confirmed by means of two-dimensional echocardiography, eliminating the need for cardiac catheterization. The ostium secundum type of defect is most common, but the sinus venosus type is associated with anomalous pulmonary venous drainage. In scimitar syndrome, the anomalous pulmonary vein can be seen on a chest radiograph, and because the anomaly is associated with a hypoplastic lung supplied by an anomalous systemic artery from the aorta, an arteriogram is appropriate. An ASD with a marked left-to-right shunt, as demonstrated by a Qp/Qs ratio greater than 1.5, should be repaired. When pulmonary vascular resistance is elevated to more than 10 to 12 Wood units/m^2 the patient is not a candidate for repair because of fixed pulmonary hypertension.

ANSWER: b

REFERENCE: *Chapter 61—Congenital Heart Disease and Cardiac Tumors: Atrial Septal Defect*

2. A 2-month-old boy is found to have congestive heart failure that manifests as tachypnea, tachycardia, and diaphoresis with poor weight gain. The physical findings suggest a ventricular septal defect (VSD). Management should include:

a. Pulmonary artery banding
b. Urgent closure if a VSD is found on echocardiography
c. Medical treatment only with digitalis and diuretics
d. If a VSD is found, repair is unlikely to be feasible because of elevated pulmonary vascular resistance
e. If a restrictive VSD is found, spontaneous closure is a possibility, and operative repair should be delayed

COMMENT: Large VSDs manifest at 6 to 8 weeks of age when a decrease in the normally elevated pulmonary vascular resistance allows an increase in the left-to-right shunt. Because approximately one half of all VSDs undergo spontaneous closure, particularly with restrictive defects, the initial management is medical. The diagnosis is confirmed by means of echocardiography and cardiac catheterization. Advanced pulmonary vascular changes usually do not occur until the child is 2 years of age. Banding is only rarely indicated for palliation of multiple complex muscular VSDs.

ANSWER: c, e

REFERENCE: *Chapter 61—Congenital Heart Disease and Cardiac Tumors: Ventricular Septal Defect*

3. The child described in question 2 undergoes cardiac catheterization, and the results confirm a VSD with a Qp/Qs ratio of 2.0 and right ventricular systolic pressure one-half systemic pressure. Which of the following statements is/are true?

a. If aortic insufficiency is detected, the defect is likely to be subpulmonic in location
b. Finding aortic stenosis in addition to the VSD is highly unlikely
c. The catheterization data indicate a restrictive type of VSD
d. If pulmonary vascular resistance decreases with tolazoline administration, it is safe to close the VSD
e. Operative closure of VSDs is possible without ventriculotomy

COMMENT: The finding of aortic insufficiency in a patient with VSD suggests prolapse of the aortic valve caused by a subpulmonic or supracristal defect. Associated aortic stenosis, mitral stenosis, and coarctation are common with VSDs. The finding of a moderate left-to-right shunt and a right ventricular pressure well below systemic levels indicates a restrictive VSD. If elevated pulmonary vascular resistance is found, the ability to respond to a vasodilator such as tolazoline indicates that the resistance is not fixed, and operative repair is possible. Operative repair of VSDs is frequently possible through an atriotomy or through the pulmonary artery.

ANSWER: a, c, d, e

REFERENCE: *Chapter 61—Congenital Heart Disease and Cardiac Tumors: Ventricular Septal Defect*

4. A 12-year-old boy is found to have an ejection systolic murmur over the aortic region with a precordial thrill and normal cardiac size on a chest radiograph. Which of the following statements is/are true?

a. A systolic ejection click signifies the stenosis is supravalvular
b. In the absence of cardiomegaly, cardiac catheterization is necessary to measure the pressure gradient
c. Development of syncope suggests an intracranial lesion
d. In valvular aortic stenosis, a pressure gradient of 80 mm Hg is an indication for operative repair regardless of symptoms
e. In membranous subvalvular aortic stenosis a pressure gradient of 40 mm Hg is an indication for operative repair

COMMENT: When a patient has findings of aortic stenosis, a systolic ejection click is evidence that the obstruction is valvular. Cardiac size does not provide an indication of the severity of the stenosis and is frequently normal. The development of angina or syncope reflects inadequate cardiac output and signifies late-stage disease. A pressure gradient greater than 75 mm Hg is an indication for an operation for valvular aortic stenosis even if the patient has no symptoms. A gradient of 30 mm Hg or more is considered sufficient for operative correction of membranous subvalvular stenosis.

ANSWER: d, e

REFERENCE: *Chapter 61—Congenital Heart Disease and Cardiac Tumors: Aortic Stenosis*

5. A 2-month-old boy who appeared healthy at birth has cyanosis and is found to have a systolic ejection murmur over the pulmonary area and a boot-shaped heart on a chest radiograph. Which of the following statements is/are true?

a. Echocardiography alone is sufficient to confirm the diagnosis of tetralogy of Fallot
b. Cyanotic spells can be appropriately managed with propranolol
c. A Blalock-Taussig shunt connects the right ventricle to the pulmonary artery
d. Increasing cyanotic spells is the most common indication for operation
e. Operative repair of right ventricular outflow obstruction is never extended across the pulmonic valve because intolerable pulmonary insufficiency would result

COMMENT: In this typical scenario of tetralogy of Fallot, echocardiography can confirm the diagnosis with no need for cardiac catheterization. Cyanotic spells are managed with supplemental oxygen, sedation with morphine, and a β-blocker such as propranolol. For a palliative increase in pulmonary blood flow, a Blalock-Taussig shunt is used to connect the subclavian artery to the pulmonary artery. Increasing cyanosis and cyanotic spells are the most common indication for operative repair. To correct the right ventricular outflow obstruction of tetralogy of Fallot, a transannular patch extending into the pulmonary artery may be needed. The pulmonary valvular insufficiency that results is well tolerated in the absence of tricuspid insufficiency or ventricular dysfunction.

ANSWER: a, b, d

REFERENCE: *Chapter 61—Congenital Heart Disease and Cardiac Tumors: Tetralogy of Fallot*

6. Within 2 hours of birth, a girl is obviously cyanotic and on a chest radiograph the heart looks like "an egg on its side." Which of the following statements is/are true?

   a. The most common cause of cyanosis this early is transposition of the great vessels (TGV)
   b. If TGV is present, echocardiography shows that the posterior vessel leaving the left ventricle is a pulmonary artery
   c. If TGV is confirmed at echocardiography, cardiac catheterization has little to add
   d. Electrocardiography (ECG) is helpful in making the diagnosis of TGV because it shows reversed dominance of the ventricles
   e. To improve mixing of pulmonary and systemic circulations, prostaglandin should be used to increase pulmonary vascular resistance

COMMENT: Transposition of the great vessels is the most common cause of cyanosis in the first week of life. This diagnosis can be confirmed with echocardiographic demonstration of a posterior pulmonary artery attached to the left ventricle. Cardiac catheterization is useful to confirm the anatomic features, detect other lesions, define coronary anatomic features, and improve cardiac mixing with balloon atrial septostomy. Electrocardiography is not helpful in the diagnosis of TGV because it shows only normal right ventricular dominance. Prostaglandin improves mixing of the circulation by means of opening the ductus arteriosus and decreasing pulmonary vascular resistance.

ANSWER: a, b

REFERENCE: *Chapter 61—Congenital Heart Disease and Cardiac Tumors: Transposition of the Great Arteries*

7. A 1-year-old boy thought to have tetralogy of Fallot is found at cardiac catheterization to have double-outlet right ventricle (DORV). Which of the following statements is/are true:

   a. Spontaneous closure of a VSD is rare
   b. Location of a VSD has little effect on the degree of cyanosis
   c. Double-outlet left ventricles do not occur
   d. Coincidental aortic stenosis with DORV is not compatible with life
   e. *Doubly committed VSD* refers to the relation between the defect and the great vessels

COMMENT: In DORV, the location of the VSD affects the direction of flow of oxygenated blood and thus determines the degree of cyanosis. The VSD rarely closes because that would result in severe decompensation or death. Double-outlet left ventricle occurs but is less common than DORV. A number of other anomalies are associated with DORV, including both valvular and subvalvular pulmonary and aortic stenosis. The VSD may be directed to either or both great vessels (doubly committed) or remote from them (noncommitted).

ANSWER: a, e

REFERENCE: *Chapter 61—Congenital Heart Disease and Cardiac Tumors: Double-outlet Right Ventricle*

8. A neonate with congestive heart failure has echocardiographic evidence of a single truncal vessel from which the pulmonary arteries arise, a VSD, and truncal valvular stenosis. Which of the following statements is/are true?

   a. The natural history of this anomaly allows only a 20% 1-year survival rate
   b. The most likely configuration of the truncal valve is bicuspid
   c. The location of the pulmonary arteries minimizes the risk of pulmonary vascular obstructive disease (Eisenmenger's syndrome)
   d. Repair of the lesion requires an extracardiac conduit
   e. Optimal timing of operative repair is at 6 to 12 months of age

COMMENT: The defect described is truncus arteriosus, which carries an 80% 1-year mortality rate if uncorrected. The truncal valve is most commonly tricuspid (65%) or quadricuspid (25%) and least likely bicuspid (9%). The large left-to-right shunt makes these patients particularly likely to develop pulmonary vascular obstruction (Eisenmenger's syndrome). Operative repair requires detachment of the pulmonary arteries, which are reconnected to the right ventricle by means of an extracardiac conduit. The optimal timing of repair is within the first 6 months of life.

ANSWER: a, d

REFERENCE: *Chapter 61—Congenital Heart Disease and Cardiac Tumors: Truncus Arteriosus*

9. A 2-month-old infant has ECG evidence of myocardial ischemia. The echocardiographic results suggest anomalous origin of the left coronary artery from the pulmonary artery. Which of the following statements is/are true?

   a. Ischemia is caused by perfusion of the myocardium with inadequately oxygenated blood
   b. Selective coronary angiography should not be attempted because of the risk of myocardial infarction
   c. Conservative treatment is preferred to allow the coronary artery to grow to a size that allows bypass construction
   d. If the infant's condition deteriorates, ligation of the coronary artery at its origin is an option
   e. The severity of the abnormality ensures that it is always detected in the first year of life

COMMENT: Anomalous origin of the left coronary artery from the pulmonary artery results in reverse flow in the coronary artery into the low-pressure system as a steal from the coronary circulation. If collaterals from the right coronary develop to allow adequate myocardial perfusion, the disorder is frequently not diagnosed until later in life when a murmur is heard. Selective coronary arteriography is appropriate to define the anatomic features and operative repair is undertaken promptly. Ligation of the anomalous coronary artery can be lifesaving but leaves the child dependent on a single vessel. Coronary bypass is preferred.

ANSWER: d

REFERENCE: *Chapter 61—Congenital Heart Disease and Cardiac Tumors: Coronary Artery Anomalies*

10. A premature infant with respiratory distress is found to have a continuous "machinery" murmur over the precordium. Which of the following statements is/are true?

   a. The most likely diagnosis is coarctation of the aorta
   b. If large pulmonary arteries are found, patent ductus arteriosus is likely
   c. To discriminate between *a* and *b*, prostaglandin administration can be used to constrict the patent ductus arteriosus
   d. If patent ductus arteriosus is found, operative repair should be delayed until the respiratory symptoms are relieved to reduce mortality rates
   e. Normal ductus closure depends on increased oxygen saturation in the pulmonary artery

COMMENT: A continuous "machinery" murmur is characteristic of patent ductus arteriosus, which typically occurs among premature infants. Normal closure of the ductus is prompted by a decrease in pulmonary vascular resistance that increases the left-to-right shunt and oxygen levels from the aorta. Indomethacin can cause ductus closure by means of cyclooxygenase inhibition, which decreases production of endogenous prostaglandins. Prostaglandin infusion would keep the ductus open. Operative closure can be done safely on even the smallest neonates and usually promptly relieves the respiratory distress.

ANSWER: b, e

REFERENCE: *Chapter 61—Congenital Heart Disease and Cardiac Tumors: Patent Ductus Arteriosus*

11. A 1-year-old girl with dyspnea and poor feeding is found to have congestive heart failure. Echocardiography shows an atrioventricular septal defect. Which of the following statements is/are true?

   a. The second heart sound has fixed splitting
   b. Despite diagnostic echocardiography, cardiac catheterization is indicated to assess pulmonary artery resistance
   c. Pulmonary arterial banding is indicated to limit pulmonary flow and allow the child to grow
   d. Atrioventricular septal defect is classified according to the morphologic features of the anterior leaflet of the common atrioventricular valve
   e. Operative repair is best performed after 2 years of age

COMMENT: Atrioventricular septal defect is a defect of endocardial cushion development that produces morphologic abnormalities of both atrioventricular valves and both atrial and ventricular septa. It is usually classified according to the morphologic features of the anterior leaflet of the atrioventricular valve. Pulmonary vascular resistance remains elevated in infancy, delaying diagnosis and producing fixed splitting of the second heart sound. Cardiac catheterization is indicated to assess pulmonary vascular resistance, but pulmonary arterial banding is no longer performed to protect the pulmonary bed. Operative repair is performed instead, preferably before the age of 6 months.

ANSWER: a, b, d

REFERENCE: *Chapter 61—Congenital Heart Disease and Cardiac Tumors: Atrioventricular Septal Defect*

12. A 9-year-old boy with hypertension has no palpable femoral pulses. Coarctation of the aorta is suspected. Which of the following statements is/are true?

 a. The most common associated abnormality is bicuspid aortic valve
 b. A chest radiograph is likely to show rib notching
 c. The cause is believed to be inflammatory aortitis
 d. In infancy, coarctation can manifest as a pink upper body and cyanotic lower body
 e. Paradoxical hypertension after operative repair indicates residual stenosis from incomplete correction

COMMENT: Coarctation of the aorta occurs just distal to the origin of the left subclavian artery and is caused by contraction of ectopic tissue from the ductus arteriosus. The most common associated abnormality is a bicuspid aortic valve. Extensive collateral development involves the mammary and intercostal arteries and produces rib notching on chest radiographs. In infancy, flow to the lower body is from the ductus arteriosus before it closes, producing differential cyanosis. The paradoxical hypertension seen postoperatively is thought to relate to sympathetic nerve stimulation and does not reflect incomplete repair.

ANSWER: a, b, d

REFERENCE: *Chapter 61—Congenital Heart Disease and Cardiac Tumors: Coarctation*

13. An infant with cyanosis has echocardiographic evidence of univentricular heart (UVH). Which of the following statements is/are true?

 a. The most common form of the disorder is a double-inlet right ventricle
 b. To be classified as a ventricle, the chamber must receive at least one half of an inlet valve
 c. This infant is a good candidate for a Blalock-Taussig shunt
 d. Optimal correction of UVH diverts all vena caval blood flow into the pulmonary arteries (Fontan procedure)
 e. In the absence of pulmonary stenosis, UVH usually manifests as congestive heart failure

COMMENT: Univentricular heart is defined by the connection of the atria to only one ventricular chamber, usually the left as a double-inlet left ventricle. A chamber must receive at least one half of an inlet valve to be considered a ventricle. The presentation of UVH depends on the pulmonary blood flow. If pulmonary stenosis is present, there is increased cyanosis, and the infant is a candidate for a Blalock-Taussig shunt. In the absence of pulmonary stenosis, pulmonary flow is excessive, and the presentation is congestive heart failure. Optimal correction of UVH diverts all vena caval flow into the pulmonary arteries as the Fontan procedure.

ANSWER: b, c, d, e

REFERENCE: *Chapter 61—Congenital Heart Disease and Cardiac Tumors: Univentricular Heart*

14. A neonate with respiratory distress has echocardiographic evidence of hypoplastic left heart syndrome (HLHS). Which of the following statements is/are true?

    a. Initial management should include prostaglandin infusion
    b. Ventilatory adjustment should maintain Paco₂ at approximately 40 mm Hg
    c. Survival depends on sustained patency of the ductus arteriosus
    d. Cardiac transplantation for HLHS requires inclusion of the donor aortic arch
    e. Reconstruction for HLHS converts the pulmonary artery into the main outlet for a functional single ventricle (Norwood)

COMMENT: A neonate with HLHS has a severely underdeveloped left ventricular and aortic arch and depends on patency of the ductus, which is facilitated by prostaglandin infusion. Ventilator adjustment to decrease supplemental oxygen and maintain Pco₂ at 40 mm Hg avoids excessive pulmonary flow. The options for treatment include cardiac transplantation, which requires a donor aortic arch and reconstruction by means of the Norwood procedure, which converts the pulmonary artery into the main outlet for a functional single ventricle.

ANSWER: a, b, c, d, e

REFERENCE: *Chapter 61—Congenital Heart Disease and Cardiac Tumors: Hypoplastic Left Heart Syndrome*

15. A 48-year-old woman with episodic syncope has echocardiographic evidence of a mass in the left atrium. Which of the following statements is/are true?

    a. Transseptal puncture should be used for definitive diagnosis
    b. If this is a primary cardiac tumor, it is most likely malignant
    c. If this is a myxoma attached to the atrial septum, the adjacent septum should be removed with it
    d. In infancy, the most common cardiac tumor is rhabdomyosarcoma
    e. The most common primary malignant tumor of the heart is angiosarcoma

COMMENT: Primary cardiac tumors commonly arise in the left atrium and can manifest as dyspnea, syncope, congestive failure, and systemic embolism. Transseptal puncture should not be used for diagnosis because of the risk of embolism. Most primary cardiac tumors are benign by a 3:1 ratio. The most common malignant tumor is angiosarcoma. Myxoma is the most common benign tumor, but it can recur, and the adjacent atrial septum should be resected with it. In infancy, the most common cardiac tumor is rhabdomyoma.

ANSWER: c, e

REFERENCE: *Chapter 61—Congenital Heart Disease and Cardiac Tumors: Primary Neoplasms of the Heart*

CHAPTER 62

VALVULAR HEART DISEASE

1. Concerning valvular heart disease, the following is/are true:

    a. Mitral stenosis is the most common lesion
    b. Of all cardiac valves, the aortic is the most anterior
    c. Stenosis is the most common lesion of the aortic valve
    d. Rheumatic heart disease is the most common cause of valve dysfunction

COMMENT: Aortic valvular stenosis is the most common type of valvular lesion followed by mitral stenosis. Anatomically, the pulmonic valve is the most anterior of the cardiac valves. Rheumatic heart disease is the most common cause of valve dysfunction and the most common cause of multivalvular disease.

ANSWER: c, d

REFERENCE: *Chapter 62—Valvular Heart Disease: Anatomy and Pathology*

2. Concerning the adaptation to cardiac valvular dysfunction, the following is/are true:

    a. Severe heart failure is more likely from acute than chronic valvular dysfunction
    b. Valvular dysfunction produces both volume and pressure afterload stress on the heart
    c. Early cardiac dilation from valve dysfunction shifts the Frank-Starling curve to depress cardiac output
    d. The LaPlace law predicts that wall stress decreases with increasing ventricular radius

COMMENT: Valvular dysfunction produces both volume and pressure overload representing afterload stress on the heart. Although cardiac reserves allow for gradual adaptation to chronic valvular dysfunction, acute dysfunction is less well tolerated and more likely to result in severe heart failure. The increase in diastolic filling which initially dilates the heart shifts the Frank-Starling curve to improve ejection and cardiac output. The LaPlace law predicts that wall stress increases with increasing ventricular radius but is inversely related to wall thickness.

ANSWER: a, b

REFERENCE: *Chapter 62—Valvular Heart Disease*

3. A 42-year-old woman has noted progressive exercise intolerance and fatigability. Examination discloses an opening snap in the mitral area suggestive of mitral stenosis. The following is/are true:

    a. Critical mitral stenosis is defined as an orifice area reduced to 2 cm²
    b. With a fixed mitral orifice, the change from sinus rhythm to atrial fibrillation has little effect on cardiac output
    c. Mural thrombi and thromboembolism are directly related to the presence of atrial fibrillation
    d. Depressed cardiac output is usually due to depressed myocardial contractility

COMMENT: Normal adults have a 4-6 cm² mitral orifice and reduction to 2 cm² is mild stenosis while reduction to 1 cm² is considered critical mitral stenosis. Even with a fixed orifice, the onset of atrial fibrillation reduces cardiac output by 20%. Mural thrombi and thromboembolism are directly related to the presence of atrial fibrillation. Mitral stenosis spares ventricular function, and the loss of cardiac output is from decreased preload.

ANSWER: c

REFERENCE: *Chapter 62—Valvular Heart Disease: Mitral Stenosis*

4. A 52-year-old man with known aortic stenosis develops angina pectoris and has a single episode of syncope. The following is/are true:

    a. Onset of angina indicates concomitant coronary artery disease independent of valvular lesion
    b. Percutaneous aortic balloon valvuloplasty should be considered since it has generally favorable results
    c. The patient is not an operative candidate since heart failure has not occurred
    d. A measured transvalvular pressure gradient greater than 50 mm Hg would be an operative indication

COMMENT: The ventricular hypertrophy which accompanies aortic stenosis increases oxygen demand while mechanical forces increase resistance to perfusion, resulting in ischemia. Only one half of these patients with angina have coronary artery disease. Percutaneous balloon valvuloplasty of the aortic valve has high complication and recurrence rates. Any such patient with symptoms has an indication for operations as would the patient with a transvalvular gradient > 50 mm Hg.

ANSWER: d

REFERENCE: *Chapter 62—Valvular Heart Disease: Management*

5. A 47-year-old male with fatigue and cardiac failure has a high-pitched, decrescendo diastolic murmur along the left sternal border and an apical diastolic rumble. His blood pressure is 148/45 mm Hg. The following is/are true:

    a. Chest radiograph will show cor bovinum
    b. The apical murmur is due to the Gallavardin phenomenon
    c. A carotid shudder would be expected
    d. Abdominal exam will show a pulsatile liver

COMMENT: This patient with aortic insufficiency has a volume loading strain on the heart which produces cor bovinum as dramatic enlargement. The apical murmur produced by turbulence with mitral forward flow mimics mitral stenosis and is called an Austin-Glint murmur. A carotid shudder occurs with aortic stenosis and a pulsatile liver is typical of tricuspid insufficiency.

ANSWER: a

REFERENCE: *Chapter 62—Valvular Heart Disease: Physical Examination*

6. The patient in the previous question with AI progresses to profound heart failure requiring medical management. The following is/are true:
   a. Perperal vasdilators are contraindicated
   b. The intraaortic balloon pump can be used to improve cardiac output
   c. Furosemide and nitroglycerin would be appropriate
   d. Valve replacement is necessary

COMMENT: Peripheral vasodilators are key to the treatment of AI favoring peripheral blood flow. The intraaortic pump is contraindicated because diastolic augmentation worsens aortic regurgitation. Both furosemide and nitroglycerin would be of value to treat the failure, but the most effective treatment requires replacement of the valve.

ANSWER: c, d

REFERENCE: *Chapter 62—Valvular Heart Disease: Medical Management*

7. A 31-year-old male drug abuser presents with fever, chills, and multiple bilateral lung abscesses. Right heart endocarditis is suspected. The following is/are true:
   a. The organisms most likely responsible are gram-negative and fungal
   b. The pulmonic valve is most likely to be affected
   c. A negative echocardiogram is useful to exclude the diagnosis
   d. Valve replacement is necessary if the native valve is excised to treat infection

COMMENT: The typical endocarditis in a drug-abuser involves fungal and gram-negative organisms which infect the tricuspid rather than the pulmonic valve. An echocardiogram is useful to confirm the presence of vegetations but it may overlook smaller ones so it cannot be used to exclude the diagnosis. Although valve replacement is usually preferable, the infected tricuspid valve can be excised without prosthetic replacement.

ANSWER: a

REFERENCE: *Chapter 62—Valvular Heart Disease: Endocarditis*

CHAPTER 63

ISCHEMIC HEART DISEASE

1. Which of the following statements is/are true concerning cardiac vascular anatomy?
   a. In 80% to 85% of cases, the posterior descending coronary artery (PDA) arises from the circumflex coronary artery
   b. The PDA gives off the atrioventricular nodal artery
   c. The great cardiac vein ascends along the right coronary artery to empty into the coronary sinus
   d. Thebesian veins drain only from the left and right ventricles

COMMENT: In 80% to 85% of cases, the circumflex coronary artery ends with branches to the left ventricle, and the PDA originates from the right coronary artery in 80% to 85% of cases. The PDA gives off the atrioventricular nodal artery, and occlusion of this vessel can result in heart block. The great cardiac vein ascends along the left anterior descending coronary artery, and the thebesian veins drain all four chambers.

ANSWER: b

REFERENCE: *Chapter 63—Ischemic Heart Disease: Coronary Circulation*

2. Which of the following statements is/are true concerning the function of the coronary circulation?
   a. Under circumstances of increased oxygen demand by the myocardium, oxygen extraction from arterial blood can increase
   b. Coronary flow is maximal during systole
   c. Adenosine is the most important metabolic regulator of coronary blood flow
   d. Sympathetic nerve stimulation constricts coronary arteries despite the need for increased cardiac output

COMMENT: Because myocardium maximally extracts oxygen from blood at rest, increased demand requires increased delivery. Systolic pressures compress intramyocardial vessels, so maximal coronary flow occurs during diastole. Adenosine, a breakdown product of adenosine triphosphate, is a vasodilator and the most important metabolic regulator of coronary blood flow. Although sympathetic nerves produce coronary vasoconstriction, the autoregulatory vasodilatory responses to increased myocardial demand overwhelm that effect.

ANSWER: c, d

REFERENCE: *Chapter 63—Ischemic Heart Disease: Regulation of Coronary Blood Flow*

3. A 42-year-old attorney who does not have symptoms undergoes a routine exercise test that has a positive result for myocardial ischemia. Which of the following statements is/are true?
   a. This is a rare event because fewer than 5% of patients with coronary artery disease have no symptoms with exercise
   b. Such a condition can progress to heart failure from ischemic cardiomyopathy
   c. Typical angina pectoris is promptly relieved by rest or relaxation
   d. Dyspnea on exertion can represent an angina equivalent

COMMENT: As many as 25% of patients with coronary artery disease found at exercise testing have no symptoms. Progressive coronary obstruction in these patients can produce heart failure from ischemic cardiomyopathy. Typical angina is relieved promptly by rest or relaxation. Ischemic reductions in ventricular contractility and compliance can produce dyspnea on exertion as an angina equivalent.

ANSWER: b, c, d

REFERENCE: *Chapter 63—Ischemic Heart Disease: Symptoms of Coronary Artery Disease*

4. Which of the following statements is/are true concerning the evaluation of a 45-year-old man with suspected coronary artery disease?
   a. Thyroid tests are included to rule out hyperthyroidism
   b. A positive result of stress electrocardiography (ECG) typically shows elevated ST segments
   c. Dipyridamole is a useful adjunct to thallium scanning because it increases coronary perfusion pressure
   d. Persisting defects on thallium scans indicate reversible myocardial ischemia

COMMENT: Diagnostic studies for coronary artery disease should help detect risk factors, such as diabetes mellitus, hyperlipidemia, and hyperthyroidism. Stress ECG typically shows downward sloping ST-segment depression. Dipyridamole is a coronary artery vasodilator that reduces systemic and coronary perfusion pressures. The persisting thallium scan defect reflects irreversibly scarred myocardium.

ANSWER: a

REFERENCE: *Chapter 63—Ischemic Heart Disease: Diagnostic Studies*

5. A 52-year-old woman with chest pain is considered for coronary arteriography because of her risk factors. Which of the following statements is/are true?
   a. All patients with typical anginal symptoms need coronary arteriography
   b. Atypical patients with borderline positive results of stress tests need arteriography
   c. Patients who need valve procedures do not need arteriography
   d. Patients with refractory heart failure awaiting cardiac transplantation need coronary arteriography

COMMENT: Patients with typical angina and ECG changes need angiography if their condition is refractory to medical management, if they are candidates for revascularization, or both. Patients with atypical signs and symptoms need angiography to confirm or exclude the diagnosis. Patients with valve disease and risk of coronary artery disease need angiography, but patients awaiting cardiac transplantation are not candidates for revascularization and do not need coronary angiography.

ANSWER: b

REFERENCE: *Chapter 63—Ischemic Heart Disease: Diagnostic Studies*

6. Which of the following statements is/are true concerning medical management of coronary artery disease?

   a. Nitroglycerin primarily dilates coronary arterioles
   b. β-Blocking agents decrease myocardial oxygen demand
   c. Calcium channel blocking agents reduce ventricular contractility
   d. Calcium channel blocking agents should not be used if there is an element of coronary vasospastic disease

COMMENT: Nitroglycerin primarily dilates venous capacitance vessels but at higher doses can produce coronary and systemic arterial dilation. β-Adrenergic blocking agents decrease myocardial oxygen demand by decreasing heart rate and contractility. Calcium channel blocking agents decrease ventricular contractility, produce vasodilation, and can protect myocytes. They are particularly effective therapy for coronary vasospastic disease.

ANSWER: b, c

REFERENCE: *Chapter 63—Ischemic Heart Disease: Medical Management*

7. After repair of an abdominal aortic aneurysm, a 66-year-old man has severe chest pain, diaphoresis, bradycardia, and hypotension. Which of the following statements is/are true?

   a. The ECG is most likely to show a prominent Q wave in lead 3 if this is a myocardial infarction (MI)
   b. If a Q wave is present, the infarct is subendocardial rather than transmural
   c. Creatine kinase measurement alone provides enough information to confirm the diagnosis of MI
   d. Because bradycardia rarely occurs with MI, another diagnosis should be considered

COMMENT: Pain is the most common symptom among patients with MI, although 20% to 25% of MIs are asymptomatic. Inferior MI involving the right coronary frequently has parasympathetic activity with bradycardia, hypotension, and a prominent Q wave in lead 3. The presence of a Q wave indicates transmural MI, which can be confirmed with measurement of the specific isoenzyme for cardiac tissue (CK-MB), because creatine kinase level can be elevated nonspecifically after stroke or an operation.

ANSWER: a

REFERENCE: *Chapter 63—Ischemic Heart Disease: Acute Myocardial Infarction*

8. Which of the following statements is/are true concerning the initial treatment of the patient with suspected acute MI in question 7?

   a. Oxygen and lidocaine should be administered prophylactically
   b. If chest pain persists, intravenous nitroglycerin should be used to limit infarct size
   c. Calcium channel blockers are of value to limit infarct size
   d. Intravenous morphine can be used but has no therapeutic effect

COMMENT: Initial treatment during early evolving MI includes oxygen, but lidocaine should be used only if arrhythmias occur. Intravenous nitroglycerin is of value to limit infarct size, but calcium channel blockers have no such benefit. Because it decreases pain and anxiety, intravenous morphine has a marked therapeutic effect in decreasing myocardial oxygen demand.

ANSWER: b

REFERENCE: *Chapter 63—Ischemic Heart Disease: Acute Myocardial Infarction; Management*

9. A 52-year-old man with chest pain and tachycardia has ECG evidence of acute MI. Which of the following statements is/are true?

   a. Thrombolytic therapy should be considered immediately because the benefit is greater the earlier it is given
   b. Of the drugs available, recombinant tissue plasminogen activator (TPA) produces better results than does streptokinase or anisoylated plasminogen streptokinase activator complex (APSAC), although it is more expensive
   c. Thrombolytic therapy requires catheterization for intracoronary administration
   d. Addition of heparin and antiplatelet drugs produces no incremental benefit

COMMENT: Thrombolytic therapy for acute MI is valuable in reducing mortality. The benefit is related to early administration. Although recombinant TPA can produce higher coronary patency rates, the results of treatment are no better than those of treatment with streptokinase or APSAC. Administration of thrombolytic drugs initially was intracoronary, but the drugs can be effective with systemic intravenous administration. There is an added benefit from heparin and antiplatelet drugs to prevent rethrombosis.

ANSWER: a

REFERENCE: *Chapter 63—Ischemic Heart Disease: Acute Myocardial Infarction; Thrombolysis*

10. Twenty-four hours after successful thrombolytic treatment, the patient described in question 9 has recurrent chest pain. Which of the following statements is/are true?

    a. Rethrombosis is most likely, and thrombolytic therapy alone should be repeated
    b. The problem could have been prevented with early elective catheterization and percutaneous transluminal coronary angioplasty (PTCA)
    c. The patient has an indication for catheterization and PTCA if single-vessel disease is found
    d. Findings of multivessel disease at catheterization indicate the need for operative bypass
    e. If operative bypass is deemed necessary, there should be a 30-day delay to allow myocardial healing

COMMENT: After thrombolytic therapy for acute MI, angina recurs in 30% to 35% of cases and is an indication for cardiac catheterization and mechanical intervention to prevent infarct extension. Prophylactic catheterization, however, has not been found to provide benefit. If the findings at catheterization show limited disease that can be controlled with it, PTCA should be performed. If multivessel disease or unfavorable anatomic features are found, operative bypass should be performed early because results are best within 30 days of MI.

ANSWER: c, d

REFERENCE: *Chapter 63—Ischemic Heart Disease: Mechanical Intervention in Acute Myocardial Infarction*

11. A 67-year-old man with documented acute MI has cardiogenic shock in 24 hours. Which of the following statements is/are true?

    a. The mortality rate for acute MI followed by cardiogenic shock is tenfold higher than that for acute MI without shock
    b. Age, ejection fraction, infarct size, and previous MI are predictors of cardiogenic shock
    c. Acute loss of more than 20% of myocardium frequently results in cardiogenic shock and death
    d. Emergency revascularization is contraindicated for a patient who has had an MI and is in cardiogenic shock

COMMENT: Cardiogenic shock is unusual after acute MI but increases the mortality rate from 4% to 65%. All of the risk factors described and a history of diabetes mellitus are predictive of cardiogenic shock. The volume of myocardium lost acutely that is associated with shock is 40%. Evidence suggests that emergency coronary bypass can be performed within 18 hours of shock to decrease the mortality rate to 7%.

ANSWER: a, b

REFERENCE: *Chapter 63—Ischemic Heart Disease: Indications for Surgery after Acute Myocardial Infarction*

12. Four days after transmural MI, a 74-year-old man has hypotension and congestive heart failure. Which of the following statements is/are true?

    a. An intraaortic balloon pump (IABP) should be used and cardiac catheterization performed
    b. Posterior infarction is most likely caused by a ventricular septal defect (VSD)
    c. A pulmonary wedge pressure tracing of prominent V waves without oxygen step-up suggests papillary muscle rupture
    d. Operative repair of a VSD after MI should be delayed to allow strengthening of the myocardium to hold sutures

COMMENT: Both VSD and rupture of the papillary muscle occur 3 to 5 days after MI and should be managed by means of an IABP, a decrease in afterload, and cardiac catheterization for diagnosis. A VSD is most common among elderly women with hypertension who have sustained anterior transmural MI. Posterior MI typically leads to papillary muscle rupture, which is diagnosed when prominent V waves are present on pulmonary wedge pressure tracings. The survival rate for both of these complications improves with early rather than late repair.

ANSWER: a, c

REFERENCE: *Chapter 63—Ischemic Heart Disease: Indication for Surgery after Acute Myocardial Infarction*

13. A 70-year-old woman with intractable angina pectoris undergoes cardiac catheterization for possible mechanical intervention. She prefers PTCA to open correction. Which of the following statements is/are true?

  a. A long symmetric lesion in the left main coronary artery would be appropriate for PTCA
  b. Multiple obstructive lesions in the same artery would be a contraindication to PTCA
  c. A focal lesion in the left anterior descending coronary artery where the vessel is 1 mm in diameter would allow PTCA
  d. Successful PTCA for a simple lesion carries less than 10% risk of recurrent stenosis

COMMENT: The ideal lesion for PTCA is focal symmetric stenosis in an epicardial vessel. However, this procedure is relatively contraindicated for extensive disease in the left main coronary, for multiple obstructive lesions in the same artery, and for vessels less than 2 mm in diameter. The rate of restenosis within the first 4 to 6 months after successful dilation for simple lesions is 20% to 40%.

ANSWER: b

REFERENCE: *Chapter 63—Ischemic Heart Disease: Mechanical Revascularization*

14. The patient in question 13 is found to have disease unsuitable for PTCA. Concerning operative revascularization by means of coronary artery bypass grafting (CABG), which of the following statements is/are true?

  a. Coronary artery bypass grafting is more effective than medical treatment for relieving angina and improving physical work capacity
  b. In CABG for unstable angina, there is no difference in late outcome between stable and unstable cohorts
  c. For CABG, the most common arterial graft is the left internal mammary artery
  d. Long-term patency improves when arterial grafts are used, but there is no difference in the early mortality rate

COMMENT: Randomized studies show that CABG is more effective than medical therapy for relieving angina, improving physical work capacity, and improving overall quality of life. When CABG is used for unstable angina, the initial complication and mortality rates are higher than for stable angina, but the late outcomes are similar. Use of arterial grafts for CABG has increased. The left internal mammary artery is used most commonly. When at least one mammary artery is used, the early mortality rate improves.

ANSWER: a, b, c

REFERENCE: *Chapter 63—Ischemic Heart Disease: Coronary Artery Bypass Surgery*

15. A 59-year-old man has undergone successful CABG with four grafts constructed but continues to have low cardiac output (less than 2 L/min per square meter) postoperatively. Which of the following statements is/are true?

a. An inotropic drug should be used initially to increase cardiac output
b. If low cardiac output persists despite optimal physiologic and pharmacologic support, an IABP should be inserted
c. Decreased cardiac filling pressures suggest the possibility of cardiac tamponade
d. When an IABP is used, the balloon is inflated during diastole

COMMENT: Initial efforts to improve cardiac output should include correction of poor oxygenation or acidosis and optimization of rhythm, preload, and afterload before an inotropic agent is used. If low cardiac output persists despite physiologic and pharmacologic support, an IABP should be inserted. It improves coronary artery perfusion by means of counterpulsation during diastole. Cardiac tamponade is heralded by increased cardiac filling pressure, narrowed pulse pressure, and pulsus paradoxus.

ANSWER: b, d

REFERENCE: *Chapter 63—Ischemic Heart Disease: Coronary Artery Bypass Surgery*

16. A 78-year-old patient who is a candidate for CABG is concerned about the risks versus benefits of the procedure. Which of the following statements is/are true?

a. Operative mortality among patients older than 70 years is more than double that of younger patients
b. If the patient is a woman, the risk is higher than it would be for a man
c. A previous CABG procedure increases the complexity and complication rate but does not alter the mortality rate
d. Results are better if there is ischemic cardiomyopathy than if there is hibernating myocardium

COMMENT: The operative mortality among patients older than 70 years was 8% in the Coronary Artery Surgery (CASS) compared with 3% among younger patients. For reasons not entirely clear, the risk of CABG is higher among women than among men. Second procedures carry a higher operative mortality because of technical difficulties, more advanced disease, and less complete revascularization. Congestive heart failure is a major determinant of poor surgical outcome, but the results are better when there is viable myocardium (hibernating) than when there is irreversible ischemic cardiomyopathy.

ANSWER: a, b

REFERENCE: *Chapter 63—Ischemic Heart Disease: Risk Factors for Operative Mortality*

CHAPTER 64

MECHANICAL CIRCULATORY SUPPORT

1. A 64-year-old man continues to have hypotension, oliguria, and mental impairment after a large MI. Which of the following statements is/are true concerning the use of intraaortic balloon pump (IABP) support?

   a. The IABP is expected to reduce infarct size
   b. The time-tension index will be decreased with an IABP
   c. Balloon deflation before systole decreases aortic compliance
   d. If percutaneous transluminal coronary balloon angioplasty (PTCA) is used, there is evidence of a lower coronary artery reocclusion rate

COMMENT: Use of an IABP for cardiogenic shock decreases myocardial oxygen demand as manifested by a lower time-tension index but does not decrease infarct size or improve outcome. Balloon deflation before systole increases aortic compliance and lowers ventricular afterload. The use of IABP after PTCA has been demonstrated to reduce the coronary reocclusion rate, presumably by increasing the rate of thrombolysis.

ANSWER: b, d

REFERENCE: *Chapter 64—Mechanical Circulatory Support: Indications for the IABP*

2. After aortic and mitral valve replacement, a 61-year-old man has ineffective ventricular function to allow weaning from cardiopulmonary bypass (CPB). Which of the following statements is/are true?

   a. Cardiopulmonary bypass should be continued for at least 12 hours to allow ventricular recovery
   b. Use of CPB is known to induce complement activation by the alternative pathway
   c. Use of extracorporeal membrane oxygenation (ECMO) is an attractive alternative because it does not activate complement
   d. An IABP would be a better alternative to CPB for this patient

COMMENT: Successful CPB is limited to 4 to 6 hours before damage to blood and perfused organs occurs because of mechanical damage to blood elements and activation of complement by the alternative pathway. Extracorporeal membrane oxygenation produces similar inflammatory responses from blood-oxygenator surface interactions. The IABP requires effective ventricular contraction to produce effective counterpulsation, so it would not be applicable in this case.

ANSWER: b

REFERENCE: *Chapter 64—Mechanical Circulatory Support: Ventricular Assist Devices and ECMO*

3. The condition of a 42-year-old woman with cardiomyopathy and chronic heart failure deteriorates to the point of consideration for a ventricular assist device (VAD) as a bridge to transplantation. Which of the following statements is/are true?

   a. For a patient to be a candidate for VAD, left atrial pressure should exceed 20 mm Hg, systolic arterial pressure should be less than 90 mm Hg, and cardiac output should be less than 1.8 L/min per square meter
   b. Decompression with a VAD can precipitate right ventricular failure
   c. Patients with a VAD have the same risk of postoperative infection as any other patient
   d. A nonpulsatile flow VAD is preferred to a pulsatile device because the nonpulsatile device produces less shearing stress on the blood

COMMENT: The criteria for use of a VAD include the hemodynamic findings of increased left atrial pressure, systolic arterial hypotension (less than 90 mm Hg), and decreased cardiac output (less than 1.8 L/min per square meter) as well as oliguria and poor tissue perfusion. Left ventricular decompression may unmask concomitant right heart dysfunction or precipitate failure because of the interaction between the ventricles. Patients with VADs are at increased risk of infection because their condition is hemodynamically unstable, and they have percutaneous foreign bodies for connection to the device. Nonpulsatile VAD requires high-speed pumping and produces substantial blood trauma.

ANSWER: a, b

REFERENCE: *Chapter 64—Mechanical Circulatory Support: Ventricular Assist Devices*

4. A 29-year-old male cardiac transplant recipient is rejecting the graft and needs prolonged mechanical support with a total artificial heart (TAH). Which of the following statements is/are true?

   a. The risk of postoperative hemorrhage is the same with the left ventricular assist device and the TAH
   b. The TAH is easier to control than is the VAD because both ventricles of the TAH can be adjusted
   c. Excision of the graft at insertion TAH would be appropriate
   d. The TAH concept involves two parallel roller pumps

COMMENT: The TAH is complicated to adjust and carries a high risk of bleeding. The control problem occurs because the blood volumes pumped by each ventricle are not in equilibrium because of the left-to-right shunt of bronchial blood and different characteristics of the great vessels. Graft excision is necessary at insertion of a TAH. The TAH concept consists of two saccular polyurethane ventricles compressed pneumatically.

ANSWER: c

REFERENCE: *Chapter 64—Mechanical Circulatory Support: Total Artificial Heart*

5. Which of the following statements is/are true concerning a permanent TAH and transcutaneous energy transmission system (TETS)?
   a. The TETS concept involves permanent transcutaneous fine wire placement connected to a rechargeable battery
   b. The TAH must be capable of providing an output of 8 L/min from each ventricle in response to everyday activities
   c. Each of the proposed permanent systems works with brushless direct-current electric motors
   d. Each proposed system responds to increased venous return with an increase in left pump output until maximum is reached

COMMENT: The concept of a long-term or permanent TAH that is tether free depends on a TETS concept of two wire coils, one inside and one outside the body without crossing the skin barrier. The requirement of the TAH is an output of 8 L/min from each ventricle, each of which is powered by a brushless direct-current electric motor. The control systems allow the TAH to function according to Starling's equation so that increased venous return increases cardiac output.

ANSWER: b, c, d

REFERENCE: *Chapter 64—Mechanical Circulatory Support: Permanent Total Artificial Hearts*

CHAPTER 65

PERICARDIUM

1. Normal functions of the pericardium include:
   a. Being essential to life
   b. Mechanical protection of the heart and serving as a barrier to infection
   c. Prevention of cardiac distention
   d. Contributing to diastolic coupling of the ventricles

COMMENT: Not all of the functions of the pericardium are well understood, and people can do well with congenital absence or surgical removal of the pericardium. Structural functions appear to include mechanical protection and anchoring of the heart, prevention of acute cardiac distention, and serving as a barrier to infection. The pericardium contributes to diastolic coupling of the ventricles. Diastolic coupling links pressure increases in the right ventricle to the left ventricle and coordinates movement of the two ventricles along their respective Starling curves. The pericardium also functions as an absorptive surface, transmitting fluid to both the thoracic duct system and the pleural spaces. The regulatory function is to act as a mechanoreceptor to govern blood pressure and heart rate. Pericardial fluid has fibrinolytic activity, which opposes clotting of the intrapericardial blood.

ANSWER: b, c, d

REFERENCE: *Chapter 65—Pericardium: Normal Physiology*

2. Correct descriptions of normal jugular venous pulsations are:
   a. The *a* wave is caused by normal atrial contraction
   b. The *c* wave is caused by bulging of the atrioventricular valve into the atrium during ventricular systole
   c. The *v* wave is caused by passive atrial filling
   d. The *x* descent represents systolic collapse
   e. The *y* descent represents the decrease in blood pressure that occurs with respiration

COMMENT: Normal jugular venous pulsations have three positive pulse waves, the *a, c,* and *v* waves, and two negative waves, the *x* and *y* descents (see Fig. 65.2). The waves result from normal atrial contraction. Its peak corresponds to S_4. The *c* wave is produced by the bulging of the atrioventricular valve into the atrium during isovolumic ventricular systole. It begins at S_1. The *x* descent (systolic collapse) is caused by downward displacement of the base of the heart during ventricular systolic and atrial relaxation. Its lowest point is in mid systole. The *v* wave is caused by passive atrial filling from the vena cava and occurs just after S_2. The *y* descent (diastolic collapse) follows opening of the atrioventricular valve and occurs during passive ventricular filling.

ANSWER: a, b, c, d

REFERENCE: *Chapter 65—Pericardium: Normal Physiology*

3. Cardiac tamponade:
   a. Is hemodynamically significant cardiac compression caused by pericardial contents
   b. Can be caused by as little as 100 to 200 mL of pericardial fluid
   c. Typically produces as inspiratory decrease in systolic blood pressure of less than 10 mm Hg
   d. Results in equalization of right atrial, left atrial, pulmonary arterial diastolic, pulmonary arterial wedge, and right and left ventricular end-diastolic pressures
   e. Results in preservation of the *x* descent and disappearance of the *y* descent

COMMENT: Cardiac tamponade can be defined as hemodynamically significant cardiac compression caused by accumulating pericardial contents (effusion, blood, pus, gas, or tumor) that evoke and defeat compensatory mechanisms. The occurrence of tamponade depends on both the volume and the rate of accumulation of pericardial contents. Rapid accumulation of a small amount of pericardial fluid (100 to 200 mL in an adult) can produce acute tamponade, whereas slow accumulation of liters of fluid can occur in a chronic effusion before tamponade occurs. Cardiac filling pressures, namely right and left atrial, pulmonary arterial diastolic and wedge, and right and left ventricular end-diastolic pressures, become equal to each other and to the pericardial pressure. The three classic signs of acute tamponade (Beck's acute cardiac compression triad) are (a) decreasing arterial pressure, (b) increasing venous pressure, (c) a small, quiet heart. Tamponade produces characteristic changes in jugular venous pulsation. The *x* descent (systolic collapse) remains, and the *y* descent (diastolic collapse) disappears. With tamponade, systolic blood pressure typically decreases more than 10 mm Hg during inspiration, or pulsus paradoxus.

ANSWER: a, b, d, e

REFERENCE: *Chapter 65—Pericardium: Cardiac (Pericardial) Tamponade*

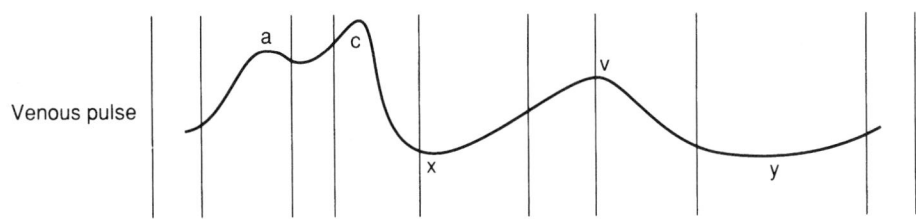

Figure 65.2

4. Pericardial constriction:

    a. Produces a rapid increase and plateau (square root sign) in the right ventricular pressure tracing

    b. Is easily differentiated from restrictive cardiomyopathy by history and physical examination

    c. Produces a preserved *x* descent and accentuated *y* descent

    d. Is controlled with pericardiocentesis

    e. Is controlled with pericardiectomy

COMMENT: Unlike cardiac tamponade, pericardial constriction produces no restriction of early diastolic filling but a sudden restriction in late diastole. Late diastolic restriction produces an early diastolic dip followed by a rapid increase and plateau (square root sign) in the right ventricular tracing (see Fig. 65.3). Jugular venous pulsations show prominent *x* and *y* descents with a *y* descent (diastolic collapse) deeper and more rapid than normal. Differentiation between pericardial constriction and restrictive cardiomyopathy can be difficult. Patients with restrictive cardiomyopathy do not have pericardial thickening. They also are more likely to have impairment of systolic ventricular function, mitral and tricuspid regurgitation, left-sided pressures higher than right-sided pressures, slower early and mid-diastolic filling, and left and right ventricular pressures that move in the same rather than opposite directions with inspiration. In some cases, pericardial or myocardial biopsy may be necessary for diagnosis. Definitive management of constrictive pericarditis is pericardiectomy.

ANSWER: a, c, e

REFERENCE: *Chapter 65—Pericardium: Pericardial Constriction*

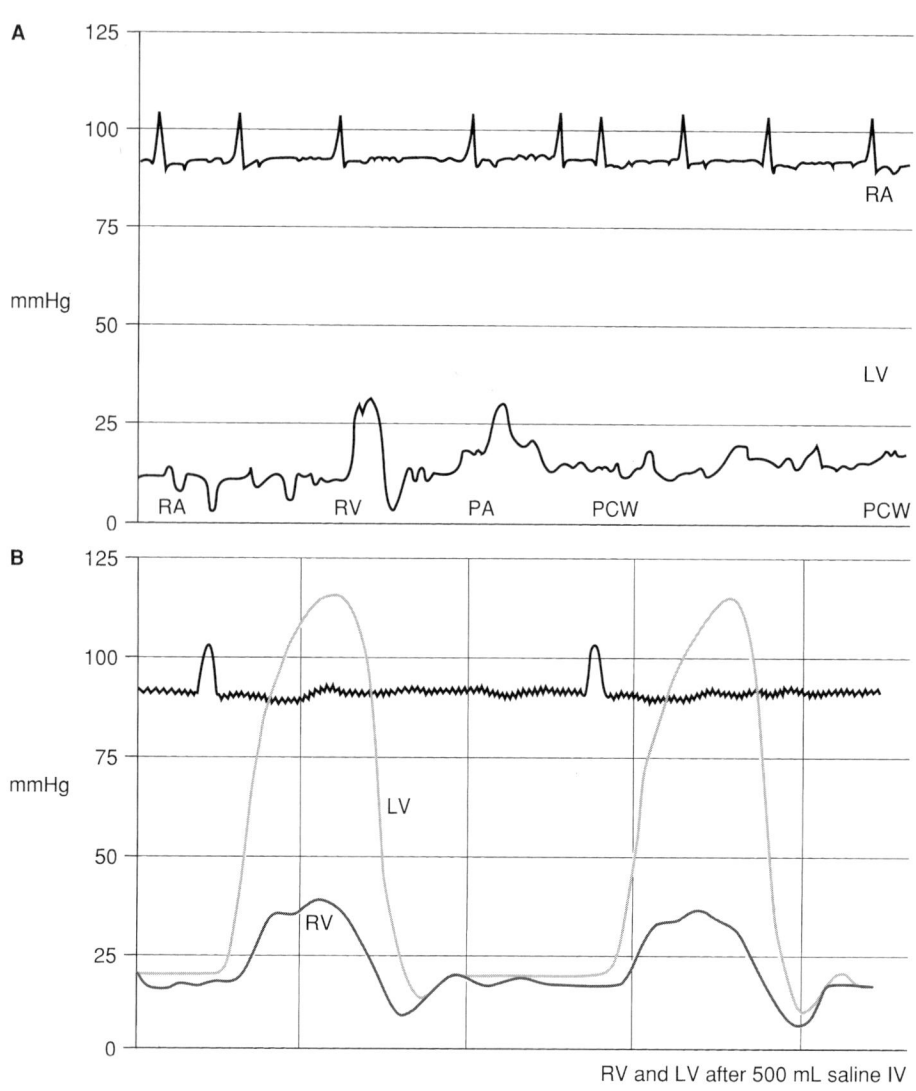

A

B

RV and LV after 500 mL saline IV

Figure 65.3

5. Potential therapies for pericarditis include
    a. Aspirin
    b. Nonsteroidal antiinflammatory drugs
    c. Steroids
    d. Pericardial drainage
    e. Pericardiectomy

COMMENT: Management of nonspecific or viral pericarditis is typically with nonsteroidal antiinflammatory drugs or aspirin. Glucocorticoids can be used as second-line therapy. Pericardiocentesis or surgical drainage may be necessary for effusions that are hemodynamically significant or unresponsive to medical therapy. Pericardiectomy is reserved for continued accumulation of fluid or late constriction.

ANSWER: a, b, c, d, e

REFERENCE: *Chapter 65—Pericardium: Pericarditis*

Section M
ARTERIAL SYSTEM
BASIC CONSIDERATIONS IN VASCULAR DISEASE

CHAPTER 66

ATHEROSCLEROSIS AND THE PATHOGENESIS OF OCCLUSIVE DISEASE

1. Which of the following statements is/are true concerning the normal structure of blood vessels?
    a. In utero, hemangioblasts give rise to both vascular conduits and hematopoietic tissue
    b. In development, smooth muscle tubes precede endothelium
    c. After birth, growth of large vessels does not change the number of elastic and smooth muscle layers
    d. Adventitia includes the external elastic lamina

COMMENT: The earliest vascular primordia in the embryo are isolated hemangioblasts that give rise to both vascular conduits and hematopoietic tissue. Endothelial cells organize at sites of vessel development followed by mesenchymal cells that form the outer layers. The number of elastic and smooth muscle layers remains constant after birth, although wall mass increases because of proliferation. The adventitia lies outside the external elastic lamina.

ANSWER: a, c

REFERENCE: *Chapter 66—Atherosclerosis and the Pathogenesis of Occlusive Disease: Normal Structure*

2. Which of the following statements is/are true concerning regulation of arterial luminal area?

   a. The main determinant of arterial diameter is blood pressure
   b. Compensatory vasodilation occurs until more than 40% of area inside the internal elastic lamina is obstructed in coronary arteries
   c. Vasodilating nitric oxide is derived from adenosine
   d. When endothelium is absent, thrombin causes vasoconstriction

COMMENT: The main determinant of arterial diameter is blood velocity as demonstrated by poststenotic dilation. This adaptation by wall relaxation is limited to 40% of the area inside the internal elastic lamina in coronary arteries. The predominant vasodilator, nitric oxide, is derived from arginine. When endothelium is absent, a number of vasodilators, including thrombin, produce vasoconstriction.

ANSWER: b, d

REFERENCE: *Chapter 66—Atherosclerosis and the Pathogenesis of Occlusive Disease: Regulation of Luminal Area*

3. Which of the following statements is/are true concerning medial and intimal thickening?

   a. Increase of wall mass is a consequence primarily of smooth muscle cell proliferation
   b. Smooth muscle cells are normally quiescent at maturity
   c. Transplanting a vein into the arterial circuit causes both endothelial and smooth muscle proliferation
   d. Heparin can suppress both proliferation and migration of smooth muscle cells

COMMENT: Endothelial proliferation does not contribute to an increase in wall mass, which is caused by proliferation of smooth muscle cells. Smooth muscle cells are normally quiescent at maturity, and proliferation and migration are inhibited by heparin. Transplanting a vein into the arterial circuit causes endothelial cell loss and smooth muscle cell proliferation.

ANSWER: a, b, d

REFERENCE: *Chapter 66—Atherosclerosis and the Pathogenesis of Occlusive Disease: Regulation of Medical and Intimal Thickening*

4. Which of the following statements is/are true concerning regulation of smooth muscle cell growth?

   a. Serum derived from plasma has substantially more growth-promoting activity than does serum from whole blood
   b. Basic fibroblast growth factor is responsible for the first wave of proliferation in experimental arterial injury
   c. The gene for platelet derived growth factor (PDGF) is nearly identical to the oncogene v-*sis*
   d. Sympathectomy promotes the increase in DNA in the media of developing arteries and in hypertension

COMMENT: The observation that serum derived from whole blood has substantially more growth-promoting activity than does serum from plasma led to the discovery of PDGF. Basic fibroblast growth factor is responsible for the first wave of proliferation in experimental carotid artery injury. The gene for PDGF is nearly identical to the oncogene v-*sis*. This finding raises the possibility that wound healing and malignant growth might have similarities of regulation. Sympathectomy inhibits an increase in DNA in the media of developing arteries and in hypertension.

ANSWER: b, c

REFERENCE: *Chapter 66—Atherosclerosis and the Pathogenesis of Occlusive Disease: Regulation of Smooth Muscle Cell Growth*

5. Which of the following statements is/are true concerning in vivo regulation of the anticoagulated state by endothelium?

   a. Heparan–antithrombin III inactivates only thrombin
   b. Thrombomodulin serves only to bind thrombin
   c. Production of von Willebrand factor inactivates platelets
   d. Endothelial cells can secrete tissue factor

COMMENT: Endothelium synthesizes heparan, which, like heparin, increases the affinity of antithrombin III for thrombin, which is inactivated along with other serine proteases, including factors VII, IX, and X. Thrombomodulin, in addition to binding thrombin, activates protein C, which binds with protein S to inactivate factor Va. On the procoagulant side, endothelial cells produce von Willebrand factor, which binds platelets, and are capable of secreting tissue factor.

ANSWER: d

REFERENCE: *Chapter 66—Atherosclerosis and the Pathogenesis of Occlusive Disease: Regulation of the Anticoagulated State*

6. Which of the following statements is/are true regarding theories of atherosclerosis?

    a. Fatty streaks in the aorta of children are not predictive of atherosclerosis or heart attacks
    b. Aging induces nonatherosclerotic thickening of the intima
    c. T lymphocytes are present in atheroma
    d. The reaction-to-injury hypothesis explains the characteristic lipid accumulation

COMMENT: It is true that fatty streaks in the aorta and coronary arteries of children are found among populations without increased incidence of atherosclerosis or heart attacks. Similarly, aging induces gradual thickening of the intima throughout the arterial tree that is not atherosclerotic. A variety of leukocytes, including T lymphocytes, are present in atheroma. The reaction-to-injury hypothesis explains smooth muscle growth in atherogenesis but does not provide an explanation for lipid accumulation or the monoclonal nature of the atherosclerotic plaque.

ANSWER: a, b, c

REFERENCE: *Chapter 66—Atherosclerosis and the Pathogenesis of Occlusive Disease: Theories of Atherosclerosis*

CHAPTER 67

NONATHEROSCLEROTIC VASCULAR DISEASE

1. A 32-year-old woman with severe hypertension is found to have renal artery changes (Fig. 67.1). Which of the following statements is/are true?

    a. Next to the renal artery, this process affects the carotid and coronary arteries most commonly
    b. In the most common variant of this disorder, the media is infiltrated with increased collagen, fibrous connective tissue, and glycosaminoglycans
    c. If similar disease is found in the carotid artery, the patient should be treated even if there are no symptoms
    d. Appropriate treatment includes percutaneous transluminal balloon angioplasty

COMMENT: Fibromuscular dysplasia is an abnormality of unknown causation primarily affecting women (90%) and the renal arteries. The carotid and iliac arteries are the next most frequently affected. Medial fibroplasia is the most common pathologic change with the pathologic findings in answer *b*. Surgical treatment is indicated only for symptomatic stenosis because many asymptomatic cases exist, the natural history of which is not known. In addition to surgical procedures, balloon angioplasty of lesions of the main renal artery is acceptable treatment.

ANSWER: b, d

REFERENCE: *Chapter 67—Nonatherosclerotic Vascular Disease: Fibromuscular Dysplasia*

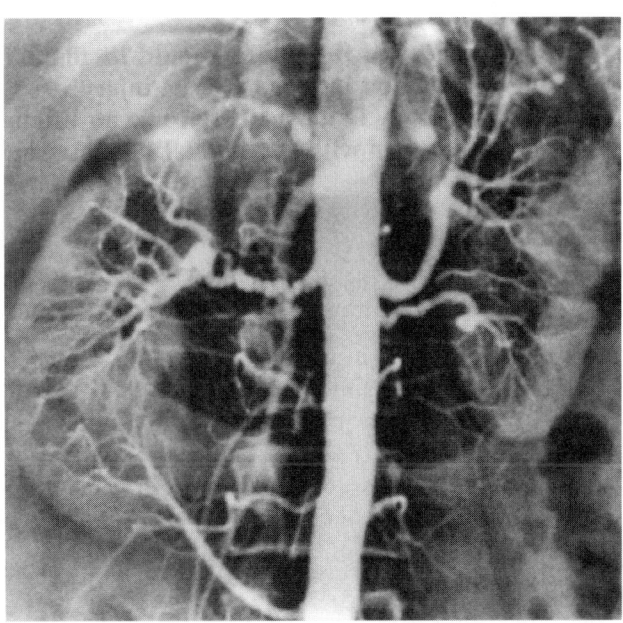

Figure 67.1

2. A 38-year-old male smoker with gangrenous changes in the toes of both feet undergoes arteriography that shows normal vessels to the popliteal trifurcation and numerous distal occlusions in small vessels. Which of the following statements is/are true?

   a. Hyperlipidemia, diabetes, and autoimmune disease must be ruled out to make the diagnosis of Buerger's disease
   b. Plethysmographic evidence of digital obstruction in all four extremities with normal proximal vessels is sufficient evidence for Buerger's disease without arteriography
   c. The most important therapy for Buerger's disease is regional surgical sympathectomy
   d. Unlike disease of the lower extremities, Buerger's involvement of the upper extremities rarely leads to amputation

COMMENT: Buerger's disease is panarteritis associated with intraluminal thrombus among young male smokers. Diabetes, hyperlipidemia, and autoimmune disease must be ruled out to fulfill the diagnostic criteria, but the diagnosis can be made at plethysmography with evidence of small-vessel obstruction in all four extremities. Cessation of all tobacco use is the most important treatment. Management is conservative. Loss of the upper extremities is rare as opposed to loss of the lower extremities.

ANSWER: a, b, d

REFERENCE: *Chapter 67—Nonatherosclerotic Vascular Disease: Buerger's Disease*

3. A 22-year-old male basketball player with back pain is found to have a dissecting aortic aneurysm. Which of the following statements is/are true?

   a. In Marfan's syndrome, a disorder of type I collagen underlies the observed cystic medial necrosis
   b. In type IV Ehlers-Danlos syndrome, little or no type III collagen is produced, and arterial rupture is likely
   c. In pseudoxanthoma elasticum, the medial elastic fibers are replaced by xanthoma cells, which calcify
   d. In arteria magna syndrome, the media is devoid of elastic tissue, and coronary artery disease is common

COMMENT: Cystic medial necrosis is associated with aortic dissection at an early age and can be caused by Marfan's syndrome with its disorder of type I collagen or type IV Ehlers-Danlos, in which little or no type III collagen is produced. In pseudoxanthoma elasticum, the medial elastic tissue is replaced by calcific deposits, and there are xanthoma-like cutaneous papules. In arteria magna syndrome, elastic tissue is absent in the media, and associated coronary artery disease is common.

ANSWER: a, b, d

REFERENCE: *Chapter 67—Nonatherosclerotic Vascular Disease: Cystic Medial Necrosis*

4. A 36-year-old woman runner who reports intermittent claudication has the arteriogram shown in Fig. 67.7. Which of the following statements is/are true?

   a. The most popular theory of origin is from a direct communication to an adjacent joint
   b. The stenotic effect of the lesion is present in all positions, differentiating it from an entrapment
   c. Percutaneous transluminal angioplasty is an acceptable form of treatment
   d. When the vessel is obstructed, cyst excision with thrombectomy is the preferred procedure

COMMENT: Adventitial cystic disease has several theories of origin, but most popular is true ganglion from an adjacent joint. Stenosis can vary depending on knee flexion or extension. Transluminal angioplasty has not been a successful method of treatment. If the vessel is obstructed, the preferred treatment is excision and replacement by autogenous vein graft.

ANSWER: a

REFERENCE: *Chapter 67—Nonatherosclerotic Vascular Disease: Adventitial Cystic Disease*

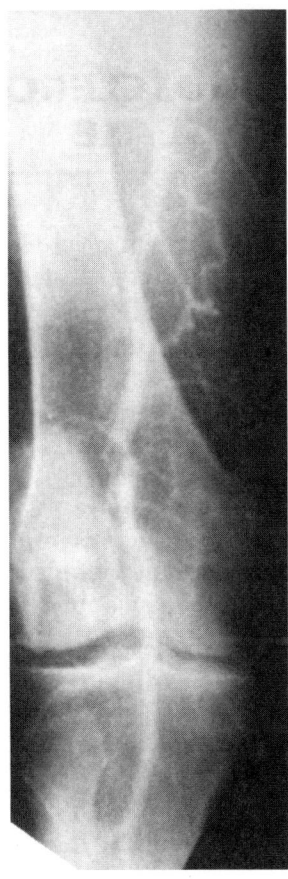

Figure 67.7

5. Ten years after irradiation of the neck for a tonsillar carcinoma, a 59-year-old woman is found to have symptomatic carotid artery disease. An arteriogram shows a 70% irregular stenotic lesion. Which of the following statements is/are true?

a. Replacement of the artery should be planned because of radiation-induced arterial injury

b. The pathologic change is most likely to be an inflammatory reaction with endothelial sloughing and thrombosis

c. If atherosclerotic disease is found, the plaque will not be different from nonirradiated plaques

d. The patient should be treated medically because of the radiation injury to the artery

COMMENT: Radiation-induced arterial injury produces three types of injury. The earliest after treatment consists of an inflammatory reaction with endothelial sloughing and thrombosis. Later fibrotic changes in the wall may produce stenosis or accelerated atherosclerosis. The latter lends itself to standard endarterectomy, and the plaque is indistinguishable from nonirradiated plaque.

ANSWER: c

REFERENCE: *Chapter 67—Nonatherosclerotic Vascular Disease: Radiation-induced Injury*

6. A 42-year-old Asian woman with a history of recurrent deep venous thrombosis has a pulsatile mass in the abdomen confirmed at ultrasound examination to be an abdominal aortic aneurysm. Which of the following statements is/are true?

a. The history and physical findings suggest Kawasaki disease

b. History and physical findings suggest polyarteritis nodosa

c. Venous thrombosis is more common than arterial disease among these patients, and the presence of an aneurysm portends a high mortality

d. Replacement of an aneurysm with a graft to manage Behçet syndrome is associated with recurrent aneurysms and thrombosis

COMMENT: Kawasaki disease is a disorder that occurs among infants and children with coronary aneurysms. Polyarteritis nodosa usually occurs among boys and men, and the inflammatory process involves small and medium-sized muscular arteries. Behçet syndrome is a form of vasculitis that produces venous thrombosis. When arterial aneurysms are present, the mortality rate approaches 20%. Because of the fragility of the arteries, recurrent aneurysm formation is likely.

ANSWER: c, d

REFERENCE: *Chapter 67—Nonatherosclerotic Vascular Disease: Immune Arteritis*

7. A 58-year-old woman has a history of severe headache, visual field loss, and transient myalgia involving the back and shoulders. Which of the following statements is/are true?

a. A tender, nodular temporal artery suggests temporal arteritis

b. The presentation is most compatible with giant cell arteritis

c. Steroids should be avoided if an operation is planned

d. Angiography is most likely to show irregular surface stenosis

COMMENT: The presentation is typical of temporal arteritis, which is a form of systemic giant cell arteritis. It is characterized by chronic inflammation of the aorta and its major branches. Glucocorticoid therapy is indicated because of its success in relieving symptoms whether or not an operation is planned. Angiographic findings in this condition show smooth rather than irregular surface stenosis.

ANSWER: a, b

REFERENCE: *Chapter 67—Nonatherosclerotic Vascular Disease: Giant Cell Arteritis Group*

8. A 23-year-old woman with fever, myalgia, and anorexia has hypertension and a cool, ischemic left arm. Angiography shows multiple areas of stenosis of the subclavian and renal arteries. Which of the following statements is/are true?

   a. Coronary angiography is indicated with a high likelihood of finding coronary disease
   b. Endarterectomy of the lesions is preferred to transluminal angioplasty
   c. The presentation is more suggestive of Behçet's disease than of Takayasu arteritis
   d. The preferred management consists of glucocorticoids

COMMENT: The presentation is most suggestive of Takayasu arteritis, which tends not to involve the coronary arteries. A variety of operations have been used to treat these patients, but endarterectomy is not recommended because of a high incidence of early failure. The preferred management is glucocorticoids.

ANSWER: d

REFERENCE: *Chapter 67—Nonatherosclerotic Vascular Disease: Giant Cell Arteritis Group*

9. A 21-year-old man with premature arteriosclerosis and mental retardation is found to have homocystinuria. Which of the following statements is/are true?

   a. The presence of mental retardation is atypical of homocystinemia
   b. The specific enzyme deficiency responsible is homocysteine methyl transferase
   c. Arteriosclerotic plaques in this condition are atypically void of lipid deposition
   d. Homocysteine exists in plasma in three forms—protein bound, mixed, and free

COMMENT: Homocystinuria reflects homocystinemia, which is associated with ectopia lentis, mental retardation, and thromboembolic disorders as well as arteriosclerosis. Three enzyme deficiencies are known to cause the disorder and deficiencies of the cofactors pyridoxine, cobalamin, and folate. Lipid deposition in plaques is characteristically absent. Homocysteine exists in plasma as the mixed disulfide homocysteine cysteine and as free and protein-bound homocysteine.

ANSWER: c, d

REFERENCE: *Chapter 67—Nonatherosclerotic Vascular Disease: Homocystinemia*

CHAPTER 68

PERIPHERAL ARTERIAL EMBOLISM

1. A 70-year-old man has sudden pain and ischemic changes in his left leg. An arterial embolus is suspected. Which of the following statements is/are true?

   a. The most likely source of an arterial embolus is intracardiac thrombus from previous myocardial infarction (MI)
   b. If atrial fibrillation (AF) is present, chronic AF is less likely to produce embolism than is paroxysmal AF
   c. The most common cause of AF is ischemic rather than rheumatic heart disease
   d. Aspirin is more effective than warfarin in the management of AF for reducing the risk of stroke and cardiovascular mortality

COMMENT: Approximately 80% to 90% of arterial emboli originate in the heart, and 66% are caused by AF. Chronic AF carries an annual risk of 3% to 6% of serious embolic complications; paroxysmal AF has a lower risk. Rheumatic heart disease once was the most common cause of chronic AF, but with its decline, ischemic heart disease has become the most common cause. Drug therapy for AF reduces the risk of stroke, but aspirin is less effective in this regard than is warfarin.

ANSWER: c

REFERENCE: *Chapter 68—Peripheral Arterial Embolism: Source and Etiology of Acute Arterial Emboli*

2. A 51-year-old man with a history of transmural MI 1 month previously has sudden occlusion of the abdominal aorta. Which of the following statements is/are true?

   a. The most likely location of MI is anterolateral
   b. Most emboli occur within 6 weeks of MI
   c. The occurrence of arterial embolism does not affect overall mortality
   d. Heparin treatment can decrease the incidence of embolism after MI

COMMENT: Acute MI with endocardial thrombus is the second most common cause of arterial embolism. It usually occurs within 6 weeks, and the most typical location at postmortem examination is anterolateral. Arterial embolism after MI is associated with an increase in mortality rate. Use of heparin after acute MI has been shown to decrease the incidence of systemic arterial embolism.

ANSWER: a, b, d

REFERENCE: *Chapter 68—Peripheral Arterial Embolism: Source and Etiology of Acute Arterial Emboli*

3. A 67-year-old man with acute popliteal arterial embolism undergoes cardiac echocardiography that does not show the source of the thrombus. Which of the following statements is/are true?

   a. The most likely noncardiac source is a thoracic aortic aneurysm
   b. Embolism is more common from femoral than popliteal arterial aneurysms
   c. Emboli from popliteal aneurysms often are clinically silent
   d. Embolism is rare from subclavian artery aneurysms

COMMENT: The most likely noncardiac source of arterial embolism is an infrarenal abdominal aortic aneurysm. Arterial embolism is more frequent from popliteal than from femoral aneurysms, and these embolic events often are clinically silent. Subclavian artery aneurysms give rise to peripheral embolism in as many as 33% of patients.

ANSWER: c

REFERENCE: *Chapter 68—Peripheral Arterial Embolism: Source and Etiology of Acute Arterial Emboli*

4. For the patient described in question 3, which of the following statements is/are true concerning the distribution of arterial emboli?

   a. Change in arterial diameter is a more important determinant of embolic site than is flow rate
   b. Aortic valvular disease is more often associated with cerebral embolism than is mitral valve disease
   c. Among embolic sites, renal emboli are least detected clinically
   d. The most common site of arterial embolus is the aortic bifurcation

COMMENT: Most arterial emboli lodge at bifurcations, where there is a sudden change in arterial diameter. Flow rate does not correlate with sites of embolism. Mitral valve disease with associated atrial fibrillation is most frequently associated with cerebral embolism. The discrepancy between clinical and autopsy evidence of embolism is significant for renal emboli—the clinical diagnosis is made in fewer than 1% of cases. The most common site of arterial embolus is the common femoral artery.

ANSWER: a, c

REFERENCE: *Chapter 68—Peripheral Arterial Embolism: Distribution of Arterial Emboli*

5. A 39-year-old woman with embolic occlusion of an iliac artery is subject to an operating room delay before perfusion can be restored. Which of the following statements is/are true?

   a. Ischemia for longer than 3 hours will result in muscle fiber autolysis
   b. The earliest ultrastructural changes of ischemia in muscle include mitochondrial swelling and loss of glycogen granules
   c. Phosphocreatine-mediated rephosphorylation of adenosine diphosphate occurs for approximately 3 hours after ischemia
   d. Capillary thrombosis is the most likely explanation for the no-reflow phenomenon

COMMENT: Skeletal muscle can tolerate ischemia by anaerobic glycolysis for up to 6 hours. The earliest ultrastructural changes in ischemic muscle include mitochondrial swelling and loss of glycogen granules. During ischemia, adenosine triphosphate levels are maintained by phosphocreatine-mediated rephosphorylation of adenosine diphosphate until phosphocreatine levels are exhausted after about 3 hours. Of the possible causes of no-reflow phenomenon, capillary obstruction by leukocytes is more likely than capillary thrombosis.

ANSWER: b, c

REFERENCE: *Chapter 68—Peripheral Arterial Embolism: Pathophysiology*

6. The clinical manifestations of the patient in question 5 include:
   a. Loss of sensation to deep pain as one of the earliest signs
   b. Paresthesia in a classic dermatome distribution
   c. Early pallor due to diminished skin blood flow and reflex vasoconstriction
   d. Involuntary muscle contraction that indicates restored flow cannot save the extremity

COMMENT: The earliest limb changes in ischemia are in sensory nerves. The sensitivity of small nerve fibers increases, and the result is loss of sensation to light touch. Sensation to deep pain, pressure, and temperature are preserved until late. The paresthesia occurs in a glove- or stocking-like distribution rather than by dermatome. Early pallor is caused by decreased blood flow and reflex vasoconstriction. Among signs of irreversible limb ischemia are complete anesthesia and involuntary muscle contraction.

ANSWER: c, d

REFERENCE: *Chapter 68—Peripheral Arterial Embolism: Clinical Manifestations*

7. An 82-year-old man with a long history of coronary and peripheral vascular disease has acute ischemia of right lower extremity. Which of the following statements is/are true?
   a. The first step in management is arteriography
   b. If intractable congestive heart failure is present, nonoperative treatment with heparin is appropriate
   c. If prolonged ischemia has occurred, reperfusion should be accompanied by sodium bicarbonate
   d. Regardless of the period of ischemia, fasciotomy should be based on the postoperative findings

COMMENT: The first step in the management of acute limb ischemia for any patient is heparin anticoagulation. If intractable heart failure is present, heparin treatment is appropriate without an operation. If prolonged ischemia has occurred, venting of the first 300 to 500 mL of venous outflow allows conservation of erythrocytes and avoidance of the consequences of high levels of potassium. If ischemia lasts more than 4 hours, four-compartment fasciotomy should be performed at the time of restoration of perfusion.

ANSWER: b

REFERENCE: *Chapter 68—Peripheral Arterial Embolism: Management*

8. Which if the following statements is/are true concerning risk and outcomes for the patient in question 7?
   a. If renal failure occurs, the mortality rate is approximately 50%
   b. If arterial embolism is confirmed, the patient should receive lifelong anticoagulation
   c. Postoperative amputation is unlikely if the embolectomy is successful
   d. Postoperative death with pulmonary embolism is unlikely

COMMENT: There has been only modest improvement in mortality and morbidity after arterial embolectomy. If renal failure occurs, the mortality rate is approximately 50%. Recurrence of arterial embolism without anticoagulation occurs among 28% to 45% of patients and justifies prolonged anticoagulation, which reduces the incidence of recurrent embolism. In addition to a high postoperative mortality rate, the amputation rate is approximately 15%. Pulmonary embolism is the second most common cause of death after embolectomy, reflecting the incidence of deep venous thrombosis among 7% to 27% of patients after arterial embolectomy.

ANSWER: a, b

REFERENCE: *Chapter 68—Peripheral Arterial Embolism: Results*

9. Two days after coronary angiography and angioplasty, a 47-year-old man with diabetes has painful blue toes on both feet. Which of the following statements is/are true?

a. It is unlikely that there is any connection between the catheterization and the extremity problem

b. The appropriate treatment is vasodilators and an antiplatelet agent

c. If both superficial femoral arteries are obstructed, the most likely cause is in situ microvascular thrombosis

d. If renal failure or pancreatitis develops, the outlook for long-term survival is poor

COMMENT: Atheroembolism is caused by plaque rupture or manipulation at catheterization and is much more frequent after catheterization than suspected clinically. Because repetitive events and additional complications are expected, prompt arteriography should be performed to delineate the possible site of origin. Excision, endarterectomy, or bypass of the site is the only effective treatment. Because plaque debris is very small, it can readily pass through collateral vessels to lodge in arterioles, and major vascular occlusion is no barrier. The kidney is the most common organ affected. If renal failure or pancreatitis develops as a sign of generalized atheroembolism, the outlook is poor—life expectancy is measured in months.

ANSWER: d

REFERENCE: *Chapter 68—Peripheral Arterial Embolism: Atheroembolism*

CHAPTER 69

ARTERIAL COMPRESSION SYNDROMES

1. A 29-year-old woman has distal necrosis of the left index finger and petechiae on two other fingers. A cervical spinal radiograph shows an bilateral elongation of the C7 transverse process. Which of the following statements is/are true?

a. An echocardiogram should be obtained

b. Selective left subclavian arteriography is indicated

c. The result of an Adson's test will likely be positive

d. Operative correction may necessitate arterial replacement

COMMENT: The presentation is typical of distal embolism from a unilateral source; therefore an echocardiogram is not necessary. The most likely source is poststenotic aneurysm formation in the subclavian artery from thoracic outlet syndrome, which can be confirmed by means of selective subclavian arteriography. With this compression, the Adson's test result is likely to be positive. With degenerative aneurysm formation, arterial replacement may be needed.

ANSWER: b, c, d

REFERENCE: *Chapter 69—Arterial Compression Syndromes: Thoracic Outlet Syndromes*

2. A 22-year-old weightlifter has pain and paresthesia in the radial dermatome distribution of the right arm with intermittent swelling and cyanosis. Which of the following statements is/are true?

a. The symptoms reflect compression of the upper portion of the brachial plexus
b. The venous compression occurs between the clavicle and the first rib
c. Thoracic outlet decompression by means of anterior scalenectomy may injure the vagus nerve
d. Subclavian venous thrombosis is not likely in this condition

COMMENT: Although thoracic outlet compression usually produces ulnar nerve paresthesia, the upper trunks can be compressed to produce radial nerve symptoms. The subclavian vein is subject to compression among the clavicle, costoclavicular ligament, and first rib. This chronic irritation often leads to subclavian venous thrombosis. Anterior scalenectomy jeopardizes the phrenic nerve rather than the vagus.

ANSWER: a, b

REFERENCE: *Chapter 69—Arterial Compression Syndromes: Thoracic Outlet Syndromes*

3. After extensive evaluation, a 52-year-old man with vertebrobasilar symptoms is found to have stenosis of the left vertebral artery at its entrance in the vertebral canal at C7. Which of the following statements is/are true?

a. The vertebral canal entry level is abnormal
b. Vertebral arterial stenosis is most likely symptomatic when there is arteriosclerotic obstruction of the opposite vertebral artery
c. Operative correction requires reimplantation of the vertebral artery
d. The vertebral artery exits the canal at C1

COMMENT: The vertebral artery usually enters the vertebral canal at C6 and exits at C2. A lower entry at C7 is more likely to be associated with compression by tendinous structures in the neck. Operative correction often requires only division of these bands or resection of osteophytes or bone. Symptomatic vertebral stenosis is most likely when the opposite vertebral artery is obstructed.

ANSWER: a, b

REFERENCE: *Chapter 69—Arterial Compression Syndromes: Vertebral Artery Compression*

4. A 21-year-old male soccer player reports pain in the left calf while running that is relieved by rest. A pulsatile mass is felt behind the knee, and distal pulses are normal. Which of the following statements is/are true?

a. Plantar flexion against resistance further suggests the diagnosis
b. Premature arteriosclerosis should be suspected
c. Bilateral arteriograms should be obtained
d. Lateral deviation of the popliteal artery confirms the diagnosis

COMMENT: Popliteal artery entrapment affects young, athletic men and can be diagnosed with disappearance of the pulse on passive dorsiflexion or active plantar flexion against resistance. Poststenotic aneurysm formation can occur and is not caused by premature arteriosclerosis. The condition frequently is bilateral, making it necessary to obtain bilateral arteriograms, which show medial rather than lateral displacement.

ANSWER: a, c

REFERENCE: *Chapter 69—Arterial Compression Syndromes: Popliteal Artery Entrapment Syndrome*

5. A 32-year-old woman has claudication of the right calf and normal distal pulses. A computed tomographic scan shows a cystic filling defect in the popliteal artery. Which of the following statements is/are true?

a. Cyst aspiration with ultrasound guidance should be attempted
b. If aspiration fails, percutaneous transluminal angioplasty should be attempted
c. Arteriography is not necessary
d. If opened, the cyst will be in the adventitia

COMMENT: Adventitial cystic disease is an uncommon cause of claudication that can lead to thrombosis and embolism. Arteriography is indicated, particularly if thrombosis or embolism is suspected. Neither cyst aspiration nor transluminal angioplasty has been successful in treatment, which requires operative evacuation of the cyst. The cyst is found beneath the adventitia.

ANSWER: d

REFERENCE: *Chapter 69—Arterial Compression Syndromes: Adventitial Cystic Disease*

6. Twenty-four hours after femoral arterial embolectomy, a 68-year-old man has pain and paresthesia in the involved leg and foot. A dorsalis pedis pulse is palpable. Which of the following statements is/are true?

a. Because a distal pulse is present, analgesics will suffice
b. Repetition of arteriography is appropriate
c. Compartment pressures in the leg should be measured
d. A compartment pressure of 35 mm Hg in this case justifies fasciotomy

COMMENT: Compartment syndrome should be suspected after ischemia and reperfusion in the lower extremity. The presence of a distal pulse does not indicate that there is capillary perfusion, and compartment pressures should be measured. The finding of a 35 mm Hg pressure is clearly abnormal and justifies fasciotomy. There is no indication for arteriography.

ANSWER: c, d

REFERENCE: *Chapter 69—Arterial Compression Syndromes: Compartment Syndromes*

CHAPTER 70

ARTERIAL HEMODYNAMICS

1. Which arterial structure bears most of the tensile load?

a. The intima
b. The elastic lamina (internal and external)
c. The media
d. The adventitia

COMMENT: The arterial wall is organized into three distinct layers—the intima, the media, and the adventitia. The intima compromises mostly endothelial cells and the internal elastic lamina. The media, which carries most of the tensile load, is primarily composed of collagen, elastin, and some smooth muscle cells arranged in bundles along the lines of greatest tension. The adventitia is primarily fibrous connective tissue, vasovasorum, and the nerve fibers that regulate medial smooth muscle cell tone.

ANSWER: c

REFERENCE: *Chapter 70—Arterial Hemodynamics: Arterial Structure and Function*

2. Which of the following is/are (an) endothelial cell function(s)?

a. Maintenance of an antithrombotic barrier
b. Production of adhesion molecules important to local inflammatory responses
c. Regulation of local hemodynamics through interaction with medial smooth muscle cells
d. Provision of tensile strength

COMMENT: Endothelial cells have an important antithrombotic function and promote hemostasis at the site of physical injury. They produce adhesion molecules important to attracting and sticking of inflammatory cells. Endothelial-medial interactions by provision of endothelium-derived relaxing factor–nitric oxide, endothelin, angiotensin II, and platelet-derived growth factors cause appropriate vasodilatory or vasoconstrictive responses in medial smooth muscle in response to a number of stimuli, including luminal shear stress. The endothelium does not contribute appreciable tensile strength.

ANSWER: a, b, c

REFERENCE: *Chapter 70—Arterial Hemodynamics: Arterial Structure and Function*

3. Which of the following statements is/are true about the physical relationships within the arterial circulation?

a. Luminal diameter decreases from central to peripheral arteries
b. Total cross-sectional area increases from central arteries to capillary beds
c. Large central arteries have a high mean blood flow velocity (20 to 30 cm/s) whereas capillaries have a low blood flow velocity (0.5 to 1.0 mm/s)
d. The cross-sectional area of the capillary bed is 800 times that of the aorta

COMMENT: The inverse relation between cross-sectional area and blood velocity is well suited to the distribution functions of the central arteries and the exchange function of the capillaries. As blood moves from the central to the peripheral circulation, the velocity of flow decreases, and the cross-sectional area available for exchange functions increases.

ANSWER: a, b, c, d

REFERENCE: *Chapter 70—Arterial Hemodynamics: Arterial Structure and Function*

4. Which of the following best explains autoregulation of blood flow (relatively constant blood flow despite changes in perfusion pressure)?
   a. The myogenic theory
   b. The metabolic theory
   c. Neurologic control integrated in the medullary cardiovascular center
   d. *a* and *b*

COMMENT: The myogenic and metabolic mechanisms of vascular control probably have complementary roles in autoregulation and during active (exercise) and reactive (postocclusive) hyperemia. The myogenic theory is that vascular smooth muscle contracts in response to stretch caused by an increase in intravascular pressure and relaxes in response to decreased stretch when perfusion pressure decreases. This feedback loop stabilizes organ blood flow by adjusting smooth muscle tone to changes in perfusion pressure. The metabolic theory is that tissue blood flow parallels metabolic activity. As the demands of tissue metabolism exceed the blood supply, metabolic byproducts accumulate and cause vasodilation of precapillary resistance vessels. Increased flow results, washes away the vasodilating metabolites, and restores baseline vascular smooth muscle tone. A number of factors, including Po_2, Pco_2, pH, and levels of adenosine, lactate, potassium, and inorganic phosphate have been implicated as metabolic autoregulators.

ANSWER: d

REFERENCE: *Chapter 70—Arterial Hemodynamics: Arterial Structure and Function*

5. Which of the following statements is/are true with respect to local control of blood volume?
   a. The sympathetic nervous system produces smooth muscle contraction and vasoconstriction
   b. The parasympathetic nervous system produces vasodilation
   c. Basal sympathetic tone is responsible for most of the total vascular resistance
   d. The density of sympathetic innervation of vascular smooth muscle is relatively constant in the various organs

COMMENT: The sympathetic nervous system has primary neural control of vascular smooth muscle tone and produces smooth muscle contraction and vasoconstriction. Neurogenic vasodilation is caused by decreased sympathetic tone, not cholinergic vasodilators. Most of the vasovascular resistance is supplied by intrinsic myogenic activity, particularly at the level of the arterioles and metarterioles. Only 15% to 20% of the peripheral resistance is the result of sympathetic activity. The density of sympathetic innervation of the vascular smooth muscle varies widely in different organs. There are only a few fibers in the cerebral and coronary arteries, whereas there is dense innervation of cutaneous arterioles.

ANSWER: a

REFERENCE: *Chapter 70—Arterial Hemodynamics: Arterial Pressure and Energy*

6. Which of the following statements is/are true with respect to the precapillary and postcapillary sphincters?
   a. Precapillary sphincters are heavily innervated by sympathetic nerves
   b. Changes in postcapillary contraction cause large changes in capillary pressure gradient and regulate the capillary filtration coefficient and the tendency to form edema
   c. Postcapillary sphincter mechanisms are sensitive to sympathetic intervention
   d. Postcapillary sphincter resistance contributes substantially to total peripheral resistance

COMMENT: There is a differential sensitivity to sympathetic stimulation between precapillary and postcapillary sphincter muscles. Postcapillary sphincter mechanisms are more sensitive to sympathetic intervention than to local metabolic effects, whereas the converse is true of precapillary sphincters. Postcapillary sphincter resistance does not contribute to the total peripheral resistance. Postcapillary contraction, however, does cause large changes in the precapillary to postcapillary pressure gradient, which regulates the capillary filtration coefficient and the tendency to accumulate edema from absorbed tissue fluid.

ANSWER: b, c

REFERENCE: *Chapter 70—Arterial Hemodynamics: Arterial Pressure and Energy*

7. Which of the following statements is/are true regarding central nervous system control of sympathetic nerve discharge?
   a. Afferent input to the medullary cardiovascular center is provided by stretch receptors in the carotid sinus, aortic arch, thyrocarotid junction, and the cardiopulmonary vascular bed
   b. The specific receptors are sensitive to blood pressure
   c. Afferent input provides sympathetic inhibition and vagal stimulation
   d. The medullary cardiovascular center is influenced by cortical-hypothalamic input

COMMENT: The medullary cardiovascular center receives afferent input from the carotid sinus, aortic arch, thyrocarotid junction, and cardiopulmonary vascular bed. These are stretch receptors influenced by distention that reflects arterial blood pressure and the degree of vascular filling. However, blood pressure and blood flow are not directly sensed by these receptors. This is important because in a calcified artery or a fibrotic plaque, where stretch or expansion is prevented, increasing arterial blood pressure does not stimulate these receptors. When the plaque-restricting blood vessel stretch is removed, such as during carotid endarterectomy, the stretch receptors cause intense stimulation, which can result in marked inhibition of sympathetic discharge and increasing vagal stimulation, which causes hypotension and bradycardia. The medullary cardiovascular center receives input from higher centers—the cerebral cortex and hypothalamus as well as the aforementioned stretch receptors.

ANSWER: a, c, d

REFERENCE: *Chapter 70—Arterial Hemodynamics: Arterial Pressure and Energy*

8. Which of the following statements is/are true regarding arterial pressure waves generated by cardiac contraction?

    a. As the pressure wave proceeds peripherally, there is an increase in pulse pressure amplitude

    b. Pulse wave reflection results in retrograde pressure and blood flow

    c. Reflected waves are caused by high resistance segments of the peripheral circulation, the distal arterioles, and arterial branches

    d. Reflected waves summate with succeeding waves and produce an increase in systolic pressure as each pressure wave proceeds peripherally

COMMENT: Systemic arterial pressure is the result of complex interaction between the cardiac pump, aortic valve, compliance of the large central arteries, peripheral vascular resistance, and total vascular volume. As the pressure wave proceeds peripherally, there is a gradual increase in pulse pressure amplitude caused primarily by reflection of pulse waves as they strike the high-resistance arterioles and arterial branch points. Reflection of pulse waves results in retrograde flow, which interacts with the next prograde wave. Summation of the two pressure waves results in amplification of systolic pressure. These effects are somewhat attenuated by the viscoelastic arterial system, but pressure does increase in the distal abdominal aorta, a factor that may contribute to the predilection of this segment of the aorta for aneurysm formation.

ANSWER: a, b, c, d

REFERENCE: *Chapter 70—Arterial Hemodynamics: Arterial Pressure and Energy*

9. Which of the following statements is/are important in determining blood viscosity?

    a. Hematocrit

    b. Plasma protein concentration

    c. Shear rate

    d. Systemic arterial blood pressure

COMMENT: Blood is a non-newtonian fluid; that is, viscosity changes with velocity of blood flow. The main determinants of blood viscosity are hematocrit, plasma protein concentration, and shear rate or blood flow velocity. These effects are particularly noticeable when the particle size becomes "large" in relation to the vessel size. Red blood cell–vessel effects become measurable when luminal diameter decreases to less than 1 mm and become important in the microcirculation when luminal diameter decreases to 100 to 200 μm.

ANSWER: a, b, c

REFERENCE: *Chapter 70—Arterial Hemodynamics: Viscosity and Laminar Blood Flow*

10. Poiseuille's law has some limitations regarding blood flow. It nevertheless is widely used for qualitative description of blood flow in the human circulatory system. Which of the following statements is/are true regarding blood flow?

    a. It is directly proportional to the pressure head

    b. It is directly proportional to viscosity

    c. It is directly proportional to radius to the fourth power

    d. It is directly proportional to tube length

COMMENT: Poiseuille's law does not precisely describe the variables in the human circulatory system because of the non-newtonian characteristics of blood, the pulsatile nature of arterial blood flow, and the tapering and elliptical cross section of nonrigid blood vessels. In general, resistance is underestimated and calculated mean blood flow is higher than appropriate. However, this law is important and qualitatively illustrates the importance of the various factors, especially small changes in the vessel diameter.

$$Q = \frac{\Delta P \pi r^4}{8l\eta}$$

ANSWER: a, c

REFERENCE: *Chapter 70—Arterial Hemodynamics: Viscous Energy Loss*

11. Which of the following statements is/are true with respect to turbulent blood flow?

    a. It causes a larger pressure gradient than can be predicted with Poiseuille's formula
    b. It can cause an audible bruit or palpable thrill
    c. It is associated with increased velocity
    d. It is associated with increased viscosity

COMMENT: Poiseuille found that at high flow rates, larger pressure gradients occurred than could be predicted with his formula. Reynolds characterized these additional energy losses and attributed them to turbulent flow. Like Poiseuille, Reynolds used long, rigid, cylindrical tubes and nonpulsatile flow. He found that when the Reynolds number exceeded 2,000 during steady flow (the critical Reynolds number) turbulence occurred. This can produce an audible noise—a bruit or a palpable thrill. Increasing velocity and decreasing viscosity causes turbulence. The Reynolds equation has the same limitations as Poiseuille's formula in describing the situation within the human circulatory system.

ANSWER: a, b, c

REFERENCE: *Chapter 70—Arterial Hemodynamics: Inertial Energy Loss*

12. Which of the following statements is/are true regarding a critical stenosis (one that reduces pressure or flow) in the arterial circulation?

    a. Pressure or flow reduction occurs at approximately a 75% to 90% reduction in cross-sectional area
    b. Pressure or flow reduction occurs at 50% to 70% reduction in diameter
    c. Stenosis not critical at low flow rates can become critical at high flow rates
    d. Higher degrees of stenosis disproportionately decrease flow

COMMENT: Experimental studies have determined that a pressure gradient or flow reduction does not occur until rather severe stenosis is reached, that is, 75% to 90% cross-sectional area, which corresponds to a 50% to 70% reduction in diameter. At higher flow velocities, stenosis that is not critical can become critical. At higher degrees of stenosis, flow and pressure reductions occur exponentially.

ANSWER: a, b, c, d

REFERENCE: *Chapter 70—Arterial Hemodynamics: Critical and Subcritical Stenoses*

13. Which of the following statements is/are true with respect to the hemodynamic contribution to aneurysm expansion and rupture?

    a. Increased arterial blood pressure increases tensile stress
    b. Internal radius increases tensile stress
    c. Saccular aneurysms are more dangerous than are fusiform aneurysms of the same internal radius
    d. A 6-cm aneurysm arising from a 1-cm aorta undergoes greater wall stress than does a 6-cm aneurysm arising from a 3-cm aorta

COMMENT: Although the factors responsible for aneurysm development are complex, the hemodynamic contribution to aneurysm expansion and rupture has been well characterized. The law of Laplace is a reasonable approximation and implies that both increased arterial blood pressure and increased internal radius are linear in proportion to wall tensile stress, whereas aneurysm wall thickness is inversely proportional to wall stress. Finite element analysis indicates that the 6-cm aneurysm arising from a 3-cm aorta has substantially less stress associated with it than the 6-cm aneurysm arising from a 1-cm aorta.

ANSWER: a, b, c, d

REFERENCE: *Chapter 70—Arterial Hemodynamics: Arterial Aneurysm*

CHAPTER 71

VASCULAR LABORATORY TESTING FOR ARTERIAL DISEASE

1. Which of the following statements is/are true regarding Doppler assessment?
   a. Conventional Doppler probes admit an ultrasonic beam in the frequency of 2 to 10 MHz
   b. The sound frequency changes in inverse proportion to the velocity of the moving particles (red blood cells) and the cosine of the angle of insonation
   c. The frequency shift is not audible
   d. More information can be obtained with spectral analysis

COMMENT: Of all of the diagnostic methods used in the noninvasive laboratory, Doppler ultrasound has the most utility. In clinical use, Doppler instruments emit an ultrasonic beam at 2 to 10 MHz. The frequency of the sound is changed in proportion to the velocity of moving particles (red blood cells) and the cosine of the angle of insonation between the beam and the velocity vector. The frequency shift is in the audible range, and listening with a pocket Doppler device provides a quick and simple method of assessing blood flow. Spectral analysis with frequency on the vertical axis, time on the horizontal axis, and amplitude changes indicated by an increasing intensity on the gray scale provides a great deal of information, particularly with respect to flow disturbance, which produces a broadening of the normally narrow bands of frequencies that parallel the flow envelope.

ANSWER: a, d

REFERENCE: *Chapter 71—Vascular Laboratory Testing for Arterial Disease: Ultrasound*

2. Which of the following statements is/are true with respect to ankle blood pressure and ankle brachial index (ABI)?
   a. An ABI less than 0.92 almost always indicates hemodynamically significant arterial disease
   b. Persons with claudication have a wide range of ABIs; the average value is 0.6 ± 0.15
   c. In limbs with rest pain, the mean ABI is typically 0.25 ± 0.13
   d. In limbs with impending gangrene, the ABI seldom exceeds 0.25 and averages approximately 0.05 ± 0.08

COMMENT: The resting ankle brachial blood pressure of a healthy person usually exceeds brachial blood pressure. Among persons with stenotic lesions that do not reduce the diameter of the arterial lumen more than 50%, there may be no change in resting ankle brachial blood pressure. An absolute ankle pressure less than 40 mm Hg always indicates severe arterial compromise regardless of the ABI. The ranges given here have been empirically derived from assessment of large numbers of patients. When the arteries cannot be compressed because of calcification, spuriously high ankle pressures may be obtained.

ANSWER: a, b, c, d

REFERENCE: *Chapter 71—Vascular Laboratory Testing for Arterial Disease: Ankle Pressures/ABI*

3. Which of the following statements is/are true regarding normal peripheral arterial flow waves?
   a. Flow is antegrade and rapidly accelerated in early systole
   b. There is a rapid deceleration phase during which velocity decreases to zero
   c. A short period of flow reversal occurs in early diastole
   d. Low-level forward flow continues through the remainder of diastole

COMMENT: The characteristic triphasic audible Doppler signal represents distinct phases—rapid acceleration in early systole, a sharp peak at maximal velocity, a rapid deceleration phase, a short flow reversal phase in early diastole caused by elastic recoil, and low-level forward flow through the remainder of diastole. Beyond an obstruction, the flow pulse becomes more rounded, the acceleration phase is less rapid, the peak is less well defined, the reverse flow component disappears, and the velocities remain above baseline throughout diastole.

ANSWER: a, b, c, d

REFERENCE: *Chapter 71—Vascular Laboratory Testing for Arterial Disease: Flow Studies*

4. Which of the following statements is/are true with respect to assessment of the carotid circulation?

   a. The external carotid artery flow pattern resembles those obtained from peripheral arteries
   b. The internal carotid artery maintains forward flow throughout the cardiac cycle
   c. Peak systolic velocity exceeding 200 cm/s suggests stenosis greater than 50%
   d. End-diastolic velocity greater than 120 cm/s suggests stenosis greater than 80%

COMMENT: The brain is a low-resistance vascular bed, and internal carotid artery blood flow is positive throughout the cardiac cycle. The external carotid artery, which supplies the muscles of the face and neck, resembles peripheral arteries. A great deal of attention has been focused on determining criteria for estimating severity of stenosis. A peak systolic velocity exceeding 130 cm/s suggests stenosis of greater than 50%. End diastolic velocity greater than 120 cm/s suggests stenosis greater than 80%. An internal carotid–common carotid peak systolic velocity ratio of 4.0 or more and an end-diastolic velocity of 100 cm/s have been proposed as criteria for identifying stenosis of 70% of the diameter of the vessel.

ANSWER: a, b, d

REFERENCE: *Chapter 71—Vascular Laboratory Testing for Arterial Disease: Flow Studies*

5. Which of the following statements is/are true with respect to transcutaneous P_{O_2} measurements?

   a. Transcutaneous P_{O_2} levels provide an index of the adequacy of tissue perfusion and depend on the quantity of oxygen delivered and that extracted to meet metabolic demands
   b. Extremity transcutaneous P_{O_2} levels are typically normalized to a well-perfused area, such as the infraclavicular skin
   c. Transcutaneous P_{O_2} levels average approximately 60 mm Hg in normal limbs
   d. Patients with limb-threatening ischemia usually have values less than 20 mm Hg and can approach zero

COMMENT: Transcutaneous P_{O_2} levels provide an index of the adequacy of tissue perfusion. They depend on the quantity of oxygen delivered by the blood and that extracted to meet metabolic demands. Because oxygen supply is a function of arterial P_{O_2}, cardiac output, and age, peripheral measurements must be compared with levels from a well-perfused central area, such as the infraclavicular skin. In normal limbs transcutaneous P_{O_2} levels average 60 mm Hg, or 90% of the infraclavicular value. Many persons with claudication have resting values in the normal range. Among patients with limb-threatening ischemia, the values usually are less than 20 mm Hg and may be zero.

ANSWER: a, b, c, d

REFERENCE: *Chapter 71—Vascular Laboratory Testing for Arterial Disease: Transcutaneous P_{O_2}*

6. Which of the following statements is/are true regarding exercise testing and reactive hyperemia among patients with peripheral vascular occlusive disease?

   a. Healthy persons walk on a treadmill at 2 mph (3.2 km/h) at a 10% grade without experiencing leg pain, and ankle pressure remains unchanged after exercise
   b. Among patients with arterial obstruction, pain usually forces cessation of walking after 2 to 3 minutes, and the ankle pressure measured immediately after exercise is diminished
   c. The time required for pressure to return to baseline usually is 2 to 3 minutes or less
   d. Reactive hyperemia can be used as a substitute for treadmill exercise

COMMENT: Healthy persons walk without pain and do not have a decrease in ankle pressure after exercise. Patients with arterial obstruction have a decrease in ankle pressure after exercise. The severity of the decrease is roughly proportional to the severity of the occlusive process. The time for pressure to return to pre-exercise levels likewise is proportional to the severity of the occlusive process. It can exceed 20 minutes in severely diseased extremities. The reactive hyperemia test is sensitive for patients who cannot exercise and can be used as a substitute for treadmill exercise.

ANSWER: a, b, d

REFERENCE: *Chapter 71—Vascular Laboratory Testing for Arterial Disease: Exercise Testing; Reactive Hyperemia*

7. Exercise testing is appropriate for which of the following patients?

   a. A patient with symptoms of intermittent claudication but normal resting ABIs
   b. A patient with rest pain, nonhealing ulcers, or gangrene
   c. A patient with a resting ankle pressure less than 30 to 40 mm Hg
   d. A patient with blue toe syndrome and readily palpable pedal pulses

COMMENT: When a patient's symptoms are compatible with claudication and the ABI is normal or nearly so, treadmill exercise is helpful in unmasking serious arterial occlusive disease. Among patients with obvious rest pain, nonhealing ulcers, or gangrene, the diagnosis of peripheral vascular disease is obvious, as it is for patients with a resting ankle blood pressure less than 30 or 40 mm Hg. Among patients with atheroemboli and palpable pedal pulses, toe brachial indices can be helpful, but exercise testing is not. A search for the source of the embolus is more appropriate.

ANSWER: a

REFERENCE: *Chapter 71—Vascular Laboratory Testing for Arterial Disease: Exercise Testing; Reactive Hyperemia*

8. Which of the following statements is/are true regarding the assessment of renal artery obstruction with duplex scanning?

   a. There is no flow reversal in early diastole in the renal artery
   b. Renal artery to aortic peak systolic velocity ratios that exceed 3.5 indicate the presence of stenosis of 60% of vessel diameter
   c. Duplex scanning regularly helps identify accessory renal arteries
   d. Duplex scanning cannot be recommended as a means for monitoring reconstruction of the renal artery

COMMENT: The kidneys are a low-resistance vascular bed. Therefore flow in the renal arteries is positive throughout the cardiac cycle, and there is no flow reversal in early diastole, as there is during assessment of peripheral arteries. A ratio of renal artery to aortic peak systolic flow that exceeds 3.5 indicates the presence of stenosis of 60% of the diameter of the vessel. Sensitivities greater than 80% and specificities greater than 90% have been reported when these criteria are used to predict stenosis of the main renal arteries. Duplex scanning, however, often does not show accessory renal arteries or segmental branch disease. It is reasonable as a screening technique for patients with suspected renal arterial hypertension and as an accurate method for monitoring after reconstruction of the renal artery.

ANSWER: a, b

REFERENCE: *Chapter 71—Vascular Laboratory Testing for Arterial Disease: Visceral Artery Obstruction*

9. Which of the following statements is/are true regarding the use of duplex scanning as a means to monitor bypass grafts?

   a. Duplex scanning is accurate and cost-effective
   b. A localized increase in systolic velocity greater than 25% compared with adjacent segments in the graft identifies a diameter reduction of at least 50%
   c. Peak systolic velocities should be less than 40 cm/s throughout the graft
   d. Arteriovenous fistulas associated with in situ bypass grafts are difficult to detect with a duplex scanner

COMMENT: Duplex scanning is an excellent way to monitor bypass grafts. It can help detect graft-threatening defects before the patient has symptoms and before the ankle pressure begins to drop. A localized increase in systolic velocity greater than 100% of that of the adjacent graft identifies a diameter reduction of more than 50%. Peak systolic velocities less than 40 cm/s are an ominous sign of markedly reduced flow. Arteriovenous fistulas are regularly recognized by their pattern of localized flow disturbances. Velocities are high at the site of the fistula and immediately proximal to the fistula and concomitantly low just distal to the fistula.

ANSWER: a

REFERENCE: *Chapter 71—Vascular Laboratory Testing for Arterial Disease: Follow-up Studies*

CHAPTER 72

DIAGNOSTIC ANGIOGRAPHY

1. Which of the following statements is/are true regarding conventional angiography?
   a. It is still the best technique to demonstrate vascular anatomy
   b. It is reliable in identification of abnormalities of the vascular wall lumen
   c. It is an appropriate guide to interventional vascular procedures
   d. Subtle differences can be inferred about the vessels, their surroundings, and the organs or tumors they supply

COMMENT: Despite the advances made with other imaging modalities and a recognized regional and systemic complication rate, transcatheter angiography is still the best method for global, high-resolution depiction of the vascular anatomic structures. It regularly identifies even small abnormalities of the vascular wall and guides most interventional vascular procedures. It remains the standard by which newer vascular imaging modalities are judged.

ANSWER: a, b, c, d

REFERENCE: *Chapter 72—Diagnostic Angiography: Technique*

2. Which of the following statements is/are true regarding the technique of diagnostic angiography?
   a. The most common vascular access is through the femoral artery by means of the Seldinger technique
   b. Aortic injections are made with a pigtail catheter, which prevents intimal laceration during catheter recoil and has numerous side holes to achieve radially uniform contrast injection
   c. Injections into branches of the aorta are made with an end-hole tip that conforms to the catheter to better depict the artery of interest
   d. Injection of too little contrast medium results in dilution, whereas injection of too much can depict irrelevant or confusing vascular anatomic structures

COMMENT: Although transbrachial and translumbar approaches to the central circulation are possible, the preferred route is transfemoral. The Seldinger technique, whereby an artery is punctured and the needle withdrawn until pulsatile blood flow is obtained and a guide wire is advanced through the needle, is the preferred means of vascular access. A central aortic injection of contrast medium usually is made before selective injections are made. These injections are made with a pigtail catheter, which is specially constructed for uniform distribution of contrast medium and to avoid intimal injury from catheter recoil. Selective injections are made after the pigtail catheter is exchanged for one with an end hole and tip that conform to the proximal course of the artery of interest. Both the volume and rate of injection of contrast material and the film speed are critical to allow optimal delineation of the vascular anatomic structures.

ANSWER: a, b, c, d

REFERENCE: *Chapter 72—Diagnostic Angiography: Technique*

3. Which of the following statements is/are true with respect to digital angiography?

   a. Digital angiography image recording is on an image intensifier rather than on film
   b. When used with various subtraction techniques, digital angiography provides high-contrast visual resolution
   c. Digital angiography provides images promptly and reduces film cost
   d. Intraarterial digital substraction angiography requires less iodinated contrast medium than does intravenous digital substraction angiography (DSA)

COMMENT: In DSA, image recording is on an image intensifier rather than on film. The image is electronically read and stored on a computer disk. As in conventional angiography, subtraction technique can enhance image resolution. Images stored on computer can be selected and recorded on film, typically several images on a single sheet of film, which greatly reduces film costs. The prompt availability of the image and the reduced film cost, as well as the smaller amounts of contrast material needed for intraarterial DSA, are the advantages of this technique.

ANSWER: a, b, c, d

REFERENCE: *Chapter 72—Diagnostic Angiography: Digital Angiography*

4. Which of the following statements is/are true with respect to helical computed tomographic (CT) angiography (spiral angiography) and magnetic resonance angiography (MRA)?

   a. Both techniques are rapidly evolving and involve sophisticated software to acquire and store images
   b. In both techniques, there is a trade-off between the resolution of the image and the size of the field
   c. Magnetic resonance angiography can be used in examination of almost all patients
   d. Picture-processing techniques, such as regions of interest, exploiting contrast threshold, and gating data acquisition are regularly used

COMMENT: Both helical CT and MRA are revolutionizing vascular imaging. Both provide reliable images with excellent resolution, particularly when the images can be limited to a focused area of interest. There is a recognized trade-off between resolution and the size of the field imaged. The vascular anatomic structures are displayed by means of computer interaction. Various techniques, including contrast thresholds, region of interest, data acquisition, and compensatory pulses can be added to the imaging train to enhance the image. These capabilities also eliminate cardiac and respiratory artifacts. Magnetic resonance angiography has a wide range of applications but is contraindicated in examinations of patients with pacemakers and with certain metallic devices adjacent to easily traumatized structures, such as the eye and the brain.

ANSWER: a, b, d

REFERENCE: *Chapter 72—Diagnostic Angiography: Helical CT Angiography; Magnetic Resonance Angiography*

5. Which of the following statements is/are correct regarding contrast media?

a. The conventional contrast medium for angiography is viscus, water soluble, and radiopaque. It can be associated with idiosyncratic anaphylactoid reactions and uncomfortable tissue responses as well as complications such as renal failure

b. Conventional contrast medium is one-tenth as expensive as nonionic agents

c. Carbon dioxide gas can be injected as a suitable contrast agent for many peripheral applications

d. Contrast medium for MRA has no documented renal toxicity

COMMENT: Contrast medium for conventional angiography is viscous, water soluble, and radiopaque. It is also toxic. Uncomfortable tissue reactions, such as pain during injection of arteries supplying the body wall, coughing during pulmonary arterial injection, and renal toxicity are widely recognized. Nonionic agents appear safer in every respect, although they have not been shown to have conclusive advantages in imaging of patients with renal failure. Nonionic agents are approximately 10 times as expensive as conventional contrast agents. Carbon dioxide gas is a suitable contrast agent for many applications. It is inherently biocompatible and is particularly useful in imaging of patients with an allergy to conventional contrast material or with renal failure. Contrast media for MRA, typically gadolinium-based compounds, are expensive but have no documented renal toxicity. Likewise, the volume of contrast medium injected is relatively small, so the risk of fluid overload is reduced.

ANSWER: a, b, c, d

REFERENCE: *Chapter 72—Diagnostic Angiography: Contrast Media*

6. Which of the following statements is/are true regarding the complications of diagnostic angiography?

a. The overall rate of serious complications is less than 1%

b. The frequency and severity of complications depend both on the experience of the angiographer and technical factors, such as the size of the catheter and sheath, the number of catheter changes, and the duration of the procedure

c. Patient factors such as uncontrolled hypertension, obesity, severe atherosclerosis, marginally compensated cardiac or renal disease, and poor coagulation status increase the risk of complications

d. Puncture site complications, catheterization, and injection complications and complications related to the administration of contrast media all contribute to the overall complication rate

COMMENT: The overall rate of serious complications of diagnostic angiography is more than 1% but is less than 5%. Puncture site complications include hematoma, dissection, pseudoaneurysm, arteriovenous fistula, thrombosis, and occasionally graft infection. Catheter and injection complications include dissection, perforation, and embolism, including stroke. Complications related to the administration of contrast medium, including renal failure, fluid overload, congestive heart failure, transverse myelitis, and anaphylactoid reaction contribute to the overall complication rate. The experience of the angiographer, technical factors, and patient factors all influence the rate of complications.

ANSWER: b, c, d

REFERENCE: *Chapter 72—Diagnostic Angiography: Complications*

7. Which of the following statements is/are true with respect to anatomy of the thoracoabdominal aorta?
    a. The anterior radiculomedullary artery (artery of Adamkiewicz) can arise anywhere from the descending thoracic to the proximal lumbar aorta and serves as a major contributor to the anterior spinal artery
    b. The celiac and superior mesenteric arteries are best depicted in the anteroposterior projection
    c. Multiple renal arteries occur in approximately 20% to 30% of cases
    d. The renal arteries are best studied in lateral projection

COMMENT: The artery of Adamkiewicz is critical to angiographers and vascular surgeons. This artery is the major blood supply to the anterior spinal artery, and transverse myelitis has occurred after injection of contrast medium. The origins of the celiac and superior mesenteric arteries arise from the ventral surface of the aorta, and thus lateral aortography is necessary to see their origins. In 20% to 30% of cases, more than one renal artery supplies a kidney. These arteries usually are smaller than the main renal artery and can arise anywhere between the body of the eleventh thoracic vertebra and the iliac artery. Because the renal arteries arise from the lateral aspect of the aorta, the orifices are best seen in the anteroposterior and slight left anterior oblique projection.

ANSWER: a, c

REFERENCE: *Chapter 72—Diagnostic Angiography: Thoracic Aorta; Abdominal Aorta*

8. Which of the following statements is/are true with respect to arterial dissection?
    a. Dissection can result from a spontaneous intimal tear that produces an intramural hematoma or from intimal trauma, usually iatrogenic
    b. Spontaneous dissections are most common in the thoracic aorta
    c. The dissection tear usually is in the transverse aortic arch
    d. The most common serious complication of dissection is rupture

COMMENT: Dissection can occur as a spontaneous intramural hematoma or as the result of intimal trauma. The trauma can be blunt or penetrating but often is iatrogenic. The thoracic aorta is the most common site of aortic dissection. Typically the tear is several centimeters above the aortic valve or just distal to the subclavian artery. In some instances, the transverse aortic arch is involved. Although rupture of the dissected aorta does occur, major morbidity results from shearing and occlusion of normal aortic branches as the intramural hematoma spirals longitudinally. Retrograde dissection can occlude coronary arteries and can cause acute aortic insufficiency, cardiac tamponade, or both.

ANSWER: a, b

REFERENCE: *Chapter 72—Diagnostic Angiography: Arterial Dissection*

CHAPTER 73

VASCULAR INFECTIONS

1. Which of the following is/are true with respect to vascular infections?

   a. The risk of infection increases with implantation of a prosthetic graft
   b. Risk increases for procedures performed under emergency conditions
   c. Vascular infection can develop months to years after implantation
   d. Vascular infection can be caused by less virulent microorganisms

COMMENT: Vascular infection is among the most challenging therapeutic problems. Although risk of infection is low, it is not negligible, and some authorities state that when both early and late infections are included more than 5% of vascular operations can be complicated by infection. Graft infection more than 4 months after implantation is relatively common and often is caused by less virulent organisms, such as *Staphylococcus epidermidis*. A prosthesis increases the risk of infection, as does an emergency procedure.

ANSWER: a, b, c, d

REFERENCE: *Chapter 73—Vascular Infections*

2. Which of the following mechanisms contribute(s) to the development of mycotic aneurysm?

   a. Direct extension from an adjacent suppurative focus
   b. Bacterial colonization of diseased arterial segments
   c. Embolism from a septic focus, such as endocarditis or septicemia
   d. Direct inoculation after an invasive vascular procedure

COMMENT: The term *mycotic aneurysm* as used in contemporary practice refers to true aneurysms as well as pseudoaneurysms caused by arterial infection. These are distinct from the simple positive culture results obtained from an aneurysmal sac. Mycotic aneurysms are fulminant infections and are commonly believed to be caused by one of the four mechanisms listed.

ANSWER: a, b, c, d

REFERENCE: *Chapter 73—Vascular Infections: Classification*

3. Which of the following statements is/are true regarding aortic graft infections?

   a. Most manifest within 6 months of graft implantation
   b. Back or groin pain, a pulsatile mass, and fever suggest the presence of an infected aortic prosthesis
   c. Most patients have a graft enteric fistula
   d. Early graft infection usually manifests with overt clinical signs of sepsis (fever, leukocytosis, bacteremia), a draining sinus, or a pulsatile mass

COMMENT: Most aortic graft infections are recognized more than 1 year after graft implantation. Approximately two thirds of cases manifest as a perigraft infection, and one third manifest as aortoenteric fistula. Early graft infections often manifest as signs of sepsis, a draining sinus track, or a pulsatile mass in the wound.

ANSWER: b, d

REFERENCE: *Chapter 73—Vascular Infections: Clinical Manifestations*

4. Normal arteries rarely become infected even during bacteremia. (An) important exception(s) is/are:

   a. Particulate embolism from a proximal septic focus
   b. Syphilitic arteritis
   c. Tuberculous arteritis
   d. Salmonella arteritis

COMMENT: Normal arteries are remarkably resistant to infection, with the above exceptions. Any injury to the vessel wall, intimal defect, or foreign material markedly facilitates the establishment of infection. The risk of infection is likewise proportional to the degree of bacterial contamination, the virulence of the underlying organism, and host resistance.

ANSWER: a, b, c, d

REFERENCE: Chapter *73—Vascular Infections: Pathophysiology of Vascular Infections*

5. Which of the following statements is/are true regarding the bacteriologic characteristics of vascular infection?

a. *Staphylococcus aureus* is the prevalent pathogen
b. Gram-negative organisms cause approximately one third of infections involving arteries, veins, or vascular grafts
c. Aneurysms infected with gram-negative organisms are at greater risk of rupture than are those infected with gram-positive organisms
d. Coagulase-negative staphylococci, especially *S. epidermidis* organisms, are frequent in late-appearing vascular prosthetic infections

COMMENT: *Staphylococcus aureus* is the prevalent pathogen in vascular graft infection, and gram-positive infections are more common overall. The prevalence of infections caused by gram-negative organisms is increasing; these organisms cause approximately one third of vascular infections. These infections are quite important because the risk of rupture is higher than that associated with infection with gram-positive organisms. The importance of coagulase-negative staphylococci, such as *S. epidermidis,* in late-presenting graft infections has been emphasized. These organisms can be quite difficult to culture because of their tendency to form surface biofilms.

ANSWER: a, b, c, d

REFERENCE: *Chapter 73—Vascular Infections: Bacteriology of Graft Infection*

6. Numerous imaging modalities have been used in an attempt to diagnose vascular infection. Which of the following computed tomographic findings suggest(s) vascular infection?

a. Well-localized vascular dilatation with a paucity of calcifications
b. Abnormal collections of fluid or air around vessels or grafts
c. Adjacent vertebral osteomyelitis or juxtaaortic retroperitoneal abscess
d. An encasing mass that obtains air

COMMENT: Contrast-enhanced computed tomography is the preferred imaging technique in evaluation for suspected infection involving the aorta, visceral arteries, or abdominal vascular grafts. All of the above findings strongly suggest vascular graft infection. Computed tomography–guided needle aspiration biopsy can be useful in identifying the infecting pathogen.

ANSWER: a, b, c, d

REFERENCE: *Chapter 73—Vascular Infections: Diagnostic Modalities*

7. Functional imaging techniques, such as radionucleotide scanning with technetium 99m–labeled leukocytes, indium 111–labeled leukocytes, and radiolabeled polyclonal human IgG antibodies, have been used extensively in the diagnosis of prosthetic graft infection. Which of the following statements is/are true with respect to these studies?

a. Results of functional studies are not reliably predictive of infection because of the low specificity of the tests
b. The results are particularly difficult to interpret in the early postoperative period
c. False-positive results can occur for hematoma, pseudoaneurysm, tumor, and other sites of inflammation
d. False-negative results are more common in late-appearing graft infection than in early infection

COMMENT: Functional imaging studies have been used in the diagnosis of prosthetic graft infections. The results, however, are not reliably predictive of infection because of the low specificity of the tests, particularly in the early postoperative period. False-positive results are relatively common, and although unusual, false-negative results do occur, particularly for late-appearing aortic graft infection complicated by aortoenteric fistula.

ANSWER: a, b, c, d

REFERENCE: *Chapter 73—Vascular Infections: Functional Imaging Studies*

8. The preferred therapy for aortic prosthetic infection is extraanatomic bypass (axillofemoral, femoral bypass) and complete excision of the aortic prosthesis. Which of the following favor(s) the use of in situ reconstructive technique?

a. Gram-negative infection
b. *Salmonella* infection
c. The absence of gross purulence and sepsis
d. Low-grade infection, as with coagulase-negative staphylococci

COMMENT: The preferred management is extraanatomic bypass and total graft excision. In certain settings, however, such as the absence of gross purulence or low-grade infection with normal adjacent arterial wall, in situ reconstruction is acceptable. In situ reconstruction is less optimal in the presence of gram-negative infection, particularly salmonella, although occasional successful outcomes have been achieved with this form of treatment.

ANSWER: c, d

REFERENCE: *Chapter 73—Vascular Infections: Principles of Management*

CHAPTER 74

BASIC ENDOVASCULAR CONSIDERATIONS AND SURGICAL TECHNIQUES

1. Angiography is planned to delineate the arterial anatomy of a 68-year-old man with diabetes, ischemic ulceration of the right great toe, and a creatinine concentration of 2.5 mg/dL. Prudent measures to help minimize the risk of further renal dysfunction include:

   a. Intravenous fluid administration to assure adequate hydration
   b. Administration of 100 mg hydrocortisone 1 hour before the procedure
   c. Arch and thoracic aortography in addition to abdominal aortography to rule out the presence of ulcerated lesions of the aortic wall, which are the likely source of the atheroemboli responsible for the renal dysfunction
   d. Use of carbon dioxide as the contrast agent
   e. Use of nonionic iodinated contrast material

COMMENT: The measures shown to minimize the risk of contrast material–induced nephropathy include prevention of dehydration and the use of non-ionic contrast material. Although the use of carbon dioxide is not associated with nephrotoxicity, it would be unusual for carbon dioxide angiography to show the reconstituted arterial anatomy to the extent that the information would be usable for operative decision making. Administration of steroids helps to minimize the severity of contrast material–related allergic reactions but has no bearing on the development of postangiography renal insufficiency. Total aortography would greatly increase the amount of contrast material used and increase the risk of renal dysfunction.

ANSWER: a, e

REFERENCE: *Chapter 74—Basic Endovascular Considerations and Surgical Techniques: Contrast Agents*

2. A 65-year-old man with disabling claudication and absent femoral pulses undergoes aortography through a left axillary artery approach. The angiogram shows an occluded distal aorta with distal reconstitution of the iliac arteries. One hour after the procedure, he reports severe arm pain, and his hand grasp strength decreases. The left radial pulse is normal. Which of the following likely explain(s) the symptoms?

   a. Right hemispheric stroke caused by catheter manipulation in the aorta
   b. Neuronal ischemia of the median nerve from embolic occlusion of the arteries of the forearm
   c. Axillary sheath hematoma
   d. Delayed contrast reaction of the nonanaphylactic type that responds to administration of steroids

COMMENT: The symptoms described include pain certainly not typical of stroke. Although it is possible to continue to have a weak radial pulse with a more proximal axillary or brachial artery occlusion (because of the good upper arm collateral network), the degree of hand ischemia would be minimal if the radial pulse were still palpable. Delayed reactions to contrast material do not manifest as pain. This patient has an axillary sheath hematoma, which can be present even without any obvious findings at physical examination. Surgical exploration for decompression should be pursued promptly.

ANSWER: c

REFERENCE: *Chapter 74—Basic Endovascular Considerations and Surgical Techniques: Risks of Arteriography*

3. Several years ago a 55-year-old man had an abrupt onset of shortness of breath and hypotension. He needed endotracheal intubation and administration of vasopressors after injection of iodinated contrast material during cardiac catheterization. Prudent measures to help prevent a recurrence of these events during an upcoming angiogram include:

   a. Administration of diphenhydramine
   b. Administration of hydrocortisone before the procedure
   c. Administration of an anxiolytic agent
   d. Use of nonionic contrast material for the study
   e. Administration of small test doses of contrast material at the beginning of the procedure to induce tolerance

COMMENT: Prospective, randomized studies have shown that administration of 100 mg hydrocortisone intravenously 12 and 2 hours before exposure to contrast material and administration of diphenhydramine substantially reduce the number of serious contrast reactions. Reduction of anxiety also decreases the frequency of contrast reactions, as does use of nonionic contrast material. There is no role for the administration of "test doses" of contrast material.

ANSWER: a, b, c, d

REFERENCE: *Chapter 74—Basic Endovascular Considerations and Surgical Techniques: Risks of Arteriography*

4. Which of the following indications is/are accepted for stent placement after iliac artery angioplasty?

   a. The presence of 40% residual stenosis after angioplasty
   b. The finding of a dissection on an angiogram after angioplasty
   c. Dilatation of a recurrent stenosis
   d. Inability of the patient to take aspirin because of long-term warfarin administration
   e. Use of the ipsilateral femoral artery for arterial access to perform the procedure

COMMENT: Generally accepted indications for stent placement after angioplasty include the presence of greater than 30% residual stenosis after angioplasty or detection of a marked dissection of the artery after balloon dilation. It is also common practice to stent a recurrent lesion after previous balloon angioplasty. Administration of warfarin or an inability to take aspirin is not an indication for stent placement. The site of arterial puncture for performance of angioplasty does not affect the indications for placement of a stent.

ANSWER: a, b, c

REFERENCE: *Chapter 74—Basic Endovascular Considerations and Surgical Techniques: Intravascular Stent Deployment*

5. The immediate technical results of an angioplasty can be assessed by means of:

   a. Angiography performed in several planes
   b. Intravascular ultrasonography
   c. Pressure measurements across the lesion dilated
   d. Angioscopy
   e. Assessment of the symptoms

COMMENT: Accepted means of assessing the technical and hemodynamic results of angioplasty include performing angiography in several planes, use of intravascular ultrasonography, and measurement of pressure gradients across the lesion. The use of angioscopy requires a blood-free field of view to achieve adequate imaging. This is not practical in most situations in which angioplasty is being performed. Assessment of symptoms is not a reasonable means of assessment of the immediate technical results of endovascular intervention.

ANSWER: a, b, c

REFERENCE: *Chapter 74—Basic Endovascular Considerations and Surgical Techniques: Overview of Basic Endovascular Techniques*

CHAPTER 75

CEREBROVASCULAR OCCLUSIVE DISEASE

1. Which of the following statements is/are true regarding cerebrovascular occlusive disease?
   a. Stroke is the third leading cause of death in the United States
   b. Morbidity is effectively eliminated with rehabilitation
   c. Changes in affect are common after stroke
   d. Most strokes are caused by emboli from a cardiac source

COMMENT: For many years, stroke has been the third leading cause of death in the United States and in other developed countries. Stroke commonly has persistent functional deficits. The severity of these deficits leads to affective disorders, including a high incidence of depression. Most (50% to 66%) strokes are caused by atherothrombotic events from extracranial arteries, 15% to 20% from cardiac sources, and an additional 15% to 20% from intraparenchymal and subarachnoid hemorrhage. The rest fall into miscellaneous categories.

ANSWER: a, c

REFERENCE: *Chapter 75—Cerebrovascular Occlusive Disease: Introduction*

2. Which of the following statements is/are true regarding surgical management of cerebrovascular disease?
   a. Symptomatic high-grade carotid stenoses (more than 75%) are effectively managed with carotid endarterectomy
   b. Asymptomatic lesions greater than 40% should be managed with prophylactic carotid endarterectomy to decrease lesion progression
   c. Elective carotid endarterectomy is routinely performed with morbidity and mortality rates less than 1%
   d. Patients at good risk with asymptomatic lesions greater than 75% benefit from carotid endarterectomy

COMMENT: Results of several large, multi-institutional trials have shown carotid endarterectomy effective in the treatment of patients with high-grade carotid stenosis with symptoms (NASCET) and without symptoms (ACAS). In the NASCET study of symptomatic stenosis, benefit was gained among patients with severe stenoses (more than 70% of luminal diameter). In the ACAS trial, the benefit was apparent for patients with stenosis greater than 60% of luminal diameter. No one has suggested a role for prophylactic carotid endarterectomy for mild stenotic disease. Some select series have had mortality and morbidity after carotid endarterectomy as low as 1%, but such reports are not representative of the collected experience, in which morbidity and mortality routinely average 3% to 5%. In some series, mortality and morbidity rates as high as 7% to 10% have been cited. The "acceptable" mortality and morbidity in contemporary series is approximately 3% to 5%.

ANSWER: a, d

REFERENCE: *Chapter 75—Cerebrovascular Occlusive Disease: Surgical Treatment*

3. Which of the following technical details regarding carotid endarterectomy is/are mandatory during carotid endarterectomy?

   a. General anesthesia
   b. Use of a shunt during carotid clamping
   c. Monitoring with electroencephalography (EEG)
   d. Patch closure with expanded polytetrafluoroethylene (Gore-Tex) or autogenous saphenous vein
   e. None of the above

COMMENT: Technical details of carotid endarterectomy vary greatly from institution to institution and surgeon to surgeon, usually with comparable results. General or regional or local anesthesia; routine, selective, or strict avoidance of shunting; monitoring with EEG; and transcranial Doppler assessment of the neurologic status of the awake patient and carotid stump pressures all have been used for monitoring. Most surgeons favor selective patching of very small carotid arteries, and patching is more common among women and in reoperations.

ANSWER: e

REFERENCE: *Chapter 75—Cerebrovascular Occlusive Disease: Surgical Therapy*

4. With respect to the symptomatic presentation of cerebrovascular disease:

   a. Symptoms almost always are pathognomonic and follow classic textbook descriptions
   b. Close correlation between symptoms and computed tomographic (CT) findings are the rule
   c. Carotid occlusion in the neck always is symptomatic
   d. Symptoms suggesting cerebrovascular disease should be investigated with noninvasive evaluation

COMMENT: Symptoms of cerebrovascular disease often are partial or incomplete syndromes. There is only a modest correlation between CT findings and clinical manifestations. Carotid occlusion in the neck can be asymptomatic. Because of the devastating consequences of missing potentially symptomatic cerebrovascular disease, all such patients need aggressive noninvasive evaluation.

ANSWER: d

REFERENCE: *Chapter 75—Cerebrovascular Occlusive Disease: Diagnosis; Noninvasive Techniques*

5. Which of the following is/are part of the evaluation for patients being considered for carotid endarterectomy?

   a. General history and physical examination with special attention to cardiovascular risk
   b. Noninvasive assessment
   c. Four-vessel pancerebral angiography
   d. Baseline CT scan or EEG

COMMENT: The main risk of carotid endarterectomy (in addition to the risk of stroke) is acute myocardial infarction. Noninvasive assessment is appropriate for all patients being considered for carotid endarterectomy, and some groups are no longer performing routine preoperative angiography. The approximately 1% risk of stroke with diagnostic cerebral angiography and the reliability of noninvasive tests have made this approach more common. Baseline CT scans, EEG, and other neurologic assessments are not routine.

ANSWER: a, b

REFERENCE: *Chapter 75—Cerebrovascular Occlusive Disease: Surgical Treatment*

CHAPTER 76

UPPER EXTREMITY OCCLUSIVE DISEASE

1. Which of the following statements is/are true with respect to upper extremity occlusive vascular disease?

    a. It is as common as lower extremity occlusive disease
    b. The overwhelming majority of cases are caused by atherosclerosis
    c. In severe bilateral hand ischemia, a systemic cause of the arterial lesion should be sought
    d. Pressure differences between the right and left brachial artery >50 mm Hg are normal

COMMENT: Clinically significant upper extremity vascular disease is distinctly less common than lower extremity occlusive vascular disease. Unlike lower extremity disease, upper extremity vascular disease entails numerous conditions. Bilateral hand ischemia is frequently caused by a systemic collagen vascular disorder. A pressure differential up to 10 mm Hg between the right and the left brachial artery is normal. Differences beyond this imply stenosis in the innominate, subclavian, axillary, or brachial artery that may or may not have clinical significance.

ANSWER: c

REFERENCE: *Chapter 76—Upper Extremity Occlusive Disease: Introduction; Clinical Examination*

2. Acute, profound hand ischemia in a young adult is most often caused by:

    a. Thoracic outlet syndrome
    b. Collagen vascular disorder
    c. Occupational injury
    d. Intraarterial injection of drugs of abuse

COMMENT: Thoracic outlet syndrome is the most common cause of severe hand ischemia among young adults. There are four possible compression sites in the thoracic outlet: (a) the costoclavicular space formed by the first thoracic rib and the clavicle, (b) the interscalene triangle, (c) the angle between the insertion of the pectoralis minor tendon and the coracoid process, and (d) the humeral head in extreme external rotation. Thoracic outlet syndrome also can be caused by bony abnormalities such as a cervical rib, an abnormal first thoracic rib, or hypertrophy of the anterior scalene muscle.

ANSWER: a

REFERENCE: *Chapter 76—Upper Extremity Occlusive Disease: Proximal Arterial Lesions*

3. Which of the following characterize(s) the diagnostic evaluation of a patient with upper extremity vascular disease?

    a. Recognition that a variety of pathophysiologic conditions can cause similar symptoms
    b. The need for an appropriately focused history, vascular examination, and noninvasive assessment
    c. Laboratory examination for systemic causes of the vascular disorder
    d. Relatively constant anatomic patterns

COMMENT: The anatomic features of the blood vessels of the upper extremity are highly variable, particularly in the region of the palmar arch, where multiple distinct patterns are recognized. Treatment must in every instance be tailored to the precise anatomic location of the obstruction and address the diverse underlying etiologic factors. The keys to recognizing the diverse causes of vascular disorders are the history, examination, noninvasive assessment, and consideration of systemic collagen vascular disorders.

ANSWER: a, b, c

REFERENCE: *Chapter 76—Upper Extremity Occlusive Disease: Clinical Examination*

CHAPTER 77

VISCERAL OCCLUSIVE DISEASE

1. Which of the following statements is/are true with respect to high-grade stenosis or occlusion of the celiac axis?

   a. It is nearly always symptomatic
   b. If unrelieved, it regularly results in visceral infarction
   c. Atherosclerosis is the cause in most cases
   d. The pancreaticoduodenal branches of the superior mesenteric artery (SMA) are major collateral vessels

COMMENT: Significant stenosis or occlusion of the celiac axis can occur from extrinsic compression by the medium arcuate ligament, from atherosclerotic occlusive disease, or from emboli, dissections, or thrombosis of a celiac aneurysm. In general, to cause symptoms or infarction, at least two of the three major visceral vessels must be compromised. The primary source of collateral vessels to the celiac artery is through the pancreaticoduodenal arcades at the head of the pancreas. Extrinsic compression of the celiac axis caused by the medium arcuate ligament is common and usually is asymptomatic.

ANSWER: d

REFERENCE: *Chapter 77—Visceral Occlusive Disease: Clinical Syndromes*

2. Ischemic events involving the intestine can cause:

   a. Toxin and mediator absorption
   b. Bacterial translocation
   c. Gastrointestinal hemorrhage on reperfusion
   d. Late stricture formation

COMMENT: Intestinal ischemia causes a variety of adverse effects. The mucosa is the most vulnerable portion of the intestinal wall. Mucosal injury allows absorption of toxins and mediators, such as tumor necrosis factor, lipopolysaccharide, and interleukin-1, and translocation of bacteria. When the circulation is restored, the damaged mucosa bleeds. Late stricture formation may result from scar formation during healing.

ANSWER: a, b, c, d

REFERENCE: *Chapter 77—Visceral Occlusive Disease: Pathophysiology of Ischemic Injury*

3. Which of the following statements is/are true with respect to noninvasive assessment of the intestinal circulation?

   a. Typical large-vessel intestinal blood flow in humans is estimated to be 500 to 1,200 mL/min
   b. After a meal, celiac artery blood flow increases dramatically, whereas estimated SMA blood flow does not increase until 90 minutes after ingestion
   c. Noninvasive studies allow ready assessment of the adequacy of the collateral circulation
   d. Intestinal viability is readily assessed with noninvasive technology

COMMENT: Resting intestinal blood flow represents 10% to 20% of cardiac output and is estimated to be between 500 and 1,200 mL/min. Duplex scanning of the celiac and superior mesenteric arteries is becoming more widely available but is compromised in the presence of marked obesity or intestinal gas. After a meal, the celiac arterial blood flow of persons who have fasted increases but usually not to a great degree. Blood flow in the SMA increases markedly 20 to 30 minutes after eating. Noninvasive technology is not useful for assessing collateral circulation or intestinal viability.

ANSWER: a

REFERENCE: *Chapter 77—Visceral Occlusive Disease: Visceral Angina*

4. Which of the following is/are true with respect to mesenteric arterial embolization?
   a. This is a distinctly uncommon cause of intestinal ischemia
   b. The embolus often arises from a cardiac source
   c. Typical symptoms have a subacute onset
   d. Laboratory tests often are pathognomonic

COMMENT: Superior mesenteric artery embolism accounts for approximately 50% of instances of acute mesenteric ischemia. The typical embolus arises from a cardiac source. Atrial fibrillation or recent myocardial infarction with mural thrombus formation is the classic source of the embolus, but any arrhythmia or anatomic cardiac defect can result in a mesenteric embolus. The onset of symptoms usually is abrupt, and the patient can often precisely localize the onset of pain. Results of laboratory tests are not pathognomonic and typically are abnormal only in advanced ischemia. Findings at the general physical examination, although not specific enough for a precise diagnosis, may indicate the underlying cardiac disorder. An irregular rate and rhythm such as occurs in atrial fibrillation, a murmur from an abnormal valve, an enlarged heart, or evidence of previous embolism, which occurs among as many as 25% of patients, may be found.

ANSWER: b

REFERENCE: *Chapter 77—Visceral Occlusive Disease: Mesenteric Embolism*

5. Which of the following is/are true with respect to SMA thrombus?
   a. The symptoms typically have a less abrupt onset than does SMA embolus, and acute symptoms can be superimposed on chronic symptoms of intestinal angina
   b. The patient has frequently undergone an extensive array of diagnostic tests addressed at the possibility of underlying gastrointestinal malignant disease or a motility disturbance
   c. The occlusive process often is quite diffuse throughout the visceral vessel, although critical occlusions tend to occur proximally
   d. Lateral aortography is essential to making the diagnosis

COMMENT: Mesenteric arterial thrombosis can occur as an acute intestinal catastrophe without antecedent symptoms or more commonly with the background of chronic intestinal angina. Such patients often have undergone extensive diagnostic evaluation, including contrast radiographic studies, endoscopy, and various scans. Such studies are appropriate for a patient with profound weight loss and abdominal pain. When the results of diagnostic studies are normal, however, the possibility of underlying mesenteric vascular occlusive disease should be considered. The occlusive process, although most critical in the proximal visceral trunks, is diffuse and widespread throughout the intestinal circulation. Lateral aortography is essential to localizing the proximal occlusive process.

ANSWER: a, b, c, d

REFERENCE: *Chapter 77—Visceral Occlusive Disease: Mesenteric Thrombosis*

6. Which of the following is/are true with respect to low-flow nonocclusive mesenteric ischemia?

   a. It appears to be increasing in frequency
   b. It is caused by vasoconstriction in the mesenteric blood vessels
   c. It tends to occur among patients who have had good ambulation
   d. It necessitates prompt surgical intervention

COMMENT: Better hemodynamic monitoring and intensive care unit practices have led to an apparent decrease in the frequency and severity of low-flow nonocclusive mesenteric ischemia. This complication typically occurs among critically ill patients in response to diminished cardiac output, shock, hypovolemia, and dehydration. The use of certain medications is known to cause to splanchnic vasoconstriction. Ergot alkaloids are well known in this regard, but almost all pressors and digitalis also decrease mesenteric blood flow. Surgery has no definitive role other than resection of necrotic intestine. The focus of therapeutic interventions is relief of vasospasm by means of optimizing hemodynamic values and volume status and when possible eliminating adverse pharmacologic agents. Papaverine and glucagon have direct vasodilatory effects and have been used to manage low-flow nonocclusive ischemia.

ANSWER: b

REFERENCE: *Chapter 77—Visceral Occlusive Disease: Low-flow Nonocclusive Mesenteric Ischemia*

7. Iatrogenic visceral ischemia:

   a. Is distinctly uncommon
   b. Occurs only as a result of surgical intervention
   c. Is rarely lethal or morbid
   d. Can be reduced by prospective attention to precipitating causes

COMMENT: Iatrogenic intestinal ischemia is certainly not rare, and it is caused by a variety of factors. Drugs such as digitalis preparations, ergotamines, and almost all pressor agents have been reported to cause intestinal ischemia. Catheter-related complications such as dissection or embolism can cause iatrogenic visceral ischemia. Aortic reconstruction is the prototypical surgical procedure associated with iatrogenic ischemia and in some reports occurs in 2% to 6% of aortic reconstructive procedures. Profound transmural infarction has an associated mortality of almost 60%, and lesser degrees of ischemia cause bloody diarrhea and stricture formation.

ANSWER: d

REFERENCE: *Chapter 77—Visceral Occlusive Disease: Iatrogenic Visceral Ischemia*

8. Other than the primary named syndromes, visceral arterial occlusion and intestinal ischemia can be caused by:

   a. Aortic dissection
   b. Collagen vascular disease
   c. Radiation
   d. Ergotism
   e. Trauma

COMMENT: Superior mesenteric artery embolization and thrombosis and low-flow nonocclusive ischemia are by far the most common causes of acute visceral arterial occlusion and intestinal ischemia. However, all of the diagnoses listed can produce intestinal ischemia and should be in the differential diagnosis once the primary causes have been excluded.

ANSWER: a, b, c, d, e

REFERENCE: *Chapter 77—Visceral Occlusive Disease: Miscellaneous Causes of Acute Visceral Ischemia*

9. At urgent exploration for intestinal ischemia, intestinal viability is commonly assessed by means of:

   a. Clinical judgment
   b. The use of an intraoperative Doppler assessment
   c. Injection of fluorescein
   d. Injection of radiolabeled microspheres
   e. Intraluminal tonometry

COMMENT: Clinical assessment, intraoperative Doppler assessment, and injection of fluorescein are regularly used to assess intestinal viability. None, however, is completely specific. The clinical algorithm is to resect all clearly necrotic intestine, leave any that is marginally viable, and perform a second look procedure within 24 to 48 hours. Other techniques to assess intestinal viability in the immediate-care setting have been described, including use of surface oximetry, radiolabeled microspheres, intraluminal tonometry, and electronic contractility monitors, but none has obtained widespread use.

ANSWER: a, b, c

REFERENCE: *Chapter 77—Visceral Occlusive Disease: Recognition of Intestinal Viability*

10. Which of the following is/are true concerning mesenteric venous thrombosis?

   a. Can be primary or secondary to hypercoagulable and inflammatory conditions
   b. Follows portacaval shunts in 15% to 20% of cases
   c. Frequently manifests as varicocele
   d. Is more common among women

COMMENT: Mesenteric venous thrombosis can be acute but is most often associated with a subacute syndrome of nonspecific abdominal pain, distention, nausea, and malaise that evolves over several days to weeks. It can be primary, that is, without recognizable cause, or secondary to an inflammatory condition, such as peritonitis or a hypercoagulable state. There is no sex predilection. Plain radiographs, computed tomography, or the venous phase of selective mesenteric angiography can depict the thrombosis. However, in most instances, the diagnosis is made intraoperatively. Large-vessel venous thrombectomy occasionally is helpful, as are the use of surgical resection of nonviable intestine and long-term anticoagulation. Systemic fibrinolytic therapy has not yet found its way into clinical utility for this condition.

ANSWER: a

REFERENCE: *Chapter 77—Visceral Occlusive Disease: Mesenteric Venous Thrombosis*

11. Which of the following is/are not true with respect to visceral angina?

   a. It typically causes midepigastric pain 30 to 45 minutes after eating
   b. It requires the involvement of at least two of the three visceral vessels
   c. Extensive weight loss occurs as a result of malabsorption
   d. Aortography, including anteroposterior and lateral views, confirms the diagnosis

COMMENT: The weight loss in visceral angina is typically considered caused by "small meal syndrome." Because eating causes abdominal pain, patients have food fear and often restrict their diets, which results in weight loss. Reproducibility of symptoms 30 to 45 minutes after eating, involvement of at least two of the three visceral vessels, and the use of lateral aortography to make the diagnosis are classic for this syndrome.

ANSWER: c

REFERENCE: *Chapter 77—Visceral Occlusive Disease: Visceral Angina*

CHAPTER 78

RENAL ARTERY OCCLUSIVE DISEASE

1. True renal arterial aneurysms are an uncommon vascular disease. Which of the following is/are true?

   a. True renal arterial aneurysms affect 0.09% of the general population
   b. 2.5% of patients with hypertension have true renal arterial aneurysms
   c. 9.2% of patients with hypertension and renal arterial fibrodysplasia have coexisting true renal artery aneurysms
   d. 10% of all patients undergoing arteriography for suspected renal parenchymal disease have true renal arterial aneurysms
   e. Men have true renal arterial aneurysms more often than do women

COMMENT: True macroaneurysms of the renal artery occur with varying frequency depending on the population being studied arteriographically. Aneurysms affect 0.09%, 2.5%, and 9.2% of the general population, the population with hypertension, and patients with arterial fibrodysplasia. Fewer than 1% of patients with renal parenchymal disease who undergo arteriography have these aneurysms. Women, because of their propensity to have medial fibroplasia, are more likely than men to have true renal arterial aneurysms.

ANSWER: a, b, c

REFERENCE: *Chapter 78—Renal Artery Occlusive Disease: Pathology of Renal Artery Occlusive Disease*

2. True renal arterial aneurysms usually are asymptomatic. Which of the following is/are true?

   a. Renal arterial aneurysms are saccular, occurring at branchings in more than 75% of cases
   b. These aneurysms are extraparenchymal in more than 90% of cases
   c. Most renal arterial aneurysms have a nonarteriosclerotic cause
   d. Thromboembolism from an aneurysm occurs in approximately 10% of cases and is a cause of renovascular hypertension
   e. Rupture of true renal arterial aneurysms occurs in 10% of cases

COMMENT: Most renal arterial macroaneurysms are saccular, having an average diameter less than 1 cm. Their origin is branchings in more than 75% of cases. More than 90% are extraparenchymal, and most are believed to arise from an elastic laminar defect. Arteriosclerosis is a secondary, not a causative event. Both thromboembolism and rupture have occurred in fewer than 3% of reported cases of true renal arterial aneurysm. Hypertension can be coincident with renal arterial aneurysms, but the aneurysm is uncommonly the cause of hypertension.

ANSWER: a, b, c

REFERENCE: *Chapter 78—Renal Artery Occlusive Disease: Pathology of Renal Artery Occlusive Disease*

3. Rupture is the most important clinical complication of a true renal arterial aneurysm. Which of the following is/are true?

   a. Rupture of renal arterial aneurysm is fatal in 10% of cases
   b. Rupture during pregnancy causes fetal death in 85% of cases and maternal death in 55% of cases
   c. Renal arterial aneurysm should be managed surgically only when associated with functionally important renal artery stenosis that causes renovascular hypertension
   d. Rupture of a renal arterial aneurysm is not likely to occur in calcified aneurysms of patients with normal blood pressure
   e. Loss of the kidney affects 50% of patients with rupture of a renal arterial aneurysm

COMMENT: Rupture of a renal arterial aneurysm occurs in less than 3% of cases and carries a 10% mortality with nearly invariable loss of the kidney among survivors. Rupture during pregnancy is more serious, causing the death of the mother in 55% of cases and of the fetus in 85%. Renal arterial aneurysm should be managed operatively when symptomatic and when the patient is a woman who may become pregnant. Large size of the aneurysm is a relative indication for operation, and calcification and normotension do not decrease the known risk of rupture.

ANSWER: a, b

REFERENCE: *Chapter 78—Renal Artery Occlusive Disease: Treatment*

4. Dissecting renal arterial aneurysms represent a heterogeneic group of diseases with a variety of causes. Which of the following is/are true?

   a. Dissecting renal arterial aneurysms rarely are bilateral
   b. Men have dissecting renal arterial aneurysms nearly ten times more often than do women
   c. Dissecting aneurysms caused by deceleration trauma and stretching of the renal artery usually have deep medial fractures
   d. Catheter-induced injury is a rare cause of dissecting renal arterial aneurysm
   e. Spontaneously occurring dissecting renal arterial aneurysm usually involves the intimal disruptions

COMMENT: Dissecting renal arterial aneurysms affect men nearly ten times more often than they do women, a reflection of the sex predilection for trauma and vascular diseases that contribute to dissection. Nearly one third of reported dissecting aneurysms are bilateral. Deceleration trauma with renal arterial stretching usually causes an intimal fracture with superficial periluminal dissection. In contrast, spontaneous dissections are deeper, involving the outer media. Catheter-induced dissection that causes renal arterial aneurysm is rare, occurring in less than 1 in 2,000 catheterizations.

ANSWER: b, d

REFERENCE: *Chapter 78—Renal Artery Occlusive Disease: Treatment*

5. A 35-year-old man involved in a head-on motor vehicle accident arrives in the emergency department with flank and back pain, hematuria, and an elevated blood pressure of 210/120 mm Hg. Renal arterial injury is suspected. Which of the following is/are true?

   a. The patient needs immediate intravenous pyelography
   b. Chronic dissecting renal arterial aneurysm can cause hypertension and renal insufficiency
   c. The patient needs early arteriography
   d. The patient needs an operation if he is found to have a hemodynamically important stenosis
   e. If the aneurysm is chronic, the patient needs an operation only if renal function deteriorates

COMMENT: Patients who may have deceleration renal arterial injury, often accompanied by dissecting aneurysm, are at high risk of loss of the kidney from ischemia. They need rapid arteriography and an operation without delay. Intravenous pyelography will not define the arterial injury, and even minor parenchymal contusions can cause lack of visualization of the kidney. Patients with chronic dissecting renal arterial aneurysm may have renovascular hypertension and renal insufficiency, the former being a valid indication for late operation.

ANSWER: c, d

REFERENCE: *Chapter 78—Renal Artery Occlusive Disease: Treatment*

CHAPTER 79

AORTOILIAC DISEASE

1. Which of the following is/are true of aortic anatomy?
   a. The abdominal aorta generally terminates at about L4, topographically the level of the umbilicus
   b. A retroaortic renal vein is present in approximately 25% of cases
   c. Multiple renal arteries are encountered in 5% to 7% of cases
   d. At the level of the renal arteries, the inferior vena cava is separated from the aorta by the renal pelvis and perirenal fat

COMMENT: The abdominal aorta begins at the aortic hiatus (T12) and continues to about L4, where it bifurcates into the common iliac arteries. This corresponds topographically to the approximate level of the umbilicus. The renal vein represents a major landmark in aortic surgery. It can be retroaortic in 5% of cases. Multiple renal arteries are encountered in 5% to 7% of cases, and at the level of the renal vein, the aorta approximates the vena cava.

ANSWER: a, c

REFERENCE: *Chapter 79—Aortoiliac Disease: Anatomy*

2. In the event of significant aortic occlusive disease, major collateral circulation includes:
   a. The internal mammary artery
   b. Intercostal and lumbar arteries
   c. Hypogastric arteries
   d. Superior mesenteric artery to inferior mesenteric artery collateral vessels

COMMENT: Both the visceral and the parietal collateral circulation compensate for major occlusive processes in the aortoiliac segment. All the structures listed are important sources of collateral circulation in the presence of aortoiliac occlusive disease.

ANSWER: a, b, c, d

REFERENCE: *Chapter 79—Aortoiliac Disease: Collateral Circulation*

3. Which of the following statements is/are true with respect to occlusion of the abdominal aorta?
   a. Most patients have profound rest pain or tissue loss
   b. The occlusive process usually involves the aortic bifurcation if the inferior mesenteric artery is patent
   c. If the inferior mesenteric artery is occluded, the occlusive process proceeds proximal to involve the infrarenal aorta
   d. This process is present in approximately 5% to 10% of patients undergoing operations for aortoiliac occlusive disease

COMMENT: Bilateral occlusion of the common iliac arteries or aortic bifurcation leads to propagation of thrombus and total occlusion of the infrarenal aorta. Complete aortic occlusion extends to the level of the inferior mesenteric artery if this vessel is patent. If the inferior mesenteric artery is occluded, the thrombus extends proximally to the juxtarenal aorta. Despite the severity of the occlusive process, the most common symptom is intermittent claudication. This process is present in 5% to 10% of patients undergoing aortoiliac reconstructive surgery.

ANSWER: b, c, d

REFERENCE: *Chapter 79—Aortoiliac Disease: Patterns of Disease and Clinical Manifestations*

4. From time to time, the clinical significance of an aortoiliac stenotic lesion is not obvious. Which of the following is/are indicative of hemodynamically significant aortoiliac occlusive disease?

   a. A resting pressure difference greater than 5 mm Hg between the distal aortic or brachial arterial pressure and common femoral arterial pressure
   b. A mean femoral arterial pressure of 80 mm Hg
   c. A decrease in femoral arterial pressure greater than 15% with reactive hyperemia induced either pharmacologically or by means of inflation of an occluding blood pressure cuff
   d. A systolic to diastolic pressure ratio greater than 2.0

COMMENT: Accurate assessment of occlusive disease usually is possible by means of traditional clinical evaluation and high-quality arteriography. From time to time determination of the hemodynamic significance of an occlusive process at each segmental level is critical in choosing the appropriate reconstructive procedure. A resting systolic pressure difference greater than 5 mm Hg or a decrease in femoral arterial pressure more than 15% from baseline with reactive hyperemia implies a hemodynamically significant inflow lesion. In general, inflow procedures are performed first.

ANSWER: a, c

REFERENCE: *Chapter 79—Aortoiliac Disease: Evaluation*

5. Which of the following is/are true with respect to aortoiliac endarterectomy?

   a. Fifty percent of patients with aortoiliac occlusive disease are eligible for this procedure
   b. Extended aortoiliofemoral endarterectomy as a straightforward technical procedure
   c. Because of increased risk of infection, it is less commonly performed than it once was
   d. Late patency rates are better than are those for aortofemoral bypass
   e. None of the above

COMMENT: Aortoiliac endarterectomy can be considered for the 5% to 10% of patients with truly localized disease (type I). Although it avoids the use of a prosthetic graft and thus has almost no risk of infection, it is considered technically more demanding than aortofemoral bypass. The long-term patency rates are not as good as those for bypass grafting in the care of patients with extensive disease.

ANSWER: e

REFERENCE: *Chapter 79—Aortoiliac Disease: Aortoiliac Endarterectomy*

6. Which of the following is/are true with respect to bypass grafts performed for aortoiliac occlusive disease?

   a. The proximal anastomosis can be either end to end or end to side
   b. The preferred site of distal anastomosis is the external iliac artery
   c. The bypass graft should originate as low as possible on the aorta
   d. The inferior mesenteric artery is routinely ligated

COMMENT: The proximal aortic anastomosis can be either end-to-end or end-to-side. End-to-end anastomosis is clearly indicated for patients with coexisting aneurysmal disease or complete aortic occlusion up to the level of the renal artery. The important principle with bypass grafting is to place the proximal anastomosis as high as possible on the infrarenal aorta. The distal anastomosis is almost always at the level of the femoral artery. This avoids the more difficult exposure of the external iliac artery in the pelvis and better allows the surgeon to manage associated occlusive disease in the common femoral artery and at the origin of the profunda femoris artery. The inferior mesenteric artery is rarely if ever ligated during aortofemoral reconstruction for occlusive disease.

ANSWER: a

REFERENCE: *Chapter 79—Aortoiliac Disease: Aortofemoral Bypass Grafts*

7. Which of the following is/are true with respect to the results of aortofemoral bypass operations?

   a. A 50% 5-year graft patency rate and 25% 10-year patency rate are the norm
   b. Perioperative mortality rates less than 5% are commonly achieved
   c. Mortality is directly related to widespread multilevel disease
   d. Anastomotic aneurysms are most common at the proximal anastomosis

COMMENT: Most large series in the modern era document 85% to 90% 5-year graft patency rates and 70% to 75% 10-year patency rates. Perioperative mortality rates well below 5% are uniformly achieved, and many centers report mortality of only 1% to 2%. The mortality risk is directly proportional to the severity of the lower extremity occlusive process. Patients with widespread multilevel disease have higher risk. Most anastomotic pseudoaneurysms occur at the femoral position.

ANSWER: b, c

REFERENCE: *Chapter 79—Aortoiliac Disease: Aortofemoral Bypass Grafts; Results*

8. Which of the following is/are true with respect to long-term complications of operations for aortoiliac occlusive disease?

   a. Graft limb occlusion occurs among 10% to 20% of patients whose cases are followed 10 years
   b. Anastomotic aneurysms occur among 20% of patients
   c. After reconstruction, cumulative long-term survival is the same as that of a healthy age- and sex-matched population
   d. Most late deaths are attributable to graft complications

COMMENT: The frequency of late complications depends on the length of the follow-up period. Ten percent to 20% of patients may have graft limb occlusion if their cases are followed for 10 years. Anastomotic pseudoaneurysms occur among 3% to 5% of patients, almost always at the femoral anastomosis. Cumulative long-term survival rates for patients with significant aortoiliac occlusive disease are 10 to 15 years less than those that may be anticipated for a healthy age- and sex-matched population. Most late deaths are attributable to coronary artery disease and its sequelae.

ANSWER: a

REFERENCE: *Chapter 79—Aortoiliac Disease: Results of Aortoiliac Surgical Revascularization*

CHAPTER 80

FEMOROPOPLITEAL AND INFRAPOPLITEAL OCCLUSIVE DISEASE

1. Which of the following is/are true with respect to the femoral artery?

   a. The femoral nerve is medial to the femoral artery
   b. The medial and lateral circumflex femoral artery typically arise from the common femoral artery
   c. Two to five inches below the inguinal ligament, the common femoral artery divides into the superficial femoral artery and the profunda femoris artery
   d. In the middle third of the leg, the profunda femoris artery enters the adductor canal (Hunter's canal)

COMMENT: The common femoral artery begins at the inguinal ligament as a direct extension of the external iliac artery. In the proximal thigh, the femoral nerve is lateral to the artery, and the femoral vein is medial. Two to five inches (5 to 12.5 cm) below the inguinal ligament, the common femoral artery divides into the profunda femoris (deep femoral) and superficial femoral arteries. The medial and lateral circumflex femoral arteries typically arise as branches of the deep femoral artery. The superficial femoral artery continues distally, passing through Hunter's canal to become the popliteal artery.

ANSWER: c

REFERENCE: *Chapter 80—Femoropopliteal and Infrapopliteal Occlusive Disease: Anatomy*

2. Which of the following is/are true with respect to the popliteal artery?

a. The popliteal artery usually is contained between the medial and lateral heads of the gastrocnemius muscle behind the knee
b. The two major branches of the popliteal artery are the anterior tibial artery and the tibioperoneal trunk
c. The peroneal artery is the main blood supply to the foot
d. The tibioperoneal trunk is the direct continuation of the popliteal artery

COMMENT: The popliteal artery emerges from the adductor canal and proceeds posteriorly behind the knee between the medial and lateral heads of the gastrocnemius muscle. It quickly divides into two major branches—the anterior tibial artery and the tibial peroneal trunk. The latter, the direct continuation of the popliteal artery, gives rise to both the posterior tibial artery and the peroneal artery. The peroneal artery courses deeply in the substance of the calf and stops just above the ankle. The anterior and posterior tibial arteries supply the foot.

ANSWER: a, b, d

REFERENCE: *Chapter 80—Femoropopliteal and Infrapopliteal Occlusive Disease: Anatomy*

3. Which of the following is the most likely artery in the lower extremity to be obstructed by atherosclerosis?

a. The popliteal artery
b. The deep femoral artery
c. The superficial femoral artery
d. The common femoral artery

COMMENT: The superficial femoral artery is the most likely artery in the lower extremity to be obstructed by atherosclerosis. The popliteal, deep femoral, common femoral, and calf arteries are involved less frequently. The occlusive process is distributed more distally among persons with diabetes.

ANSWER: c

REFERENCE: *Chapter 80—Femoropopliteal and Infrapopliteal Occlusive Disease: Collateral Circulation*

4. Which of the following is/are true with respect to intermittent claudication?

a. Resting blood flow is typically within the normal range
b. Fixed obstruction precludes normal augmentation of flow in response to exercise
c. Symptoms are produced one level above and one level below the site of arterial obstruction
d. Most patients with claudication have multilevel disease

COMMENT: Moderate arterial obstruction produces no change in resting blood flow but restricts the ability of arterial flow to increase normally in response to exercise. The site of the symptoms is always one level distal to the site of arterial obstruction. Most patients with symptoms confined to claudication have dominant arterial obstruction at a single site.

ANSWER: a, b

REFERENCE: *Chapter 80—Femoropopliteal and Infrapopliteal Occlusive Disease: Pathophysiology*

5. Which of the following is/are true regarding the course of infrainguinal arteriosclerosis?

a. Approximately 50% of persons with claudication need limb amputation
b. Persons with claudication and an ankle-brachial index (ABI) less than 0.5 are as likely to need revascularization as those with a higher ratio
c. Infrainguinal atherosclerosis is an important predictor of life expectancy
d. Among patients undergoing reoperation for limb-threatening ischemia, the 5-year survival rate is approximately 70%

COMMENT: Less than 10% of persons with claudication ever need amputation of an ischemic limb. However, the presence and severity of lower extremity ischemia are more readily and accurately assessed by quantitative means in a noninvasive laboratory as well as by clinical assessment. Patients with claudication and an ABI less than 0.5 are approximately 3.5 times as likely to need revascularization as those with higher ABIs. Life expectancy is directly proportional to the severity of lower-extremity ischemia. Among patients with mild claudication, the 5-year survival rate is 97.4%. Among patients who need operations for claudication, the 5-year survival rate is 80%. It decreases to 48% among patients with limb-threatening ischemia and is only 12% among patients who need reoperations for limb-threatening ischemia.

ANSWER: c

REFERENCE: *Chapter 80—Femoropopliteal and Infrapopliteal Occlusive Disease: Natural History of Limb Threatening Atherosclerosis*

6. Which of the following is/are true with respect to exercise and lower-extremity vascular disease?

   a. Improvement in walking distance in a structured exercise program results from increased collateral development
   b. Ankle brachial indices parallel improvement in walking distance
   c. Increased oxygen extraction and decreased venous lactate level are characteristic
   d. Most patients who have a benefit notice it within 8 to 12 weeks

COMMENT: It was formerly assumed that improvement in walking distance resulted from increased collateral development, but this is not the case, and most patients do not have improvement in ABI after exercise training. They do have improvement in metabolic efficiency and extract more oxygen and produce less lactate with the same amount of exercise. Eight to 12 weeks typically is sufficient to notice the benefits.

ANSWER: c, d

REFERENCE: *Chapter 80—Femoropopliteal and Infrapopliteal Occlusive Disease: Exercise*

7. Which of the following is/are true with respect to pharmacologic management of lower-extremity ischemia?

   a. In large vessels, the important flow characteristic is viscosity
   b. In the microcirculation, cellular deformability is a critical determinant of blood flow
   c. Vasodilators have proved effective in the management of lower-extremity ischemia
   d. No properly constructed clinical trials exist to document the benefits of any pharmacologic intervention in lower-extremity occlusive disease

COMMENT: Vasodilators are not approved for use in the United States for management of lower-extremity ischemia. The most important flow characteristic in large vessels is blood viscosity. In the microcirculation, cellular deformability is critical. Erythrocytes are typically 6 to 8 μm in diameter, and leukocytes are 6 to 15 mm, whereas capillaries are typically 4 to 5 μm in diameter. Deformability is important in terms of capillary perfusion capacity, and pentoxifylline affects blood viscosity, cellular deformability, and cellular aggregation. A number of prospective, double-blind trials in the United States and Europe have shown that this drug increases treadmill walking distance among approximately one half of persons with claudication.

ANSWER: a, b

REFERENCE: *Chapter 80—Femoropopliteal and Infrapopliteal Occlusive Disease: Pharmacologic Therapy*

8. Which of the following is/are true regarding bypass grafting in the lower extremities?

   a. Reversed saphenous vein is the preferred method of reconstruction
   b. Prosthetic bypasses work as well as saphenous vein as long as the bypass is confined to the popliteal artery
   c. Alternative vein sources, such as arm, lesser saphenous, and superficial femoral veins, have been successfully used for lower-extremity reconstruction
   d. Reconstruction below the level of the malleolus is unlikely to succeed

COMMENT: Bypasses for management of infrainguinal atherosclerosis has been expanded to include almost any conceivable site. Saphenous vein remains the best conduit, and either the in situ or reverse saphenous vein technique can be used. Saphenous vein has a clear advantage over a prosthesis in almost all sites, including bypasses to the popliteal artery. When necessary, autogenous vein reconstruction with alternative vein sources can be performed. Bypass to the pedal arteries is routinely performed with excellent patency and limb salvage.

ANSWER: c

REFERENCE: *Chapter 80—Femoropopliteal and Infrapopliteal Occlusive Disease: Vein Bypass Graft*

9. Which of the following is/are true with respect to lower-extremity bypass?
   a. Survival is strongly influenced by the indication for operation
   b. Long-term patency is related to the quality of the vein conduit, the site of distal anastomosis, and the indication for operation
   c. In situ techniques are clearly preferable
   d. The long-term limb salvage rate after 5 years is approximately 25%

COMMENT: Survival after lower-extremity venous bypass is most strongly influenced by the indication for operation because the severity of the systemic atherosclerotic process is accurately mirrored by the severity of the atherosclerosis of the lower extremity. Persons with claudication have significantly better survival rates than do patients treated for limb-threatening ischemia. The long-term patency of venous grafts is directly related to the quality of the vein conduit, the site of the distal anastomosis, the original indication for operation, and the experience and skill of the operating team. Despite considerable controversy, there seems little difference in patency between reversed or in situ techniques, and either technique results in a long-term limb salvage rate of approximately 80%.

ANSWER: a, b

REFERENCE: *Chapter 80—Femoropopliteal and Infrapopliteal Occlusive Disease: Complications*

CHAPTER 81

LOWER EXTREMITY AMPUTATION

1. Which of the following is/are true with respect to the indications for amputation?
   a. The most common cause of lower-extremity amputation is osteogenic sarcoma
   b. The aggressive limb salvage technique of arterial reconstruction has reduced the need for amputation
   c. Among patients with unreconstructable vascular disease and unremitting rest pain or wet gangrene, amputation is acceptable as a primary procedure
   d. When a graft fails, amputation is inevitable

COMMENT: The most common indication for amputation in the United States is chronic irreversible ischemia secondary to atherosclerotic occlusive disease or diabetes. This can cause gangrene, unremitting rest pain, and invasive infection. Amputation for tumor, congenital deformity, or trauma is much less common. Aggressive arterial reconstruction techniques, including in situ bypass, composite grafting, and the distal origination of bypass grafts from the profunda femoris (deep femoral) or popliteal artery, sometimes with veins harvested from remote sites, has resulted in salvage of limbs that would previously have been amputated. Amputation is not inevitable after late graft failure, but primary amputation remains an appropriate procedure in the care of patients with wet gangrene or unreconstructable disease.

ANSWER: b, c

REFERENCE: *Chapter 81—Lower Extremity Amputation: Indications*

2. Which of the following aid(s) in the selection of the appropriate level of amputation?

    a. Physical assessment
    b. Doppler segmental blood pressures
    c. Transcutaneous oxygen measurements
    d. Laser Doppler findings

COMMENT: Selection of the appropriate amputation level is guided by the basic principle of removing all necrotic, painful, and dysfunctional tissue while ensuring primary wound healing and maximal potential for rehabilitation. In practice, most decisions regarding the level of amputation are made with a combination of clinical assessment and relatively simple tests such as Doppler determination of segmental arterial blood pressure. A blood pressure of 55 mm Hg at the knee or 60 to 75 mm Hg in the low thigh usually is predictive of healing of a below-knee amputation. Both transcutaneous oxygen determination and measurement of skin blood flow with a laser Doppler device have gained increased acceptance. Other techniques, such as isotope clearance, fluorescein injection, and photoplethysmography or thermography, have not yet received widespread acceptance.

ANSWER: a, b, c, d

REFERENCE: *Chapter 81—Lower Extremity Amputation: Choice of Level of Amputation*

3. Which of the following is/are true with respect to below-knee amputation?

    a. Primary healing occurs in 85% to 90% of such procedures
    b. The mortality is less than 1%
    c. Technical features include a fish-mouth incision and tibial weight bearing
    d. Walking with a below-knee prosthesis requires a 200% increase in energy expenditure

COMMENT: Despite occasional reports of relatively low mortality, the average reported mortality for below-knee amputation is 10% to 12%, reflecting the serious underlying systemic illnesses common among such patients. Primary healing occurs in approximately 85% to 95% of cases. The standard operative technique entails use of a long posterior flap. The end of the stump is not a weight-bearing surface. Walking with a below-knee prosthesis regularly requires a 30% to 60% increase in energy expenditure. Walking with an above-knee prosthesis may require a 100% increase in energy expenditure.

ANSWER: a

REFERENCE: *Chapter 81—Lower Extremity Amputation: Below-knee Amputation*

CHAPTER 82

PATHOGENESIS OF ANEURYSMS

1. Excluding intracranial aneurysms, the most common site of aneurysm formation is:

    a. Thoracic aorta
    b. Infrarenal abdominal aorta
    c. Superior mesenteric artery
    d. Common femoral artery

COMMENT: The most common location for aneurysms is the infrarenal abdominal aorta. Superior mesenteric arterial and femoral arterial aneurysms are distinctly uncommon. Thoracic aortic aneurysms are intermediate in frequency. Overall, abdominal aortic aneurysm (AAA) ranks fifteenth as a cause of death in the United States, and the incidence appears to be increasing.

ANSWER: b

REFERENCE: *Chapter 82—Pathogenesis of Aneurysms: Incidence*

2. Which of the following statements is/are true with respect to the epidemiology of AAA?

a. Autopsy studies indicate a prevalence range between 1.8% and 6.6%
b. There are 200,000 deaths per year of AAA
c. The apparent incidence of aneurysms has increased dramatically over the last 30 years
d. The male to female ratio of AAA is approximately 10:1

COMMENT: Approximately 15,000 deaths per year are caused by AAA. The prevalence has increased dramatically over the last 30 years; in autopsy series, it ranges from 1.8% to 6.6%. At least a portion of this increase may be due to better diagnostic imaging modalities and the aging population. The increase in the incidence of AAA occurred despite an overall decrease in the rate of coronary artery disease and stroke. This finding suggests aneurysmal disease of the aorta may have a different cause from atherosclerotic stenotic disease. Contemporary reports of the male to female sex ratio for AAA range from 2:1 to 8:1, most authors suggesting a male to female ratio of approximately 4:1.

ANSWER: a, c

REFERENCE: *Chapter 82—Pathogenesis of Aneurysms: Incidence*

3. Which of the following statements is/are true with respect to AAA?

a. White men have a threefold higher incidence than do black men
b. Patients with a family history of AAA among first-degree relatives are more likely to have AAA
c. The peak prevalence of AAA is 10 to 15 years later among women than it is among men
d. Patients with AAA tend to be taller and older than typical patients with atherosclerosis and occlusive disease

COMMENT: Better epidemiologic studies with population-based inquiries, family studies, and other epidemiologic techniques have shown a genetic component to AAA. Patients with a family history in a first-degree relative are much more likely to have AAA than are control patients. White men have an incidence of AAA threefold higher than that among black men or women. Patients with AAA tend to be taller and older than are typical patients with atherosclerotic occlusive disease. The peak prevalence is 10 to 15 years later among women than it is among men.

ANSWER: a, b, c, d

REFERENCE: *Chapter 82—Pathogenesis of Aneurysms: Incidence*

4. Which of the following characterize(s) the histologic and histochemical features of AAA?

a. A decrease in the amount of elastin
b. Marked adventitial inflammatory cell infiltration
c. More immunoglobulin in extracts from aneurysms than in normal aorta
d. Decrease in elastin content directly correlates with the size of the aneurysm

COMMENT: Unlike occlusive disease, in which medial elastin tissue is often well preserved, AAA is associated with a noteworthy decrease in the amount of elastin. Conspicuous inflammatory infiltration in the adventitia is found at histologic examination, as are more immunoglobulins in extracts of the aortic aneurysmal wall. The decrease in elastin content does not correlate with the size of the aneurysm and appears to be essentially complete at a relatively early stage of aneurysm development.

ANSWER: a, b, c

REFERENCE: *Chapter 82—Pathogenesis of Aneurysms: Arterial Structure*

5. Which of the following is/are true with respect to aortic elastin?

a. Numerous studies have confirmed deficiency of elastin within aortic aneurysms; however, the amount of collagen has been found to be normal, decreased, or increased
b. Human tissues do not generate much new elastin after the first decade of life
c. Vessels treated with elastase dilate and become less compliant
d. Glycine makes up one third of the amino acids of elastin

COMMENT: Most human tissues do not generate much new elastin after the first decade of life. Most studies of aortic aneurysm have shown there is a decrease in the amount of elastin. The amount of collagen has been found to be normal, increased, or decreased, most likely because fibroblasts have substantial ability to synthesize new collagen to repair deficiencies. In ex vivo models of human iliac arteries, vessels treated with elastase dilated and became stiffer. The human aorta also has been found to become less compliant with age. Glycine is the most common amino acid in elastin, composing approximately one third of all the amino acid residues.

ANSWER: a, b, c, d

REFERENCE: *Chapter 82—Pathogenesis of Aneurysms: Biochemistry*

6. Which of the following statements is/are true regarding elastin in aortic tissue?
   a. Elastin is arranged in layers
   b. The number of lamellae in the abdominal aorta of humans is disproportionately low for the load that it must bear (compared with other mammalian species)
   c. The estimated half-life of elastin is approximately 70 years
   d. Elastin is synthesized solely by mesothelial cells

COMMENT: Elastin is synthesized by many mesenchymal cells, such as smooth muscle cells, chondroblasts, mesothelial cells, fibroblasts, and myofibroblasts. Its half-life is approximately 70 years, and little de novo synthesis occurs after the first decade of life. The typical arrangement of elastin fibers is in lamellae separated by smooth muscle cells. This pattern is found in all mammalian species, but the human abdominal aorta has a disproportionately low number of lamellae for the load that it carries.

ANSWER: a, b, c

REFERENCE: *Chapter 82—Pathogenesis of Aneurysms: Biochemistry*

7. Which of the following is/are true with respect to aortic collagen?
   a. Glycine, proline, and hydroxyproline are the major amino acid constituents of collagen
   b. The backbone of a collagen molecule is the left-handed helix called an *α chain*
   c. The tensile strength of collagen is four times greater than that of elastin
   d. Elastin bears the load at small diameters, but as arterial diameter increases, collagen increasingly bears the load and prevents further progression and aneurysmal expansion

COMMENT: In a normal aorta, elastin bears much of the pressure load. However, as the aorta degenerates and arterial diameter increases, collagen bears an increasing portion of the load and prevents further dilation and aneurysmal expansion. Collagen is substantially stronger than elastin in terms of tensile strength but it is much less resilient. The major amino acid constituents of collagen include glycine, proline, and hydroxyproline organized into an α chain.

ANSWER: a, b, c, d

REFERENCE: *Chapter 82—Pathogenesis of Aneurysms: Biochemistry*

8. Which of the following is/are true with respect to fibrillin, an important structure of the extracellular matrix?
   a. Fibrillin acts as the scaffolding for the deposition of elastin during elastogenesis
   b. Fibrillin mutations cause Marfan's syndrome
   c. The gene for fibrillin is located in the long arm of chromosome 15
   d. Fibrillin is important in the pathogenesis of AAA

COMMENT: Recognition that fibrillin serves as scaffolding for the deposition of elastin during elastogenesis and that the gene for fibrillin is located on the long arm of chromosome 15 and is responsible for Marfan's syndrome has caused investigators to consider its role in AAA disease, but this is not yet established.

ANSWER: a, b, c

REFERENCE: *Chapter 82—Pathogenesis of Aneurysms: Thoracic Aortic Aneurysms*

9. Which of the following is/are true regarding extracellular matrix proteins?
   a. Elastase activity is increased in AAA tissue
   b. Collagenase activity is increased in AAA tissue
   c. Matrix metalloproteinases are present in tissue from AAA
   d. The level of tissue plasminogen activator has been found to be elevated in AAA

COMMENT: Increased collagenase activity in AAA was found in 1980 and increased elastase activity in 1982. Since then, many investigators have confirmed these results. Leukocyte, pancreatic, and smooth muscle elastase all have been implicated. The story with collagenases is a little less clear, but most investigators believe levels of these substances are elevated as well. Matrix metalloproteinases 1 through 9 are a family of extracellular proteinases that digest components of the matrix, including collagen, elastin, fibronectin, laminae, and proteoglycans. Level of tissue plasminogen activator has been found to be elevated in AAA. Plasmin is known to degrade extracellular matrix, and it appears that plasmin may have a role in the pathogenesis of AAA.

ANSWER: a, b, c, d

REFERENCE: *Chapter 82—Pathogenesis of Aneurysms: Extracellular Matrix*

10. Which of the following findings suggesting inflammation have a role in AAA?

   a. Increased concentrations of T and B lymphocytes and macrophages in the adventitia

   b. Recognition that levels of interleukin-1β and TNFα are higher in AAA extracts than in control substances

   c. A specific IgG immunoglobulin directed against aortic wall antigen

   d. Control of aneurysm size with administration of aspirin

COMMENT: Although aspirin administration has several beneficial effects in vascular disorders, it has not been implicated in the pathogenesis of AAA. At histologic examination, T and B lymphocytes and macrophages often have been found in the adventitial layer of aortic aneurysms. The lymphocytes are known to secrete cytokines, including interferon-γ, tumor necrosis factor α, and the interleukins. These factors can increase the proteolytic activity of macrophages and thereby potentiate aneurysmal dilation and rupture. These findings have been detected in "garden variety" AAA—they are not specific to inflammatory AAA.

ANSWER: a, b, c

REFERENCE: *Chapter 82—Pathogenesis of Aneurysms: Inflammatory Changes*

CHAPTER 83

EXTRACRANIAL CAROTID, INNOMINATE, SUBCLAVIAN, AND AXILLARY ARTERY ANEURYSMS

1. A 58-year-old male smoker reports small, painful, dark blue spots on the tips of the first and fifth fingers of his left hand. Blood pressure in his left arm is 20 mm Hg less than that in the right arm at rest. The patient also has a left supraclavicular bruit. Duplex ultrasound examination confirms a left subclavian artery aneurysm with thrombus. Which of the following is least useful as a diagnostic test?

   a. Posteroanterior and lateral chest radiographs

   b. Computed tomography of the chest

   c. Pulse volume recordings of the left hand

   d. Arch arteriography

   e. Magnetic resonance imaging of chest

COMMENT: Each of the options other than c adds to the needed information to plan management of this lesion. Chest radiographs may show a cervical or abnormal first rib. Computed tomography of the chest also may show this abnormality and give anatomic information regarding the aneurysm that duplex ultrasound examination cannot provide. Most surgeons would consider arch arteriography mandatory before treating a patient for this condition. Magnetic resonance imaging and magnetic resonance angiography have proved extremely useful in the care of many patients and may prove to be the diagnostic tests of choice in the coming years. Pulse volume recordings of the left hand are not of use in evaluation and management at this time in this case.

ANSWER: c

REFERENCE: *Chapter 83—Extracranial Carotid, Innominate, Subclavian, and Axillary Artery Aneurysms: Diagnosis and Evaluation*

2. Arch arteriography of the patient in question 1 shows a poststenotic aneurysm originating in the middle portion of the subclavian artery and tapering quickly within the mid to distal intrathoracic subclavian artery. Which of the following treatments is most likely to give this patient long-term recovery from this condition?

   a. Endovascular stent placement
   b. Anticoagulation
   c. Resection of diseased artery and interposition graft with synthetic graft
   d. Resection of diseased artery, cervicodorsal sympathectomy, and interposition synthetic graft
   e. Resection of diseased artery, first rib resection, and interposition synthetic graft

COMMENT: Resection of the diseased artery and offending first rib with interposition grafting are essential in the treatment of this patient. If there is no evidence of narrowing caused by a cervical or prominent first rib and the aneurysm appears to be atherosclerotic, resection without rib resection would be the best procedure. Cervicodorsal sympathectomy has a limited role in persistent severe ischemia with chronic pain. Although endovascular stenting has been found technically feasible, its long-term effectiveness has not been established in the management of this condition.

ANSWER: e

REFERENCE: *Chapter 83—Extracranial Carotid, Innominate, Subclavian, and Axillary Artery Aneurysms: Surgical or Endovascular Treatment*

3. For the patient described in questions 1 and 2, which of the following would not be an appropriate approach to the mid-subclavian pathologic lesion?

   a. Combined supraclavicular and infraclavicular approaches
   b. Left posterolateral thoracotomy
   c. Median sternotomy
   d. Left transaxillary approach
   e. Isolated left infraclavicular approach

COMMENT: Because the aortic arch runs posteriorly near the takeoff of the left subclavian artery, median sternotomy generally does not provide easy access to the left subclavian artery. Any of the other approaches can be used depending on exact location of the aneurysm and the surgeon's preference.

ANSWER: c

REFERENCE: *Chapter 83—Extracranial Carotid, Innominate, Subclavian, and Axillary Artery Aneurysms: Surgical or Endovascular Treatment*

4. Which of the following maneuvers is/are not appropriate in exposure of the distal internal carotid artery during repair of a carotid artery aneurysm?

   a. Nasotracheal intubation
   b. Subluxation of the jaw
   c. Division of the posterior belly of the digastric muscle
   d. Division of the glossopharyngeal nerve
   e. Division of the stylomandibular ligament

COMMENT: Each of these maneuvers may be necessary in exposing a difficult, distal internal carotid artery except division of the glossopharyngeal nerve. This nerve generally runs with or directly behind the posterior belly of the digastric muscle. Injury to the glossopharyngeal nerve is the most morbid of all cranial nerve injuries. The risk of cranial nerve injury is accepted to be somewhat higher in repair of carotid artery aneurysms, and cranial nerve dysfunction may be the presenting symptom for such patients.

ANSWER: d

REFERENCE: *Chapter 83—Extracranial Carotid, Innominate, Subclavian, and Axillary Artery Aneurysms: Carotid Artery Aneurysm*

CHAPTER 84

THORACIC AORTIC ANEURYSMS

1. Which of the following statements is/are true with respect to thoracic aortic aneurysms?
   a. Unlike abdominal aortic aneurysm (AAA), which is increasing in frequency, the incidence of thoracic aortic aneurysm appears to be declining
   b. Involvement of the descending aorta is more common than involvement of the ascending aorta
   c. The natural history of thoracic aortic aneurysm has been well described
   d. It has been possible to manage thoracic aortic aneurysm for only approximately the last 30 years

COMMENT: Thoracic aortic aneurysm appears to be increasing in frequency, as are AAAs. There is an approximately 3:1 male to female ratio. That many patients have a family history of thoracic aortic aneurysm suggests a genetic component. The descending aorta is the most common site of thoracic aneurysm. Unlike AAA, the natural history of these aneurysms remains only vaguely defined. In a series of 600 patients described before operative repair was possible, two thirds died as result of the aneurysm. Until recently, however, inability to precisely measure thoracic aortic aneurysms has limited natural history studies. Finally, many developments in vascular surgery occurred in the early 1950s, including the first AAA repair, the first carotid endarterectomy, and the first report of successful resection of a thoracic aortic aneurysm.

ANSWER: b

REFERENCE: *Chapter 84—Thoracic Aortic Aneurysms: Arteriosclerotic Aneurysms*

2. With respect to Marfan syndrome which of the following is/are true?
   a. It is an autosomal recessive disorder
   b. Abnormalities of fibrillin, the main component of extracellular microfibrils, have been detected and are caused by a defective gene on the long arm of chromosome 15
   c. The aneurysms in Marfan syndrome begin more proximally than do arteriosclerotic aneurysms, that is, at the level of the aortic annulus, and involve the coronary sinuses as well as the supracoronary aorta
   d. If the person is not treated, Marfan syndrome reduces life expectancy approximately 10 years

COMMENT: Marfan syndrome is a severe, autosomal dominant disorder with variable clinical manifestations. The defective gene for fibrillin is located on the long arm of chromosome 15. The connective tissue disorder is widespread and involves the aortic annulus rather than arising at the level of the sinotubular ridge as do atherosclerotic aneurysms. This is important because it often requires replacement of the aortic valve and implantation of the coronary arteries. Historical series have made it abundantly clear that untreated patients with Marfan syndrome have markedly reduced life expectancies. Fewer than one half of patients live past the age of 45 years, and more than 90% of deaths have cardiovascular causes.

ANSWER: b, c

REFERENCE: *Chapter 84—Thoracic Aortic Aneurysms: Marfan Syndrome*

3. Which of the following statements with respect to aortic dissection is/are true?

    a. Acute dissection of the thoracic aorta is more common than a ruptured AAA
    b. Timely diagnosis is critical because the mortality is 1% to 2% per hour during the first 24 to 48 hours after acute dissection
    c. If the dissection is not diagnosed, the mortality rate for ascending aortic dissection approaches 90% at 3 months
    d. Most such patients receive prompt diagnoses

COMMENT: The incidence of acute aortic dissection is approximately twice that of ruptured AAA. Acute aortic dissection can manifest with protean signs and symptoms and mimic other, more common illnesses. This results in a delay in diagnosis and often in excessive mortality. The mortality is 1% to 2% per hour during the first 24 to 48 hours; if dissection is not diagnosed the mortality is fully 90% within 3 months. Even in the modern era, one third of cases of dissection go undiagnosed.

ANSWER: a, b, c

REFERENCE: *Chapter 84—Thoracic Aortic Aneurysms: Aortic Dissections*

4. Which of the following is the best diagnostic modality for aortic dissection?

    a. Contrast enhanced dynamic computed tomography or magnetic resonance imaging
    b. Biplanar aortography
    c. Multiplanar transesophageal echocardiography
    d. Whichever test is most readily and rapidly available at the institution

COMMENT: All of these diagnostic modalities have sufficient accuracy to establish the diagnosis. Given the 1.5% to 2% hourly mortality of acute aortic dissection, it is imperative that prompt diagnosis be made and treatment instituted. Whichever test is most readily available should be used.

ANSWER: d

REFERENCE: *Chapter 84—Thoracic Aortic Aneurysms: Aortic Dissections*

5. Which of the following is/are true with regard to traumatic thoracic aortic disruption?

    a. The most common site of injury is just distal to the ligamentum arteriosum
    b. Eighty percent to 90% of patients who sustain this injury die at the time of the acute event
    c. Among survivors, the aortic adventitia and pleura temporarily contain the hemorrhage
    d. Traumatic disruption of the aorta can occur with no other signs of serious chest trauma

COMMENT: Decelerating trauma resulting in thoracic aortic disruption is common, and most patients (80% to 90%) die immediately. Among the others, the rupture is partially contained by the aortic adventitia and pleura, but the risk of subsequent hemorrhage is real. The most frequent site of rupture is just distal to the ligamentum arteriosum. Early diagnosis and early operative repair are indicated in most instances.

ANSWER: a, b, c, d

REFERENCE: *Chapter 84—Thoracic Aortic Aneurysms: Miscellaneous Conditions*

CHAPTER 85

THORACOABDOMINAL ANEURYSMS

1. Which of the following statements is/are true regarding thoracoabdominal aortic aneurysm (TAAA)?

   a. Reliable epidemiologic data on TAAA are available
   b. The natural history of untreated TAAA is precisely known
   c. In the only large series of patients with untreated TAAA, 68% of untreated patients died, and of these 57% died of aneurysm rupture
   d. As with abdominal aortic aneurysm, available data suggest that TAAA develops from loss of elastin

COMMENT: Because of the relatively low prevalence of these lesions, reliable epidemiologic and natural history data are not available. Many of the estimates are based on autopsy studies from urban areas and reflect a selected referral pattern. The available data suggest that untreated TAAA eventually ruptures and causes death. Only 19% of patients with untreated TAAA survive 5 years, whereas 60% of those undergoing TAAA repair survive 5 years. Histochemical and histopathologic studies of TAAA have not been done.

ANSWER: c

REFERENCE: *Chapter 85—Thoracoabdominal Aneurysms: Magnitude of the Problem*

2. Which of the following is/are true regarding clinical manifestations of TAAA?

   a. Small TAAAs (less than 5 cm in diameter) usually are asymptomatic
   b. The cephalic extent of the aneurysm may be indistinct in the upper abdomen
   c. Most patients have symptoms when first encountered
   d. Occasionally symptoms and compression of adjacent structures or distal embolization can occur

COMMENT: Although approximately three fourths of patients with TAAA have symptoms when first encountered and almost one half have frank rupture, small TAAAs of less than 5 cm in diameter usually are asymptomatic. At physical examination, the cephalic extent of the aneurysm usually is not palpable. Compression of adjacent viscera or renal arteries occasionally produces atypical symptoms, as can embolization or thrombosis.

ANSWER: a, b, c, d

REFERENCE: *Chapter 85—Thoracoabdominal Aneurysms: Clinical Manifestations*

3. Which of the following is/are true regarding the operative management of TAAA?

   a. Current management favors the graft inclusion technique

   b. A posterolateral thoracoabdominal incision is used to gain access to the aorta

   c. Management of the visceral vessels usually allows the celiac, superior mesenteric, and right renal arteries to be reimplanted as a single button. The left renal artery occasionally can be included with the other three visceral vessels, but most often it is reimplanted separately

   d. The distal anastomosis is performed after reperfusion of the viscera

COMMENT: The graft inclusion technique has largely replaced bypass with multiple side arms. This remains a formidable surgical procedure. Multiple technical requirements for anesthesia, blood bank, and experienced nursing exist. The standard surgical approach is through a posterolateral thoracoabdominal incision. The aorta is exposed in either the retroperitoneal or the retroperitoneal-transperitoneal approach. A variety of adjuvants to enhance spinal cord perfusion and visceral perfusion have been advocated. Few have demonstrated efficacy. After completion of the proximal anastomosis in an end-to-end manner, the visceral patch is performed with the celiac, superior mesenteric, and right renal arteries. The left renal artery is reimplanted separately. If the anatomy is favorable, all four visceral vessels occasionally can be anastomosed in a single patch. Perfusion of the viscera is performed before completion of the distal anastomosis.

ANSWER: a, b, c, d

REFERENCE: *Chapter 85—Thoracoabdominal Aneurysms: Operative Technique*

4. Which of the following statements is/are true regarding the results of operative repair of TAAA?

   a. The overall mortality rate is between 9% and 15% but increases dramatically for emergency procedures and for aneurysms of maximal extent

   b. Major complications include postoperative bleeding, respiratory insufficiency, renal failure, and spinal cord ischemia

   c. The rate of occurrence of neurologic deficits for types I, II, III, and IV TAAA are as high as 12%, 27%, 46%, and 3%

   d. Reimplantation of intercostal arteries effectively eliminates neurologic complications

COMMENT: Results of operative repair have improved, but clinical reports of elective repair of TAAA often describe operative mortality rates of 10% to 15%, the more extensive aneurysms having even higher mortality. For emergency operations, the operative mortality rate approaches 50%. Major complications include postoperative bleeding, respiratory insufficiency, renal failure, and spinal cord ischemia in addition to all of the other predictable complications of major vascular reconstruction. Paralysis remains an unpredictable, unpreventable, and uncontrollable complication. Opinion is divided regarding the utility of intercostal reimplantation. A host of other adjuvant measures have been proposed to protect the spinal cord. None has met with universal success.

ANSWER: a, b, c

REFERENCE: *Chapter 85—Thoracoabdominal Aneurysms: Results*

CHAPTER 86

ABDOMINAL AORTIC ANEURYSMS

1. Which of the following is/are associated with risk of development of abdominal aortic aneurysm (AAA)?
   a. Smoking
   b. Family history of first-degree relative with an AAA
   c. Heart transplant
   d. History of intracranial aneurysms
   e. Portal hypertension

COMMENT: The multiple risk factors for the development of AAA include age, sex, smoking history, hypertension, hyperlipidemia, and family history. The Aneurysm Detection and Management (ADAM) Veterans Affairs Cooperative Study Group reported that smoking was the strongest risk factor associated with AAAs larger than 4 cm in diameter (odds ratio 5.57; 95% confidence interval 4.24–7.31) among the 73,451 veterans screened. Johansen and Koepsell reported that the incidence of AAA was 19.2% among first-degree relatives of patients with aneurysms, but only 2.4% among the first-degree relatives of the control patients with atherosclerosis of the abdominal aorta. The prevalence of AAA and the rate of expansion both are high among recipients of heart transplants. A history of intracranial aneurysm and portal hypertension are not independent risk factors for aortic aneurysm.

ANSWER: a, b, c

REFERENCE: *Chapter 86—Abdominal Aortic Aneurysms: Pathogenesis and Risk Factors*

2. Which of the following statements regarding the natural history of AAA and its management is/are true?
   a. The risk of rupture is inversely related to diameter
   b. The overall mortality of a ruptured AAA is 50%
   c. Operative mortality is equivalent for symptomatic and asymptomatic intact AAAs
   d. All AAAs should be repaired electively regardless of size
   e. Operative repair of an asymptomatic, intact AAA is a prophylactic operation

COMMENT: The decision to offer surgical repair of an asymptomatic, intact AAA is based on weighing the natural history of an AAA against the risk of operation. The goal of this prophylactic surgical therapy remains to lower the chance of death of ruptured AAA. The risk of AAA rupture is directly related to size. A general rule is that the annual rupture risk is 5% for a 5-cm aneurysm, 10% for a 6-cm aneurysm, and 20% for a 7-cm aneurysm. Approximately 50% of patients with a ruptured AAA die before reaching the hospital. Approximately 50% of those operated on die. This corresponds to an overall mortality rate of ruptured AAAs of approximately 80%, although this may be an underestimate. The operative mortality rate for intact symptomatic aneurysms among patients undergoing emergency repair is approximately 20%, significantly higher than the rate for intact asymptomatic aneurysms (mortality approximately 4%).

ANSWER: e

REFERENCE: *Chapter 86—Abdominal Aortic Aneurysms: Clinical Presentation and Diagnosis; Operative Indications*

3. Which of the following statements is/are true in relation to the presentation and evolution of AAA?

a. Most patients have compressive symptoms due to the mass effect of the aneurysm
b. Abdominal ultrasound remains the most cost-effective test to evaluate for ruptured AAA
c. Computed tomography (CT) is the contemporary standard for determining aneurysm suitability for endovascular repair
d. Angiography provides consistent overestimates of AAA diameter because of parallax magnification effects
e. Indications for angiography before elective repair of AAA include concomitant lower extremity occlusive disease, suspicion of renovascular hypertension, or presence of a horseshoe kidney

COMMENT: The overwhelming majority of patients with AAA have no symptoms. Most aneurysms are found incidentally during abdominopelvic imaging studies. The sensitivity of abdominal ultrasound examination for detecting AAA is good, and the results are reproducible. However, ultrasound scans usually do not allow reliable differentiation between a ruptured aneurysm and an intact aneurysm. Computed tomography is sensitive in the detection of both intact and ruptured aneurysms. It is excellent for determining the proximal and distal extent of an aneurysm and in detecting involvement of the iliac vessels, a limitation of ultrasound examination. Computed tomography also is the current standard used to determine the suitability of an aneurysm for endovascular repair. Angiography depicts the lumens of vessels. Abdominal aortic aneurysm frequently is filled with laminated thrombus, through which there is a vessel lumen of closer to normal caliber. A "lumenogram" produced with contrast medium reflects the patent lumen rather than the true lumen and thus gives an underestimate of the actual size of the aneurysm. Preoperative arteriography in conjunction with CT may be helpful to patients undergoing endovascular aneurysm repair to appropriately size the graft. Preoperative arteriography can be helpful to a subset of patients undergoing standard open repair who have aortoiliac occlusive disease, poorly controlled hypertension or renal insufficiency, symptoms of chronic mesenteric ischemia, and renal anomalies, including horseshoe kidney.

ANSWER: c, e

REFERENCE: *Chapter 86—Abdominal Aortic Aneurysms: Clinical Presentation and Diagnosis*

4. Which of the following statements is/are true regarding the contemporary therapeutic considerations and options for management of AAA?

a. Good risk patients with AAAs larger than 5 cm in diameter and a life expectancy of at least 2 years should be offered elective repair
b. Patients may be offered endoluminal repair but only under a U.S. Food and Drug Administration (FDA) approved investigational device protocol
c. Hospital length of stay, operative blood loss, and costs are equivalent for standard open and endoluminal repair of AAA
d. Endovascular repair of AAA has been shown to prevent aneurysm rupture in the long term and is comparable with standard repair
e. All patients with symptomatic or ruptured AAAs should undergo surgical repair provided quality of life and life expectancy are reasonable

COMMENT: Patients at good risk with intact, asymptomatic AAAs larger than 5 cm in diameter need repair if they have a life expectancy greater than 2 years and a reasonable quality of life. Two endovascular devices have been approved by the FDA for implantation in patients with AAA to decrease the risk of premature death of ruptured aneurysm. The results of initial trials of the various endovascular devices suggest that the hospital and intensive care unit length of stays are decreased, the operative blood loss is less, and that the recovery time in terms of return to normal daily activities is markedly improved after endovascular repair. However, these reported decreases in total length of stay and intensive care unit length of stay have not resulted in decreases in the hospital costs primarily because of the dramatic price differential of the grafts (endovascular much more expensive than conventional). The trials have established that the devices can be safely deployed and that aneurysm rupture can be prevented during short- to intermediate-term follow-up periods. However, the long-term outcome of use of these devices in both mechanical stability and ability to prevent aneurysm rupture remains unresolved. There have been reports of aneurysms rupturing during the follow-up period despite successful endovascular repair. All patients with symptomatic or ruptured AAAs need operative repair unless they have underlying medical conditions that preclude long-term survival or their quality of life is not sufficient to justify the intervention.

ANSWER: a, e

REFERENCE: *Chapter 86—Abdominal Aortic Aneurysms: Choice of Standard or Endoluminal Repair*

5. Match each endoleak type with the appropriate description:
   a. Type I
   b. Type II
   c. Type III
   d. Type IV
   1. Patent lumbar artery
   2. Bleeding through pores in graft material
   3. Leak at proximal attachment site
   4. Delayed distal limb migration with leak at distal anastomosis
   5. Leak between components of a modular endograft

COMMENT: Endoleaks are arterial blood flow perfusion of the aneurysm outside the lumen of the endograft and within the aneurysmal sac. They have been classified as types I through IV according to the mechanism of the leak. Type I leak occurs at the proximal or distal attachment site. Type II leak occurs when the collateral circulation originates from the lumbar or inferior mesenteric artery. Type III leaks are caused by fabric tears or problems at the graft interfaces in the modular devices. Type IV leaks are transgraft and reflect the porosity of the graft and the presence of needle holes.

ANSWER: 1. b, 2. d, 3. a, 4. a, 5. c

REFERENCE: *Chapter 86—Abdominal Aortic Aneurysms: Endovascular Repair of Intact Abdominal Aortic Aneurysms*

6. Endovascular repair of AAA is associated with which of the following?
   a. 25% chance of necessitating a secondary remedial procedure
   b. 3% chance of early or late endoleak
   c. Need for long-term surveillance with imaging studies
   d. Strict device-specific AAA and iliac artery anatomic requirements for patient selection
   e. Continued aneurysm expansion, although risk of rupture is eliminated by exclusion from direct arterial blood flow

COMMENT: The initial clinical experience with endovascular repair has emphasized that long-term follow-up evaluation with serial imaging is mandatory. It has been reported that approximately 25% of patients need some type of remedial procedure. Computed tomographic scans are optimal for assessing aneurysm size, and anteroposterior and lateral abdominal radiographs for assessing graft configuration. Both CT and color flow duplex ultrasonography are effective and are potentially complementary in the evaluation of endoleaks. An acceptable algorithm includes appropriate imaging immediately postoperatively and 3 months, 6 months, 12 months, and every 6 to 12 months thereafter. A metaanalysis of 23 publications describing repair of endovascular aneurysm that encompassed 1,189 patients showed a 24% endoleak rate. The most common site of leakage was the distal attachment.

The most important concern about an endoleak is that the pressure transmitted to the aneurysm wall is sufficient to increase size or cause a rupture. Use of the endovascular approach is currently limited by the anatomic configuration of the aneurysm and iliac arteries. For example, the neck of the infrarenal abdominal aorta artery should be 16 to 26 mm in diameter and more than 1 cm in length without excessive angulation. The ideal outcome after endovascular repair is that the aneurysm shell shrink or regress over time. Aneurysms that continue to enlarge after endovascular repair present increased risk of rupture and mandate further intervention. Aneurysms that remain stable in size may reflect an occult endoleak and warrant careful follow-up evaluation.

ANSWER: a, c, d

REFERENCE: *Chapter 86—Abdominal Aortic Aneurysms: Complications and Outcome*

7. Which of the following statements is/are true regarding the preoperative evaluation and optimization of patients undergoing elective repair of AAA?

a. Perioperative β blockade improves outcome
b. Routine pulmonary function tests improve outcome
c. Coronary arterial occlusive disease is uniquely uncommon among these patients, who tend to have aneurysmal rather than occlusive disease
d. For typical infrarenal aortic aneurysms, preoperative imaging with ultrasound alone is sufficient and avoids the radiation and contrast exposure associated with CT
e. Preoperative angiography is indicated before repair for patients with renal anomalies or suspected renal vascular hypertension

COMMENT: Patients undergoing elective repair of AAA need therapeutic β blockade unless this therapy is contraindicated. Several randomized, controlled studies have shown that β-blockade decreases the incidence of cardiac events after vascular surgery in both the perioperative period and the long term. Routine pulmonary function tests and arterial blood gas measurements are not indicated, although they can be beneficial in the care of selected patients with advanced chronic obstructive pulmonary disease. The presence of chronic obstructive pulmonary disease often complicates postoperative ventilator management, but it is unusual that pulmonary disease would be sufficiently severe to preclude operation. History and physical examination alone are sufficient to identify this small subset of patients. The prevalence of coronary artery disease among patients undergoing AAA repair is high. Hertzer et al., in a landmark publication, reported that 25% of 1,000 patients undergoing evaluation for peripheral vascular surgery (cerebrovascular occlusive disease, lower extremity arterial occlusive disease, AAA) had severe, surgically correctable lesions at cardiac catheterization; 6% had severe, uncorrectable disease, and only 8% had no evidence of disease. The incidence of surgically correctable disease was highest among patients undergoing evaluation for AAA. Abdominal ultrasound examination is insufficient as the sole imaging study before aneurysm repair in light of the inability to accurately depict the proximal extent of the aneurysm and involvement of the iliac vessels. Preoperative arteriography is necessary for patients undergoing endovascular repair if CT findings alone are insufficient and for the subset of patients undergoing standard repair with renal anomalies or occlusive disease in the renal, mesenteric, or aortoiliac vessels.

ANSWER: a, e

REFERENCE: *Chapter 86—Abdominal Aortic Aneurysms: Operative Indications*

8. Standard maneuvers for elective open repair of intact infrarenal AAA include which of the following?

   a. Permissive hypothermia to decrease the basal metabolic rate of the lower extremities during clamping
   b. Exclusive use of the transperitoneal approach in operations on patients with abdominal wall stomas to allow direct dissection of the bowel under direct vision
   c. Reimplantation of the inferior mesenteric artery only if vigorous backbleeding is encountered after the aneurysmal sac is opened
   d. Implantation of a bifurcated aortobifemoral prosthetic graft for reconstruction if either common iliac artery is larger than 2.0 cm in diameter
   e. Abandonment of the repair if sigmoid colotomy is made before graft implantation, even if the patient has undergone mechanical preoperative bowel preparation

COMMENT: During aneurysm repair, strategies to maintain core body temperature should be initiated. The room temperature should be increased, warming devices should be attached to all intravenous infusion lines, and either a recirculating alcohol blanket or forced air blanket applied to the patient. Abdominal aortic aneurysm can be repaired through several different incisions or approaches, including midline, retroperitoneal, or transverse (supraumbilical straight, infraumbilical straight, infraumbilical curvilinear, bilateral subcostal). The various incisions and approaches must be viewed as complementary because none is perfect for every clinical scenario. The retroperitoneal approach is optimal for patients with multiple previous abdominal incisions and the proverbial "hostile abdomen" and those with abdominal wall stomas, suprarenal aneurysms, inflammatory aneurysms, horseshoe kidneys, or redo aortic procedures.

The retroperitoneal approach is limited by the inability to adequately assess the intraperitoneal structures and the limited access to the right renal artery and right iliac vessels. When patent, the inferior mesenteric artery should be reimplanted into either the body of the graft or the left limb. Seeger et al. reported that routine reimplantation of the inferior mesenteric artery decreased the rate of colonic infarction and death after aortic reconstruction. Under most circumstances, common iliac arteries larger than 2.0 cm in diameter should be considered aneurysmal and replaced. This usually requires replacing the entire common iliac artery with the distal anastomosis at the iliac (not femoral) bifurcation, although it is possible to replace only the proximal common iliac artery if the aneurysmal changes are isolated. Common iliac arteries smaller than 2.0 cm in diameter have a relatively benign natural history and do not need to be replaced. Only a small percentage become aneurysmal and necessitate treatment.

Aortobifemoral bypass grafts should be reserved for the small subset of patients who truly have concomitant aneurysms and severe occlusive disease. Although aortobifemoral bypass is easier to perform than aortobiliac bypass, the risks in terms of wound complications and graft infections are significantly greater. If the colon is injured before the aneurysm repair, the defect in the colon should be fixed and the aneurysm repair aborted. If the small bowel is injured before the aneurysm repair, the same course should likely be followed, although this decision requires clinical judgment. The risk of infecting the aortic graft is the main justification for aborting aneurysm repair in this setting.

ANSWER: e

REFERENCE: *Chapter 86—Abdominal Aortic Aneurysms: Operative Indications*

9. Match each description with the appropriate endovascular device:

 a. AneuRx
 b. Ancure
 c. Both
 d. Neither
 1. FDA approved for AAA exclusion in care of selected patients
 2. Externally supported with a nitinol exoskeleton
 3. Circumferential hooks at proximal and distal ends to facilitate attachment
 4. Entirely percutaneous delivery system

COMMENT: Two endograft devices have been approved by the FDA for implantation in the care of selected patients with AAA. The Aneurex device is made of a polyester graft completely externally supported with a nitinol exoskeleton. The radial forces of the self-expanding nitinol exoskeleton facilitate attachment at the proximal and distal ends of the graft. Both tube and bifurcated systems are available in the Ancure device. They are made of a polyester graft with circumferential hooks at the proximal and distal ends that facilitate attachment to the vessel walls, but the graft is not supported by an exoskeleton. Both devices are placed by means of femoral artery cutdown.

ANSWER: 1. c, 2. a, 3. b, 4. d

REFERENCE: *Chapter 86—Abdominal Aortic Aneurysms: Endovascular Repair of Intact Abdominal Aortic Aneurysms*

10. Which of the following clinical circumstances and operations are reasonable approaches for an otherwise healthy 60-year-old man?

 a. Isolated 4-cm common iliac artery aneurysm managed by means of aortobiliac prosthetic graft reconstruction
 b. 5.5-cm AAA with a 1-cm thick wall, medial deviation of the ureters, and chronic back pain requiring narcotics managed by means of AAA repair by the retroperitoneal approach
 c. 5-cm AAA and nearly obstructing cancer of the left colon managed by means of staged repair of AAA and colonic lesion with colectomy performed first
 d. 7 cm suprarenal AAA with renovascular hypertension from left renal artery stenosis managed by means of a retroperitoneal approach to AAA repair and simultaneous left renal revascularization
 e. 3.5-cm AAA with horseshoe kidney managed by means of elective repair after angiography by a retroperitoneal approach

COMMENT: All are reasonable approaches except e. The principles of management of asymptomatic, isolated iliac artery aneurysms are comparable with those for AAA. Operative repair is justified when the risk of rupture offsets the risk of repair. Because of the poorly defined natural history, the size criteria to justify repair of isolated iliac artery aneurysm remains unclear. Aneurysm rupture has been reported for aneurysms smaller than 2 cm in diameter, although it is rare for aneurysms smaller than 3 cm to rupture. It is generally recommended that patients at low risk undergo operative repair for isolated iliac (common or internal) artery aneurysms larger than 3 cm. Inflammatory AAAs constitute approximately 5% of all AAAs. The difference between the inner and outer diameters of the aorta ranges from 1 to 5 cm. Patients with inflammatory AAAs frequently have back or abdominal pain or both.

Open repair of inflammatory AAA is complicated by the fact that the adjacent structures, including the duodenum, colon, and ureters, may be involved in the inflammatory process and may be densely adherent to the aortic wall. These problems can be avoided by means of repairing the aneurysm through a retroperitoneal approach. The general recommendation for patients with AAA and an additional intraabdominal surgical problem is to address the more imminent problem first—in this case, the nearly obstructing colonic lesion. The left retroperitoneal approach with incision of the diaphragm and its crus offers good exposure of the distal thoracic aorta and left renal artery. However, exposure of the right renal artery and right iliac artery bifurcation is more challenging from this approach. In view of the low annual rupture risk of a 3.5-cm AAA, most surgeons would advocate "watchful waiting" (counseling on rupture symptoms and serial imaging) for such a small aneurysm.

ANSWERS: a, b, c, d

REFERENCE: *Chapter 86—Abdominal Aortic Aneurysms: Additional Considerations*

CHAPTER 87

SPLANCHNIC ARTERY ANEURYSMS

1. Splenic artery aneurysm is the most common aneurysm affecting the splanchnic arteries. Which of the following statements is/are true?

   a. Grand multiparity is associated with splenic artery aneurysm
   b. Factors contributing to splenic artery aneurysm include portal hypertension and arterial fibrodysplasia
   c. Splenic artery aneurysm is common among recipients of liver transplants
   d. Splenic artery aneurysm is multiple 75% of the time
   e. The aneurysm usually affects the distal main splenic artery

COMMENT: One half of splenic artery aneurysms affecting women have been related to six or more completed pregnancies and the hormonal and hemodynamic effects of pregnancy on the vasculature. Nearly 10% of patients with portal hypertension and approximately 4% of those with renal arterial fibrodysplasia have these aneurysms. The former disease may account for the common presence of splenic artery aneurysm among recipients of orthotopic liver transplants. These aneurysms usually occur at branchings beyond the main splenic artery and are multiple in 20% of patients.

ANSWER: a, b, c

REFERENCE: *Chapter 87—Splanchnic Artery Aneurysms: Splenic Artery Aneurysm*

2. Rupture of a splenic artery aneurysm is the most serious complication. Which of the following statements is/are true?

   a. Rupture of a splenic artery aneurysm usually is into the peritoneal cavity with exsanguinating hemorrhage
   b. The operative mortality for rupture of a splenic artery aneurysm is 25%
   c. Rupture of a splenic artery aneurysm during pregnancy occurs in the third trimester among 69% of patients
   d. Fewer than 2% of splenic artery aneurysms rupture
   e. Splenic artery aneurysms that rupture during pregnancy cause 95% fetal and 75% maternal mortality

COMMENT: Rupture of a previously asymptomatic (bland) splenic artery aneurysm affects less than 2% of patients. It usually occurs first into the lesser sac, where the hemorrhage is tamponaded before free exsanguinating hemorrhage occurs into the peritoneal cavity (double rupture phenomenon). The reported operative mortality for aneurysm rupture is 25%, with the exception of rupture during pregnancy, which has a 95% fetal and 75% maternal mortality. Rupture during pregnancy is most common (69%) during the third trimester.

ANSWER: b, c, d, e

REFERENCE: *Chapter 87—Splanchnic Artery Aneurysms: Splenic Artery Aneurysm*

3. Hepatic artery aneurysms account for 20% of all splanchnic artery aneurysms. Which of the following statements is/are true?

a. Hepatic artery aneurysms are extrahepatic in 80% of cases and intrahepatic in 20% of cases
b. Hepatic artery aneurysms have a reported 3% rupture rate
c. Rupture of a hepatic artery aneurysm carries a 90% mortality rate
d. Hepatic artery rupture into the biliary tract causes biliary colic, hematemesis, and jaundice
e. Ligation of a hepatic artery aneurysm is the preferred treatment

COMMENT: Hepatic artery aneurysms affect the extrahepatic arteries in 80% of cases. In recent times, rupture of 20% of these aneurysms has occurred with a 35% mortality. Rupture occurs with equal frequency into the peritoneal cavity and biliary tract, the latter causing hematobilia, which is characterized by biliary colic, hematemesis, and jaundice. The preferred treatment is an arterial reconstructive procedure. Resection of the aneurysm after arterial ligation may be appropriate if hepatic ischemia is not apparent with temporary hepatic artery clamping.

ANSWER: a, d

REFERENCE: *Chapter 87—Splanchnic Artery Aneurysms: Hepatic Artery Aneurysm*

4. The clinical spectrum of superior mesenteric artery aneurysms has changed little since the 1950s. Which of the following statements is/are true?

a. Infection from a cardiac course is the most common cause of superior mesenteric artery aneurysm
b. Superior mesenteric artery aneurysm with mural dissection often leads to intestinal ischemia
c. Rupture of superior mesenteric artery aneurysm has a mortality approaching 90%
d. Superior mesenteric artery aneurysm is inappropriately managed by means of ligation and aneurysmorrhaphy
e. Most reported superior mesenteric artery aneurysms are asymptomatic

COMMENT: Aneurysm of the superior mesenteric artery continues to be caused most commonly by infectious endocarditis, with many aneurysmal vessels undergoing dissection involving the proximal artery and its inferior pancreaticoduodenal and middle colic branches. The occlusive nature of these dissections often leads to chronic intestinal ischemia. Rupture is uncommon, but when it occurs the mortality rate is 50%. The most often reported surgical procedures used to manage superior mesenteric artery aneurysm have been ligation and aneurysmorrhaphy, although direct revascularization with venous grafts when possible is favored.

ANSWER: a, b

REFERENCE: *Chapter 87—Splanchnic Artery Aneurysms: Superior Mesenteric Artery Aneurysm*

5. Intact celiac artery aneurysms usually are asymptomatic or are associated with vague abdominal discomfort. Which of the following statements is/are true?

a. Celiac artery aneurysms in contemporary times are most often caused by arteriosclerosis
b. Rupture of celiac artery aneurysms occur in 80% of cases
c. Celiac artery aneurysms that rupture cause a 50% mortality
d. Celiac artery aneurysms are managed successfully by means of operation in 90% of cases
e. Aneurysmectomy with arterial ligation is the preferred management of celiac artery aneurysms

COMMENT: Celiac artery aneurysm affect men and women equally. It is caused most often by medial degeneration, and arteriosclerosis is a secondary event. Rupture has accompanied 13% of recently reported aneurysms, carrying a mortality of 50%. Operative therapy is successful in 90% of cases. Arterial reconstruction of the celiac artery is the preferred procedure.

ANSWER: d

REFERENCE: *Chapter 87—Splanchnic Artery Aneurysms: Celiac Artery Aneurysm*

6. Gastric and gastroepiploic artery aneurysms usually are encountered among patients older than 50 years, who often have a history of peptic ulcer disease. Which of the following statements is/are true?

a. Gastric and gastroepiploic artery aneurysms are multiple in 50% of patients
b. Gastric and gastroepiploic artery aneurysms usually are symptomatic
c. Rupture of gastric and gastroepiploic artery aneurysms has occurred in 90% of reported cases
d. Rupture of gastric and gastroepiploic artery aneurysms cause gastrointestinal bleeding twice as often as intraperitoneal bleeding
e. Intramural gastric or gastroepiploic artery aneurysms are best resected with distal gastrectomy

COMMENT: Gastric artery aneurysms are 10 times more common than gastroepiploic artery aneurysms. Most of these aneurysms are solitary and result from perimedial inflammation or medial degeneration. In many reported cases, the clinical presentation may have been overstated. Most aneurysms have been symptomatic. Ninety percent have ruptured, bleeding into the gastroduodenal tract twice as often as into the peritoneal cavity, causing the deaths of 50% of patients. Management of intramural aneurysms usually entails resection of a small portion of the stomach with the aneurysm.

ANSWER: b, c, d

REFERENCE: *Chapter 87—Splanchnic Artery Aneurysms: Gastric and Gastroepiploic Artery Aneurysms*

7. Intestinal branch (jejunal, ileal, and colic artery) aneurysms affect older patients with a variety of underlying medical diseases. Which of the following statements is/are true?

   a. Intestinal branch aneurysms are multiple in 90% of cases
   b. Abdominal pain has been present in most reported cases
   c. Rupture of intestinal branch aneurysms has occurred in 90% of cases
   d. Rupture carries a mortality of 80%
   e. Intestinal branch aneurysm is the most common cause of abdominal apoplexy

COMMENT: Aneurysms of the jejunal, ileal, and colic arteries are uncommon, and the health risks may be overstated in the literature. In most reports, the patients have had abdominal pain. These aneurysms are multiple 10% of the time. Rupture affects 30% of these intestinal branch aneurysms and causes death in 20% of cases. Rupture has been described as the most common cause of abdominal apoplexy. Arterial ligation with or without aneurysmectomy usually is successful, as is resection of the involved bowel in the case of intramural aneurysm.

ANSWER: b, e

REFERENCE: *Chapter 87—Splanchnic Artery Aneurysms: Jejunal, Ileal, and Colic Artery Aneurysms*

8. Most peripancreatic (pancreaticoduodenal, pancreatic, and gastroduodenal) artery aneurysms are associated with pancreatitis-related vascular necrosis or vessel erosion by an adjacent pancreatic pseudocyst. This adds to the risk of managing these aneurysms. Which of the following statements is/are true?

   a. These aneurysms affect men four times more often than they do women
   b. 60% of gastroduodenal and 30% of pancreaticoduodenal artery aneurysms are related to pancreatitis
   c. Pancreaticoduodenal artery aneurysms have a propensity to occur at branchings of collateral vessels in patients with celiac artery occlusions
   d. Inflammatory peripancreatic artery aneurysm ruptures 75% of the time
   e. Rupture of these aneurysms carries a mortality approaching 50%

COMMENT: Pancreaticoduodenal, pancreatic, and gastroduodenal artery aneurysms are grouped together because of their close relations to pancreatic inflammatory disease. Because pancreatic inflammatory disease is more common among men than among women, these aneurysms are four times more likely to affect men than they are women. Pancreatitis is associated with 60% of gastroduodenal and 30% of pancreaticoduodenal artery aneurysms. These inflammatory aneurysms rupture 75% of the time, with a mortality of 50%. Pancreaticoduodenal artery aneurysm at branchings of the collateral vessels between the superior mesenteric artery and the celiac artery, in cases of occlusion of the latter vessel, is much less hazardous than peripancreatic inflammatory aneurysm.

ANSWER: a, b, c, d, e

REFERENCE: *Chapter 87—Splanchnic Artery Aneurysms: Pancreaticoduodenal, Pancreatic, and Gastroduodenal Artery Aneurysms*

9. Gastroduodenal artery aneurysms often are difficult to diagnose and manage. Which of the following statements is/are true?

  a. Rupture of gastroduodenal artery aneurysms occurs into the peritoneal cavity more often than into the gastrointestinal tract
  b. Gastroduodenal artery aneurysms related to pancreatitis should never be managed by means of arterial ligation within the aneurysmal sac
  c. Pseudocyst-related false aneurysms can be most safely managed by means of arterial ligation and cyst drainage or pancreatectomy
  d. Transcatheter embolization of pancreatitis-related aneurysms carries a high risk of infection
  e. Gastroduodenal artery aneurysm managed by means of transcatheter ablation rarely is complicated by rebleeding

COMMENT: Gastroduodenal artery aneurysm ruptures into the gastrointestinal tract more often than into the peritoneal cavity. Because of the hazards of dissecting around an inflamed pancreas, control of blood flow into an aneurysm is best obtained by means of arterial ligation within the aneurysmal sac or pseudocyst that has eroded into the artery. In the latter cases, the cyst must be drained if not removed with partial pancreatectomy. Transcatheter embolization of these aneurysms is a common temporizing measure but carries a risk of infection that accounts, in part, for the frequent cases of rebleeding among these patients.

ANSWER: c, d

REFERENCE: *Chapter 87—Splanchnic Artery Aneurysms: Pancreaticoduodenal, Pancreatic, and Gastroduodenal Artery Aneurysms*

10. Which one of the following, in decreasing order, is the correct frequency of splanchnic arterial aneurysm?

  a. Splenic, gastroduodenal, and hepatic arterial aneurysms
  b. Hepatic, pancreaticoduodenal, and superior mesenteric arterial aneurysms
  c. Splenic, hepatic, and celiac arterial aneurysms
  d. Superior mesenteric, jejunal-ileal-colic, and celiac arterial aneurysms
  e. Hepatic, gastroduodenal, and gastric arterial aneurysms

COMMENT: The relative frequency of aneurysms affecting the different splanchnic arteries has remained constant since the 1950s. An exception is disruption of small intrahepatic arteries associated with blunt trauma and discovered on computed tomographic scans obtained soon after injury. These small pseudoaneurysms may be the most common contemporary splanchnic artery aneurysm, but most undergo spontaneous thrombosis and are of little clinical importance.

ANSWER: c

REFERENCE: *Chapter 87—Splanchnic Artery Aneurysms*

CHAPTER 88

RENAL ARTERY ANEURYSMS

1. Renal arterial occlusive disease is the most common cause of surgically correctable hypertension. Which of the following statements is/are true?

   a. The most common cause of renal failure is renal arterial occlusive disease

   b. Renal arterial occlusive disease becomes functionally important with 80% stenosis

   c. Aortic spillover arteriosclerosis is the most common form of renal arterial occlusive disease

   d. Renal arterial occlusive disease is most commonly caused by arterial fibrodysplasia

   e. Renal arterial occlusive disease among children is most commonly caused by occult trauma

COMMENT: The most common cause of renovascular hypertension and the most common form of renal arterial occlusive disease are aortic arteriosclerosis that extends into the proximal renal artery, so-called spillover disease. Hemodynamic and functional significance occur as the stenosis exceeds 80% and causes renin-mediated blood pressure elevations. Impairment of renal function is an uncommon consequence of renal arterial occlusive disease. Arterial fibrodysplasia and developmental stenosis are the most common renal arterial occlusive diseases among middle-aged women and children, respectively.

ANSWER: b, c

REFERENCE: *Chapter 88—Renal Artery Aneurysms: True Renal Artery Aneurysms*

2. Renin production and release increase in severe renovascular occlusive disease. Which of the following statements is/are true?

   a. The direct and indirect effects of renin account for blood pressure elevations in renovascular hypertension

   b. Renin is a proteolytic enzyme that acts on angiotensinogen to form angiotensin I

   c. Renin is removed from the circulation primarily by the kidney

   d. Renin has a half-life of 20 to 30 minutes

   e. Renin exists in a relative steady state in the peripheral circulation

COMMENT: Renin enters the circulation as a consequence of severe renal arterial stenosis. There it acts as an enzyme to convert angiotensinogen, an α_2 globulin produced in the liver, to angiotensin I. Conversion of angiotensin I to angiotensin II is the primary cause of blood pressure elevations in renovascular hypertension owing to direct vasoconstrictive action and an indirect increase in aldosterone production. Renin has a half-life of 20 to 30 minutes and acts in a steady state dependent on sodium and fluid balance. It is degraded in the liver.

ANSWER: a, b, d, e

REFERENCE: *Chapter 88—Renal Artery Aneurysms: True Renal Artery Aneurysms*

3. Angiotensin II activity is central in causing renovascular hypertension. Which of the following statements is/are true?

   a. Angiotensin II is an octapeptide formed from angiotensin I by angiotensin-converting enzyme (ACE)

   b. Angiotensin II has a half-life of 20 to 30 minutes

   c. The vasoconstrictive agent in renovascular hypertension is angiotensin II

   d. Sodium retention is enhanced by angiotensin II

   e. Angiotensin II enhances the release of renin

COMMENT: Angiotensin II is formed by ACE cleavage of two amino acids from the decapeptide angiotensin I. It has a direct vasoconstrictive effect with a half-life of 4 minutes, enhances sodium retention with increased aldosterone production, and provides for a negative feedback to reduce renin release.

ANSWER: a, c, d

REFERENCE: *Chapter 88—Renal Artery Aneurysms: True Renal Artery Aneurysms*

4. A 70-year old man has a blood pressure of 220/115 mm Hg while undergoing two-drug therapy. Arteriographic studies show bilateral arteriosclerotic renal arterial occlusive disease. Which of the following statements is/are true?

   a. Sixty percent of reported cases of renovascular hypertension are due to arteriosclerotic renal arterial disease
   b. Men have renal arterial arteriosclerosis twice as often as do women
   c. Renal arterial arteriosclerosis represents aortic spillover disease in 80% of cases
   d. Renal arterial arteriosclerotic occlusive disease is bilateral in 75% of patients
   e. Excentric fibrous plaques account for most advanced renal arterial occlusive lesions

COMMENT: Arteriosclerotic renal arterial occlusive disease accounts for 95% of cases of renovascular hypertension. It affects men twice as often as it does women, although both sexes are of similar ages when the disease manifests itself. This disease is bilateral 75% of the time, representing aortic spillover disease in 80% of patients. Advanced lesions manifest as complex arteriosclerotic plaques with necrosis, hemorrhage, calcification, and evidence of luminal thrombus.

ANSWER: b, c, d

REFERENCE: *Chapter 88—Renal Artery Aneurysms: True Renal Artery Aneurysms*

5. A 40-year-old woman has fatigue and occipital headaches. She is found to have a blood pressure of 190/115 mm Hg. Arteriographic studies reveal renal artery stenosis suggestive of arterial fibrodysplasia. Which of the following statements is/are true?

   a. The categorization of arterial fibrodysplasia includes intimal fibroplasia, medial fibroplasia, perimedial dysplasia, dissection, and aneurysm
   b. The intimal type affects younger patients without a sex predilection
   c. The medial type usually affects women between the ages of 35 and 45 years
   d. The medial type is bilateral in 60% of cases
   e. The perimedial type is primarily a disease of excessive elastic tissue

COMMENT: Arterial fibrodysplasia is categorized by the primary vessel wall layer involved—the intima, media, or perimedial-adventitial region. Dissections and aneurysms are considered secondary complications of the former lesions. Intimal disease usually manifests as focal narrowing in young patients. Medial fibroplasia occurs as a string-of-beads lesion among 35- to 45-year-old women and is bilateral in 60% of cases. Perimedial dysplasia occurs in which accumulation of elastic tissue causes serial stenosis without aneurysmal dilatation.

ANSWER: b, c, d, e

REFERENCE: *Chapter 88—Renal Artery Aneurysms: True Renal Artery Aneurysms*

6. Developmental renal arterial stenosis is the third most common cause of renovascular hypertension. Which of the following statements is/are true?

   a. Ninety percent of renal arterial occlusive lesions associated with pediatric renovascular hypertension are developmental
   b. Developmental renal artery stenosis occurs at the same embryonic time as fusion of the two dorsal aortas
   c. When associated with coarctation of the abdominal aorta, developmental disease usually affects solitary renal arteries to each kidney
   d. Developmental renal arterial stenotic lesions are true hypoplastic vessels
   e. Developmental renal arterial stenosis manifests as branch stenosis

COMMENT: Developmental renal arterial stenosis is a unique disorder affecting slightly fewer than one half of children with renovascular hypertension. It occurs because of a mesenchymal abnormality present when the two dorsal aortas fuse and the metanephric vessels disappear. This results in hourglass-shaped hypoplastic renal arteries at their aortic origins. When stenosis occurs with coarctation of the abdominal aorta, several renal arteries to each kidney usually are affected.

ANSWER: b, d

REFERENCE: *Chapter 88—Renal Artery Aneurysms: True Renal Artery Aneurysms*

7. A 50-year-old man with uncontrolled hypertension has arteriographic evidence of severe right renal arterial stenosis and mild left renal arterial stenosis. Which of the following are evidence of renovascular hypertension in this patient?

   a. Arteriographic evidence of collateral vessels circumventing renal artery stenosis
   b. Peak systolic velocities of 180 to 200 cm/s in the main renal artery at ultrasonography
   c. Renal vein renin ratios comparing the right to the left greater than 1.48
   d. Renal to systemic renin indices that total more than 0.48
   e. Delay in the contrast-enhanced appearance of the right-side collecting system and washout on a hypertensive intravenous pyelogram

COMMENT: Arteriographic demonstration of collateral vessels supports the existence of renal arterial stenosis causing a pressure gradient sufficient to stimulate renin release from the kidney. Results of hypertensive intravenous pyelography are abnormal among some patients with proven renovascular hypertension, as in this case, but are of limited value in the presence of bilateral disease or with isolated unilateral segmental renal arterial stenosis. Ultrasonography is useful in showing abnormally elevated peak systolic velocities but may not reveal occluded accessory renal arteries. Renin assays are useful in equivocal cases to document the presence of hyperreninemia when ratios exceed 1.48 or the sum of bilateral indices exceeds 0.48.

ANSWER: a, b, c, d, e

REFERENCE: *Chapter 88—Renal Artery Aneurysms: True Renal Artery Aneurysms*

8. An 8-year-old patient has high-grade ostial stenosis of the left renal artery and severe hypertension while undergoing three-drug therapy. Which of the following statements is/are true?

   a. Pediatric renal arterial stenosis usually is not controlled with percutaneous transluminal angioplasty (PTA)
   b. Children with renovascular hypertension may need aortic reconstruction in the presence of coarctation of the abdominal aorta
   c. Pediatric renal arterial stenosis is optimally managed by means of aortic reimplantation of the normal renal artery beyond the ostial stenotic lesion
   d. Pediatric renal arterial stenosis is appropriately managed by means of aortorenal bypass with a venous graft
   e. Compared with other age groups, children have the poorest operative results

COMMENT: Developmental ostial stenosis among children is hypoplastic and is not appropriate for PTA. It is best managed by means of aortic reimplantation of the transected and spatulated normal renal artery beyond the stenosis. Venous graft reconstruction is not favored in the treatment of children because of late aneurysmal changes. Aortoplasty or thoracoabdominal bypass may be necessary for simultaneous management of coexistent coarctation of the abdominal aorta. The cure rate after surgical intervention for renovascular hypertension among children is better than for all other age groups with this disease.

ANSWER: a, b, c

REFERENCE: *Chapter 88—Renal Artery Aneurysms: True Renal Artery Aneurysms*

9. A 40-year-old woman with severe hypertension has classic medial fibroplasia of the right renal artery. Which of the following statements is/are true?

   a. Medial fibroplasia can be managed successfully with PTA when the stenosis is limited to the main renal artery
   b. Surgical therapy for medial fibroplasia has a better than 90% rate of salutary outcome
   c. Aortorenal venous bypass is appropriate when the disease affects both the main renal artery and its first-order branchings
   d. Medial fibroplasia can be managed by means of ex vivo reconstruction for complex disease involving multiple segmental branches
   e. Operative dilation can be useful in the management of concomitant intraparenchymal segmental disease during bypass procedures for disease of the main renal artery

COMMENT: Renovascular hypertension due to medial fibroplasia limited to the main renal artery is most often managed by means of PTA, although surgery would benefit more than 90% of these patients. Aortorenal bypass is appropriate in the treatment of patients with disease that extends into branches. Intraoperative dilation often is used for simultaneous control of distal segmental lesions. Ex vivo reconstruction is reserved for patients with extensive complex disease not amenable to in situ revascularization.

ANSWER: a, b, c, d, e

REFERENCE: *Chapter 88—Renal Artery Aneurysms: True Renal Artery Aneurysms*

10. A 70-year-old man has severe hypertension due to bilateral 90% arteriosclerotic narrowing of the renal artery and mild renal insufficiency during three-drug therapy, including an ACE inhibitor. Which of the following statements is/are true?

    a. Aortic spillover renal arterial arteriosclerosis can be successfully managed with PTA without stenting in 30% to 50% of cases
    b. Arteriosclerosis of the renal artery occurring as aortic spillover disease can be successfully managed by means of PTA with stenting in 50% to 80% of cases
    c. Arteriosclerotic stenosis should not be managed by means of aortorenal endarterectomy when multiple arteries to each kidney are affected with ostial disease
    d. Arteriosclerotic renovascular hypertension is likely to be successfully managed by means of surgical intervention in 70% to 90% of cases
    e. Arteriosclerotic renal artery disease should be managed by means of hepatorenal or splenorenal revascularization only in cases of hostile aorta

COMMENT: Arteriosclerotic renovascular hypertension due to bilateral renal arterial stenosis among elderly patients can be managed operatively with an anticipated 70% to 90% benefit, albeit with morbidity and mortality that exceed those of PTA. In general, PTA is successful in 30% to 50% of cases without stenting and 50% to 80% with stenting. Although aortorenal bypass is the most common operation, aortorenal endarterectomy is most useful for disease of several renal arteries to each kidney. Nonanatomic bypass is indicated when aortic exposure would be difficult because of hostile aorta or when clamping the aorta would be hazardous, such as in an operation on a patient with coronary artery disease and precarious cardiac function.

ANSWER: a, b, d

REFERENCE: *Chapter 88—Renal Artery Aneurysms: True Renal Artery Aneurysms*

CHAPTER 89

FEMORAL AND POPLITEAL ANEURYSMS

1. Which of the following statements is/are true with respect to peripheral (femoropopliteal) arterial aneurysms?

    a. Three percent of patients with aortoiliac aneurysms have a peripheral arterial aneurysm
    b. Seventy percent of patients with peripheral aneurysms have a concomitant abdominal aortic aneurysm (AAA)
    c. The male to female ratio for these aneurysms is 3:1 to 4:1, the same as for AAA
    d. The incidence of femoral and popliteal aneurysms has been defined with precision

COMMENT: Femoral and popliteal arterial aneurysms are much less common than is AAA. Their exact incidence has not been well defined. The male to female ratio for femoral and popliteal aneurysms is 20:1, distinctly different form the 3:1 to 4:1 ratio for AAA. Most patients, with peripheral arterial aneurysm, approximately 70%, have concomitant AAA. The converse is not true; only 3% of patients with aortoiliac aneurysm have peripheral aneurysms.

ANSWER: a, b

REFERENCE: *Chapter 89—Femoral and Popliteal Aneurysms: Incidence*

2. Which of the following statements is/are true with respect to femoral and popliteal arterial aneurysms?

   a. These lesions frequently are symptomatic
   b. When symptomatic, the aneurysm manifests as lower extremity ischemia due to thrombosis or distal embolization
   c. Rupture and approximately 50% mortality are common outcomes of these aneurysms
   d. Femoral and popliteal aneurysms are approximately equal in propensity for complications

COMMENT: Femoral and popliteal aneurysms frequently are asymptomatic incidental findings during a routine physical examination. When symptomatic, the aneurysm commonly manifests as lower extremity ischemia due to thrombosis or distal embolization. Local pain due to enlargement and irritation of adjacent structures occasionally occurs. Edema can be caused by compression of adjacent veins. Popliteal aneurysm poses considerably more risk to the viability of the lower extremity than does femoral arterial aneurysm.

ANSWER: a, b

REFERENCE: *Chapter 89—Femoral and Popliteal Aneurysms: Femoral Artery Aneurysms*

3. Which of the following statements is/are true with respect to anastomotic pseudoaneurysms caused by disruption of the suture line between the graft and the host artery?

   a. After aortofemoral bypass, the femoral anastomotic site more commonly has a pseudoaneurysm than does the aortic anastomotic site
   b. Six percent of femoral Dacron polyester graft anastomoses have pseudoaneurysms as opposed to 1% of autogenous venous anastomoses
   c. Anastomotic aneurysms are typically an early complication of bypass
   d. Twenty percent of femoral arterial anastomoses have a pseudoaneurysm

COMMENT: Three percent of all femoral anastomoses are complicated by pseudoaneurysm formation, whereas only 0.2% of aortic anastomoses have this complication. Use of Dacron polyester results in a 6% incidence of femoral pseudoaneurysm; autogenous saphenous vein causes pseudoaneurysm in fewer than 1% of cases. Finally, anastomotic aneurysm is a late complication of bypass procedures, occurring after a mean interval of 6 years.

ANSWER: a, b

REFERENCE: *Chapter 89—Femoral and Popliteal Aneurysms: Anastomotic Aneurysms*

4. Which of the following statements is/are true with respect to catheter-induced pseudoaneurysm?

   a. The incidence of catheter-induced pseudoaneurysm is approximately 0.05% of diagnostic catheterizations and as high as 10% of more complex procedures
   b. Confirmation of the clinical suspicion of a catheter-induced pseudoaneurysm can be obtained by means of computed tomography, magnetic resonance imaging, ultrasonography, or color flow duplex technique
   c. With ultrasound-guided compression, most patients, including those undergoing anticoagulation, can have successful thrombosis of the pseudoaneurysm
   d. Surgical therapy is mandatory for catheter-induced pseudoaneurysms that are acutely expanding, compressing adjacent nerves, or compromising overlying skin

COMMENT: Approximately 0.05% of diagnostic catheterizations and approximately 0.4% of more complex procedures are complicated by pseudoaneurysm formation. Direct focal application of pressure usually seals the defect. The diagnosis is suspected when a pulsatile groin mass is found after femoral arterial catheterization. Computed tomography, magnetic resonance imaging, ultrasonography, or duplex scanning readily delineates the mass. With ultrasound-guided compression, thrombosis of the pseudoaneurysm occurs among 86% of patients undergoing anticoagulant therapy and 98% of those not taking anticoagulants.

ANSWER: b, c, d

REFERENCE: *Chapter 89—Femoral and Popliteal Aneurysms: Catheter-induced Pseudoaneurysms*

5. Which of the following statements is/are true with respect to popliteal arterial aneurysm?

   a. Fifty percent to 70% of patients have bilateral popliteal aneurysms
   b. Seventy percent of patients have concomitant AAA
   c. Most aneurysms are asymptomatic at the time of diagnosis
   d. The risk of complications is directly related to the size of the aneurysm

COMMENT: The high incidence of bilaterality and concomitant AAA has been found in almost all series of patients with popliteal arterial aneurysm. Approximately one half the patients have symptoms such as claudication, rest pain, or gangrene when they come to medical attention. Blue toe syndrome, a popliteal mass, leg pain, and phlebitis due to compression of adjacent venous structures also are common. Even very small popliteal arterial aneurysms can induce symptoms.

ANSWER: a, b

REFERENCE: *Chapter 89—Femoral and Popliteal Aneurysms: Clinical Manifestations*

CHAPTER 90

VASCULAR MALFORMATION AND ARTERIOVENOUS FISTULA

1. The presence of a congenital arteriovenous fistula in the extremity shunts blood away from the high resistance capillary bed. Temporary occlusion of the fistula results in one or more of the following changes, referred to as the Nicoladoni-Branham sign:

   a. Bradycardia
   b. Tachycardia
   c. Hypertension
   d. Hypotension

COMMENT: Patients with large peripheral AV fistulae are adapted to chronically low peripheral resistance. Occlusion of the fistula results in a sudden increase in the peripheral resistance, in turn causing an increase in the blood pressure. The resulting hypertension stimulates the aortic and carotid baroreceptors, causing a vagus-mediated bradycardia.

ANSWER: a, c

REFERENCE: *Chapter 90—Vascular Malformation and Arteriovenous Fistula: Physiologic Changes Resulting from Arteriovenous Malformations*

2. The presence of a high-flow arteriovenous fistula or large hemangioma can result in one or more of the following systemic abnormalities:

   a. Activation of the renin-angiotensin-aldosterone system
   b. Osmotic diuresis and salt wasting
   c. High output cardiac failure
   d. Thrombocytosis and consumption coagulopathy

COMMENT: Increased venous return to the heart as a result of a peripheral AV fistula results in elevated right atrial pressure and increased cardiac output. As a result of a chronic elevation in the cardiac output, a clinical condition similar to congestive heart failure occurs, termed "high output" heart failure. Physiologic hypotension resulting from bypass of the peripheral capillary bed results in stimulation of the renin-angiotensin-aldosterone system. Fistula ligation will reverse this phenomenon resulting in a profound osmotic diuresis. Kaposiform hemangioendotheliomas can cause platelet trapping (thrombocytopenia) and consumption coagulopathy, referred to as the Kasabach-Merritt syndrome.

ANSWER: a, c

REFERENCE: *Chapter 90—Vascular Malformation and Arteriovenous Fistula: Physiologic Changes Resulting from Arteriovenous Malformations*

3. Progressive enlargement in the size of congenital arteriovenous malformations occurs as result of one or more of the following:

   a. Malignant transformation
   b. Platelet trapping
   c. Rapid endothelial cell proliferation and differentiation
   d. Dilatation and elongation of preexisting vascular channels due to high volume of blood flow

COMMENT: Congenital AV malformations (AVM) do not represent a true neoplasm. Endothelial cells of AVM are well differentiated and do not harbor a malignant potential. An increase in size may result from elongation and tortuosity of preexisting vascular pathways.

ANSWER: d

REFERENCE: *Chapter 90—Vascular Malformation and Arteriovenous Fistula: Classification and Embryologic Development*

4. A 67-year-old man underwent cardiac catheterization via the right common femoral artery. The results of the cardiac evaluation were normal but a thrill and bruit were subsequently noted over the right groin. The patient had 4+ pedal pulses and was in no apparent distress. A duplex evaluation of the catheterization site revealed a communication between the femoral artery and vein. The correct management of this complication is:

a. Surgical repair of the fistula
b. Ultrasound guided thrombin injection
c. Ultrasound guided compression of the fistula tract until thrombosis is noted
d. Duplex follow-up as an outpatient, since the majority of these spontaneously resolve.

COMMENT: Iatrogenic trauma resulting in an AV fistula is often subclinical and goes unnoticed. The presence of a palpable thrill or bruit is often the first sign of the fistulous communication. In the absence of symptoms (local or systemic) the majority of these can be observed and are noted to disappear on subsequent evaluation.

ANSWER: d

REFERENCE: *Chapter 90—Vascular Malformation and Arteriovenous Fistula: Classification and Embryologic Development*

5. Multiple capillary hemangiomas of the face and trunk are noted in a 2-year-old infant since birth. The mother is anxious, as she is definite that there is an increase in the size and number of the lesions. The best therapy for the child at this point is/are:

a. Subcutaneous administration of angiogenesis inhibitors (interferon alfa 2a, 2b)
b. Topical injection of triamcinolone (corticosteroids)
c. Reassure the mother that therapy is unnecessary at this point
d. Carbon dioxide laser vaporization
e. Systemic prednisone (2 to 3 mg per kilogram body weight)

COMMENT: The majority of capillary hemangiomas in neonates disappear within the first few months of birth. Persistent multiple hemangiomas often respond dramatically to systemic corticosteroid therapy. Major side effects such as hypertension and growth retardation are reversed on discontinuation of the drug.

ANSWER: e

REFERENCE: *Chapter 90—Vascular Malformation and Arteriovenous Fistula: Management*

6. A 52-year-old female patient is seen in the clinic complaining of an enlarging soft compressible bluish mass over the left thigh. She received therapy at an another institution with multiple attempts at transcatheter embolization of the "feeding" vessels of this mass. Failure of inflow vessel occlusion to reduce the mass may be a result of which one or more of the following:

a. Localized lymphedema from coil material
b. Presence of multiple feeding vessels
c. Malignant transformation
d. Development of collateral circulation due to local ischemia produced by inflow occlusion
e. Enlargement due to venous reflux into the hemangioma

COMMENT: Cavernous hemangiomas typically have multiple feeding vessels and are seldom limited to a single tissue plane. Transcatheter embolization of the "feeding vessels" produces local ischemia stimulating neovascularization and recurrence of the lesion. Definite therapy requires surgical excision or coil embolization and sclerosis of the hemangioma directly. Inflow vessel embolization may be used to decrease the blood flow to the lesion as an adjunct to surgical excision, to decrease operative blood loss.

ANSWER: b, d

REFERENCE: *Chapter 90—Vascular Malformation and Arteriovenous Fistula: Management*

7. A 9-year-old boy is noted to have port wine stains in the distribution of the first division of the trigeminal nerve. Associated clinical features may include:

a. Mental retardation
b. Epilepsy
c. Retinal angiomatosis
d. Cerebellar ataxia

COMMENT: The typical features of Sturge-Weber syndrome include the triad of port wine stains, epilepsy (90%), and mental retardation (60%). Intractable seizures may require radical procedures such as hemispherectomy before permanent damage develops.

ANSWER: a, b

REFERENCE: *Chapter 90—Vascular Malformation and Arteriovenous Fistula: Arteriovenous Malformations as a Part of Complex-combined Malformations*

8. The typical triad of Klippel-Trenaunay syndrome (Fig. 90.1) includes all **except:**

   a. Varicose veins
   b. Arteriovenous communication
   c. Capillary malformations
   d. Soft tissue or bony hypertrophy

COMMENT: The presence of associated multiple AV communications is called the Parks-Weber syndrome. KTS is a syndrome complex that includes varicose veins, port-wine stains, and limb hypertrophy, but may not manifest all three findings in every case. Capillary hemangiomas and local hypertrophy are obvious in Fig. 90.1 but varicose veins are absent.

ANSWER: b

REFERENCE: *Chapter 90—Vascular Malformation and Arteriovenous Fistula: Arteriovenous Malformations as a Part of Complex-combined Malformations*

Section N
VENOUS AND LYMPHATIC SYSTEMS

CHAPTER 91

VENOUS PHYSIOLOGY AND VENOUS THROMBOEMBOLISM

1. Which of the following statements is/are true concerning veins in the lower extremities?

   a. Large venous lakes are present in the gastrocnemius muscle
   b. The superficial femoral vein is the proximal extension of the popliteal vein
   c. The left common iliac vein is compressed between the spine and the left common iliac artery
   d. Normal venous return from the calf depends on the competence of (a) valve(s) in the popliteal vein

COMMENT: In the lower extremity, large venous lakes are present in the soleal muscles. The popliteal vein continues proximally as the superficial femoral vein. The left common iliac vein is compressed between the spine and the crossing of the right common iliac artery. Normal venous return depends on the competence of the valves primarily in the popliteal vein.

ANSWER: b, d

REFERENCE: *Chapter 91—Venous Physiology and Venous Thromboembolism: Venous Anatomy*

2. Which of the following statements is/are true concerning venous physiology?

a. When a person is upright, venous pressure in the foot is expected to exceed 100 mm Hg
b. Venous flow is at its maximum during peak inspiration
c. Venous claudication is caused by dysfunction of the calf muscle pump
d. The normal valve sinus is wider than the diameter of the vein

COMMENT: In the erect position, hydrostatic pressure is added to resting kinetic venous pressure and is expected to exceed 100 mm Hg in the foot. Venous flow is at its minimum during peak inspiration. Venous claudication syndrome occurs with exercise owing to obstruction of the iliofemoral venous segment and resulting venous hypertension. The normal valve sinus is wider than the diameter of the vein. Distention of the valve places tension on valvular commissures and enhances their competency.

ANSWER: a, d

REFERENCE: *Chapter 91—Venous Physiology and Venous Thromboembolism: Venous Physiology*

3. An obese 40-year-old woman has prominent varicose veins in both legs and a history of venous thrombosis during a previous pregnancy. Which of the following statements is/are true?

a. Preferred treatment is injection sclerotherapy
b. If pain is present, the patient is a candidate for operative excision of the varices
c. Optimal surgical management of varicose veins is high ligation and stripping of the saphenous venous system
d. Photoplethysmography of reflux can help predict the success of removal of varicose veins and the need for postoperative elastic support

COMMENT: For this patient, the preferred treatment is graded elastic stocking support, periodic elevation of the legs, and exercise. If pain is present, it may be caused by chronic venous insufficiency or obstruction, and a venous ultrasound duplex examination of the deep venous system is indicated. The classic procedure of high ligation and stripping of the saphenous vein has been replaced by selective removal of the vein. Reflux testing with photoplethysmography can help predict the success of removal of varicose veins and the need for postoperative elastic support.

ANSWER: d

REFERENCE: *Chapter 91—Venous Physiology and Venous Thromboembolism: Disorders of the Superficial Veins*

4. A 47-year-old man with chronic postthrombotic edema of the left leg has an irregular nonhealing ulcer above the medial malleolus. Which of the following statements is/are true?

a. The cause of the ulceration is extension of venous thrombosis to the superficial capillary bed
b. The ulcer is certain to be infected and merits antibiotic treatment
c. The underlying perforating veins are likely incompetent
d. Isolated incompetence of the saphenous vein can produce such a situation

COMMENT: The presentation indicates chronic venous insufficiency with stasis ulceration caused by sustained venous hypertension. The pathophysiologic characteristics include leukocyte capillary trapping, an inflammatory reaction, and scarring of the subcutaneous tissues with ischemia of the skin. The stasis ulcer can be managed with an occlusive dressing, Unna boot, and elastic support without antibiotics. The location is typical for stasis ulcer because of adjacent underlying incompetent perforator veins. Such a situation also occurs with isolated saphenous vein incompetence.

ANSWER: c, d

REFERENCE: *Chapter 91—Venous Physiology and Venous Thromboembolism: Disorders of the Deep Veins*

5. If the patient in question 4 does not improve with conservative treatment, which of the following is/are true?

   a. The explanation is most likely arterial insufficiency
   b. The optimal diagnostic study is air plethysmography
   c. Occlusive dressings impair formation of granulation tissue
   d. Ascending phlebography is the optimal study of venous valve function

COMMENT: Failure of healing of a chronic stasis venous ulcer is caused by refractory venous hypertension rather than by arterial insufficiency. Air plethysmography is the optimal diagnostic study because it provides quantitative information about several areas of extremity function. Occlusive dressings are oxygen impermeable, and because wound angiogenesis is inversely proportional to ambient oxygen tension, granulation tissue forms quickly. Ascending phlebography provides useful anatomic information, but descending phlebography is necessary to assess valvar function.

ANSWER: b

REFERENCE: *Chapter 91—Venous Physiology and Venous Thromboembolism: Disorders of the Deep Veins*

6. A 38-year-old woman with history of left iliofemoral deep venous thrombosis has refractory edema and severe pain in the leg with ambulation. Which of the following statements is/are true?

   a. Phlebography is an essential diagnostic study
   b. Arteriography is necessary to rule out arterial insufficiency
   c. If proximal venous obstruction is found, saphenopopliteal bypass should be performed
   d. If the patient has no saphenous vein, she can be treated with a prosthetic venous bypass

COMMENT: The description indicates venous claudication, most likely due to chronic obstruction of the iliac vein, which can be confirmed with phlebography. Arteriography is not indicated because there is no evidence of arterial insufficiency. If proximal venous obstruction is found, femorofemoral bypass is indicated rather than saphenofemoral bypass, which would only bypass an obstructed superficial femoral vein. Prosthetic graft material has been used successfully for this purpose.

ANSWER: a, d

REFERENCE: *Chapter 91—Venous Physiology and Venous Thromboembolism: Disorders of the Deep Veins*

7. A 57-year-old woman with chronic venous insufficiency and a nonhealing stasis ulcer does not improve after ligation of perforator veins. Which of the following statements is/are true?

   a. Only further conservative treatment is appropriate
   b. Skin grafting is optimal if there is good granulation tissue after ulcer excision
   c. If valvar incompetence is demonstrated, femoral valvuloplasty should be considered
   d. If no valve tissue is seen, autologous valvar transplantation to the popliteal region should be considered

COMMENT: A nonhealing stasis ulcer is not likely to be relieved with any treatment short of relief of hydrostatic pressure. Ulcer excision with skin grafting also will fail, but construction or repair of venous valves has resulted in a respectable percentage of favorable results. Valvuloplasty, banding, and plication venous wall all have advocates, but autologous valve transplants has been successful in the highest percentage of cases when placed in the popliteal position.

ANSWER: c, d

REFERENCE: *Chapter 91—Venous Physiology and Venous Thromboembolism*

CHAPTER 92

CHRONIC VENOUS DISEASE

1. Which of the following statements is/are true of the normal venous system of the lower extremity?

   a. It can be devoid of venous valves
   b. Collateral veins have no valves
   c. The superficial venous system is composed of the greater saphenous vein, lesser saphenous vein, and superficial femoral vein
   d. The deep venous valves normally close in less than 0.5 seconds when evaluated with a rapidly inflating-deflating pneumatic calf cuff
   e. The left common iliac vein is crossed by the right common iliac artery

COMMENT: Aplasia of the venous valves in the lower extremity, although rare, has been described. Failure of collateral vein valves has dire hemodynamic consequences and is not a normal finding. The superficial femoral vein is not a part of the superficial system—a critical distinction if acute thrombosis involves this vein because its involvement is consistent with deep venous thrombosis (DVT). Deep venous valves normally close rapidly within less than 0.5 seconds. The right common iliac artery crosses the left common iliac vein and can actually be a cause of external obstruction or intraluminal webs as a result of scarring.

ANSWER: a, d, e

REFERENCE: *Chapter 92—Chronic Venous Disease: Pathophysiology and Etiology*

2. The standard ambulatory intravenous pressure measurement study allows direct hemodynamic evaluation of the venous system during exercise. Which of the following statements is/are true regarding this study?

   a. Ten steps generally more than halve the standing venous pressure measured in the foot
   b. After exercise, baseline standing venous pressure is reached only after more than 20 seconds of rest
   c. Ambulatory venous pressure (AVP) has no association with the appearance of clinical sequelae
   d. The standing intravenous pressure in the foot at rest is in great part determined by the patient's height
   e. Nonfunctioning venous valves result in a venous refilling time of less than 20 seconds

COMMENT: The standing intravenous pressure exercise study provides a direct, invasive measurement of what is occurring in the venous system of the lower extremity. When the patient stands, the pressure in the foot approximates the pressure generalized by a column of blood extending from the heart to the catheter and generally reflects the height of the patient. With exercise of 10 toe raises, AVP should be less than one-half that during standing at rest (<45 mm Hg). Venous refilling time is greater than 20 seconds if there is no venous valvar insufficiency. The higher the AVP over 45 mm Hg, the greater is the risk of venous ulceration. Therefore, AVP does correlate with the appearance of clinical sequelae.

ANSWER: a, b, d, e

REFERENCE: *Chapter 92—Chronic Venous Disease: Venous Function Measurement*

3. Which of the following epidemiologic statements accurately describes chronic venous disease?

   a. Obstructive venous disease is the main hemodynamic problem in 25% of cases
   b. Venous insufficiency accounts for approximately 85% of cases of chronic venous disease
   c. It is estimated that 6 million persons in the United States have moderate to severe chronic venous disease
   d. Chronic venous disease is more commonly a result of superficial rather than deep venous disease
   e. Deep venous valvar insufficiency is almost exclusively due to DVT

COMMENT: It is estimated that 6 million persons in the United States have serious chronic venous disease. Fewer than 15% of cases are caused by an obstructive process, whereas more than approximately 85% are caused by venous insufficiency. Whether considering patients with any signs of chronic venous disease or only those with ulceration, superficial disease is more commonly the problem than is deep disease. Deep venous valvar insufficiency can be a primary problem (e.g., floppy valves, wall dilatation) in 30% to 60% of reported cases. Therefore DVT is not the exclusive cause of deep venous insufficiency.

ANSWER: b, c, d

REFERENCE: *Chapter 92—Chronic Venous Disease: Pathophysiology and Etiology*

4. A patient classified as $C_{6,S}$ E_S A_D P_R could have which of the following?

   a. A venous ulcer
   b. Past DVT
   c. Greater saphenous disease
   d. Deep venous obstruction
   e. Hemodynamic reflux

COMMENT: A proper classification of chronic venous disease is required for proper reporting and comparison of treatment options. Only recently has this concept gained widespread acceptance. $C_{6,S}$ describes a patient with symptomatic venous ulcers. E_S describes a patient with a known etiologic factor, such as DVT. The anatomic classification D signifies deep venous disease rather than superficial or perforator disease. The hemodynamic or pathophysiologic problem is reflux rather than obstruction. In the treatment of patients with chronic venous disease, the class should be recorded at each visit to provide a method of comparison over time and between treatment regimens.

ANSWER: a, b, e

REFERENCE: *Chapter 92—Chronic Venous Disease: Clinical Signs and Symptoms*

5. A patient arrives in the office with the diagnosis of varicose veins and previous medial malleolar venous ulceration. The air plethysmographic study shows a venous filling index (VFI) of 7 mL/s without an above-knee tourniquet. With a tourniquet, the VFI is 1.9 mL/s. The outflow fraction is 50%, and the ejection fraction 70%. The venous duplex evaluation shows all veins to be easily compressible. The deep venous valves have a reflux time of 0.2 seconds, and the greater saphenous vein has retrograde flow of 1.5 seconds after calf compression. Which of the following is the most appropriate surgical therapy?

   a. Sclerotherapeutic injection of all apparent varicose veins
   b. Endoscopic perforator vein ligation to prevent recurrent venous ulceration
   c. Further studies to determine the proper deep venous valve or valves to repair
   d. High ligation and stripping of the greater saphenous vein
   e. Further evaluations to determine the area or areas of obstruction and consideration of an appropriate venovenous bypass

COMMENT: The patient described has major axial greater saphenous incompetence. This clinical scenario is not unusual in that isolated saphenous venous reflux can result in the entire spectrum of disease from mild edema to skin changes and ulceration. There has been a misconception that deep or perforative disease must be present for this to occur. Normalization of the air plethysmographic VFI with tourniquet occlusion of the saphenous vein and a reflux time longer than 1 second at duplex evaluation of the saphenous valves is consistent with this diagnosis. The presence of major saphenous reflux results in an unacceptable recurrence rate after sclerotherapy. The other operative approaches deal with an incorrect venous system or mistaking reflux for an obstructive problem.

ANSWER: d

REFERENCE: *Chapter 92—Chronic Venous Disease: Diagnostic Evaluation*

6. A descending venogram (Fig. 92.6) performed during a Valsalva maneuver is obtained for a patient with a $C_{5,S}$ E_S A_D P_R classification. Which of the following statements is/are true?

   a. The venogram shows grade 3 or higher venous insufficiency
   b. The need for surgical intervention depends on the general health of the patient, the degree of disability present, and the presence or absence of valves in the lower extremity
   c. This patient may need deep venous valvar surgery
   d. Air plethysmographic study would show a VFI >2 mL/sec
   e. If surgery is necessary in the venous system shown, one can expect a long-term clinical success rate of 40% to 70% at 5 years in the prevention of recurrent ulcer

COMMENT: The descending venogram shows grade 3 or higher reflux with blood cascading down past the popliteal area during a Valsalva maneuver. Choice *b* is false because a venous valve in the lower extremity is not needed for valvar transplantation. If the patient has severe symptoms, a surgical approach to alleviate deep venous insufficiency can be considered. Because a VFI >2 mL/sec is consistent with venous insufficiency, this abnormality would be found in evaluation of this patient. The range of clinical success shown is consistent with the data in the literature for autogenous venous valve repair (valvuloplasty, transposition, or transplantation).

ANSWER: a, c, d, e

REFERENCE: *Chapter 92—Chronic Venous Disease: Diagnostic Evaluation*

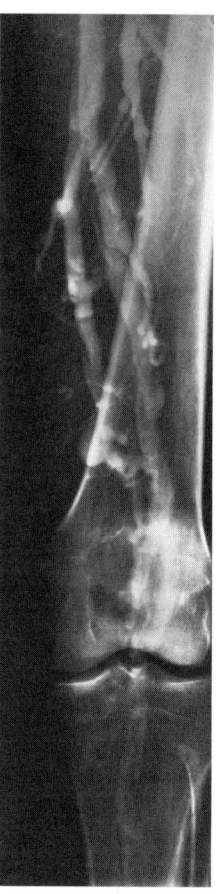

Figure 92.6.

7. When an operative approach to deep venous valvar insufficiency is considered, which of the following factors is/are important to clinical success?

   a. The presence of a floppy venous valve
   b. A grade 3 or 4 reflux as found at descending venography
   c. The reflux status of the profunda femoris (deep femoral) vein
   d. The long-term competence of the valve reconstruction
   e. The technique of valve repair—valvuloplasty versus transposition versus transplantation

COMMENT: A floppy venous valve often can be repaired by means of valvuloplasty of the valve cusps. It has the longest historical follow-up and best overall results at a 70% rate of valve competence with similar clinical success. If any valve repair fails, recurrent symptoms are the norm. The transposition operation and transplantation are more challenging and have slightly less gratifying results (approximately 50% clinical success at 5 years). One must correct all major axial reflux in the thigh to prevent recurrent symptoms. This is true of reflux in the deep and superficial femoral and greater saphenous veins. Most surgeons will not operate for reflux in the deep system if the descending venogram grade is less than 3. A lesser degree of reflux does not appear to affect the sensitive "gaiter" area. Therefore the symptoms are difficult to correlate with reflux.

ANSWER: a, b, c, d, e

REFERENCE: *Chapter 92—Chronic Venous Disease: Venous Valve Repair or Replacement*

CHAPTER 93

LYMPHATIC SYSTEM DISORDERS

1. Which of the following statements is/are true concerning the development and anatomy of the lymphatic vessels?

   a. There is disagreement about whether lymphatic vessels arise from the venous system or by means of fusion of mesenchymal spaces
   b. Lymphatic vessels collect more than 50% of the circulating albumin every 24 hours
   c. Lymphatic vessels have a highly permeable basement membrane
   d. Cystic hygroma occurs only in the neck and mediastinum

COMMENT: Embryologists disagree about whether lymphatic vessels arise from the venous system or from mesenchymal spaces. Lymphatic vessels must collect the more than 50% of circulating albumin lost to the extravascular spaces every 24 hours. Lymphatic vessels have no basement membrane. Cystic hygroma can occur in the abdomen as well as the neck and thorax.

ANSWER: a, b

REFERENCE: *Chapter 93—Lymphatic System Disorders: Anatomy and Function*

2. A 54-year-old woman with chronic lymphedema after a radical mastectomy has pain and red streaks on the involved upper extremity. Which of the following statements is/are true?

   a. The most likely cause is coliform infection
   b. Lymphangiography should be performed
   c. The most serious complication of this disorder is late development of lymphoma
   d. Intravenous antibiotics are appropriate treatment

COMMENT: Lymphangitis in chronic lymphedema is most often caused by streptococci. There is no indication for lymphangiography. The most serious late complication of the disorder is lymphangiosarcoma. In the management of lymphangitis, intravenous antibiotics are most appropriate.

ANSWER: d

REFERENCE: *Chapter 93—Lymphatic System Disorders: Pathophysiology*

3. A 39-year-old woman with recent onset of bilateral edema of the lower extremities seeks evaluation. Which of the following statements is/are true?

   a. Rubbery edema involving the feet is not likely due to venous disease
   b. The diagnosis should be confirmed by means of lymphangiography
   c. If findings on a venous duplex scan are normal, the patient can be treated for lymphedema
   d. Aspiration of tissue fluid to measure protein content is appropriate

COMMENT: Unlike hydrostatic venous edema, lymphedema is rubbery and nonpitting and involves the feet. Lymphangiography is only rarely used for diagnosis, and aspiration of tissue fluid for protein measurement is unnecessary. If the findings on the venous duplex scan are normal, the patient can be assumed to have lymphedema.

ANSWER: c

REFERENCE: *Chapter 93—Lymphatic System Disorders: Diagnosis*

4. After a gunshot wound to the chest, a 24-year-old man has a chylous fluid collection on the right side. Which of the following statements is/are true?

   a. Initial management should be thoracostomy tube drainage
   b. An elemental diet and administration of medium-chain triglycerides are appropriate
   c. As long as the lung is expanded, operative correction can be delayed 4 to 6 weeks
   d. If operative correction is undertaken, the duct can be visualized readily and ligated

COMMENT: Initial management of a traumatic chylothorax includes a thoracostomy tube. The combination of an elemental diet with administration of medium-chain triglycerides reduces lymphatic drainage. Even if the lung is expanded, it is advisable to proceed with operative correction if drainage persists for longer than 1 week. Because the duct is difficult to visualize at operation, it is advisable to use dye or preoperative administration of milk to improve visualization.

ANSWER: a, b

REFERENCE: *Chapter 93—Lymphatic System Disorders: Trauma*

5. A 15-year-old girl has had progressive unilateral leg swelling with signs suggesting lymphedema. Which of the following statements is/are true?

a. This is most likely secondary lymphedema
b. The most likely diagnosis is lymphedema tarda
c. Initial management should be with firm elastic stockings
d. The patient is not a candidate for a lymphaticovenous connection procedure

COMMENT: The presentation is characteristic of lymphedema praecox, which is a primary rather than a secondary lymphedema. Optimal management is pneumatic compression to reduce the size of the extremity followed by use of firm elastic stockings to maintain the control. The best candidates for a lymphaticovenous connection procedure are patients with secondary lymphedema and dilated lymphatic vessels rather than those with primary lymphedema.

ANSWER: d

REFERENCE: *Chapter 93—Lymphatic System Disorders: Management of Lymphedema*

Section O
PEDIATRICS

CHAPTER 94

NEONATAL AND PEDIATRIC PHYSIOLOGY

1. Which of the following statements is/are true regarding premature infants?

a. Complications of prematurity account for approximately 85% of fetal deaths
b. Prematurity is defined by the World Health Organization as birth before 35 weeks of gestation
c. Infants with intrauterine growth retardation have physiologic problems more dependent on birth weight than on gestational age
d. Preterm infants are at higher risk of hypocalcemia and hypoglycemia than are term infants

COMMENT: Prematurity is defined by the World Health Organization as a gestational age at birth of less than 37 weeks. Complications of prematurity account for approximately 85% of fetal deaths. These deaths are commonly caused by perinatal asphyxia, respiratory failure, and infection. The term *intrauterine growth retardation* describes a pathophysiologic process that results in restriction of fetal growth. Fetal, placental, or maternal abnormalities are common. These infants are a heterogeneous population and tend to have neonatal problems related more to gestational age than to birth weight. These problems include asphyxia, hypoglycemia, hypothermia, hypocalcemia, pulmonary hemorrhage, necrotizing enterocolitis, and other complications related to specific syndromes or congenital anomalies.

ANSWER: a, d

REFERENCE: *Chapter 94—Neonatal and Pediatric Physiology: Growth and Metabolism*

2. Which of the following statements is/are true regarding the nutritional requirements of infants?

a. Total daily water requirement is estimated to be 94 mL per 94 kcal ingested
b. Resting energy expenditure is approximately twice that of an adult
c. The highest rate of nitrogen retention with parenteral nutrition occurs among infants given approximately 40% of calories as carbohydrate and the rest as fat
d. The protein requirement for a newborn infant is approximately 2.5 g/kg per day

COMMENT: Taking all factors into account, total daily water requirements for a term infant are estimated to be 94 mL per 94 kcal ingested, assuming an insensible loss of 50 mL/kg per day and a growth requirement of approximately 15 mL/kg per day. The energy expenditure of healthy neonates is approximately twice that of normal adults (50 kcal/kg per day versus 25 kcal/kg per day).

In most circumstances, high carbohydrate to low fat ratios in parenteral nutrition result in high rates of energy expenditure and decreased nitrogen retention. Low carbohydrate to high fat ratios result in excessive fat deposition. A balanced ratio (approximately 40% carbohydrate) provides the highest rate of nitrogen retention and is consistent with the proportion of carbohydrate in breast milk and with the estimates of minimal carbohydrate needs determined with isotope infusion studies. A consensus statement by the World Health Organization and the United Nations University estimates the protein requirement at 2.5 g/kg per day for an infant and 1.25 g/kg per day for a 1-year-old child. For preterm infants, the protein need ranges from 2.5 to 3.9 g/kg per day if the weight is less than 2.5 kg.

ANSWER: a, b, c, d

REFERENCE: *Chapter 94—Neonatal and Pediatric Physiology: Growth and Metabolism*

3. For a 22-kg infant, the daily maintenance fluid requirement is approximately which of the following?

a. 194 mL
b. 1,250 mL
c. 1,550 mL
d. 1,700 mL
e. 1,850 mL

COMMENT: Maintenance fluid requirements are shown in Table 94.4. Maintenance requirements of sodium are about 2 to 3 mEq/kg daily in term infants and potassium requirements are approximately 2 mEq/kg daily. The composition of the intravenous fluids is generally D_5 ¼ normal saline solution or D_5 ½ normal saline solution with 10 mEq/L potassium chloride.

ANSWER: c

REFERENCE: *Chapter 94—Neonatal and Pediatric Physiology*

Table 94.4. **HOLLIDAY-SEGAR METHOD FOR ESTMATING FLUID REQUIREMENTS**

Weight (kg)	Fluid requirement (mL/d)
0–10	100/kg
10–20	1,000 + 50/kg over 10
>20	1,500 + 20/kg over 20

4. A term infant 48 hours of age suddenly has hypoxemia, irritability, and glucose and temperature instability. Which of the following statements is/are true?

   a. Empiric antibiotic coverage for β-hemolytic streptococci and *Escherichia coli* organisms should be initiated

   b. Intravenous infusion of prostaglandin E_1 should be initiated immediately

   c. Exogenous surfactant should be given immediately

   d. The mortality risk for this child is approximately 50%

COMMENT: This infant has the classic findings of neonatal sepsis. This is defined as a generalized bacterial infection accompanied by a positive blood culture result during the first month of life. Early-onset sepsis occurs during the first week of life and is caused primarily by maternal organisms, such as β-hemolytic streptococci, *E. coli* organisms, or *Listeria monocytogenes* organisms. The mortality rate for early-onset sepsis is approximately 50%. Late-onset sepsis is caused primarily by hospital-acquired organisms such as *Staphylococcus epidermidis, Staphylococcus aureus,* or *Pseudomonas* species. The mortality rate for this entity is approximately 20%.

The signs and symptoms of neonatal sepsis are subtle and nonspecific. Early signs include lethargy, irritability, temperature instability, change in the respiratory pattern, and changes in feeding pattern. Hematologic findings include thrombocytopenia, leukocytosis, and leukopenia. Hemodynamic manifestations occur late. Presumptive therapy should be based on the suspected organism but often includes ampicillin or an antistaphylococcal agent plus an aminoglycoside.

Infusion of prostaglandin E_1 is inappropriate because it is used to treat patients with duct-dependent congenital heart disease. Exogenous surfactant is unlikely to be helpful in the care of a term infant who has previously been well and can be expected to begin the illness with a normal complement of pulmonary surfactant.

ANSWER: a, d

REFERENCE: *Chapter 94—Neonatal and Pediatric Physiology*

5. Which of the following statements is/are true about pulmonary surfactant?

   a. Endogenous surfactant deficiency is the most important physiologic problem among preterm infants with infant respiratory distress syndrome

   b. Surfactant function can be restored to normal with administration of aerosolized phosphatidylcholine

   c. Exogenous surfactant replacement has been shown to reduce mortality among preterm infants with infant respiratory distress syndrome

   d. Surfactant is produced by type I alveolar epithelial cells

COMMENT: The pulmonary surfactant complex decreases surface tension and stabilizes the alveolus, even at low lung volumes. It is a complex material secreted by type II alveolar epithelial cells. It is composed of 80% to 90% phospholipid (primarily phosphatidylcholine) and unique surfactant-associated proteins (10%). Surfactant proteins appear to play a critical role in the organization of the phospholipid molecules, and they modify the surface-active properties of the lipids. Phospholipid synthesis and expression of surfactant proteins increase with advancing gestational age. Concentrations of surfactant in the amniotic fluid have been used for many years to predict pulmonary maturity. Surfactant deficiency is the primary factor in the pathophysiologic mechanism of neonatal respiratory distress syndrome. The use of exogenous surfactant replacement therapy is under investigation for the management of neonatal respiratory distress and has been shown to reduce mortality in a variety of specific circumstances involving preterm infants. Several commercially available preparations are available and are undergoing clinical investigation.

ANSWER: a, c

REFERENCE: *Chapter 94—Neonatal and Pediatric Physiology: Respiratory Physiology and Support*

CHAPTER 95

PEDIATRIC HEAD AND NECK

1. Branchial cleft remnants most often manifest as which of the following clinical problems?

   a. Infection
   b. Airway obstruction
   c. Hemorrhage
   d. Malignant degeneration
   e. Pain

COMMENT: The more common second branchial cleft anomalies typically manifest as a pinpoint opening on the anterior border of the sternocleidomastoid muscle. Attention is drawn to the defect often by the appearance of small drops of clear fluid at the orifice or by occurrence of infection in the tract itself. Less frequently, a mass may manifest anterior to the upper portion of the sternocleidomastoid muscle and represent a cyst derived from this tract. Infection is a more common problem in the older age group. Airway obstruction and hemorrhage are rare manifestations. Pain usually is caused by infection. Malignant degeneration is reported but is exceedingly rare. Treatment consists of surgical excision. If infection is present, a course of antibiotics is administered first.

ANSWER: a

REFERENCE: *Chapter 95—Pediatric Head and Neck: Branchial Cleft Remnants*

2. Proximity to which of the following structures places it at risk during surgical excision of a second branchial cleft remnant?

   a. Internal carotid artery
   b. External carotid artery
   c. Hypoglossal nerve
   d. All of the above
   e. None of the above

COMMENT: Operative excision of a second branchial cleft remnant begins with an elliptical transverse incision at the sinus opening and cephalic dissection of the tract to its farthest extent, generally reaching the floor of the tonsillar pillar. The dissection is kept directly on the track to avoid injury to contiguous structures, such as the internal jugular vein, the internal or external carotid artery (between which it passes), and the hypoglossal nerve. The operation almost always can be performed through a single incision if the track is kept under traction and digital pressure is exerted through the tonsillar fossa. Dissection of the sinus tract can be facilitated by means of passing a fine silver probe or piece of heavy nylon suture through the length of the track.

ANSWER: d

REFERENCE: *Chapter 95—Pediatric Head and Neck: Branchial Cleft Remnants*

3. Other than the history and physical examination, which of the following studies is considered an essential feature of the preoperative evaluation of a patient for suspected thyroglossal duct cyst?

a. Cervical ultrasonography
b. Thyroid scan
c. Measurement of serum levels of triiodothyronine and thyroxine
d. Needle aspiration
e. None of the above

COMMENT: A thyroglossal duct cyst is typically a midline structure connected to the foramen cecum at the base of the tongue. It is pulled proximally and superiorly as the tongue protrudes. It can be superior to or inferior to the hyoid bone and occasionally is slightly off the midline. Because in rare instances the thyroglossal cyst contains the patient's only thyroid tissue, some surgeons have recommended a technetium 99m radioisotope thyroid scan before excision. However, excision of the cyst is indicated regardless, because infection of the cyst is likely, and the dysgenetic thyroid tissue in the cyst has malignant potential. For these reasons, patients with suspected thyroglossal duct cysts need routine surgical excision. Preoperative ultrasonography, thyroid scan, measurement of triiodothyronine and thyroxine levels, and needle aspiration are not necessary. If thyroid tissue is found in the cyst at pathologic examination, and postoperative thyroid function tests confirm there is no remaining thyroid, tissue and replacement therapy can be prescribed.

ANSWER: e

REFERENCE: *Chapter 95—Pediatric Head and Neck: Thyroglossal Duct Cyst*

4. Standard therapy for acute epiglottitis in a child is:

a. Tracheostomy
b. Intravenous antibiotic treatment in an intensive care unit
c. Endotracheal intubation in the operating room and intravenous antibiotic therapy
d. Indirect laryngoscopy and intravenous administration of antibiotics
e. Intravenous administration of steroids and antibiotics

COMMENT: Acute epiglottitis is a common cause of acquired airway obstruction in the pediatric age group. *Haemophilus influenzae* type B is nearly always the causative organism. Most children are in toxic condition at presentation with an elevated temperature and increased heart and respiratory rates. Prolonged inspiratory stridor that worsens in the supine position is characteristic. The child usually sits erect, is anxious and drooling, and becomes increasingly exhausted with air hunger. No attempt should be made to visualize the larynx outside of the operating room for fear of sudden airway occlusion. Standard therapy is short-term endotracheal intubation performed in the operating room with general anesthesia. The inflammatory process resolves rapidly with intravenous antibiotics. Intubation is seldom needed for more than 3 days. In the past, tracheostomy was the standard therapy, but comparative reviews have shown that short-term endotracheal intubation is associated with less morbidity and fewer complications.

ANSWER: c

REFERENCE: *Chapter 95—Pediatric Head and Neck: Airway Obstruction*

5. Suppurative cervical lymphadenitis in a 3-year-old child is commonly related to which of the following organisms?

    a. *Staphylococcus aureus* organisms
    b. Atypical mycobacterial organisms
    c. Streptococcal organisms
    d. Lymphoma with secondary pyogenic organisms
    e. Organisms from a cat scratch

COMMENT: The diagnosis of acute suppurative lymphadenitis related to bacterial pathogens is generally straightforward. There often is accompanying infectious illness. The lymph nodes enlarge rapidly and are tender, and erythema of the overlying skin is present. Fever and an elevated white blood cell count with a left shift usually are present. Fluctuant nodes can be aspirated. Streptococci and *S. aureus* are the most common organisms. The initial course of antibiotic therapy is directed at these organisms. If the adenopathy does not resolve in 2 to 3 weeks, the patient likely needs excisional biopsy. Atypical mycobacteria, cat scratch disease, and infection with *Mycobacterium tuberculosis* are more uncommon than is bacterial lymphadenitis. These diseases do not typically produce tenderness or systemic signs. Lymphoma with secondary pyogenic infection is similarly uncommon.

ANSWER: a, c

REFERENCE: *Chapter 95—Pediatric Head and Neck: Lymphadenopathy*

CHAPTER 96

PEDIATRIC CHEST

1. Which of the following statements is/are true regarding congenital chest wall deformities?

    a. Children with pectus excavatum deformities typically have physiologically insignificant limitation of exercise tolerance
    b. The rate of recurrence after operative repair of a pectus excavatum deformity is between 5% and 15%
    c. Pectus carinatum is the most common congenital chest wall defect
    d. The most common indication for operative repair of congenital chest wall deformities is restoration of normal appearance

COMMENT: The most common congenital chest wall deformity is pectus excavatum, representing approximately 90% of the total. Approximately 5% to 7% of the lesions are pectus carinatum, and a variety compose the remainder. Most children with pectus excavatum have no symptoms. There have been numerous efforts to document associated cardiac and pulmonary abnormalities. Objective data show that although there are minor demonstrable cardiopulmonary abnormalities, these do not appear to be appreciably improved by surgery, and they are generally not limiting physiologically. The importance of repair, however, should not be minimized in a largely adolescent population. The repair is technically straightforward but involves moderate morbidity. The minimally invasive repair (Nuss technique) has achieved substantial acceptance. The long-term results are good. The recurrence rate is between 5% and 15% in most institutions with a large number of patients who have participated in long-term follow-up evaluations.

ANSWER: a, b, d

REFERENCE: *Chapter 96—Pediatric Chest: Chest-Wall Deformities*

2. Of the following malformations of the tracheo-bronchial tree, which is most likely to be asymptomatic when discovered?

   a. Intralobar pulmonary sequestration
   b. Extralobar pulmonary sequestration
   c. Congenital cystic adenomatoid malformation
   d. Congenital lobar emphysema

COMMENT: Intralobar pulmonary sequestration and cystic adenomatoid malformations typically manifest as either neonatal respiratory distress or infection related to inadequate clearance of secretions. Given enough time, nearly all of these lesions become infected. Congenital lobar emphysema is characterized by air-trapping within an otherwise normal lung. This typically manifests as respiratory distress, which ranges from mild to life threatening. Hemodynamic instability necessitating emergency thoracotomy occasionally is present.

Extralobar sequestration typically is a mass of disorganized pulmonary parenchymal tissue within its own investing pleura outside the normal lung parenchyma. This does not communicate with the normal tracheobronchial tree. Infection is rare, and although hemorrhage, arteriovenous shunting, mediastinal compression, and an occasional malignant tumor can occur, these lesions are typically asymptomatic and often are discovered at a prenatal ultrasound examination. Excision is recommended for each of these lesions and typically involves lobectomy.

ANSWER: b

REFERENCE: *Chapter 96—Pediatric Chest: Congenital Cystic Disease of the Lung*

3. The definitive evaluation for a child with a suspected congenital cystic abnormality of the tracheobronchial tree is best performed with which of the following?

   a. Rigid bronchoscopy
   b. Computed tomography (CT) or magnetic resonance imaging (MRI)
   c. Chest radiograph
   d. Angiography
   e. Barium esophagography

COMMENT: Plain-film radiography is the first imaging study performed and remains a cornerstone of the diagnosis and follow-up evaluation of this group of lesions. The use of additional imaging provides a definitive diagnosis and allows planning for the surgical approach. Computed tomography and magnetic resonance imaging can separate cystic from solid components in a radiopaque lung mass. These are the most definitive diagnostic studies available. Magnetic resonance imaging has reconstructive capabilities that obviate angiography. Intravenous contrast enhancement during CT provides similar anatomic information. Ultrasonography is less expensive, more readily performed, and in selected cases as sensitive.

Angiography is not used because alternative imaging strategies provide similar information at lower cost with less morbidity. Barium esophagography is helpful in diagnosis for children with dysphagia, but that is a rare presentation of these lesions. Bronchoscopy is rarely helpful for these lesions and for infants and small children carries the risk of general anesthesia and positive pressure ventilation. In the care of children with congenital lobar emphysema and cystic adenomatoid malformation, hyperinflation after positive pressure overinflation induces mediastinal compression and causes a surgical emergency. For these reasons, CT or MRI is considered the best definitive diagnostic imaging study after the initial chest radiograph.

ANSWER: b

REFERENCE: *Chapter 96—Pediatric Chest: Congenital Cystic Disease of the Lung*

4. Which of the following is the most common primary lung tumor among infants and children?

a. Pulmonary blastoma
b. Squamous cell carcinoma
c. Endobronchial carcinoid
d. Leiomyoma
e. Metastatic osteogenic sarcoma

COMMENT: Bronchial adenoma is the most common primary lung tumor in childhood. Nevertheless, it is quite rare. The typical lesion is a low-grade adenocarcinoma, such as endobronchial carcinoid, cylindroma, mucoepidermoid tumor, or bronchomucous gland adenoma. Carcinoid tumors are the most common bronchial adenomas and represent over 80% of the total.

Although common among adults, bronchogenic carcinoma of the lung is extremely rare in childhood. A review of the world literature in 1993 revealed only 49 such patients. Pulmonary blastoma is a rare malignant lung tumor composed of cells that resemble fetal lung. The incidence is highest among adults, although the tumor does occur among children. Benign tumors of the lung also are rare in childhood. The most common of these are pulmonary hamartoma or chondroma. Others include leiomyoma, leiomyoblastoma, and mucus gland adenoma. Metastatic osteogenic sarcoma is more common than any primary lung tumor but is by definition a secondary metastatic lesion and therefore not the correct answer to the question posed here.

ANSWER: c

REFERENCE: *Chapter 96—Pediatric Chest: Thoracic Tumors in Children*

5. A newborn infant has coughing, choking, and cyanosis with the first feeding. He also has excessive drooling. What are the important associated anomalies that must be sought before surgical intervention?

a. Right-sided aortic arch
b. Hydrocephalus
c. Genitourinary obstruction
d. Congenital heart disease

COMMENT: This child has a classic history for esophageal atresia and has a very high (85% or more) probability of having distal tracheoesophageal fistula. The simplest way to establish the diagnosis is to attempt to pass a catheter through the mouth or nose into the stomach. If the tube encounters obstruction, a plain radiograph should document the atresia.

Patients with esophageal atresia and tracheoesophageal fistula frequently have associated anomalies. This incidence is approximately 30% to 50% in most reports. Anomalies vary from minor skeletal deformities to uncorrectable cardiac defects. The most common associated anomalies are cardiac and gastrointestinal, especially imperforate anus (10%). Vertebral, genitourinary, and limb anomalies also occur. Approximately 5% of patients with esophageal atresia have a right-sided aortic arch. This is an important technical issue because the usual approach is right thoracotomy. This should be changed to left thoracotomy in the presence of this finding. There is no association with hydrocephalus.

ANSWER: c

REFERENCE: *Chapter 96—Pediatric Chest: Esophageal Atresia/Tracheoesophageal Fistula*

6. Which of the following is most common after primary esophagoesophagostomy for esophageal atresia with a distal tracheoesophageal fistula?

   a. Anastomotic leak
   b. Esophageal stricture
   c. Recurrent tracheoesophageal fistula
   d. Gastroesophageal reflux
   e. Tracheomalacia requiring aortopexy

COMMENT: The preferred approach to esophageal atresia with a distal tracheoesophageal fistula in a patient without other problems is extrapleural right thoracotomy with division of the tracheoesophageal fistula and primary esophagoesophagostomy. No gastrostomy is ordinarily used. The results with this approach are better than those with a staged approach. Three serious complications are related to the esophageal anastomosis—leak, stricture, and recurrent fistula. The incidence of leak varies from 10% to 20% depending on the type of anastomosis and the degree of tension. A distinct advantage of extrapleural anastomosis is the predictable resolution of these leaks if adequately drained. Similarly, the stricture rate varies between 10% and 25%, again depending on the type of anastomosis. Many infants need one or two dilations, but few have serious long-term problems. The incidence of recurrent esophageal fistula is difficult to determine because few authors emphasize this technical problem, but it appears to be approximately 10% in most reports.

Gastroesophageal reflux due to dysmotility of the distal esophagus is a serious problem and occurs to some degree among almost all of these patients. A large number of these infants, 25% to 30% or more, are refractory to medical therapy and need surgical fundoplication. Tracheomalacia is a complication of the malformation, not of the repair. This appears to result from inadequate cartilaginous tracheal rings at the level of the fistula. The reported incidence is as high as 25% in recent series. Most infants with tracheomalacia improve with growth and time, but a small percentage have severe respiratory difficulty, which necessitates surgical aortopexy.

ANSWER: d

REFERENCE: *Chapter 96—Pediatric Chest: Esophageal Atresia/Tracheoesophageal Fistula*

7. Infants with a double aortic arch most commonly have which of the following problems?

   a. Dysphagia
   b. High-output cardiac failure related to patent ductus arteriosus
   c. Positional hyperemia and edema of the right upper extremity
   d. Symptomatic tracheal compression

COMMENT: Double aortic arch is the most common type of complete vascular ring. It arises from the ascending aorta and bifurcates, one arch passing on either side of the trachea and the esophagus. The symptoms of complete vascular rings are caused by compression of the trachea, the esophagus, or both. A child with a double aortic arch generally has the most serious symptoms, and most patients have symptoms in infancy. The typical clinical features are symptomatic tracheal compression, which includes inspiratory wheezing, coughing, noisy breathing, shortness of breath, stridor, and frequent bouts of pneumonia. Feeding problems can become apparent when solid foods are started, but this is less common than is tracheal compression. The most important screening test is a barium swallow radiographic study; results of CT or MRI are definitive. Angiography and endoscopy usually are not helpful. Any patient who is symptomatic from a vascular ring should be treated surgically.

ANSWER: d

REFERENCE: *Chapter 96—Pediatric Chest: Vascular Rings*

8. Which of the following statements is/are true regarding congenital diaphragmatic hernia?
   a. The incidence of right-sided and left-sided lesions is equal
   b. Malrotation is to be expected
   c. Left-to-right shunting through a patent ductus arteriosus is a serious but expected physiologic consequence of pulmonary hypoplasia
   d. Survival rates of 65% to 75% have been reported
   e. Congenital heart disease is present among approximately 20% of these infants

COMMENT: During organogenesis, closure of the right hemidiaphragm normally precedes that of the left. This asynchronous closure and the presence of the liver on the right account for the finding that 85% to 90% of congenital diaphragmatic hernias involve the left hemidiaphragm. Malrotation is an expected finding with diaphragmatic hernia because intestinal herniation into the thorax normally precedes fixation of the intestine to the posterior body wall. Pulmonary hypertension is an important feature of congenital diaphragmatic hernia. Right-to-left shunting through a patent ductus arteriosus is present in almost all of these children. Fifteen percent to 25% of infants with diaphragmatic hernia have an associated anomaly, the most important being cardiovascular abnormalities. Although ventricular septal defect and aortic coarctation are most common, almost all anomalies of the heart and great vessels have been reported. Cardiac echocardiographic screening examinations therefore are routine. Survival rates as high as 75% to 90% among selected patients at high risk with congenital diaphragmatic hernia have been reported in several large clinical series since the mid 1980s.

ANSWER: b, d, e

REFERENCE: *Chapter 96—Pediatric Chest: Congenital Abnormalities of the Diaphragm*

9. Which of the following ventilation strategies is the best initial approach to care of a neonate with a left congenital diaphragmatic hernia and the following postductal arterial blood gas values: Pao_2, 50 mm Hg; $Paco_2$, 60 mm Hg; pH 7.35?
   a. High-frequency jet ventilation
   b. Permissive hypercapnia with conventional pressure controlled ventilation
   c. Extracorporeal membrane oxygenation (ECMO)
   d. Induced respiratory alkalosis
   e. Inhaled nitric oxide with conventional volume-controlled ventilation

COMMENT: Management of congenital diaphragmatic hernia emphasizes permissive hypercapnia with any necessary mode of respiratory support. Pressure-controlled ventilation ordinarily is the initial mode of support. The purpose is to reduce the iatrogenic lung injury associated with high-pressure mechanical ventilation. The latter problem, barotrauma-induced lung injury, has reduced enthusiasm for induced respiratory alkalosis. Although alkalosis sometimes can be achieved, the price often is prohibitive mean and peak airway pressures. High-frequency jet ventilation, ECMO, and inhalation of nitric oxide are evolving strategies that may be useful but are reserved for use after this initial strategy is unsuccessful.

ANSWER: b

REFERENCE: *Chapter 96—Pediatric Chest: Congenital Abnormalities of the Diaphragm*

10. There is an emerging consensus that surgical repair of congenital diaphragmatic hernia is best done:

a. As an emergency procedure at the bedside to eliminate the risks of transporting an unstable neonate
b. During ECMO
c. When extubation is possible
d. Within the first 48 to 72 hours of life

COMMENT: Infants with diaphragmatic hernia have considerable variation in the degree of respiratory distress, and the degree of distress dictates timing of repair. Infants traditionally were rushed to the operating room in an emergency for reduction of the herniated viscera and diaphragmatic closure. Because effective preoperative decompression of the intestine usually is possible and because it has become clear that the underlying pulmonary hypoplasia is not reversed by an emergency operation, this sense of urgency is no longer accepted. Most surgeons now commit themselves to a period of preoperative stabilization to confirm the diagnosis and optimize medical care. The current recommendation is that operative repair be undertaken when the patient is in stable condition at a level of ventilatory support that soon allows extubation, regardless of the means of support used. This means that repair is done at or after the end of cardiopulmonary bypass, if bypass has been necessary. The results of a delayed approach appear at least equivalent and in several series better than with emergency or early repair. The concept is that it is desirable to defer operative injury to a time when the neonatal pulmonary vascular bed is less vulnerable to vasospasm.

ANSWER: c

REFERENCE: *Chapter 96—Pediatric Chest: Congenital Abnormalities of the Diaphragm*

CHAPTER 97

PEDIATRIC ABDOMEN

1. Which of the following statements is/are true regarding gastroschisis?

a. Primary fascial closure can be achieved in only about 25% of cases
b. The incidence of associated anomalies is approximately 40% to 50%
c. The overall survival rate is approximately 80% to 90%
d. When the diagnosis is known prenatally, planned cesarean section is the safest method of delivery

COMMENT: Gastroschisis is a full-thickness defect of the abdominal wall with herniation of a variable amount of uncovered intestine. Prenatal diagnosis has enabled diagnosis of gastroschisis before delivery. Prospective evaluation comparing vaginal delivery with elective cesarean section has shown no difference in outcome. Careful vaginal delivery generally remains the birthing method of choice. Unlike omphalocele, which is commonly (50% of cases) associated with other anomalies, other structural anomalies are associated with gastroschisis in approximately 10% of patients.

Primary fascial closure after reduction of the herniated viscera is the best surgical option; this is possible in the care of 60% to 70% of infants. Care must be taken not to generate excessive intraabdominal pressure when performing primary abdominal wall closure. In general, an intraabdominal pressure less than 20 cm water is well tolerated. If the herniated viscera cannot be reduced primarily, a polymeric silicone (Silastic) pouch is constructed to temporarily contain the extraabdominal bowel, and a series of partial reductions are begun. This approach combined with adequate nutritional support by means of total parenteral nutrition yields survival rates of at least 80% to 90% in most contemporary series of gastroschisis.

ANSWER: c

REFERENCE: *Chapter 97—Pediatric Abdomen: Gastroschisis*

2. Which of the following are typical causes of neonatal intestinal obstruction?

a. Intussusception
b. Meconium ileus
c. Hirschsprung's disease
d. Meckel diverticulum
e. Incarcerated hernia

COMMENT: Neonatal bowel obstruction is defined as intestinal obstruction that develops in the first 30 days of life. The cardinal manifestation is bilious vomiting, often in conjunction with abdominal distention. Common causes are reviewed in Table 97.1. Meconium ileus and Hirschsprung's disease are classic causes of neonatal intestinal obstruction. Incarcerated inguinal hernia is the most common cause of neonatal intestinal obstruction. Hernia usually does not present diagnostic difficulty. Simple inspection of the groin yields an obvious diagnosis. Intussusception, although a cause of distal bowel obstruction in infants, does not usually become a consideration until at least 3 to 6 months of age. Intestinal obstruction related to Meckel diverticulum is generally related to intussusception or volvulus associated with a band from the Meckel diverticulum to the abdominal wall. Both of these events tend to occur later than the neonatal period.

ANSWER: b, c, e

REFERENCE: *Chapter 97—Pediatric Abdomen: Neonatal Intestinal Obstruction*

3. Which of the following statements is/are true regarding duodenal atresia?

a. Twenty percent to 40% of infants with duodenal atresia have trisomy 21
b. When duodenal atresia is associated with annular pancreas, division of the pancreas at the site of obstruction is curative
c. Bilious vomiting is typical because the obstruction usually is distal to the ampulla of Vater
d. Reconstruction is best achieved with Roux-en-Y duodenojejunostomy

COMMENT: Twenty percent to 40% of infants with congenital duodenal obstruction have trisomy 21. Because this syndrome is not always apparent during the physical examination, a routine karyotype should be obtained. Preoperative echocardiographic ultrasound examination is appropriate to evaluate the possibility of associated congenital heart disease. Feeding intolerance and bilious vomiting in the first 24 to 48 hours of life are characteristic. The malformations typically are distal to the ampulla of Vater, thus the infants present with bilious vomiting and proximal duodenal and gastric distention. Malformation proximal to the ampulla of Vater causes nonbilious vomiting, and this possibility must not be ignored.

Bypass of the obstructing lesion generally is the best approach whether or not atresia or annular pancreas is responsible. Division of an annular pancreatic band is inappropriate for two reasons: (a) the duodenum almost always is atretic; (b) division of this pancreatic tissue divides the accessory pancreatic duct within it, creating the real possibility of pancreatic fistula. Construction of a duodenostomy that minimizes the length of defunctionalized duodenum usually is preferred. The procedure used is diamond-shaped duodenostomy. Simple duodenojejunostomy without a Roux-en-Y anastomosis sometimes is necessary for lesions in the distal duodenum (Fig. 97.13).

ANSWER: a, c

REFERENCE: *Chapter 97—Pediatric Abdomen: Congenital Duodenal Obstruction*

4. A 1,500-g neonate born after 30 weeks of gestation is fed at 2 weeks of age. He has abdominal distention, bilious vomiting, and guaiac-positive stool. A plain radiograph of the abdomen shows pneumatosis intestinalis. Which of the following statements is/are true?

a. An emergency barium upper gastrointestinal (GI) radiographic series should be obtained to rule out malrotation
b. The child needs a nasogastric tube placed and broad-spectrum intravenous antibiotics, and sequential abdominal radiographs should be obtained
c. The likelihood of intestinal perforation is greater than 50%
d. The expected survival rate is approximately 70%

COMMENT: The clinical history is classic for neonatal necrotizing enterocolitis (NEC), an idiopathic clinical condition characterized by mucosal intestinal injury that can progress to transmural bowel necrosis. This condition typically occurs among critically ill, preterm infants and is characterized by abdominal distention, bilious vomiting, and either occult or gross blood in the stool. In this setting, pneumatosis intestinalis is pathognomonic. When the diagnosis is suspected on clinical grounds and the findings on a plain radiograph, contrast imaging should not be performed because it can complicate or contribute to the problems of perforation. The child in this case has an unequivocal history, and an upper GI series would be inappropriate.

One half of all infants with NEC have birth weights less than 1,500 g, and 80% of these infants weigh less than 2,500 g at birth. The incidence is approximately 1 to 2 in 1,000 live births. Neonatal necrotizing enterocolitis is the most common surgical emergency among neonates in North America. The initial treatment of infants with NEC is nasogastric decompression, broad-spectrum antibiotics, and correction of hypoxemia, hypotension, acidosis, fluid or electrolyte disorders, and other reversible medical problems. As many as 90% of infants with NEC can be treated successfully without a surgical procedure, but this figure is widely variable among institutions because of differences in referral and practice patterns. Intestinal perforation is characterized by pneumoperitoneum and is an indication for operation. Although the incidence of perforation is variable, it generally is less than 20% to 40%. The overall survival rate among neonates with NEC is approximately 60% to 70% for both operative and nonoperative management. This represents a substantial improvement from the 20% to 30% survival probability when the entity was first recognized in the late 1960s.

ANSWER: b, d

REFERENCE: *Chapter 97—Pediatric Abdomen: Necrotizing Enterocolitis*

5. Which of the following statements is/are true regarding an infant with meconium ileus?
   a. The probability is 100% that he will have cystic fibrosis (CF)
   b. Nonoperative therapy resolves this problem for approximately two thirds of patients
   c. The average life expectancy is approximately 26 to 28 years for this infant
   d. The findings on the plain radiograph (Fig. 97.23A) are an absolute operative indication

COMMENT: Meconium ileus is characteristic obstruction of the small intestine among neonates with CF. Ten percent to 20% of infants with CF initially have meconium ileus. All infants with meconium ileus have CF. Cystic fibrosis is characterized by a transport defect of epithelium that results in impermeability of the chloride ion and therefore water. Inspissated secretions in the pancreas and intestine cause obturator obstruction of the terminal ileum from meconium in the neonate. Approximately two thirds of these infants have simple meconium ileus; the others have complications such as proximal volvulus, perforation, or atresia. These latter problems may be associated with the development of a meconium cyst. In this instance, speckled calcifications on a plain radiograph or ultrasound scan establish the diagnosis. The radiograph in Fig. 97.23 shows a meconium pseudocyst, which is consistent with intraperitoneal spillage of meconium from intestinal perforation. This finding necessitates surgical exploration.

Sixty percent to 70% of infants with simple meconium ileus can be treated by means of enema instillation of one of several irrigation solutions into the obstructed terminal ileum. Saline solution, hyperosmolar contrast agents, dilute *N*-acetylcysteine, and a variety of other solutions have been used successfully. After resolution of the obstruction, most institutions report survival rates as high as 70% to 100%. The average life expectancy for patients with CF is well into the third decade of life. It is primarily determined by the course of pulmonary disease rather than the gastrointestinal problems. A number of important medical advances, including the realistic prospect of gene therapy, are foreseeable for these infants.

ANSWER: a, b, c, d

REFERENCE: *Chapter 97—Pediatric Abdomen: Meconium Ileus*

6. A 3-week old infant undergoes a barium upper GI radiographic series to evaluate vomiting. The duodenojejunal flexure is found to the right of the midline and is more caudal and anterior than a normal ligament of Treitz. The child has spontaneous reflux of barium to the level of the midthoracic esophagus. Which of the following is/are recommended?
   a. Barium enema radiographic examination
   b. Emergency laparotomy
   c. A trial of histamine H_2 receptor blockade, and cisapride therapy
   d. Upper GI endoscopy
   e. Overnight pH probe analysis

COMMENT: This child has malrotation and is at risk of midgut volvulus because of the imaging findings. Malrotation typically produces incomplete obstruction of the duodenum with a corkscrew or coiled appearance in the third or fourth portions of the duodenum. Malposition of the duodenojejunal junction establishes the diagnosis. This includes a location to the right of the midline. Failure to achieve normal posterior and cephalad fixation is typical. The small bowel is situated in the right part of the abdomen, and the colon and cecum are on the left. Attempts at radiographic differentiation of malrotation with or without volvulus are unreliable and therefore hazardous. This child has gastroesophageal reflux likely caused by partial duodenal obstruction due to malrotation. None of the alternatives other than emergency laparotomy is appropriate. There is no role for nonoperative management of malrotation in a neonate. Assessment, resuscitation, and preoperative preparation should be conducted concurrently as the child is prepared for laparotomy. This urgency is necessary because a delay of hours can represent the difference between viable and infarcted midgut at laparotomy. Fifty percent to 75% of cases of malrotation are discovered in the first month of life, and about 90% occur among children younger than 1 year.

ANSWER: b

REFERENCE: *Chapter 97—Pediatric Abdomen: Malrotation*

7. Which of the following statement is/are true regarding Hirschsprung's disease?

a. Suction rectal biopsy almost always provides enough information for diagnosis if the specimen includes submucosa

b. Hirschsprung's disease is caused by a sex-linked dominant gene

c. The endorectal pull-through is demonstrably superior to other forms of surgical construction

d. Ninety percent or more of patients have excellent or good functional results after reconstructive surgery

e. The most important cause of mortality in contemporary practice is enterocolitis

COMMENT: The incidence of Hirschsprung's disease is approximately 1 case per 5,000 live births. There is no racial predilection, but there is a marked male-to-female (4:1) preponderance. Most cases are sporadic, but long-segment or total colonic aganglionosis and female sex are strongly associated with familial disease. Data suggest an association with the *ret* protooncogene. The genetic basis of Hirschsprung's disease is under investigation. It appears that several genes, including those located on chromosomes 10, 13, 22, and possibly others, are involved. The condition is neither sex linked nor dominant. There is a rare association with the multiple endocrine neoplasia syndromes, particularly medullary carcinoma of the thyroid.

The accuracy of suction rectal biopsy was 100% in several large series in which the biopsy was performed correctly, that is, included submucosa, and the specimen was examined by an experienced pediatric pathologist. The examination must include a search for ganglion cells and evaluation of the axons of the myenteric neurons with either conventional staining techniques or histochemical staining for acetylcholinesterase.

Definitive operations for congenital aganglionosis depend on resection or bypass of the distal aganglionic rectum with a low rectal anastomosis to normally innervated pulled-through proximal intestine. Selection among operations depends more on a surgeon's individual training and preference than on demonstrable differences in outcome. Although endorectal pull-through is a widely practiced and popular procedure, it is not demonstrably superior to the procedures described by Duhamel or Swenson. Eighty percent to 90% or more of patients have excellent or normal bowel function after reconstructive surgery for Hirschsprung's disease when evaluated after 5 years, regardless of the procedure used.

The primary remaining cause of death directly attributable to Hirschsprung's disease itself is enterocolitis. When it occurs, enterocolitis is typical among infants or neonates for whom the diagnosis has been delayed. Postoperative enterocolitis does occur, but it tends to be substantially less virulent than neonatal Hirschsprung's enterocolitis. Undiagnosed neonatal Hirschsprung's enterocolitis can lead to death from overwhelming sepsis in 12 to 24 hours.

ANSWER: a, d, e

REFERENCE: *Chapter 97—Pediatric Abdomen: Congenital Aganglionosis (Hirschsprung's Disease)*

8. Which of the following is/are the most likely cause(s) of hemodynamically significant lower GI bleeding in a 6-month-old boy?

   a. Meckel diverticulum
   b. Henoch-Schönlein purpura
   c. Intussusception
   d. Crohn's colitis
   e. Hemolytic uremic syndrome

COMMENT: All of the choices are possible causes of lower GI bleeding in a 6 month old; intussusception and a bleeding Meckel diverticulum are the most common. Upper GI hemorrhage with distal passage of blood also should be considered. It is not discussed in detail here because sampling of a nasogastric aspirate is a relatively easy and reliable means of differentiating these problems. The amount of blood loss associated with intussusception usually is minor, but the associated vomiting and bowel obstruction can cause volume depletion with hemoconcentration. Hemorrhage usually is more profuse with Meckel diverticulum. Infectious diarrhea occurs among this age group. The signs and symptoms include fever and ileus with bloody diarrhea. The diagnosis is confirmed with stool examination for leukocytes and cultures for specific pathogens. The causes of lower GI hemorrhage among infants and children by age group are presented in Table 97.2.

ANSWER: a, c

REFERENCE: *Chapter 97—Pediatric Abdomen: Gastrointestinal Hemorrhage*

9. Which of the following is the most common liver tumor of childhood?

   a. Hemangioma and hemangioendothelioma
   b. Hepatoblastoma
   c. Hepatocellular carcinoma
   d. Mesenchymal hamartoma

COMMENT: Primary liver tumors are uncommon in children. Of these, about one-third are benign and two-thirds are malignant (Table 97.11). The most common presenting feature of liver tumors is an asymptomatic abdominal mass. The diagnostic evaluation usually is an initial ultrasound examination followed by either computed tomography or magnetic resonance imaging for definitive diagnosis. The relative incidence of liver tumors is shown in Table 97.3.

Hepatoblastoma is the most common liver tumor of childhood. Most hepatoblastomas are discovered within the first 2 years of life. Although these are large and may necessitate primary chemotherapy, a 65% to 75% survival rate can be achieved with resection that yields histologically clear margins of resection.

ANSWER: b

REFERENCE: *Chapter 97—Pediatric Abdomen: Tumors of the Liver*

10. A 6-week-old infant with jaundice has biliary atresia. Which of the following statements is/are true?

   a. Portoenterostomy is the initial procedure of choice
   b. Primary liver transplantation with either a reduced-size cadaveric graft or a graft from a living related donor is the procedure of choice
   c. Approximately two thirds of patients treated with portoenterostomy eventually have chronic liver disease sufficient to necessitate liver transplantation
   d. Because biliary atresia has pathogenic components of acute and chronic inflammation, antiinflammatory therapy is known to delay the onset of liver failure

COMMENT: Biliary atresia is an idiopathic process in which the extrahepatic bile ducts are replaced in whole or in part with dense fibrous tissue containing evidence of both acute and chronic inflammation. There is an intrahepatic component as well. Although antiinflammatory therapy is of theoretical interest, no data suggest that antiinflammatory pharmacologic therapy will influence the course of liver disease associated with biliary atresia.

The approach to the usual infant with biliary atresia discovered within the first 90 days of life is to confirm the suspected diagnosis by means of cholangiography at laparotomy and to proceed with portoenterostomy. In general, one third of these infants do well on a long-term basis, one-third have prompt failure, and the others have chronic liver disease that becomes a problem more slowly. Therefore, approximately two thirds of these patients have chronic liver disease for which liver transplantation is a reasonable alternative. Hepatic transplantation is best considered a necessary and complementary approach to portoenterostomy for infants with biliary atresia. Data support its use if portoenterostomy fails or in the care of older infants with established cirrhosis when they come to medical attention. Growth failure, hepatic synthetic failure, and sequelae of portal hypertension are indications to proceed with transplantation.

ANSWER: a, c

REFERENCE: *Chapter 97—Pediatric Abdomen: Biliary Atresia*

11. The operative procedure of choice for managing the most common type of choledochal cyst is which of the following?

    a. Cyst gastrostomy
    b. Cyst jejunostomy
    c. Excision with Roux-en-Y hepatojejunostomy
    d. Transduodenal marsupialization
    e. Endoscopic sphincterotomy

COMMENT: The most common choledochal cyst is a type I cyst—80% to 90% of the total in most reports. These are characterized by fusiform dilatation of the choledochus itself. These cysts typically involve the entire common bile duct with only mild dilatation of the common hepatic duct and a normal intrahepatic system. Management of this lesion always is surgical. Internal drainage procedures without cyst resection (e.g., cyst duodenostomy, cyst gastrostomy, and cyst jejunostomy) were routinely performed for type I choledochal cysts until the 1970s. The rate of failure (e.g., stricture, recurrent cholangitis, stone formation, pancreatitis) ranged from 30% to 75%, depending on the length of the follow-up period and the type of procedure. As these late complication rates became apparent, the risk of bile duct adenocarcinoma in the residual cyst also became widely recognized. Therefore, the preferred operative management of type I choledochal cyst is total transmural excision with Roux-en-Y hepatojejunostomy. Adults with severe inflammation and fibrosis occasionally need intramural cyst dissection that leaves the posteromedial (outer) wall of the cyst in situ to protect the adjacent portal vein and hepatic artery.

ANSWER: c

REFERENCE: *Chapter 97—Pediatric Abdomen: Congenital Cystic Disorder of the Biliary Tract*

12. The risk of development of adenocarcinoma of the biliary tract in a patient with a choledochal cyst left in situ is approximately:

    a. Less than 1%
    b. 3% to 5%
    c. 10% to 15%
    d. Greater than 25%

COMMENT: Adenocarcinoma of the biliary tract develops among 3% to 5% of patients who have choledochal cysts. Although this represents a small number of patients, the total number reported exceeds 50 times and the incidence is approximately 1,000 times that of the healthy population. Carcinoma can develop as early as the adolescent years, in marked contrast to the incidence among the healthy population, in which a presentation in the fifth or sixth decade of life is typical. Neoplastic transformation of the dysplastic biliary cyst epithelium can be caused by chronic inflammation. Consideration of this problem has contributed to the current emphasis on surgical excision of these cysts.

ANSWER: b

REFERENCE: *Chapter 97—Pediatric Abdomen: Congenital Cystic Disorder of the Biliary Tract*

13. The most common cause of acute pancreatitis in childhood is:

    a. Pancreas divisum
    b. Cholelithiasis
    c. Trauma
    d. Valproic acid therapy
    e. Annular pancreas

COMMENT: Although pancreatitis among adults usually is related to cholelithiasis or ingestion of alcohol, pediatric causes are considerably more varied. Fifty percent to 70% of cases of acute pancreatitis among children are idiopathic or posttraumatic. Trauma is the single most common cause of acute pancreatitis in childhood. Cholelithiasis is an important cause for the adolescent population and for children with hematologic disorders. Annular pancreas normally is associated with duodenal atresia and produces neonatal duodenal obstruction but not acute pancreatitis. Pancreas divisum is an anatomic variation present in 10% to 15% of healthy children that is occasionally the cause of acute pancreatitis. Valproic acid is an important anticonvulsant used in pediatric neurology. One of its possible complications is development of acute pancreatitis or necrotizing pancreatitis. Fortunately, this effect is rare because it often is lethal.

ANSWER: c

REFERENCE: *Chapter 97—Pediatric Abdomen: Acute Pancreatitis*

14. A 6-week-old child has generalized seizures, a serum glucose level of 30 mg/dL, and concurrent hyperinsulinemia. The priority is which of the following?

    a. Permanent central venous access and glucose infusion
    b. Administration of cortisone and corticotropin
    c. Computed tomography of the abdomen to look for islet cell adenoma
    d. Urgent pancreatic resection

COMMENT: Most cases of hyperinsulinemia in the first 2 years of life are caused by nesidioblastosis, a condition associated with excessive and diffuse formation of neoislets from primitive pancreatic ductal cells. Hyperinsulinemia secondary to islet cell adenoma or carcinoma or islet cell hyperplasia is more common among older children. Infants with nesidioblastosis, such as the one described here, typically have symptomatic hypoglycemia, seizures, and hyperinsulinemia. An insulin-to-glucose ratio (insulin in IU/mL divided by glucose in mg/dL) greater than 0.5 with fasting is highly suggestive.

Infants with nesidioblastosis are treated initially medically with maintenance of blood glucose levels above 40 mg/dL. This treatment is best provided by means of infusion of hypertonic glucose solutions through a permanent central venous catheter. Diazoxide, cortisone, and corticotropin and streptozocin also have been used to manage hypoglycemia.

Definitive management of nesidioblastosis may necessitate pancreatic resection. This requires pancreatectomy, usually estimated at 95% to 99% with splenic and duodenal preservation. After 90% to 95% pancreatectomy, more than 90% of infants with nesidioblastosis have permanent euglycemia. Computed tomography of the abdomen to search for adenoma is an appropriate diagnostic maneuver, but it is not the priority.

ANSWER: a

REFERENCE: Chapter 97—Pediatric Abdomen: Endocrine Lesions of the Pancreas

15. Meckel diverticulum can present with which of the following signs or symptoms?

    a. Hemorrhage
    b. Intussusception
    c. Volvulus
    d. Patent omphalomesenteric duct
    e. Right lower quadrant peritoneal findings

COMMENT: The most frequent congenital anomaly of the GI tract is Meckel diverticulum. The prevalence is approximately 2% of the general population, and many diverticula remain asymptomatic. Estimates of the frequency with which symptoms develop among persons with Meckel diverticula vary from 4% to 30%, but it is clear that the risk diminishes substantially with age. Approximately one half of persons with diverticula that become symptomatic are younger than 2 years. Hemorrhage, acute diverticulitis, perforation, and small-bowel obstruction or intussusception are classic presenting scenarios for a child with Meckel diverticulum (Table 97.6). Figure 97.43 shows the various anatomic abnormalities and the associated clinical presentations. These presentations include Meckel diverticulitis, which is almost indistinguishable from acute appendicitis.

ANSWER: a, b, c, d, e

REFERENCE: Chapter 97—Pediatric Abdomen: Meckel's Diverticulum and Related Disorders

16. The most common cause of pyogenic liver abscess among children is which of the following?

    a. Perforated appendicitis
    b. Blunt liver injury
    c. Immunocompromised host
    d. Percutaneous liver biopsy
    e. Omphalitis

COMMENT: In the preantibiotic era, pyogenic hepatic abscesses occurred most frequently after perforated appendicitis. This complication is rarely seen today. Chronic granulomatous disease of childhood is a principal condition associated with hepatic abscess. This disease is the result of deficient oxidant-mediated bacterial killing by circulating granulocytes. In the pediatric age group, 40% of pyogenic liver abscesses occur among children with chronic granulomatous disease, and another 30% among children with other immunodeficiencies, most commonly leukemia. Other rare causes of liver abscesses among pediatric patients are umbilical vein catheter-induced infection, omphalitis, and other biliary disease. Pyogenic liver abscess after blunt liver injury or percutaneous liver biopsy is a distinctly rare event.

ANSWER: c

REFERENCE: Chapter 97—Pediatric Abdomen: Hepatic Infections

17. You are asked to recommend therapy for a 2-year-old without symptoms who swallowed a small alkaline watch battery 4 hours ago. A plain radiograph shows the intact battery in the intestine beyond the stomach. The best course of therapy is:

a. Immediate laparotomy, enterotomy, and removal of the battery
b. Enteroscopy with extraction
c. Laparoscopy with ultrasound localization and extraction
d. Administration of cathartics and a follow-up plain radiograph in 48 hours if the child continues to have no symptoms

COMMENT: Passage of an ingested foreign body beyond the gastroesophageal junction is associated with a 95% probability of uneventful distal transit. The character of the foreign body is largely irrelevant, but batteries, particularly alkaline disk batteries, present a potentially serious hazard to children and may necessitate an aggressive approach. A number of reports have documented the unique risk of intestinal perforation resulting from disruption of the battery casing and associated spillage of the toxic contents. Although some experts advocate routine immediate removal, this does not appear necessary. If the battery is endoscopically accessible in the esophagus, it should be removed when recognized. Cathartics and enemas may help expedite passage of batteries found when already in the small or large bowel. Delay for more than a few days, evidence of casing rupture on a plain radiograph, or symptoms of any kind necessitate extraction. Despite the risks, most batteries pass without these sequelae.

ANSWER: d

REFERENCE: *Chapter 97—Pediatric Abdomen: Foreign Bodies*

CHAPTER 98

PEDIATRIC GENITOURINARY SYSTEM

1. The ureteral bud arises from the

a. Gartner duct
b. Metanephric blastema
c. Mesonephric duct
d. Müllerian duct

COMMENT: The mesonephric, or wolffian duct, gives rise to the urethral bud between the 4th and 6th weeks of gestation. This bud joins the metanephric blastema and induces nephron formation. The müllerian duct gives rise to the female genital tract. The Gartner duct is a mesonephric duct remnant in women.

ANSWER: c

REFERENCE: *Chapter 98—Pediatric Genitourinary System: Nephric System*

2. In a patient with a right pelvic kidney, the right adrenal gland is usually:

a. In the left upper quadrant
b. Next to the kidney in the right hemipelvis
c. In the normal position in the right renal fossa
d. Absent

COMMENT: The adrenal gland develops separately from the kidney and is therefore found in its normal position despite anomalies in renal position.

ANSWER: c

REFERENCE: *Chapter 98—Pediatric Genitourinary System: Renal Ectopy*

3. A causative factor in the development of multicystic dysplastic kidney is thought to be:

a. Failure of ureteral bud contact
b. Contralateral renal agenesis
c. Congenital absence of the vas deferens
d. Ureteral reflux

COMMENT: Failure of the ureteral bud to properly contract and induce transformation of the developing metanephric blastema is probably the causative factor in such cases. Multidysplastic kidney is the most common type of renal cystic disease. This anomaly represents a severe form of renal dysplasia with complete replacement of renal parenchyma by different sized cysts (Fig. 98.1)

ANSWER: a

REFERENCE: *Chapter 98—Pediatric Genitourinary System: Nephric System*

4. The best predictor of upper urinary tract damage in children with spinal dysraphism is:

   a. Leak-point pressure greater than 40 cm water
   b. Presence of vesicoureteral reflux
   c. Spinal cord injury above L5
   d. Presence of anterior myelomeningocele

COMMENT: An elevated leak-point pressure is the most important independent predictor of upper tract deterioration. At a bladder pressure of 40 cm water, the ureterovesical junction is presumed no longer to protect the upper tracts from transmission of this pressure. Even without reflux or hydronephrosis, without intervention these patients are likely to have renal damage. Abnormal development of the spinal column affecting spinal cord function (myelodysplasia) is the most common cause of neurogenic bladder among children. Myelomeningocele accounts for more than 90% of open spinal dysraphic states. Bladder dysfunction usually results in urinary incontinence, although a poorly compliant bladder with a leak-point pressure greater than 40 cm water can cause vesicoureteral reflux and hydronephrosis, which lead to deterioration of renal function. Urinary continence de-

pends on bladder capacity and bladder outlet (bladder neck and urethral sphincter) resistance. The most important contribution affecting treatment of these children was the introduction of clean intermittent catheterization to facilitate timely bladder emptying. Evaluation of infants by means of urodynamic studies, renal ultrasonography, and voiding cystourography helps identify those at risk of renal damage.

The primary goals in the care of children with neurogenic bladder are maintenance of safe intravesical pressure, achievement of urinary continence, and preservation of renal function. If anticholinergic therapy with or without clean intermittent catheterization is unsuccessful in achieving these goals, surgical reconstruction is necessary. Owing to the high incidence of gradual upper tract deterioration and the serious sequelae of altered body image after cutaneous urinary diversion, incontinent diversion is no longer considered an acceptable alternative to reconstruction in pediatrics. The goals of reconstructive surgery are to achieve a large capacity, low pressure reservoir, adequate bladder outlet resistance, and easy access for catheterization. A variety of donor tissues sources, including bowel segments, stomach, and ureter, are available for bladder augmentation (Fig. 98.7). Potential complications of enterocystoplasty include electrolyte abnormalities, spontaneous perforation of the bowel segment, and tumor formation. Bladder outlet resistance can be increased by means of bladder neck reconstruction, implantation of an artificial urinary sphincter, urethral or bladder neck suspension, submucosal injection of collagen, or a combination of these procedures. A Mitrofanoff neourethra (appendiceal or ileal) usually is necessary to provide bladder access for decompression and continence and is highly successful in even the most devastating cases (Fig. 98.8).

Neurogenic bladder is frequently accompanied by refractory fecal incontinence. This can severely compromise care with respect to urinary tract infection, incontinence, and achieving independent self-care. When preoperative conventional therapy (dietary modification, timed toileting, cathartics, bulking agents, and enemas) is unsuccessful to control complete evacuation of the colon, an antegrade continence enema, performed through a continent cecostomy with appendix or tapered ileum, is an option (Fig. 98.9). The antegrade continence enema procedure has been successfully used in the management of intractable fecal incontinence, even in association with the most debilitating childhood rectourogenital anomalies.

ANSWER: a

REFERENCE: *Chapter 98—Pediatric Genitourinary System: Neurogenic Bladder*

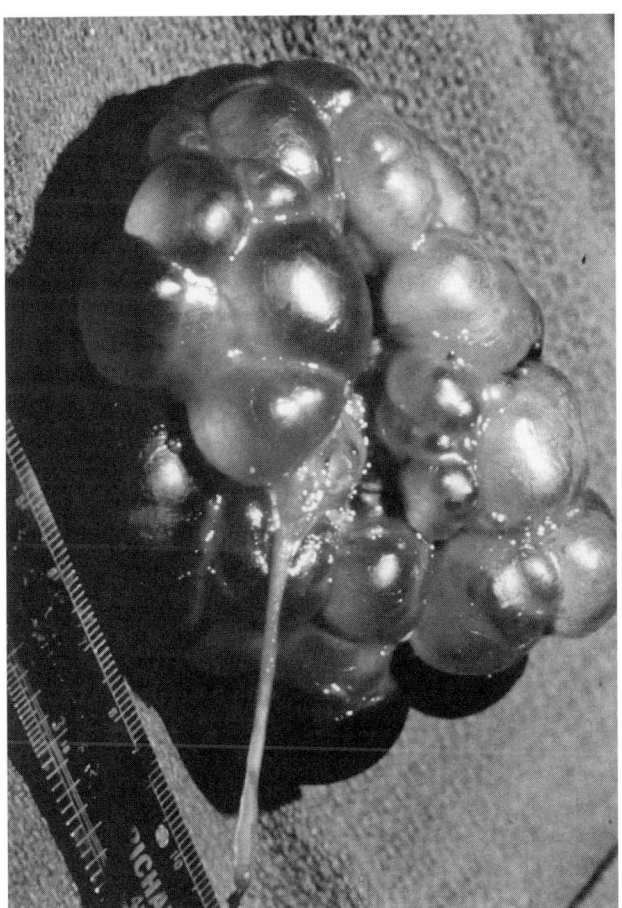

Figure 98.1.

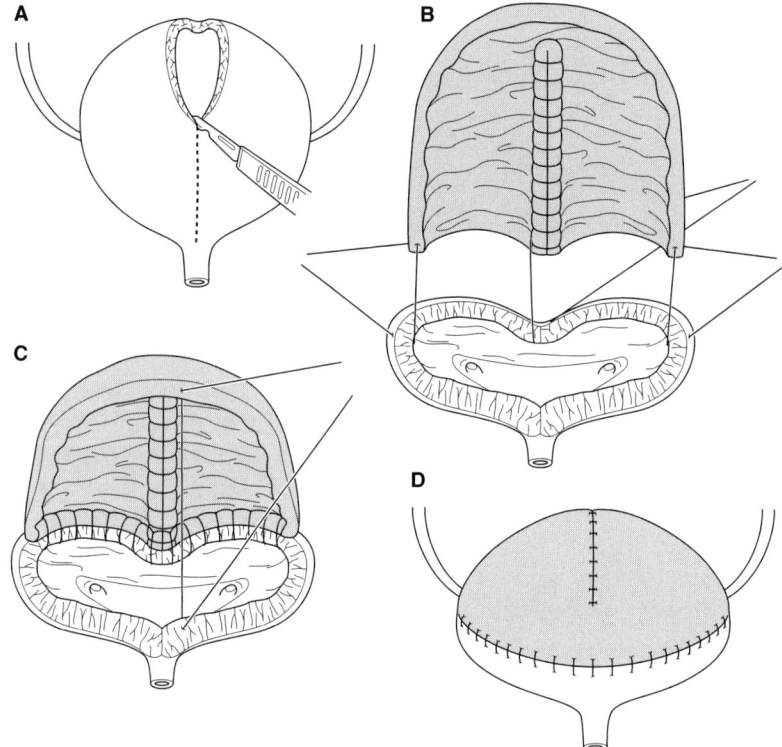

Figure 98.7.

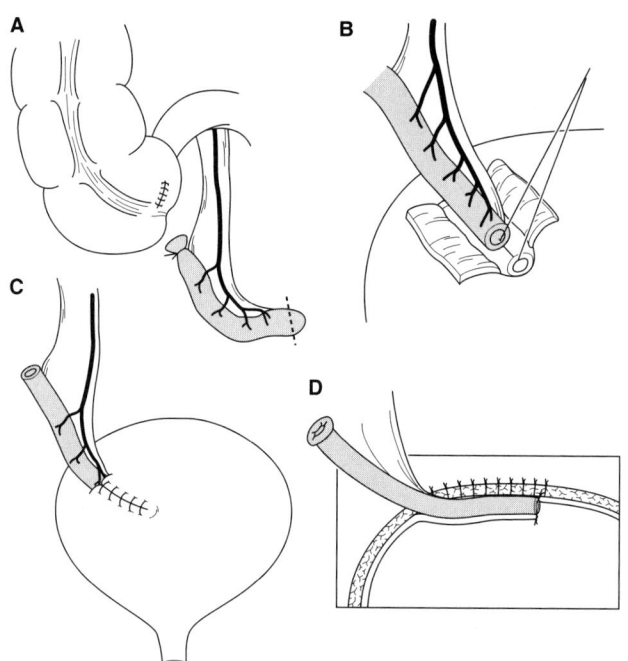

Figure 98.8.

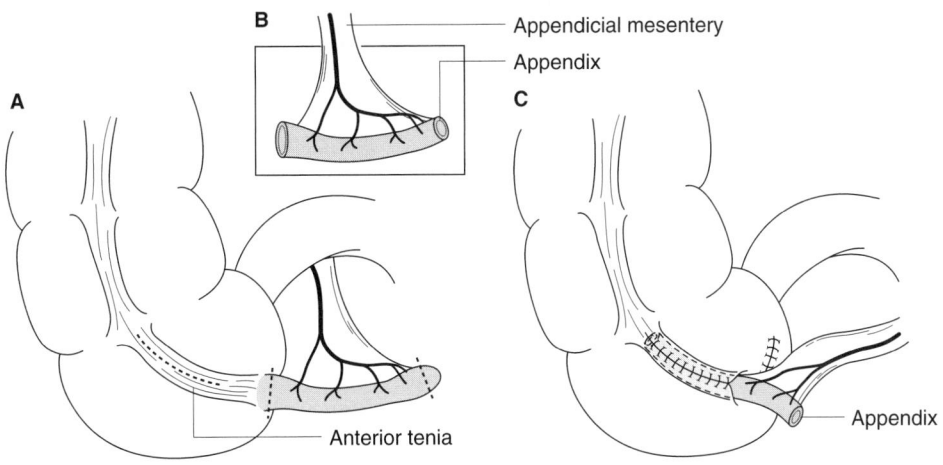

Figure 98.9.

5. A 3-day-old male infant arrives in the emergency department in respiratory distress. He has a dribbling urinary stream. Abdominal ultrasound examination reveals bilateral hydronephrosis and a dilated, thick-walled bladder. The most appropriate initial management is:

a. Cystoscopy
b. Catheter placement
c. Percutaneous nephrostomies
d. Suprapubic tube placement

COMMENT: The child most likely has posterior urethral valves causing bladder outlet obstruction and bilateral hydronephrosis. Immediate management must include urethral catheterization to decompress the obstructed bladder. Posterior urethral valves are the most common obstructive urethral lesions in male infants and represent a membrane or mucosal leaflet within the prostatic urethra. The diagnosis usually is suspected among neonates because of abnormal findings on prenatal ultrasound examinations and the presence of hydronephrosis (bilateral hydronephrosis, distended bladder) and oligohydramnios. Some patients are found to have flank masses, ascites, and urinary retention. Older children usually have voiding symptoms, urinary tract infection, or hematuria. Voiding cystourethrography provides enough information for a diagnosis in most cases, although cystoscopy may be necessary in an equivocal setting. Patients with marked bilateral hydronephrosis need screening for renal insufficiency, and nuclear scintigraphy may be indicated to rule out ureteral obstruction and renal dysplasia.

Temporary urinary drainage with a urethral catheter (feeding tube) can be performed for critically ill patients. Otherwise, primary endoscopic valve ablation is the preferred approach and can be performed safely in most instances. Initial temporary cutaneous vesicostomy sometimes is useful. High upper urinary tract diversion may on rare occasions be necessary in the care of infants with a rising creatinine level despite lower tract drainage. Long-term follow-up care is necessary with special attention to development of a poorly compliant, high-pressure bladder. Careful urodynamic evaluation and timely management of the "valve bladder" with anticholinergics, clean intermittent catheterization, and highly selective vesical reconstruction, including enterocystoplasty, as well as prevention of urinary tract infection, ensure the best chance for successful prevention and management of chronic renal failure.

ANSWER: b

REFERENCE: *Chapter 98—Pediatric Genitourinary System: Anomalies of the Urethra; Posterior Urethral Valves*

6. A newborn infant is found to have clitoromegaly, XX karyotype, and hyponatremia at birth. The most likely cause is:

   a. Androgen insensitivity
   b. 21-Hydroxylase deficiency
   c. 5-α-Reductase deficiency
   d. True hermaphroditism

COMMENT: The most common cause of female pseudohermaphroditism is congenital adrenal hyperplasia, which is most commonly associated with an error of metabolism in the 21-hydroxylase enzyme in the adrenal zona fasciculata. This results in accumulation of androgens and a decrease in mineralocorticoids and cortisol and produces masculinization of the external genitalia and electrolyte imbalances. Congenital adrenal hyperplasia results from a deficiency in the enzymes responsible for the synthesis of mineralocorticoids and glucocorticoids. The result is overproduction of adrenal androgens. A deficiency of 21-hydroxylase is present among 95% of patients with congenital adrenal hyperplasia. All of these patients are genetically female (46,XX karyotype, ovarian gonads) with masculinization of the external genitalia ranging from an enlarged clitoris to a normal-appearing male phallus with complete labial fusion. These patients are potentially fertile regardless of the degree of virilization.

A high index of suspicion allows early diagnosis of this condition and initiation of hormone replacement (glucocorticoids and mineralocorticoids) to prevent adrenal insufficiency, salt-wasting syndrome, and continued virilization. Because internal müllerian structures are always present, these children are reared as girls and feminizing genitoplasty is performed. If the vagina enters the urogenital sinus distal to the external urinary sphincter, cutback or flap vaginoplasty can be combined with clitoroplasty (reduction and relocation of the clitoris with preservation of glandular sensation) and labioplasty in a single procedure (Fig. 98.10). If the vagina enters the urogenital sinus more proximally, a pedicled skin flap, vaginal pull-through, or segmental bowel interposition vaginoplasty is deferred to a later date.

ANSWER: b

REFERENCE: *Chapter 98—Pediatric Genitourinary System: Ambiguous Genitalia; Female Pseudohermaphroditism*

7. Cryptorchid testis should be managed surgically:

   a. For cosmetic reasons alone
   b. Before the patient reaches 5 years of age
   c. To decrease the risk of cancer in the contralateral testis
   d. Before the patient reaches 1 year of age

COMMENT: Permanent damage to the germinal epithelium has usually occurred by 1 year of age. Orchiopexy after this time will not preserve function in this testicle. The incidence of cancer in the ipsilateral testis is not reduced by orchiopexy. However, orchiopexy does facilitate the process of lifelong follow-up evaluation and self-examination of the testis.

Descent of the testis from its original position near the kidney into the cooler scrotum is necessary for its normal development and production of fertile sperm. Various mechanisms, including gubernacular traction and intraabdominal pressure, have been proposed to be responsible for testicular descent, but endocrine factors of the hypothalamic-pituitary-testicular axis also have an important role in this process. Between the 12th and 17th weeks of gestation, the testis undergoes transabdominal migration to a location near the internal inguinal ring. It is not until the 7th month of gestation that transinguinal migration of the testis to its final position takes place.

True undescended testes fail to reach the scrotum despite following a normal line of descent. Ectopic testes follow the usual course of descent until they emerge from the external inguinal ring but are then misdirected to an ectopic position (superficial inguinal pouch, perineal, femoral, transverse scrotal). Although approximately 3.4% of term male infants have undescended testes, 30% of premature infants have this anomaly. By the end of the first year, the incidence of cryptorchidism is approximately 1% and remains at this level thereafter. Most cryptorchid testes that descend during the first year of life do so within the first 3 months after birth. The diagnosis of cryptorchidism relies on gentle and patient genital examination. Relaxation of the patient and warming of the examiner's hand aid in successful examination. Reexamination of the child in the cross-legged position also may reveal the gonad.

A functional classification of cryptorchidism that provides a practical approach to therapy is based on whether the testis is palpable or impalpable (20%). Although endocrine testing is reliable in predicting bilateral anorchidism, radiologic means, including abdominal sonography, computed tomography, magnetic resonance imaging, or gonadal arteriography, are inaccurate in localization of nonpalpable testes. Diagnostic laparoscopy provides the diagnosis of vanishing testis through identification of blind-ending spermatic vessels or accurate localization of the intraabdominal testis in this situation. Undescended testes must be differentiated from retractile testes that may reside above the scrotum but with careful positioning can be made to stay within the lower scrotum without continuous traction.

Although correction of undescended testes eliminates any coexisting inguinal hernia (found in 95% of all cases) and prevents possible testicular injury or torsion (the risk of which is increased among these patients), the central issues in treating these patients revolve around future fertility and the risk of testicular neoplasia. There is increased risk of testicular carcinoma in undescended testes, and orchidopexy facilitates self-examination and early detection of cancer. Because the germ cell count of an infant with undescended testis deteriorates after 1 year of life, correction of cryptorchidism is indicated between 6 and 12 months of age. For palpable undescended testes, routine inguinal orchidopexy is successful for most patients. For high intraabdominal testes, testicular microsurgical autotransplantation provides the highest success rate among different surgical options.

ANSWER: d

REFERENCE: *Chapter 98—Pediatric Genitourinary System: Anomalies of the Male Genitalia; Cryptorchidism*

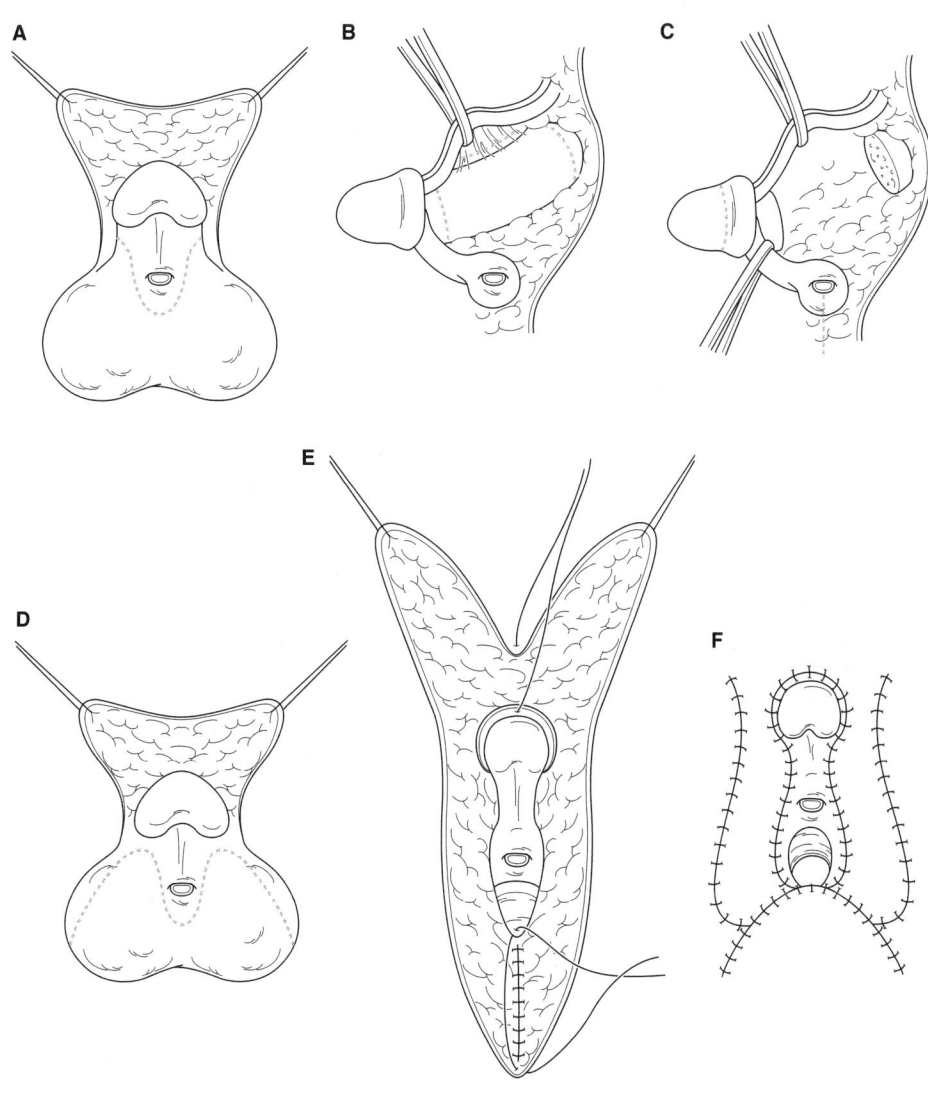

Figure 98.10.

8. A solid, tender, 2-cm by l-cm mass in the right hemiscrotum is found in a newborn boy. This likely represents:

a. Testicular tumor
b. Torsion of the spermatic cord
c. Streak gonad
d. Testicular rhabdomyosarcoma

COMMENT: The most likely diagnosis is prenatal testicular torsion. The tumors rarely manifest as tenderness and are uncommonly identified during the neonatal period. Prenatal torsion presents with a firm, hard scrotal mass that does not transilluminate. The infant otherwise has no symptoms. Salvage of the testis is extremely rare, but timely surgical exploration is indicated to anchor the contralateral testis, because bilateral (synchronous or asynchronous) neonatal testicular torsion has been described. Among older boys, sudden onset of severe testicular pain followed by scrotal swelling is the classic presentation of testicular torsion.

At physical examination, a swollen, tender testis with shortening of the cord is noticed. If testicular torsion is suspected, immediate surgical exploration of the scrotum is indicated. Normal findings at exploration of the scrotum are more acceptable than loss of a testis that might have been salvaged. When suspicion of testicular torsion is low, color Doppler ultrasonography of the scrotum or a testicular nuclear scan can be helpful to differentiate torsion from acute epididymitis. At surgical exploration, the testis is untwisted and examined for viability. A frankly necrotic testis is removed, and viable gonads (return of color, return of Doppler flow, signs of arterial blood after incision of tunica albuginea) are fixed to the scrotal wall to prevent subsequent torsion. Exploration and anchoring of the contralateral testis, which can be done through the same incision, are mandatory to prevent subsequent torsion. Manual detorsion of the twisted testis usually is difficult because of acute pain during manipulation. If manual detorsion is successful (and confirmed with color Doppler ultrasonography for a patient with complete resolution of symptoms), definitive surgical fixation of the testes should be performed as an urgent rather than an emergency procedure before the patient leaves the hospital.

ANSWER: b

REFERENCE: *Chapter 98—Pediatric Genitourinary System: Anomalies of the Male Genitalia; Torsion of the Testis and Appendages*

CHAPTER 99

CHILDHOOD TUMORS

1. Which of the following statements is/are true regarding neuroblastoma?

a. Neuroblastoma is the most common abdominal malignant tumor of childhood
b. Approximately 80% of cases of neuroblastoma are diagnosed before the patient is 4 years of age
c. N-*myc* oncogene copy number in neuroblastoma tissue is inversely related to survival probability
d. *trk* Protooncogene expression in neuroblastoma tissue is inversely related to survival probability
e. All of the above

COMMENT: Neuroblastoma is the most common extracranial solid tumor and the most common abdominal malignant tumor of childhood. The incidence is approximately 8 to 10 per million children younger than 15 years of age. The incidence is uniform throughout the world. This results in approximately 500 new cases reported each year in the United States. The median age at diagnosis is approximately 2 years, and 80% of children are younger than 4 years of age at diagnosis. The N-*myc* oncogene, the function and mechanism of action of which remain the subject of investigation, has been shown empirically to be a useful predictor of survival and risk. Patients with increased copies of the N-*myc* gene have a poor prognosis. Most authorities consider a copy number more than 10 to be significant. The *trk* protooncogene is a component of the high-affinity nerve growth factor receptor and is expressed in human neuroblastoma tissue. Expression of *trk*-A is inversely correlated with N-*myc* amplification and is associated with lower stage at diagnosis and improved prognosis.

ANSWER: a, b, c

REFERENCE: *Chapter 99—Childhood Tumors: Neuroblastoma*

2. Common sites of neuroblastoma metastasis are which of the following?

    a. Lung
    b. Regional lymph nodes
    c. Bone marrow
    d. Cortical bone
    e. Liver

COMMENT: Neuroblastoma metastasizes to both regional lymph nodes and distant sites, most frequently bone marrow or cortical bone. The liver and lungs are rarely the site of metastatic spread. Cortical bone involvement manifesting as positive findings on a bone scan is a particularly poor prognostic indicator. Most patients have locally advanced disease at the time of diagnosis.

ANSWER: b, c, d

REFERENCE: *Chapter 99—Childhood Tumors: Neuroblastoma*

3. Which of the following are considered low-risk features among patients with neuroblastoma?

    a. Age younger than 1 year
    b. Stage 2A and 2B disease (International Staging Criteria)
    c. Stage 4S disease (International Staging Criteria)
    d. Neuron-specific enolase plasma level less than 100 ng/mL
    e. None of the above

COMMENT: Risk status is determined for patients with neuroblastoma by means of a number of characteristics elaborated since the mid 1970s (Table 99.3).

ANSWER: a, b, c, d

REFERENCE: *Chapter 99—Childhood Tumors: Neuroblastoma*

4. Which of the following syndromes is/are associated with the development of Wilms' tumor?

    a. Beckwith-Wiedemann syndrome (hemihypertrophy, macroglossia, aniridia)
    b. Neurofibromatosis
    c. Denys-Drash syndrome (pseudohermaphroditism, glomerulopathy)
    d. Gonadal dysgenesis
    e. Hemolytic uremic syndrome

COMMENT: A number of syndromes are associated with the development of Wilms' tumors. When present, they necessitate routine periodic screening (Table 99.4). There is no known association between hemolytic uremic syndrome and development of Wilms' tumor.

ANSWER: a, b, c, d

REFERENCE: *Chapter 99—Childhood Tumors: Table 99.4*

5. Patients with Wilms' tumors most frequently have which of the following when they come to medical attention?

    a. Bilateral metachronous lesions
    b. Bilateral synchronous lesions
    c. An extrarenal primary lesion
    d. A multicentric primary lesion
    e. A unifocal, unilateral lesion

COMMENT: It is currently hypothesized that Wilms' tumor arises from primitive metanephric blastema and that individual tumors often contain not only primitive metanephric cells but also cartilage, skeletal muscle, and squamous epithelium. Most tumors arise unifocally within the kidney, but approximately 7% of unilateral Wilms' tumors are multicentric. The proportion of synchronous bilateral tumors among all patients with nephroblastoma ranges from 4.4% to 7.0%, whereas that of metachronous tumors is 1.0% to 1.9%. Wilms' tumors are equally distributed with regard to the left and right side and can occur with no apparent connection to the kidneys. Extrarenal Wilms' tumor usually occurs in the retroperitoneal area, but other reported sites include the pelvis, scrotum, and inguinal region.

ANSWER: e

REFERENCE: *Chapter 99—Childhood Tumors: Wilms' Tumor*

6. Which of the following approaches is considered standard care for most patients with Wilms' tumor in the United States?

    a. Doxorubicin hydrochloride (Adriamycin) and vincristine therapy followed by surgical resection
    b. Needle biopsy followed by either chemotherapy or resection depending on the histologic findings
    c. Primary surgical resection followed by chemotherapy
    d. Radiation therapy if the lesion is judged unresectable at computed tomography or magnetic resonance imaging

COMMENT: The standard of care of patients with Wilms' tumor in the United States is initial surgical resection. Exceptions to this rule include extensive intracaval tumors that necessitate cardiopulmonary bypass for extraction, obviously unresectable tumors with documented invasion of contiguous structures, and possibly bilateral tumors, especially if it is unclear which side is most heavily involved. All patients with resectable Wilms' tumor receive postoperative chemotherapy with the possible exception of those with stage 1 favorable histologic features younger than 24 months of age at diagnosis who have tumors that weigh less than 250 g at resection. Chemotherapy followed by surgical resection is practiced in Europe with outcomes roughly equal to those in the United States, but this approach has the disadvantage of changing the surgical and pathologic staging that forms the basis of the national Wilms' tumor studies and is the cornerstone of treatment in the United States. Needle biopsy has a limited role for unusual presentations of Wilms' tumor because the diagnosis is generally apparent with modern imaging techniques. Radiation therapy is not a primary mode of therapy for Wilms' tumor under contemporary national Wilms' tumor treatment protocols.

ANSWER: c

REFERENCE: *Chapter 99—Childhood Tumors: Wilms' Tumor*

7. Which of the following statements is/are true regarding renal tumors of childhood and adolescence?

    a. Clear cell sarcoma is considered a variant of Wilms' tumor with a poor prognosis
    b. Clear cell sarcoma of the kidney has a high rate of metastasis to bone
    c. Rhabdoid tumors can arise in the kidney, mediastinum, or brain
    d. Childhood rhabdoid tumors of the kidney carry an excellent prognosis

COMMENT: Clear cell sarcoma of the kidney is considered a distinct histopathologic and clinical entity from Wilms' tumor. It has an age distribution similar to that of Wilms' tumor but a markedly worse prognosis. It is characterized by a proclivity to metastasize to bones and has been called *bone-metastasizing renal tumor of childhood*. Relapse and death occur among 75% of patients, and more than one-half die within 1 year of diagnosis. Aggressive systemic chemotherapy is recommended for all stages of the disease. Postoperative radiation to the tumor bed also is recommended regardless of stage.

Rhabdoid tumors are rare malignant lesions that most commonly involve the kidney in childhood but also can occur primarily in the mediastinum or brain. Outcome is particularly poor, and there is no proven chemotherapy regimen. Rhabdoid tumors of the kidney occur in infancy with a median age at presentation of 13 months. Survival rates are almost zero, and even patients with stage I disease fare poorly. Aggressive therapy is warranted, including surgical resection, local radiation therapy, and systemic chemotherapy.

ANSWER: b, c

REFERENCE: *Chapter 99—Childhood Tumors: Non-Wilms' Renal Tumors of Childhood and Adolescence*

8. A 1-month-old female infant is brought for evaluation of a friable polypoid mass prolapsing through the vaginal introitus. The presumptive diagnosis is:

 a. Ectopic ureterocele
 b. Rectal prolapse
 c. Congenital adrenal hyperplasia with ambiguous genitalia
 d. Embryonal rhabdomyosarcoma

COMMENT: Vaginal and cervical primary rhabdomyosarcoma often prolapses through the vaginal orifice as a friable polypoid mass and can hemorrhage. Botryoid tumors are of the embryonal subtype but grow into a hollow space, such as the vagina or bladder, so they acquire a characteristic "grape-like" appearance. Other patterns of rhabdomyosarcoma include alveolar and pleomorphic morphologic features. The incidence of rhabdomyosarcoma is biphasic with one peak in infancy followed by the second in the adolescent years. The nature of presentation is site dependent. This patient has a classic presentation of vaginal botryoid rhabdomyosarcoma. The emphasis is to perform a thorough pretreatment evaluation that completely defines the extent of local tumor and the regional and distant sites of metastases.

ANSWER: d

REFERENCE: *Chapter 99—Childhood Tumors: Rhabdomyosarcoma*

9. Which of the following statements is/are true regarding rhabdomyosarcoma?

 a. Surgical resection of the primary tumor results in cure of approximately 80% to 90% of all patients
 b. Currently recommended therapy includes complete resection of primary tumors before chemotherapy for small noninvasive lesions or after documented response with more formidable primary tumors
 c. Alveolar histologic findings are a favorable prognostic finding
 d. The overall survival rate is approximately 50%

COMMENT: In the early 1970s, surgical resection of the primary tumor was the mainstay of therapy for rhabdomyosarcoma but resulted in an overall survival rate of only approximately 20%. This improved to approximately 50% with the addition of chemotherapy. Survival is stage dependent. If all cases (both high and low risk) are included, the overall survival rate for rhabdomyosarcoma is approximately 50%. It is recommended that complete resection of primary tumors should be undertaken either before chemotherapy for small, noninvasive lesions or after documented response with more formidable primary tumors. In certain situations in which chemotherapy results in complete or very good tumor regression, external beam radiation can be used as a primary means of local control. Debilitating or disfiguring surgery is performed only if residual tumor is present after both chemotherapy and therapeutic irradiation. Alveolar histologic features are associated with a particularly poor prognosis for rhabdomyosarcoma.

ANSWER: b, d

REFERENCE: *Chapter 99—Childhood Tumors: Rhabdomyosarcoma*

10. Hepatoblastoma is a childhood liver tumor characterized by:

a. Multicentricity
b. Cirrhosis in the uninvolved liver
c. Long-term survival if an unresectable tumor is subjected to cytoreductive chemotherapy
d. Jaundice

COMMENT: Children with hepatoblastoma most commonly have an abdominal mass or diffuse abdominal swelling. The child is typically in good health, and the lesion is found by an observant parent or a clinician at routine examination. Weight loss and other symptoms are unusual. Results of liver function tests usually are normal or nonspecifically altered. Jaundice is uncommon. The most useful tumor marker is serum α-fetoprotein level, which is elevated in approximately 90% of cases.

Hepatoblastoma usually manifests as a single, pseudoencapsulated lesion that often reaches large proportions before becoming apparent. The umbilical fissure generally is not breached. Multicentricity occurs in less than 20% of cases, and cirrhosis of the surrounding liver is unusual. Multicentricity and associated cirrhosis are typical of hepatocellular carcinoma. Complete surgical resection remains the most important objective of therapy for hepatoblastoma. At presentation, approximately 60% of patients with hepatoblastoma have resectable tumors. Chemotherapy is the main treatment option available for unresectable tumors. Over the last decade, it has become apparent that some of these tumors can be rendered resectable with preoperative chemotherapy.

ANSWER: c

REFERENCE: *Chapter 99—Childhood Tumors: Hepatic Tumors*

Section P
MUSCULOSKELETAL SYSTEM

CHAPTER 100

ORTHOPEDIC SURGERY

1. The most important structural component of connective tissue is collagen. Which of the following statements is/are true concerning types of collagen?

a. All collagen is fiber forming
b. Type I collagen is the most abundant in the human body
c. Type II collagen is found in cartilage
d. The basement membrane collagens, type IV and V, do not form regular fibers

COMMENT: At least 15 separate collagen molecules have been identified, each with a specific confirmation associated with a unique kinetic or mechanical property. The collagens can be categorized into two major groups—fiber-forming collagen and collagen that does not form regular fibers. The fiber-forming types of collagen are I, II, and III. Type I collagen is the most abundant in the human body and is the dominant constituent in tendons, ligaments, bone, skin, vessel walls, and scar and granulation tissue. Type II collagen is present in cartilage, and type III collagen is present in tendon and ligament sheaths as well as in muscle, skin, blood vessel walls, and scar tissue. The other types of collagen do not form regular fibers and include the basement membrane collagens, types IV and V.

ANSWER: b, c, d

REFERENCE: *Chapter 100—Orthopedic Surgery: Soft Tissues*

2. Which of the following statements is/are true concerning soft-tissue repair?

   a. The first stage involves a formation of granulation tissue
   b. The initial pattern of collagen fibers and the degrees of waviness are random and therefore not as functional as the normal structure
   c. Early immobilization, regulated physical stimulation, and good vascular supply are beneficial to healing
   d. Normal physiologic loading conditions impair wound remodeling

COMMENT: The healing of soft tissue occurs in stages. The first stage involves granulation tissue, in which the collagen fibers are oriented in a random pattern and the degree of waviness also is random. This tissue is not as functional as the more optimal normal structure. In time, the soft tissue is remodeled to produce an architecture more nearly that of normal intact tissue. Factors associated with beneficial effects on healing include early immobilization, regulated physical stimuli, and good vascular supply. Remodeling or adaptation of soft tissues also has been shown to occur under normal physiologic loading conditions. There are reports that training effects increase the properties of tissues and metabolically active cells incorporated within the matrix.

ANSWER: a, b, c

REFERENCE: *Chapter 100—Orthopedic Surgery: Soft Tissues*

3. Which of the following statements is/are true concerning types of bone in the human body?

   a. Trabecular and cortical bone differ in chemical, molecular, and cellular components
   b. Primary bone must be formed on existing surfaces
   c. Woven bone reflects a highly organized microstructural organization
   d. Secondary osteonal bone is the primary constituent of adult cortices

COMMENT: Two major types of bone are present in the human body—trabecular and cortical. Although the chemical, molecular, and cellular components are similar, the organization of these components at the ultrastructural and microstructural levels leads to considerable differences in mechanical and metabolic activities. The microstructural organization of bone can be classified into three types—primary bone, secondary bone, and woven bone. The most important characteristic of primary bone is that it must be formed on existing surfaces. The surfaces can be cartilaginous or preexisting bone. This bone is highly organized and has excellent mechanical properties. Secondary osteonal bone is the primary constituent of adult cortices. The final microstructural type of bone is woven bone. Although the collagen matrices in lamellar and osteonal bone are precisely organized and provide maximal mechanical properties with minimal material, woven bone is composed of disorganized yet highly mineralized tissue and is expressed in the course of fracture or damage repair. It has the advantage of being quickly deposited but the disadvantage of having fewer mechanical properties than highly ordered primary and secondary bone.

ANSWER: b, d

REFERENCE: *Chapter 100—Orthopedic Surgery: Bone and Joint Infections in Adults*

4. Which of the following statements is/are true concerning bone remodeling?

   a. Remodeling can occur only on the surface of trabeculae
   b. The remodeling process takes approximately 120 days in an adult
   c. Trabecular bone remodeling occurs up to 10 times faster than cortical bone remodeling
   d. Bone modeling involves bone formation without resorption

COMMENT: After initial development and deposition, bone is remodeled in an effort to produce optimal alignment and structure. This process involves the resorption by osteoclasts followed by deposition of nonmineralized matrix (osteoid) by osteoblasts. During mineralization, the osteoblasts become entrapped in their matrix and serve as the resulting bone cells (osteocytes). This remodeling can occur on the surface of trabeculae, on the surface of cortical bone, and intercortically. It proceeds as a method of normal turnover to provide access to minerals needed for normal homeostasis. Under normal circumstances, the process takes approximately 120 days in an adult. Trabecular bone remodels at a rate 5 to 10 times that of cortical bone remodeling, probably because of its porosity and greater surface to volume ratio. It is important to differentiate bone remodeling from modeling. Bone remodeling involves resorption of existing bone followed by formation within the resorption cavity. Modeling describes the phenomenon of bone formation without resorption. This modeling can occur only through deposition of woven bone and during fracture healing.

ANSWER: b, c, d

REFERENCE: *Chapter 100—Orthopedic Surgery: Bone and Joint Infections in Adults*

5. Which of the following statements is/are true concerning the biologic mechanisms of fracture repair?

   a. The mechanisms involved depend primarily on the stability of the fracture
   b. The first material formed by osteoblasts at the fracture site is woven bone
   c. Callus increases the cross-sectional area of the injury and weakens the structure
   d. Woven bone provides a permanent microstructure in the area of a fracture

COMMENT: After initial inflammation and neovascularization of an area of fracture, the repair continues by a combination of mechanisms—endochondral ossification, direct bone apposition, and primary healing involving acceleration of the normal remodeling process directed across a stable, securely reduced fracture line. The occurrence and distribution of these mechanisms depends primarily on the stability of the fracture during management and secondarily on the fracture location. The more unstable the fracture, the more endochondral is the repair process and the greater is the cross-sectional area of the callus. The biologic processes are driven by the need to establish mechanical integrity as quickly as possible. The first material formed by osteoblast at the fracture site is woven bone. Although woven bone has inferior mechanical properties compared with lamellar bone, it can be laid down rapidly and at high density. The laws of mechanics dictate that an increase in cross-sectional area as produced by surrounding callus greatly increases the resistance of the structure to bending or torsional loads. An increase in unit diameter of the cross section increases the strength of the structure by the fourth power of the diameter change. Therefore, even if callus is made of an inferior material, the cross-sectional attributes more than compensate for the inferior substance. Once the fracture is stabilized by means of initial woven bone proliferation, secondary remodeling occurs.

ANSWER: a, b

REFERENCE: *Chapter 100—Orthopedic Surgery: Orthopedic Disorders*

6. Which of the following statements is/are true concerning the management of diaphyseal fractures?

    a. The use of intramedullary rods allows early weight bearing and minimal immobilization
    b. The infection rate with intramedullary fraction fixation devices is minimal
    c. Results of the use of intramedullary rods are better for fractures of the femoral shaft than of the tibia
    d. Loss of limb length is inevitable with segmented or comminuted fractures

COMMENT: Management of diaphyseal fractures, particularly tibial, femoral, and humeral fractures, entails use of intramedullary fracture fixation devices. The use of intramedullary rods allows early weight bearing and requires minimal immobilization of the joints above and below the fracture. Little long-term remodeling (loss of bone) has been documented. Rehabilitation is rapid, and blood loss is minimized. For simple transverse or oblique closed fractures, the infection rate is nearly zero. When used to manage segmented or comminuted fractures or other unstable fractures with proximal and distal bone loss, the interlocking allows surgical reestablishment of the bone compartment and therefore limb length. The device can maintain length until the fracture is healed. Although this technique is the optimal management of most fractures of the femoral shaft, application of these same principles to the tibia has not resulted in such dependable results.

ANSWER: a, b, c

REFERENCE: *Chapter 100—Orthopedic Surgery: Orthopedic Disorders*

7. Principles to be considered with the use of open reduction and internal fixation include:

    a. Anatomic reduction and fixation stability
    b. Maintenance of maximal soft tissue coverage and interposition between the device and skin surface
    c. Development of fixation constructs that minimize load shielding of the underlying bone
    d. Maximal maintenance of periosteal and vascular tissue without compromising stability

COMMENT: When open reduction and internal fixation treatment are chosen, the following principles should be considered: (a) maximal maintenance of periosteal and vascular tissues without compromising stability; (b) anatomic reduction and fixation stability; (c) the use of high-strength, biocompatible implants; (d) the development of fixation constructs that minimize load shielding of the underlying bone; and (e) maintenance of maximal soft-tissue coverage and interposition between the device and skin surface.

ANSWER: a, b, c, d

REFERENCE: *Chapter 100—Orthopedic Surgery: Orthopedic Disorders*

8. Which of the following statements is/are correct concerning total joint replacement arthroplasty?

   a. Total knee and hip prostheses have a life expectancy of approximately 10 years

   b. The most important failure of total joint arthroplasty is aseptic mechanical loosening at the interface between the bone, cement, and implant

   c. Biologic tissue ingrowth into a prosthesis worsens long-term results

   d. Rigid fixation at the time of implantation is important to secure tissue ingrowth

COMMENT: Technologic advances in both biomaterials and manufacturing have led to dramatic improvement in total joint replacement surgery. These advances have improved the longevity of artificial joints, particularly hip and knee prostheses, which are by far the most common. Despite these advances, the procedure is still considered primarily for elderly patients. Total knee and hip prostheses have a fixation life expectancy of approximately 15 years or more in many patients. The most important failure of total joint arthroplasty is aseptic mechanical loosening at the interface between the bone, cement, and implant. Factors that contribute to loosening include excessive weight, high activity level, component misalignment, and breakdown of the cement interface. An advance that has had clinical success is the use of porous surface coated prostheses that promote biologic tissue ingrowth and fixation of the implants. These implants are designed to be inserted surgically into carefully prepared bone under conditions of interference fit (tight intimate contact). It is proposed that significant bone tissue infiltration into the porous surface will begin within 8 to 12 weeks and that after an appropriate amount of time (perhaps 1 year), long-term equilibrium bone remodeling will result in a well-fixed bone ingrowth phase that will last for years. Two factors are important to secure fixation. First, the implant must be fixed rigidly within the bone during the initial ingrowth period. Second, the local mechanical environment must promote a positive remodeling response of the supporting trabecular bone.

ANSWER: b, d

REFERENCE: *Chapter 100—Orthopedic Surgery: Mechanically Damaged Joints*

9. Which of the following statements is/are true concerning operative arthroscopy?

   a. Arthroscopy is unquestionably the most effective method of diagnosis and management of knee ligament injuries

   b. Arthroscopic repair allows almost immediate rehabilitation

   c. Despite advances, an anterior cruciate ligament tear will essentially end any high-level sports activity

   d. The presence of loose osteochondral fragments necessitates open arthrotomy

COMMENT: Arthroscopy is unquestionably the most effective method for the diagnosis and management of injuries to the knee ligaments. Previously there was no certainty that there was a torn ligament, or how many, or whether the tears were complete. With arthroscopy, ligament injuries can be diagnosed with certainty the day of injury or soon thereafter and reparative surgical treatment initiated. Complete tears of the anterior cruciate ligament are devastating. The arthroscope allows immediate and certain diagnosis of an anterior cruciate ligament tear and is a valuable tool in operative reconstruction of function. With small external incisions, special drilling guides, and an arthroscope, strong bone-ligament-bone grafts can be placed in an anatomic location. Considerable increased stability often is achieved, allowing patients to return to high-level sports activity. The small incision, clear visualization of the interior of the joint, and ability to perform definitive surgical correction with minimal damage to other structures often allows immediate rehabilitation. Muscular atrophy due to extensive immobilization and prohibition of weight bearing is prevented. Loose fragments from minuscule injuries can be removed easily with an arthroscope. If the fragments are too large for removal with standard small, delicate arthroscopy instruments, small direct arthrotomy can be performed and arthroscopically directed open removal of loose fragments easily accomplished. Loose bodies that previously had to be removed by means of open arthrotomy are more easily managed with arthroscopic instrumentation.

ANSWER: a, b

REFERENCE: *Chapter 100—Orthopedic Surgery: Mechanically Damaged Joints*

10. Serum proteins that have been found to influence bone induction include:

   a. Platelet-derived growth factor
   b. Transforming growth factor-β
   c. Osteogenin
   d. Fibroblast growth factor

COMMENT: A number of proteins have been found to directly or indirectly influence bone induction. Platelet-derived growth factor from platelets and macrophages has been shown to induce migration and mitosis of mesenchymal cells in wounds and to enhance cartilage and bone formation in adult rats. Fibroblast growth factor is a mitogenic and angiogenic protein that favors new bone formation, particularly if neovascularization is required. Transforming growth factor-β is secreted from bone cell cultures. This protein appears to be naturally released from platelets at the time of a fracture and stimulates proliferation of osteoblasts and increases their production of collagen. A purified and partially sequenced regulator from bovine bone matrix called *osteogenin* has been isolated. This substance can induce cartilage and bone formation and has an important controlling role in the development of de novo bone in muscle and subcutaneous tissues.

ANSWER: a, b, c, d

REFERENCE: *Chapter 100—Orthopedic Surgery: Growth Factors and Other Small-protein Cytokines*

Section Q

NERVOUS SYSTEM

CHAPTER 101

NERVOUS SYSTEM

1. A 29-year-old woman is brought to the emergency department 2 hours after a fall from her horse. The patient apparently was unconscious after the accident but is awake when she arrives and reporting only a "headache." Physical examination reveals bilateral bruising around the eyes and cerebrospinal fluid (CSF) rhinorrhea. A detailed neurologic examination reveals no focal deficits, and computed tomography documents a basilar skull fracture with no other injuries. The most appropriate management with regard to CSF rhinorrhea would be:

   a. Initiation of aerosolized antibiotic therapy
   b. Immediate surgical exploration with a fascial patch graft to close the defect
   c. Immediate decompression of CSF with a closed lumbar drainage catheter
   d. Bilateral nasal packing with sterile gauze
   e. Expectant management

COMMENT: Traumatic CSF rhinorrhea or otorrhea should be managed expectantly. Cerebrospinal fluid leaks typically stop within the first 7 to 10 days after injury. Persistent leaks can be managed with lumbar CSF drainage to seal the leak by means of decreasing CSF volume and intracranial pressure. If this therapy fails, surgical exploration and oversewing of the defect with a fascial patch graft are indicated. Fewer than 5% of patients need surgical repair. Prophylactic antibiotics are no longer used because prospective studies have not shown appreciable benefit from their use.

ANSWER: e

REFERENCE: *Chapter 101—Nervous System: Trauma; Skull Fracture*

2. The clinical scenario of a suddenly comatose patient with a history of head trauma 20 hours ago associated with brief loss of consciousness immediately after injury followed by a lucid interval and no neurologic symptoms is classic for:

a. Epidural hematoma
b. Traumatic rupture of a cerebral arteriovenous malformation
c. Acute subdural hematoma
d. Subacute subdural hematoma
e. Subdural hygroma

COMMENT: Epidural hematoma classically follows a blow to the head that causes a brief period of unconsciousness. After the patient regains consciousness, there may be a lucid interval during which there are no abnormal neurologic symptoms or signs. As a hematoma between the inner table of the skull and the dura mater enlarges, hemispheric compression occurs and causes coma. Epidural hematoma usually arises from a tear of the middle meningeal artery or one of its branches and typically is associated with fracture of the temporal bone. Arterial bleeding strips the dura from the undersurface of the bone and produces still more bleeding because the small bridging veins from the dura to the skull are torn.

ANSWER: a

REFERENCE: *Chapter 101—Nervous System: Trauma; Epidural Hematoma*

3. An injury resulting in acute transection of the spinal cord at the level of C7 would result in which of the following findings below the level of the lesion?

a. Areflexia, spasticity, anesthesia, and autonomic paralysis
b. Hyperreflexia, flaccidity, anesthesia, and autonomic paralysis
c. Areflexia, flaccidity, anesthesia, and autonomic paralysis
d. Areflexia, flaccidity, anesthesia, and autonomic spasticity
e. Hyperreflexia, flaccidity, anesthesia, and autonomic paralysis

COMMENT: Transection of the spinal cord leads to a complete spinal cord lesion, signifying total loss of function below the level of injury. Acute transection is characterized by areflexia, flaccidity, anesthesia, and autonomic paralysis below the level of the lesion. Arterial hypotension is present when the transection is above T5 because of loss of sympathetic vascular tone.

ANSWER: c

REFERENCE: *Chapter 101—Nervous System: Trauma; Spinal Cord Injury*

4. A 50-year-old man is brought to the emergency department by paramedics after a motor vehicle accident in which his car was struck from behind by another vehicle traveling approximately 30 miles per hour (48 km/h). Neurologic examination reveals bilateral loss of motor function and pain sensation in the upper extremities with relative preservation of motor function and sensation in the lower extremities. Plain radiographs of the cervical spine reveal no fracture or dislocation. These findings are most consistent with a diagnosis of:

a. Anterior spinal artery syndrome
b. Central cord syndrome
c. Brown-Sequard syndrome
d. Spinal shock
e. Factitious paralysis

COMMENT: Patients with incomplete spinal cord lesions have some neurologic function below the level of injury. Central cord syndrome is characterized by bilateral loss of motor function and pain and loss of temperature sensation in the upper extremities with relative preservation of these functions in the lower extremities. The distal upper extremities are more severely affected because the most medial portions of the corticospinal and spinothalamic tracts subserve these areas. These findings often are present after hyperextension injury to the cervical spine with or without fracture. Anterior spinal artery syndrome involves bilateral loss of motor function, pain, and temperature sensation below the level of the lesion with sparing of position and vibratory and light touch sensation. This lesion occurs with occlusion of the anterior spinal artery and leads to bilateral ischemia in the anterior and lateral columns. Brown-Sequard syndrome involves ipsilateral loss of motor function and position and vibratory sensation with contralateral loss of pain and temperature sensation below the level of injury.

ANSWER: b

REFERENCE: *Chapter 101—Nervous System: Trauma; Spinal Cord Injury*

5. In acute meningitis occurring after closed head trauma with CSF rhinorrhea, the most common causative organism is:

a. *Streptococcus pneumoniae*
b. *Staphylococcus epidermidis*
c. *Staphylococcus aureus*
d. *Escherichia coli*
e. *Candida albicans*

COMMENT: Meningitis occurring after closed head trauma with either a skull fracture or CSF rhinorrhea is most often caused by *S. pneumoniae*. Meningitis that develops after a penetrating wound or a neurosurgical procedure usually is caused by staphylococcal, streptococcal, or gram-negative organisms. Ventricular shunt and reservoir infections leading to meningitis are more likely due to *Staph. epidermidis* or *Staph. aureus*.

ANSWER: a

REFERENCE: *Chapter 101—Nervous System: Trauma; Skull Fracture*

6. High-grade astrocytoma:
    a. Is a rare intracranial tumor
    b. Is primarily a brain tumor of children
    c. Although malignant histologically, is a well encapsulated tumor
    d. Has a poor prognosis with an average survival time of approximately 12 months, despite surgery and adjuvant therapy
    e. Arises from the glial cells that line the ventricular system

COMMENT: High-grade astrocytoma (grades III and IV) is the most common primary intracranial tumor, constituting 35% to 45% of all adult brain tumors and 50% of all gliomas. Age at discovery ranges from 45 to 65 years. The frontal and temporal regions are most commonly involved. Because of their infiltrative nature, many of these high-grade neoplasms involve both cerebral hemispheres by invading across the corpus callosum and are called *butterfly gliomas*. The histologic features of these malignant lesions are sheets of anaplastic cells with bizarre nuclei, numerous mitoses, endothelial proliferation, and abundant necrosis. Patients have a short history of headache, focal neurologic deficit, changes in mental status, or seizures (typically weeks in duration). The tumors are readily seen on computed tomographic scans as low-attenuation lesions with marked peritumoral edema and mass effect. Ninety-six percent show enhancement with intravenous administration of contrast material. Despite aggressive surgery, radiation therapy, and chemotherapy, which can extend survival and improve quality of life, these tumors are nearly uniformly fatal. Although younger patients tend to do better, the average survival time with surgery and adjuvant therapy is approximately 12 months.

ANSWER: d

REFERENCE: *Chapter 101—Nervous System: Neoplasms; Astrocytoma*

7. A 70-year-old man arrives for his yearly physical and reports that 1 week ago he had a 48-hour period in which he was unable to move his right upper extremity. He noticed no other symptoms, and this temporary hemiparesis resolved. A detailed neurologic examination reveals no residual deficit. This acute loss of motor function can best be classified as:
    a. Transient ischemic attack
    b. Reversible ischemic neurologic deficit
    c. Amaurosis fugax
    d. Vertebrobasilar insufficiency
    e. Completed stroke with resolution

COMMENT: Most ischemic episodes last seconds to minutes; rarely do they last longer than 30 minutes. A neurologic deficit that resolves within 24 hours is a transient ischemic attack. An ischemic deficit that lasts 24 hours to 1 week is called a reversible ischemic neurologic deficit. Ischemic deficits that last longer than this are considered completed strokes. Transient cerebral ischemia in the carotid circulation usually consists of temporary hemianesthesia, hemiparesis, or aphasia. Amaurosis fugax is transient loss of vision in one eye, usually in the form of an ascending or descending shade effect. Ischemia in the vertebrobasilar system can consist of transient diplopia, dizziness, dysarthria, dysphagia, weakness, numbness, loss of vision, or even loss of memory.

ANSWER: b

REFERENCE: *Chapter 101—Nervous System: Cerebrovascular Disease*

8. For a patient with known lumbar disk disease, the most urgent indication for surgical intervention would be:
    a. A second episode requiring narcotics for pain management
    b. A positive result of a straight leg raise test
    c. Symptoms of neurogenic claudication
    d. Acute sphincter dysfunction
    e. Diagnostic confirmation of lumbar radiculopathy by means of electromyography

COMMENT: Surgical management of lumbar disk disease is reserved for patients with an acute or progressive neurologic deficit, chronic disabling pain, or both. The acute onset of weakness or sphincter disturbance constitutes an emergency and demands prompt diagnosis and an early operation.

ANSWER: d

REFERENCE: *Chapter 101—Nervous System: Degenerative Spine Disease; Lumbar Spine*

Section R

GENITOURINARY SYSTEM

CHAPTER 102

MALE ANATOMY AND PHYSIOLOGY

1. Benign prosthetic hypertrophy (BPH) is the most common cause of bladder outlet obstruction in older men. Which of the following statements is/are true concerning this condition?

   a. Urinary flow rate in men with urinary obstruction is usually less than 50 mL in five seconds

   b. Medications such as α1-adrenergic blockers and 5-α-reductase inhibitors provide an alternative for surgical therapy for BPH

   c. A careful history with respect to a patient's medications is important to rule out a pharmacologic cause for bladder outlet obstructive symptoms

   d. Transurethral resection of the prostrate (TURP) remains the only surgical option

COMMENT: Although BPH is by far the most common cause of bladder outlet obstruction in men older than 50-years of age, assorted other conditions may be associated with similar symptoms including urethral stricture, prostrate cancer, neurogenic bladder, bladder calculus, prostatitis, bladder-neck contraction and bladder cancer. History and physical examination combined with appropriate laboratory testing represents the cornerstone of diagnosis. Medication should be reviewed in all patients to discern whether any may be associated with voiding dysfunction. Agents that depress bladder muscle contractility (e.g., anticholinergic agents, anti-spasmodic drugs and anti-depressant drugs) or increase bladder outlet resistance (e.g., sympathomimetics) are known to disturb normal micturition. The urinary flow rate, represented by the amount of urine voided during a timed period, is a simple, valuable tool. Normal men have five-second volumes exceeding 75 mL, whereas men with urinary obstruction have flows less than 50 mL in five seconds. The management of BPH has rapidly expanded in recent years to include a variety of medical and surgical options. Both surgical prostectomy (i.e., transurethral resection of prostrate) or open surgical enucleation of the adnomenous tissue through suprapubic, retropubic or peroneal incisions have been long available and remain the standard interventions in the setting of significant anatomic urinary obstruction with risks of bladder decompensation. The preferred approach allows an assessment of the condition of the patient and the size and configuration of the prostrate gland. USDA approval has been given to medications that appear increasingly attractive to use particularly when lower urinary tract symptoms provide primary indication for intervention. These include α1-adrenergic blockers (e.g., doxazosin, terazosin and tamsulosin) and 5-α-reductase inhibitors (e.g., finasteride).

ANSWER: a, b, c

REFERENCE: *Chapter 102—Male Anatomy and Physiology: Lower Urinary Tract*

2. Which of the following are common organic cause of erectile dysfunction?

a. Medications
b. Endocrine disorders
c. Peripheral vascular disease
d. Surgery to the pelvis or retroperitoneum
e. Alcohol abuse

COMMENT:

Table 102.2. COMMON ORGANIC CAUSES OF ERECTILE DYSFUNCTION

Category	Examples
Systemic disorders	Atherosclerosis, hypertension, peripheral vascular disease, diabetes mellitus, renal failure
Neurogenic disorders	Diabetes, cardiovascular accidents, Parkinson's disease, multiple sclerosis
Endocrine disorders	Hypogonadism, hyperprolactinemia, hyperthyroidism, hypothyroidism
Penile disorders	Peyronie's disease, priapism
Injuries	Perineal, pelvic, or nervous system trauma; radiation or surgery to the pelvis or retroperitoneum
Medications	Antihypertensives, antidepressants, antiandrogens, nonsteroidal antiinflammatory drugs
Substances of abuse	Alcohol, tobacco, recreational drug

ANSWER: a, b, c, d, e

REFERENCE: *Chapter 102—Male Anatomy and Physiology*

3. Which of the following statements is/are true concerning male infertility?

a. Male factors contribute to only the minority of cases
b. The presence of a varicocele may contribute to male infertility
c. Semen analysis is the cornerstone of male infertility evaluation
d. Oligospermia is usually treated empirically with clomiphene citrate

COMMENT: Infertility, defined as the inability to conceive a pregnancy within one year of unprotected sexual intercourse, affects approximately 15% of couples in the United States. Male factors are thought to contribute to approximately half of the instances. An informative and cost-effective initial evaluation should begin with a complete history-taking, physical examination and appropriate laboratory tests. Physical examinations should focus on the genitalia. Scrotal contents should be carefully assessed to evaluate whether the testes are abnormal and whether a varicocele is present. Semen analysis represents the cornerstone of male infertility evaluation. Therapy in the field of male infertility is evolving towards identifying a treatable cause and rationally initiating therapy that has a high likelihood of success. Oligospermia (low sperm count) usually receives empiric treatment with clomiphene citrate to raise gonadotropin levels and, in theory, stimulate the testes to function better. Varicocelectomy through laparoscopic ligation or open microsurgical techniques has in some instances improved sperm counts and function, supported by the hypothesis that varicoceles cause disordered, scrotal temperature regulation and retrograde flow of adrenal hormones and renal toxins.

ANSWER: b, c, d

REFERENCE: *Chapter 102—Male Anatomy and Physiology: Male Genitalia and Reproductive System*

4. Which of the following statements is/are true concerning types and characteristics of kidney stones?

   a. Calcium oxalate stones, which are radiopaque, are the most common stone type

   b. Cystine stones, which are radiolucent, occur only in patients with a rare congenital defect called cystinuria

   c. Uric acid stones are radiolucent

   d. Eighty percent of renal stones are calcium-containing and therefore radiopaque

COMMENT:

Table 102.5. TYPES OF KIDNEY STONES

Stone composition	Frequency (x)	Degree of radiopacity
Calcium stones (total)	82	Opaque
Calcium oxalate ± calcium phosphate	75	Very opaque
Pure calcium phosphate	7	
Magnesium ammonium phosphate	12	Opaque
Uric acid	7	Lucent
Cystine	2	Slightly opaque

ANSWER: a, c, d

REFERENCE: *Chapter 102—Male Anatomy and Physiology: Urolithiasis*

5. Which of the following statements is/are true concerning the treatment of urolithiasis?

a. Most renal stones require some form of intervention, either operative or non-operative
b. Shock wave lithotripsy is a procedure choice for renal stones greater than 2 cm in size
c. A staghorn calculus is considered appropriate for percutaneous nephrolithotomy and not lithotripsy
d. Ureteroscopy is seldom successful for distal ureteral calculi

COMMENT: Most stones (less than 6mm) pass spontaneously and can be followed conservatively. In an emergency setting, intravenous hydration and analgesics are usually sufficient to treat the acute attack. The patient can be discharged with out-patient urology follow-up when pain and associated symptoms have been controlled. The chance of spontaneous stone passage is related to stone size and anatomic features of the upper urinary tract. Extracorporeal shock wave lithotripsy (SWL) is the procedure of choice for renal stones less than 2 cm in size. Treatment-related failure and complication rates increase significantly for larger and staghorn calculi. Patients who have failed SWL therapy or possess factors making success of SWL unlikely (e.g., staghorn calculus, lower pole location, cystine composition) should be considered for percutaneous stone removal. Percutaneous nephrolithotomy has the ability to both fragment and remove stones without depending on spontaneous passage of fragments. Ureteroscopy is used as either a primary or adjunctive therapy for stones in any location. Rigid or semi-rigid retrograde ureteroscopy is successful in over 95% cases of distal ureteral calculi.

ANSWER: c

REFERENCE: Chapter 102—Male Anatomy and Physiology: Urolithiasis

6. Absolute indications for immediate intervention for urolithiasis include:

a. Obstructive polynephritis
b. Deteriorating renal function
c. Anuria due to ureteral obstruction
d. Large ureteral stones (greater than 7 mm)

COMMENT:

Table 102.7. INDICATIONS FOR IMMEDIATE INTERVENTION

Absolute
Obstructive pyelonephritis (true emergency)
Unremitting pain
Deterioration of renal function
Anuria due to ureteral obstruction
  Bilateral stones
  Solitary kidney
Relative
Large ureteral stones (>7 mm) that are unlikely to pass spontaneously
Occupational requirements (i.e., airline pilot)
Transplant kidney

ANSWER: a, b, c

REFERENCE: Chapter 102—Male Anatomy and Physiology

7. Which of the following is not considered a risk factor for the development of urothelial carcinoma?

a. Radiation exposure
b. Tobacco exposure
c. Heavy-metal exposure
d. Aniline dye exposure

COMMENT:

Table 102.13. FACTORS ASSOCIATED WITH THE DEVELOPMENT OF UROTHELIAL TUMORS

Aniline dyes
2-Naphthylamine
Nitrosamines
Cyclophosphamide
Acrolein
Phenacetin
Schistosomiasis (e.g., Schistosoma haematobium)
Chronic irritation (stones or hardware such as a catheter)
Radiation exposure
Tobacco exposure

ANSWER: c

REFERENCE: Chapter 102—Male Anatomy and Physiology: Urothelial Carcinoma

8. The treatment of bladder carcinoma is dependent on the stage of the tumor. Which of the following statements is/are true concerning treatment options?
   a. Superficial urothelial carcinomas of the bladder are generally treated with endoscopic local resection
   b. Adjuvant chemotherapy is used primarily for recurrent superficial bladder cancers
   c. Muscle-invasive transitional cell carcinoma of the bladder in a male is treated with a radical cystoprostatectomy
   d. Reconstruction following radical cystoprostatectomy precludes the use of a continent neobladder

COMMENT: Treatment options for superficial urothelial carcinomas include endoscopic local resection with or without intravesical chemotherapy. The use of adjuvant intravesical chemotherapy is largely restricted to recurrent superficial transitional cell carcinomas and carcinoma in situ. Muscle-invasive transitional cell carcinomas are most appropriately treated with radical cystoprostatectomy in men or anterior exenteration in women, provided the patient is a reasonable surgical candidate. Radical surgery involves removal of the local-regional lymph nodes, the bladder, prostate seminal vesicles and a portion of the vas deferens. The urinary system therefore must be diverted either into a continent neo-bladder or through an intestinal conduit to a cutaneous stomal apparatus.

ANSWER: a, b, c

REFERENCE: *Chapter 102—Male Anatomy and Physiology: Urothelial Carcinoma*

9. Renal cell carcinoma accounts for 3% of adult solid tumors. Which of the following statements is/are true concerning this neoplasm?
   a. The classic triad of flank pain, flank fullness or mass and hematuria is a common presentation
   b. All renal cysts should be considered pre-malignant and require intervention
   c. Extended lymphadnectomy is an important component of radical nephrectomy for renal cell carcinoma
   d. Laparoscopic surgery is an option in patients with renal cell carcinoma

COMMENT: Proposed risk factors associated with the development of renal cell carcinoma include renal cystic disease, exposure to lead or cadmium, asbestos, high-fat diet, obesity, hypertension and tobacco exposure. Renal cystic masses detected by CT are confirmed by ultrasound for evaluation of any solid components. The risk of cancer progression in complex renal cysts has been clearly identified and classified. Class 1 and class 2 cysts which are either simple cysts or minimal complex cysts with curvilinear calcification and thin septa have a very low malignant potential and are typically followed. More complex cysts may require surgical exploration and resection. The widespread use of routine radiographic imaging has resulted in a marked increase in the number of incidentally discovered renal masses (approximately 40%–50%) with the result in migration to a lower-stage disease discovery. As a result, the class triad of flank pain, flank fullness or mass and hematuria now occurs in less than 10% of patients diagnosed with renal cell carcinoma. The introduction of radical nephrectomy for renal cell carcinoma in the 1960s resulted in the dramatic increase in 5-year survival rates. Traditionally, a radical nephrectomy procedure is performed through a flank incision and involves the removal of the kidney, adrenal gland and proximal ureter en bloc and with Gerota's fascia. The role of an extended nephrectomy is limited and it is usually not performed. A recent development has been to use laparoscopy for performing a radical or even a partial nephrectomy. Early data regarding outcomes from this approach show a significant decrease in morbidity without compromising disease-free survival.

ANSWER: d

REFERENCE: *Chapter 102—Male Anatomy and Physiology: Renal Neoplasms*

10. Which of the following statements is/are true concerning the treatment of prostate cancer?

    a. Older men with low-volume disease may be observed without surgery
    b. Radical retropubic prostatectomy, although excellent for surgical control of localized prostate cancers, is associated with high incidence of urinary incontinence and erectile dysfunction
    c. After treatment, PSA (prostrate specific anagen) levels is the most sensitive indicator of freedom of disease
    d. Hormonal therapy is a mainstay of palliative treatment for advanced prostate cancer

COMMENT: Because advanced prostate cancer remains essentially incurable, the diagnosis and treatment of localized prostate cancer (clinical stages T1 and T2) represents a unique opportunity for cure. However, just because a cancer can be cured does not mean a cure is necessary. Small-volume, latent prostate cancer in older men may not affect overall health because of the long natural history of the disease and the limited life expectancy of older men. Therefore, watchful waiting is an appropriate alternative for older men with limited disease. Patients with local, but clinically significant disease, require intervention. There are two conventional modes of therapy—radiation and surgery. Of the radiation-based options, the most commonly used method consists of external beam radiation, typically with a conformal apparatus. Brachytherapy using radioactive implants has been also gaining widespread popularity. Surgical therapy of local prostate cancers most commonly performed as an anatomically radical retropubic prostatectomy. This procedure has resulted in significantly reduced morbidity in terms of recovery of urinary continence and maintenance of erectile function. Outcomes from the Medicare population suggests that morbidity is higher in older men. After treatment, PSA is the most sensitive indicator of freedom of disease. An undetectable PSA after surgery indicates eradication of cancer. Similarly, a stable PSA (not rising) of less than 0.5 ng/mL after radiation therapy is thought to be consistent with disease-free state. Hormonal therapy is the mainstay of palliative treatment for advanced prostate cancer. Current options for hormonal therapy include orchiectomy, LH-releasing hormone agonists and anti-androgen therapy.

ANSWER: a, c, d

REFERENCE: *Chapter 102—Male Anatomy and Physiology: Prostate Cancer*

11. Risk factors for the development of testicular cancer include:

    a. Black race
    b. Cryptorchism
    c. Family history
    d. Smoking history

COMMENT:

Table 102.20.	**RISK FACTORS FOR THE DEVELOPMENT OF TESTICULAR CANCER**
Age	
Pediatric	Nonseminomatous tumor (e.g., yolk sac tumors)
Young adults	Seminoma > nonseminomatous tumors
Geriatric	Spermatocytic seminoma, lymphoma
Race (whites at highest risk)	
Cryptorchidism	
Family history	
HIV infection/AIDS (lymphoma)	
Presence of carcinoma in situ (e.g., testicular biopsy for infertility)	
Prior history of testicular cancer in contralateral testis	
Occupational risks (nonseminomatous tumors only)	
Miners, oil and gas workers, leather workers, food and beverage processing workers, janitors, and utility workers	

ANSWER: b,c

REFERENCE: *Chapter 102—Male Anatomy and Physiology: Testis cancer*

12. Which of the following statements is/are true concerning the diagnosis and treatment of testicular cancer?

a. Seminomas are the most common type of testicular tumors and are noted to secrete α-feto protein (AFP)

b. Choriocarcinoma is known to secrete β-human chorionic gonadotropin (β-HCG)

c. Orchiectomy for testicular cancer should be performed through a transscrotal incision

d. Seminomas are highly radiosensitive and should receive adjuvant radiation therapy to the paraaortic and to the paracaval nodes

COMMENT: Metastatic testicular carcinoma is a highly lethal disease. Because the testes contain both germ cells and supportive cells, tumors derived from the testes can occur from either source. Seminomas are the most common type of testicular tumors, although mixed tumors are common. Non-seminomatous tumors may secrete certain marker proteins that allow both pre-operative and post-operative assessment. Endodermal sinus cancer is known to secrete α-fetoprotein (AFP) and choriocarcinoma is known to secrete β-HCG. Pure seminomas do not secrete AFP but may secrete β-HCG in up to 10% of cases. Thus, if these tumor markers are elevated before surgery, they are useful markers to follow after surgery for recurrence or progression.

Initial treatment and definitive diagnosis occur contemporaneously by orchiectomy through an inguinal surgical incision. Transscrotal orchiectomy carries the theoretic risk of altering the lymphatic drainage and is discouraged. Once a definitive diagnosis is made, staging can be completed. Radiographic staging requires a CT scan of the chest, abdomen and the pelvis, with oral and intervenous contrast. Seminomas are known to be highly radiosensitive. Thus, patients with stage I or II seminomas are treated with adjuvant radiotherapy to the paraaortic and paracaval areas below the diaphragm, as well as the ipsilateral inguinal and pelvic regions. Non-seminomatous tumors are less radiosensitive and thus require either surgical resection or chemotherapy, or both. Because of advances in chemotherapy, metastatic testis cancer is still considered a treatable disease. Survival rates greater than 70% are reported in patients with advanced disease and greater than 90% for lower-stage disease.

ANSWER: b, d

REFERENCE: *Chapter 102—Male Anatomy and Physiology: Testis Cancer*

CHAPTER 103

FEMALE GENITAL TRACT

1. The ureter is vulnerable to injury during pelvic surgery at several characteristic sites. They all include all except which of the following?

a. As the ureter runs through the pararectal space towards the perineum

b. As the ureter enters the pelvis on top of the bifurcation of the common iliac artery

c. At the site of the ureter entering the bladder wall

d. As the ureter runs under the uterine artery

COMMENT: Gynecologic pelvic surgery is the most common source of iatrogenic ureteral injury. The position of the ureter may be distorted by inflammation or neoplasms, but it is recognized that the ureter is most often injured in three important positions: as the ureter enters the pelvis under the infindibulopelvic ligament and on top of the bifurcation of the common iliac artery, as the ureter runs below the uterine artery as that vessel enters the uterus, and at the ureter entrance into the bladder wall.

ANSWER: a

REFERENCE: *Chapter 103—Female Genital Tract: Surgical Anatomy*

2. Which of the following is true regarding the management of major vulvar gland (i.e., Bartholin's) infections?

   a. These infections are rarely associated with a sexually-transmitted disease
   b. Surgical therapy is nearly always necessary and should therefore be seen as primary therapy
   c. Marsupialization is the surgical procedure of choice
   d. When resection is necessary, the procedure should be performed immediately to prevent further recurrence

COMMENT: Bartholin's gland infections are usually associated with a sexually-transmitted disease, usually gonorrhea. Appropriate initial management includes antibiotics and topical therapy (sitz baths). Surgical intervention is indicated in persistent or recurrent cases, with marsupialization being the procedure of choice. In cases where, marsupialization fails, resection of the gland is necessary. This is best done when the tissues are not acutely inflamed, to minimize scarring and ensure complete resection of the gland.

ANSWER: c

REFERENCE: *Chapter 103—Female Genital Tract: Vulva*

3. Which of the following statements describing vulvar intraepithelial neoplasia is true?

   a. VIN represents a premalignant lesion in the continuum towards adenocarcinoma
   b. The majority of VIN lesions have detectable human papillomavirus DNA
   c. Recurrence after excisional or laser vaporization treatment is rare, occurring in less than 5% of patients
   d. VIN occurs as the end result of chronic inflammation and is often associated with significant comorbid disease (diabetes mellitus, chronic steroid use)

COMMENT: VIN, like other premalignant lesions of the female genital tract, represents an early step in the continuum towards squamous cancer of the vulva. VIN appears to result from chronic inflammation and occurs in patients with significant comorbid disease. Like cervical cancer, HPV infection is thought to be a risk factor, though viral DNA is identified in the minority of cases. Excisional therapy or laser vaporization may be effective in controlling disease, but recurrence is common (30%–40%) and careful surveillance is required.

ANSWER: d

REFERENCE: *Chapter 103—Female Genital Tract: Vulva*

4. A 65-year-old woman presents complaining of pain in her right adnexa. Physical examination is notable for mild abdominal distention with probable ascites. Pelvic exam reveals a fixed, tender mass in the right adnexa. What is the most appropriate treatment option for this patient?

   a. Referral to a medical oncologist for systemic chemotherapy
   b. Exploratory staging laparotomy, confirmation of tissue diagnosis, radical hysterectomy
   c. Laparoscopy and biopsy to confirm diagnosis
   d. Observation with repeat exam in 3 months

COMMENT: This patient presents with a typical presentation of ovarian cancer. Unfortunately, the treatment is often delayed due to lack of recognition or the misconception that little can be done for patients with advanced disease. The most important variable for patient prognosis with ovarian cancer is the ability to debulk as much disease as possible at the time of surgery. This is best accomplished with radical hysterectomy, accompanied by bowel resection, omentectomy, peritoneal stripping, and hepatic resection when indicated. Even patients with ascites and positive cytology can have survival rates of greater than 50% if the disease is otherwise confined to the involved adnexa. Systemic chemotherapy is of minimal if any benefit in patients without surgical debulking.

ANSWER: b

REFERENCE: *Chapter 103—Female Genital Tract: Ovary*

5. Risk factors for endometrial cancer include all except which of the following?

   a. Obesity
   b. Late menarche
   c. Nulliparity
   d. Atypical endometrial hyperplasia

COMMENT: Several important risk factors have been identified for endometrial cancer, many of which are associated with prolonged unopposed estrogen exposure. They include, nulliparity, late menopause, unopposed estrogen use, tamoxifen, and obesity. Obesity greater than 50 pounds over ideal body weight is associated with a tenfold increase in risk of endometrial cancer. Atypical endometrial hyperplasia may progress to endometrial cancer if untreated.

ANSWER: b

REFERENCE: *Chapter 103—Female Genital Tract: Uterus*

6. Established therapies for uterine fibroids includes:

   a. Gonadotropin-releasing hormone antagonists
   b. Hysterectomy
   c. Hysteroscopic myomectomy
   d. Selective embolization
   e. All of the above

COMMENT: All of these therapies are accepted alternatives for the treatment of uterine fibroids. Medical therapy with GnRH antagonists will shrink up to 70% of leiomyomata that are less than 7 to 9 cm by up to 70% in volume. However, these medications have significant side effects from estrogen withdrawal and are not good long-term treatments. They can be very useful in the short term to arrest bleeding and shrink fibroids prior to surgery. Surgical options include hysterectomy or myomectomy. Myomectomy may be performed laparoscopically, hysteroscopically, or via laparotomy. The advantage of myomectomy is the ability to maintain fertility, but uterine rupture is a potential fatal complication that can occur with subsequent pregnancy. Selective embolization is currently gaining acceptance as an effective therapy, but long-term follow-up is not available.

ANSWER: a, b, c

REFERENCE: *Chapter 103—Female Genital Tract: Uterus*

7. Choose the correct statement describing cervical neoplasia.

   a. Approximately 50%–60% of women with a minimally abnormal Pap smear (ASCUS or LGSIL) may be found to have an associated precancerous lesion (CIN II or III)
   b. Occult cancers may be found in 3%–10 % of patients with CIN II or III after excision
   c. Adenocarcinomas account for 45%–50% of cervical cancers
   d. Cervical cancer that presents without detection by Pap smear is most often asymptomatic, accounting for its advanced stage at presentation

COMMENT: Cervical cancer is the second leading cause of cancer death in women in the developing world, where Pap smear screening in not widely used. Pap screening in this country has minimized the morbidity and mortality from cervical cancer in the United States, but the management of premalignant lesions and abnormal smears remains a large task for the gynecologic surgeon. There are approximately 3.5 million minimally abnormal Pap smears in the United States annually, and 15%–20% of women will be found to have an associated premalignant lesion. Excisional therapy of these lesions will further uncover occult cancers in 3%–10% of patients, which speaks to the importance of a systematic evaluation of abnormal Pap smears. Most cervical cancers are squamous cells cancers and are associated with HPV infection, while adenocarcinomas account for 15%–25% of cases. Patients who are diagnosed with cervical cancer without Pap screening are most often symptomatic, with 75% of these women developing abnormal bleeding, pain, or vaginal discharge.

ANSWER: b

REFERENCE: *Chapter 103—Female Genital Tract: Cervix*

CHAPTER 104

THE PREGNANT PATIENT

1. Which of the following laboratory values is/are affected by pregnancy?

   a. Hemoglobin
   b. White blood cell count
   c. Alkaline phosphatase
   d. Total bilirubin

COMMENT: Maternal blood volume increases markedly during pregnancy. This serves to meet the demands of the hypertrophied uterus and conceptus while protecting the mother against the deleterious effects of inferior vena cava compression and impaired venous return. The red blood cell mass does not expand to the same degree as plasma volume, which leads to dilutional anemia with values as low as 11 g/dL in late pregnancy. The peripheral white blood cell count generally increases during pregnancy owing to decreased polymorphonuclear leukocyte chemotaxis and adherence. Total alkaline phosphatase activity almost doubles during pregnancy. Most of this increase is attributed to placental isozymes, which can be differentiated by heat stability up to 65°C. Total bilirubin levels do not change during pregnancy, and levels remain stable unless affected by hepatobiliary disease.

ANSWER: a, b, c

REFERENCE: *Chapter 104—The Pregnant Patient: Physiologic Changes of Pregnancy that Mimic Disease*

2. Computed tomography during pregnancy:

   a. Always leads to fetal demise
   b. Causes teratogenesis 75% of the time
   c. Should be avoided at all costs
   d. Increases the risk of childhood cancer

COMMENT: Abdominal computed tomography delivers a dose of 2,000 to 3,000 mrad to the conceptus. Although this dosing increases the risk of childhood cancer, the risk of spontaneous abortion or teratogenesis is low. Avoiding imaging studies with ionizing radiation is ideal during pregnancy, but these studies are not contraindicated if critical diagnostic information can be obtained.

ANSWER: d

REFERENCE: *Chapter 104—The Pregnant Patient: Imaging Modalities*

3. Appendicitis during pregnancy:
   a. Should be managed medically because of the risk of surgically induced premature labor
   b. Is a surgical emergency
   c. Rarely occurs and should be considered only after gynecologic causes of symptoms are eliminated
   d. Can be diagnosed and managed laparoscopically

COMMENT: Appendicitis occurs in 1 of 1,500 pregnancies and is the most common nonobstetric indication for surgery during pregnancy. This diagnosis should be immediately considered when any pregnant patient has abdominal pain. Surgical intervention is the only form of treatment. Because of uterine interference with omental migration, perforated appendicitis is difficult to wall off and results in peritonitis with a high rate of preterm labor and fetal loss. Laparoscopy for both diagnosis and appendectomy is safe during pregnancy.

ANSWER: b, d

REFERENCE: *Chapter 104—The Pregnant Patient: Appendectomy*

4. Colorectal cancer discovered during pregnancy:
   a. Can be diagnosed with sigmoidoscopy
   b. Is an early, localized lesion
   c. Can be managed conservatively until after birth
   d. Is increasing in frequency

COMMENT: Colon cancer is rare during pregnancy, but the prevalence may be increasing because of advancing maternal age and delay in pregnancy until later in life. Most cancers occur below the peritoneal reflection and are easily evaluated by means of sigmoidoscopy. Biopsy by means of sigmoidoscopy also is easy. Colorectal cancer usually manifests as locally advanced disease because of a delay in diagnosis among this young patient population. Cancer discovered in the first half of pregnancy should be resected because of the risk of metastasis and obstruction if treatment is delayed until fetal maturity.

ANSWER: a, d

REFERENCE: *Chapter 104—The Pregnant Patient: Colorectal Cancer During Pregnancy*

5. Conditions that can be diagnosed and managed in utero include:
   a. Congenital diaphragmatic hernia
   b. Severe combined immunodeficiency
   c. Obstructive uropathy for posterior urethral valves
   d. Myelomeningocele

COMMENT: Expansion of prenatal diagnostic modalities has paved the way for fetal surgery. Prenatal intervention for congenital diaphragmatic hernia, obstructive uropathy, myelomeningocele, and numerous other conditions offers the potential to correct the anatomic defect before end-organ damage occurs. Intrauterine hematopoietic stem cell transplantation can correct hemoglobinopathy and immunodeficiency while avoiding the postnatal morbidity of these conditions.

ANSWER: a, b, c, d

REFERENCE: *Chapter 104—The Pregnant Patient: Fetal Surgery*

Section S

SKIN AND SOFT TISSUE

CHAPTER 105

CUTANEOUS NEOPLASMS

1. Which of the following statements is/are true concerning the epidemiologic and etiologic aspects of malignant melanoma?
   a. The incidence of melanoma has increased more rapidly than that of any other cancer
   b. Populations residing closer to the equator have a higher incidence of melanoma
   c. Dysplastic but not congenital nevi carry increased risk of development of melanoma
   d. There is no familial predisposition to melanoma

COMMENT: The incidence of melanoma in the United States is approximately 30,000 new cases annually. Melanoma represents 3% of all newly diagnosed cancers. Most important, the incidence of melanoma has increased faster than that of any other cancer. The typical patient with melanoma has a fair complexion and the tendency to sunburn rather than tan, even after a relatively brief exposure to sunlight. Melanoma occurs infrequently among blacks and Asians, suggesting that skin pigment plays a protective role. Melanoma rates are subject to large geographic and ethnic variation, mainly because of the inverse correlation with latitude and the degree of skin pigmentation. Specifically, populations that reside closer to the equator have a higher incidence of melanoma. The reasons for the increasing incidence of melanoma are not clear but may be increased exposure to ultraviolet radiation from the sunlight that reaches the earth's surface.

Factors in addition to environmental factors are associated with increased risk of development of melanoma. Three to five percent of patients who have had one melanoma have another one. Another group at increased risk of development of melanomas is persons with dysplastic nevi. Dysplastic nevi are acquired lesions of the skin that have characteristics distinguishing them from common nevi. They are generally larger and can appear anywhere on the body, although they are most frequent on the trunk. Another risk factor associated with the development of melanoma is congenital nevi. A congenital nevus is a melanocytic nevus present at birth. Large congenital nevi can vary greatly in size, can occupy a large portion of the body surface, and carry an estimated lifetime risk of development of melanoma of between 5% and 20%. It is unclear to what extent melanoma develops in small and medium-sized congenital nevi. It is estimated that approximately 8% to 12% of cutaneous melanomas occur among persons with a familial predisposition. Most evidence indicates an autosomal dominant mode of transmission for hereditary melanoma with variable penetrance.

ANSWER: a, b

REFERENCE: *Chapter 105—Cutaneous Neoplasms: Melanoma; Epidemiology and Etiology*

2. Which of the following statements is/are true concerning the characteristic appearance and presentation for malignant melanoma?
   a. Variation in color, primarily a bluish tint, is of particular concern for a pigmented lesion
   b. Angular indentation or notching is frequently present at the perimeter of the lesion
   c. Irregular elevations of the surface are characteristic
   d. Ulceration of a pigmented lesion is pathognomonic of melanoma

COMMENT: Melanoma has a characteristic appearance that can lead to early detection if careful attention is paid to certain features. First, there often is a variation in color in which brown or black lesions contain shades of red, white, or blue. Of all the colors, shades of blue are the most ominous. Second, angular indentation or notching frequently is present at the perimeter of the lesion. Third, irregular elevation of the surface is characteristic. Another indication of possible malignant growth is enlargement, darkening, bleeding, or ulceration of a pigmented lesion. None of these clinical signs is pathognomonic because these features can be present in a number of benign lesions.

ANSWER: a, b, c

REFERENCE: *Chapter 105—Cutaneous Neoplasms: Melanoma; Clinical Diagnosis and Classification*

3. Which of the following statements is/are true concerning major categories of malignant melanoma?
   a. Lentigo maligna melanoma is a nonaggressive type of melanoma that occurs most commonly among older women
   b. Superficially spreading melanoma accounts for about 70% of cutaneous neoplasms with a peak incidence in the fifth decade of life
   c. Nodular melanoma, the most aggressive type, occurs most commonly among women
   d. Acral lentiginous melanoma occurs exclusively among white persons

COMMENT: According to growth patterns and clinical characteristics, melanoma can be classified into four major categories—lentigo maligna melanoma, superficial spreading melanoma, nodular melanoma, and acral lentiginous melanoma. Lentigo maligna melanoma constitutes 10% to 15% of cutaneous melanomas and is the least aggressive of the four types. It typically occurs on sun-exposed areas of the head and neck and the dorsum of the hands. The median age at diagnosis is 70 years, and the tumor appears to be more prevalent among women. Superficial spreading melanoma accounts for 70% of cutaneous melanomas and is intermediate in malignancy compared with the other types. These lesions generally arise in a preexisting nevus. The peak incidence is in the fifth decade of life, and there is equal distribution between sexes. Nodular melanoma occurs among approximately 15% to 30% of patients with cutaneous melanoma and is the most aggressive of the four types of melanoma. The median age at diagnosis is 50 years, and the lesions occur twice as often among men as among women. The tumor commonly originates from uninvolved skin rather than arising from preexisting nevus. Acral lentiginous melanoma is a distinct clinicopathologic variant of melanoma that occurs on the palms, soles, and subungual locations. These lesions occur among only 2% to 8% of whites with melanoma but among a much higher percentage (35% to 60%) of dark-pigmented people such as blacks, Hispanics, and Asians.

ANSWER: a, b

REFERENCE: *Chapter 105—Cutaneous Neoplasms: Melanoma; Clinical Diagnosis and Classification*

4. Which of the following statements is/are true concerning staging and prognostic factors for melanoma?
   a. In the Clark classification, melanoma is sorted according to depth of invasion in relation to histologically defined layers of the skin
   b. The classification of Breslow, which is based on the thickness of the primary tumor, is not as useful as Clark level of invasion
   c. The location of the melanoma does not affect prognosis
   d. Ulceration within a melanoma appears to be associated with a better prognosis because of early detection

COMMENT: A great deal of information is available regarding various factors that correlate with clinical outcome among patients with melanoma. One of the most important prognostic features of cutaneous melanoma relates to microstaging of the primary tumor. Two methods have been described to assess different aspects of microstaging. Clark and associates described a system to classify melanoma according to depth of invasion. They described five levels of invasion related to histologically defined layers of the skin. The other microstaging method used routinely was originally described by Breslow. In this method, the thickness of the primary tumor is measured with an oculomicrometer from the top of the granular layer to the base of the tumor. Most investigators have documented an inverse correlation between tumor thickness and survival. Several studies have demonstrated that tumor thickness conveys more prognostic information than does the determination of Clark level of invasion. Within the same Clark levels of invasion, one can find gradations of tumor thickness that have independent prognostic significance. In addition, the measurement of tumor thickness is often more reproducible and less subjective than determining the Clark level of invasion.

Several other factors have been reported to be significant predictors of survival among patients with localized melanoma. The anatomic location of melanoma has been shown to be a significant independent prognostic indicator among patients with clinically localized disease. Several studies have shown that patients with melanoma of the extremities, excluding the hands and feet, have a better survival rate than do those with lesions on the trunk or the head and neck. Among patients with melanoma of the extremities, those with lesions on the hands and feet have considerably worse outcomes than do patients with lesions on other sites on the extremities. Several studies have shown that women with melanoma have a better survival rate than do men, although this may be related to different distribution sites of melanoma on men and women. The presence of ulceration within a melanoma also appears to be associated with a poorer prognosis. Finally, genetic markers may be more important as prognostic factors in the future. The presence of abnormal DNA content (DNA aneuploidy) determined by means of flow cytometry has been reported to have an unfavorable prognosis among patients with localized melanoma.

ANSWER: a

REFERENCE: *Chapter 105—Cutaneous Neoplasms: Melanoma; Staging and Prognostic Factors*

5. Which of the following statements is/are true concerning biopsy of a lesion believed to be melanoma?
   a. A margin of 5 mm should be obtained in the biopsy of all suspicious lesions
   b. Punch biopsy has no role in the evaluation of lesions believed to be melanoma
   c. Frozen section should be performed at primary biopsy to indicate immediate treatment
   d. Full-thickness biopsy to the adipose tissue is required for any lesion believed to be melanoma

COMMENT: For melanoma, tumor thickness is the single most important variable that most accurately determines therapy and prognosis. Full-thickness biopsy to the adipose tissue is required for any lesion believed to be melanoma. If the melanoma is transected with partial-thickness shave biopsy, the ability to obtain accurate measurement of tumor thickness is lost. Therefore superficial shave biopsy is never recommended for a suspicious pigmented lesion. Excisional biopsy with 1- to 2-mm margins is the preferred biopsy method for suspect lesions to provide the pathologist a total specimen for histologic interpretation and microstaging. A formalin-fixed, paraffin-embedded permanent section should be used for biopsy diagnosis of primary cutaneous melanoma to accurately determine tumor thickness and other histopathologic prognostic variables. Frozen sections do not have a role in the microstaging of primary melanoma. For suspect lesions too large for complete excision or anatomically located where the amount of skin is critical in terms of functional or cosmetic results, incisional biopsy can be performed with either a scalpel or a punch tool 4 to 6 mm in diameter. Several punch biopsies can be obtained from different areas for lesions with multiple morphologic features.

ANSWER: d

REFERENCE: *Chapter 105—Cutaneous Neoplasms: Melanoma; Treatment of Primary Melanoma*

6. The traditional approaches to management of melanoma have been challenged. Which of the following statements is/are true concerning the primary management of melanoma?

a. Thin melanoma, less than 1 mm thick, can be safely excised with a 1-cm margin
b. Intermediate-thickness melanoma, 1.0 to 4.0 mm, should be managed with at least a 3-cm margin
c. Therapeutic lymph node dissection in the care of patients with stage III disease can result in cure for as many as one third of patients
d. Prospective, randomized studies have clearly shown the value of elective lymph node dissection in the care of patients with melanoma of the extremities

COMMENT: After confirmation of the diagnosis of malignant melanoma, appropriate surgical management is indicated. For thin melanoma, excision of normal skin 0.5 cm around the lesion or previous biopsy site is acceptable for local control. For invasive cutaneous melanoma, wide excision of the primary tumor or biopsy site has been advocated for optimal control. Limited excision, such as excisional biopsy, is associated with local recurrence rates in the 30% to 60% range. The routine approach once was to excise all primary melanomas with a 3- to 5-cm margin, which often necessitated a split-thickness skin graft for coverage. It now is clear that less than the traditional wide local excision is adequate for the surgical management of some cases of melanoma. In a prospective study patients with primary melanoma less than 2 mm thick were randomized to undergo excision with 1-cm margins versus greater than 3-cm margins. No patient with a tumor less than 1 mm thick had a local recurrence, regardless of the excision margin. Although three local recurrences were reported in the group of patients with melanoma 1 to 2 mm thick, all of whom had undergone narrow excision, the disease-free and overall survival rates were not different between the two groups after a mean follow-up period of almost 5 years. A prospective, randomized study was performed to evaluate the efficacy of 2-cm versus 4-cm margins for intermediate thickness melanoma measuring 1.0 to 4.0 mm. The results of that study showed a 2-cm margin is sufficient to manage intermediate-thickness melanoma. For lesions more than 4 mm thick, excision margins of at least 3 cm should be considered the standard approach.

Surgical excision of metastatic lesions to regional lymph nodes is the only therapeutic modality that has potential for cure. Surgical excision of clinically positive lymph nodes is called *therapeutic lymph node dissection*. In several reported series, the 5-year survival rate among patients who underwent lymphadenectomy for clinically positive involved nodes (American Joint Committee on Cancer stage III) ranged from 13% to 39%. Elective lymph node dissection, which is performed to excise clinically normal appearing regional lymph nodes because of the risk of occult or microscopic metastasis, is an extremely controversial issue. Results of retrospective studies have been unclear. Results of two large prospective studies addressing the issue of elective lymph node dissection have been reported. In neither case was improvement in survival observed among patients treated by means of elective lymph node dissection for melanomas of an extremity.

ANSWER: a, c

REFERENCE: *Chapter 105—Cutaneous Neoplasms: Melanoma; Treatment of Primary Melanoma*

7. Which of the following statements is/are true concerning the management of disseminated melanoma?

    a. There is no role for surgical excision of recurrent melanoma for either survival benefit or palliation

    b. Melanoma is generally not responsive to radiation therapy

    c. Melanoma tends to respond well to a number of chemotherapeutic regimens

    d. Trials of immunotherapy at the National Cancer Institute have led to some encouraging results for this treatment of patients with disseminated melanoma

COMMENT: Melanoma can disseminate to any organ. The most common sites of recurrence are skin, subcutaneous tissues, and distant lymph nodes, followed by visceral metastasis. Common visceral sites of metastasis, in order of decreasing frequency, are lung, liver, brain, bone, and gastrointestinal tract. Surgical excision of recurrent melanoma can be effective palliation for patients with isolated recurrences in the skin, central nervous system, lung, or gastrointestinal tract. Resection of isolated metastatic lesions is generally not considered curative but can lengthen the disease-free survival period. Melanoma can respond to radiation therapy, which is commonly used for palliation of bone pain caused by metastatic disease or brain metastasis. Melanoma is responsive to few chemotherapeutic drugs. Even the best response to single agents is in the range of 10% to 20%. Complete responses are rare. No evidence indicates that combination chemotherapy offers any better results than use of the single agent dacarbazine (DTIC).

Immunotherapy entails administration of cytokines, such as interferons and interleukins, to patients to modulate the immune response. The most impressive results with immunotherapy for melanoma have been associated with the use of interleukin-2. In trials at the National Cancer Institute, adoptive immunotherapy in which patients receive antitumor reactive cells known as lymphokine-activated killer T cells or tumor-infiltrating lymphocytes in combination with high-dose interleukin-2 and cyclophosphamide has led to a good response rate among patients with advanced melanoma.

ANSWER: d

REFERENCE: *Chapter 105—Cutaneous Neoplasms: Melanoma; Treatment of Disseminated Melanoma*

8. More than 1 million cases of non-melanoma skin cancer are diagnosed in the United States each year. Which of the following statements is/are true concerning the cause of these cases of cancer?

    a. Prolonged exposure to ultraviolet light is the most common cause of non-melanoma skin cancer

    b. There is no association between skin cancer and viral infection

    c. Radiation exposure usually is associated with invasive squamous cell carcinoma (SCC) or basal cell carcinoma (BCC) within 5 years of exposure

    d. Non-melanoma skin cancer can develop in areas of trauma and scarring

COMMENT: Non-melanoma cutaneous malignant tumors, including BCC and SCC, are the most common type of malignant tumors among humans. The ratio of BCC to SCC is approximately 4:1. Both BCC and SCC are induced by chronic exposure to ultraviolet light, which is the most common cause of non-melanoma skin cancer. These cancers are the predominant neoplasms of the head, neck, and hands, where sun exposure is common. Chemical carcinogens have been implicated as etiologic agents that contribute to the formation of skin cancer. Human papillomavirus has been implicated in the formation of SCC among humans. The degeneration of chronic radiodermatitis into invasive SCC or BCC is well described. Typically there is at least a 20-year latency period between radiation exposure and the development of the malignant lesion. Squamous cell carcinoma and BCC also can develop in the areas of trauma, scars, and chronic scarring disorders.

ANSWER: a, d

REFERENCE: *Chapter 105—Cutaneous Neoplasms: Nonmelanoma Skin Tumors*

9. Which of the following statements is/are true concerning the presentation of non-melanoma skin cancers?

   a. Basal cell carcinoma rarely metastasizes

   b. BCC is seldom associated with serious morbidity

   c. Most cases of BCC manifest as an ulcerated well-circumscribed nodule

   d. The initial clinical feature of SCC is an erythematous papulonodule with overlying keratotic crusting or ulceration

   e. Ulcerative SCC arising from actinic damaged skin follows an aggressive pattern

COMMENT: Basal cell carcinoma is the most common form of skin cancer. Although BCC rarely metastasizes, it is characterized by slow but relentless, destructive local invasion resulting in high morbidity without treatment. The most common subtype of BCC is the ulcerative well-circumscribed nodular variety. Squamous cell carcinoma is the second most common type of skin cancer and is derived from epithelial keratinocytes. Because these tumors can deeply invade surrounding structures or metastasize to regional lymph nodes, they must be recognized and managed aggressively. Squamous cell carcinoma causes approximately 2,500 deaths per year in the United States. The initial clinical feature of SCC usually is an erythematous papulonodule with overlying keratotic crust or ulceration. Ulcerative SCC is an aggressive malignant lesion of the skin that typically occurs with a simple ulceration with raised borders. These tumors can arise in actinic damaged skin, solar keratosis, and cutaneous horns, burn scars, or chronic wounds. When these tumors spread to regional lymph nodes, the prognosis is poor—a 5-year survival rate less than 50%. If the tumors arise in chronic wounds or burn scars, they exhibit particularly aggressive behavior. Many patients have regional lymphatic spread when they come to medical attention. In contrast, tumors that arise in actinic, damaged skin have a less aggressive pattern. This is particularly true of the hand, where SCC often is indolent and grows slowly.

ANSWER: a, c, d

REFERENCE: *Chapter 105—Cutaneous Neoplasms: Nonmelanoma Skin Tumors*

10. Which of the following statements is/are true concerning the surgical management of non-melanoma skin cancers?

   a. Curettage and electrodesiccation, cryosurgery, and radiation are inferior to surgical resection for low-risk skin cancer

   b. Surgical margins for low-risk SCC and BCC should be at least 2 cm

   c. Elective lymph node dissection for clinically negative lymph nodes for SCC is not indicated

   d. Elective lymph node dissection is frequently indicated for BCC

COMMENT: Skin biopsy for diagnosis is important before therapy for any skin cancer. Most cases of non-melanoma skin cancer are small, low-risk lesions that can be managed with a 90% to 95% cure rate with standard techniques, including curettage and electrodesiccation, cryosurgery, radiation, and surgical excision. Most skin tumors can be removed with elliptical excision following the skin tension lines. Margins for both low-risk SCC and BCC are adequate at 1 cm or less. Regional lymphadenectomy is an important component of the surgical procedure if clinically positive nodes are evident. The diagnosis of metastatic squamous cell carcinoma can be made with fine-needle aspiration. Elective lymph node dissection for clinically negative regional SCC is not indicated unless the tumor extends to the parotid capsule or the lesion is large and contiguous with a draining nodal basin. Basal cell carcinoma rarely metastasizes and should not be managed with regional lymph node dissection.

ANSWER: c

REFERENCE: *Chapter 105—Cutaneous Neoplasms: Nonmelanoma Skin Tumors*

11. Which of the following statements is/are true concerning Mohs surgical management of skin cancer?

    a. The procedure involves precise anatomic delineation of the extent of tumor by means of histologic interpretation of frozen section
    b. Mohs surgery results in high cure rates for all skin cancers
    c. The technique is particularly important for tumors in areas where conservation of normal tissue is important, such as the face
    d. Mohs surgery is useful to patients at high risk of local recurrence

COMMENT: Mohs micrographic surgery is a technique most useful for the management of high-risk non-melanoma skin cancer. After removal of all gross tumor, the surgeon excises a thin layer of tissue approximately 2 to 3 mm wide at the deep and lateral margins. The tissue is immediately processed for frozen section to define the precise anatomic location of any residual tumor, which is reexcised until all margins are tumor free. A Mohs surgeon can microscopically track subclinical tumor extension. This method results in the highest cure rate with maximal preservation of normal tissue. In general, Mohs surgery should be considered for: (a) non-melanoma tumors associated with a high risk of recurrence after conventional treatment, and (b) tumors for which conservation of normal tissue is important. Tumors for which maximal conservation of tissue may be important include tumors of the eyelid, nose, ear, lip, digits, and genitalia and tumors among young patients. Mohs surgery does not result in higher cure rates over conventional techniques for small, low-risk lesions.

ANSWER: a, c, d

REFERENCE: *Chapter 105—Cutaneous Neoplasms: Nonmelanoma Skin Tumors*

CHAPTER 106

SARCOMAS OF BONE AND SOFT TISSUE

1. Which of the following statements is/are true concerning the epidemiologic characteristics of soft tissue sarcoma?

    a. A history of trauma is clearly associated with a predisposition to development of sarcoma
    b. The contrast agent Thorotrast has been associated with the development of hepatic angiosarcoma
    c. There is no association among humans between infection and the development of sarcoma
    d. A genetic predisposition is associated with retinoblastoma and some forms of neurofibrosarcoma

COMMENT: Most cases of sarcoma occur among patients who have no identifiable predisposing factors—genetic or environmental. Although a history of trauma often is recalled by patients with soft tissue sarcoma, traumatic injury does not seem to predispose to development of sarcoma. Radiation exposure is clearly linked to the development of sarcoma. The radioactive substance thorium dioxide (Thorotrast) was widely used as a contrast agent for radiologic procedures in the 1940s and 1950s. After a latency period of 18 to 36 years, hepatic angiosarcoma occurs with extremely high frequency among patients who have received Thorotrast. Certain chemicals that are not radioactive have been implicated as causing sarcoma. These include arsenic and vinyl chloride, both of which are associated with hepatic angiosarcoma. Infection with human immunodeficiency virus (HIV-1) is also associated with a marked increase in the incidence of an otherwise extraordinarily rare lesion, Kaposi's sarcoma. It is unclear, however, whether the predilection to development of these sarcomas is caused by a specific carcinogenic effect of the virus or to the underlying immunodeficiency caused by the HIV infection. Neurofibromatosis type I (von Recklinghausen's disease) is a condition with a genetic predisposition to development of sarcoma. An estimated 5% of patients with neurofibromatosis have sarcoma during their lifetime. Almost all these tumors are neurofibrosarcoma and generally arise from preexisting neurofibromas. A genetic predisposition to sarcoma also exists among patients with retinoblastoma.

ANSWER: b, d

REFERENCE: *Chapter 106—Sarcomas of Bone and Soft Tissue: Epidemiology*

2. Advances in molecular biology have provided tools for analyzing histologic type, prognosis, and the cause of sarcoma. Which of the following statements is/are true concerning the molecular biologic characteristics of bone and soft tissue sarcoma?

a. The RB1 gene is a recessive oncogene, or tumor suppressor gene, which requires both alleles to be inactivated before malignant transformation can occur
b. The RB1 gene is associated only with the development of retinoblastoma
c. Abnormalities in the p53 gene are associated with both the inherited Li-Fraumeni syndrome and sporadic sarcoma
d. The MDR1 (multidrug resistance) gene is found in greater numbers of untreated sarcomas than in most other tumor types

COMMENT: The finding of a linkage between familial retinoblastoma and sarcoma led toward research to find specific genetic changes responsible for the observed susceptibility to development of sarcoma. Retinoblastoma has been associated with a gene defect in the retinoblastoma gene (RB1) on the long arm of chromosome 13. RB1 is a recessive oncogene, or tumor suppressor gene, which means that both alleles must be inactivated before malignant transformation can occur. Patients with familial retinoblastoma inherit one inactivated RB1 gene. The RB1 gene appears to affect more than retinoblastoma development. RB1 also may play a role in the pathogenesis of certain types of nonfamilial soft tissue sarcoma.

Molecular biologic principles are again seen with the alterations in the p53 gene associated with the Li-Fraumeni syndrome. This familial cancer syndrome involves early-onset breast cancer, sarcoma, and a variety of other malignant tumors. Patients with Li-Fraumeni syndrome inherit a defective copy of the p53 gene, another essential growth regulatory gene. Abnormalities of the p53 gene also are common in sporadic cases of sarcoma. In one study, investigators found p53 abnormalities in approximately 60% of osteosarcomas and malignant histiocytomas as well as approximately 32% of other sarcomas. Another important genetic change in some sarcomas is the presence of the MDR1 (multidrug resistance) gene, which is present in greater numbers of untreated sarcomas than most other tumor types. The presence of this gene has been correlated in vitro with resistance to a number of cytotoxic drugs, many of which are routinely used in chemotherapy for sarcoma.

ANSWER: a, c, d

REFERENCE: *Chapter 106—Sarcomas of Bone and Soft Tissue: Molecular Biology*

3. Which of the following statements is/are true concerning biopsy of a soft tissue tumor?

   a. A 5-cm soft tissue mass on the extremity after minor local trauma can be safely observed
   b. The incision for biopsy of an extremity mass should be transverse to the long axis of the extremity
   c. Fine-needle aspiration cytologic examination has little role in the diagnosis of soft tissue sarcoma
   d. Core needle biopsy frequently causes hematoma and dissemination of tumor cells
   e. Core needle biopsy can be used for direct determination of the histologic type and grade of sarcoma in more than 90% of cases

COMMENT: Benign soft tissue tumors far outnumber their malignant counterparts. Because of this, prolonged delay before definitive treatment begins is common among patients with sarcoma. Patients rarely have persistent soft tissue masses from either chronic traumatic hematomas or pulled muscles. Only in the setting of clear local trauma should these diagnoses be entertained. If a soft tissue mass arises in a patient with no history of trauma or persists 6 weeks after local trauma, biopsy should be performed. Biopsy should be performed for almost all soft tissue masses larger than 5 cm and for any new, enlarging, or symptomatic lesions. Properly performed, timely surgical biopsy is the critical first step in the multimodality treatment approach. Improperly performed, it can markedly complicate the care of a patient with sarcoma and occasionally even eliminate treatment options. Excisional biopsy should be reserved for small soft tissue masses for which the likelihood of malignancy is low and for which complete excision would not jeopardize subsequent treatment in the event a sarcoma is found. For all other soft tissue masses, incisional biopsy is indicated. For lesions on the extremities, the incision should be oriented along the long axis of the extremity. Any biopsy site should be placed directly over the tumor, at the point where the lesion is closest to the surface, and there should be no raising of flaps or disturbance of tissue planes superficial to the tumor.

Fine-needle aspiration cytologic examination has a role in the diagnosis of some soft tissue lesions. Computed tomography (CT)–guided fine needle aspiration has proved helpful in the diagnosis of intraabdominal retroperitoneal tumors but is rarely needed for sarcoma of the extremities. Even experienced cytologists, however, often are unable to discern the grade and histologic type of sarcoma from an aspirate. Core needle biopsy, however, has been found to show both the histologic type and grade of sarcoma in more than 90% of cases. Fears that core needle biopsy would result in a large number of hematomas, resulting in dissemination of tumor cells, appear to be groundless.

ANSWER: e

REFERENCE: *Chapter 106—Sarcomas of Bone and Soft Tissue: Diagnosis and Staging of Soft-tissue Sarcomas*

4. Which of the following statements is/are true concerning the staging and prognostic importance of sarcoma of bone or soft tissue?

   a. The histologic grade of a tumor has little prognostic significance
   b. Tumor size is an important prognostic indicator for sarcoma
   c. More superficial tumors have a more favorable prognosis than do deeper tumors
   d. Once a tumor reaches 5 cm in diameter (T2) there is no worsening in prognosis associated with increased size

COMMENT: Because of the prognostic importance of histologic grade, the staging of the primary tumor is based on both clinical and histologic information. The usual TNM classification is modified according to a GTNM system in which the histologic grade of the tumor is considered. This staging classification is clinically useful because it separates patients into groups with clearly different prognoses. Next in prognostic importance to tumor grade is tumor size. The larger the primary sarcoma, the greater is the risk of metastatic disease and of death. In the GTNM system, T1 tumors are 5 cm in diameter or smaller, and T2 tumors are larger than 5 cm. Although the GTNM cutoff is 5 cm, tumors larger than 10 cm have an even worse prognosis. It is also recognized that superficial tumors (those entirely above the deep or muscular fascia of the body) have a more favorable prognosis.

ANSWER: b, c

REFERENCE: *Chapter 106—Sarcomas of Bone and Soft Tissue: Diagnosis and Staging of Soft-tissue Sarcomas*

5. Which of the following statements is/are true concerning a patient with soft tissue sarcoma of an extremity?

   a. Both CT and magnetic resonance imaging (MRI) should be performed to evaluate the lesion
   b. Angiography would be particularly useful in the evaluation of this lesion
   c. Chest CT should be performed for all patients
   d. Liver metastasis is common among such patients; therefore abdominal CT should be routinely performed
   e. Radionucleotide bone scans should be obtained routinely to find local invasion by tumor and metastatic disease

COMMENT: The initial evaluation of a patient with sarcoma of an extremity must provide information about the extent of the primary tumor. Computed tomography and MRI are the most important studies for assessing the extent of resectability of soft tissue sarcoma regardless of the site of origin. These studies allow definition of the primary tumor in relation to bone, muscle, neurovascular structures, and adjacent organs—critical information for planning of treatment. Both CT and MRI can provide this information. In most cases, either study is sufficient. The choice is based on availability, cost, and the experience of the radiologist. Each study has advantages and disadvantages, however, and these should be considered on a case-by-case basis. Plain radiographs and radionucleotide bone scans occasionally provide useful information regarding invasion of bone by tumor, but these studies usually do not play an important role in the evaluation for primary soft tissue sarcoma. Sarcoma has a characteristic angiographic appearance—prominent neovascularity and displacement of normal vessels. Angiography, however, rarely is necessary for extremity lesions, although it may be more important in retroperitoneal tumors.

For all patients with newly diagnosed soft tissue sarcoma, a chest radiograph and chest CT are appropriate to search for pulmonary metastases. For intraabdominal or retroperitoneal tumors, CT that includes the liver should be added. Distant metastatic disease is present in as many as 25% of patients with soft tissue sarcoma at presentation. By far the most common site of metastasis is the lung. Among patients with sarcoma who have metastatic lesions, the lungs are involved more than 75% of the time. Liver involvement is rare except in cases of intraabdominal and retroperitoneal sarcoma, in which it represents the second most common site of distant spread. Some patients have bone or central nervous system metastasis; however, these lesions are uncommon among patients who do not already have lung metastasis. Therefore radionucleotide bone scans and CT or MRI of the head are not indicated in the absence of symptoms of metastatic involvement.

ANSWER: c

REFERENCE: *Chapter 106—Sarcomas of Bone and Soft Tissue: Diagnosis and Staging of Soft-tissue Sarcomas*

6. Which of the following statements is/are true concerning treatment of a patient with soft tissue sarcoma of an extremity?

  a. Radical amputation is no longer considered an option for most patients with sarcoma of an extremity
  b. Wide local excision of soft tissue sarcoma usually includes resection of the entire muscle compartment
  c. Postoperative radiation therapy after wide surgical excision should involve irradiation of the entire circumference of the extremity
  d. Preoperative radiation therapy is of primary value in the management of tumors larger than 10 cm in diameter
  e. The use of a multiagent chemotherapy regimen that includes doxorubicin hydrochloride can improve disease-free survival after high-grade sarcoma of an extremity

COMMENT: The most common site of origin of sarcoma is the lower extremity. Radical amputation of at least one joint space above the most proximal end of the tumor once was advocated for treatment of most patients. With the advent of multimodality approaches, limb-sparing resection can be performed for 90% of patients. The local recurrence rate has been reported to be 10% or less. Radical amputation is reserved for patients who are not suitable candidates for limb-sparing approaches, usually because of bony invasion or large tumor size. Wide local excision of sarcoma of an extremity involves gross total removal of the tumor with a wide margin of normal tissue. No attempt is made to resect an entire muscle compartment; rather, a margin of 3 to 5 cm of normal tissue is obtained proximally and distally. On the lateral and deep margins, at least one grossly uninvolved fascial plane is resected en bloc with the tumor whenever possible.

Most patients undergoing surgical excision receive additional therapy to improve the likelihood of local control. This additional therapy usually includes radiation. Postoperative radiation therapy after wide surgical excision provides excellent local control of primary sarcoma of the extremities up to 10 cm in size. Results of a randomized trial of amputation versus wide local excision and radiation therapy validated the concept of limb-sparing surgery combined with postoperative radiation therapy. In general, a dose of 6,000 cGy or greater is needed to ensure local control. At this dose, the entire circumference of the extremity must not be irradiated, or massive lymphedema will result. Experience with postoperative radiation therapy for tumors of the extremity larger than 10 cm in diameter has shown a high incidence of local failure. Therefore for tumors larger than 10 cm or for fixed sarcoma of an extremity, limb-sparing therapy necessitates preoperative management of the tumor in most cases. Radiation alone or with chemotherapy is a reasonable preoperative approach for these patients. A prospective, randomized trial of multiagent therapy including doxorubicin after surgery has shown improved disease-free survival among patients with high-grade sarcoma of an extremity (but not sarcoma on the trunk or retroperitoneal sarcoma). The toxicity of such regimens can be substantial.

ANSWER: a, d, e

REFERENCE: *Chapter 106—Sarcomas of Bone and Soft Tissue: Management of Extremity Soft-tissue Sarcomas*

7. Which of the following statements is/are true concerning retroperitoneal sarcoma?

a. The prognosis for retroperitoneal sarcoma compares favorably with that of sarcoma of the extremities
b. Wide excision of all gross tumor can be achieved for most patients and seldom requires resection of adjacent organs
c. Excellent local control rates with postoperative radiation for retroperitoneal sarcoma usually can be obtained
d. Postoperative adjuvant chemotherapy shows no benefit for patients with retroperitoneal sarcoma

COMMENT: Retroperitoneal sarcoma accounts for approximately 15% of all sarcomas and approximately 55% of all retroperitoneal tumors. Advances in multimodality therapy for sarcoma of the extremities have not been matched by similar progress in the management of retroperitoneal tumors. Most patients with retroperitoneal sarcomas die of the disease, frequently with local recurrent tumor as the main or sole site of failure. Unlike the situation with sarcoma of the extremities, even patients with low-grade retroperitoneal sarcoma usually die of progressive tumor. The poor outcome of retroperitoneal sarcoma is related in part to inability to diagnose these tumors at an early stage.

The wide margins of resection routinely obtained for sarcoma of the extremities are difficult to achieve in the retroperitoneum. Complete excision of all gross tumor is essential for long-term disease-free survival, but this is achievable in only 50% of cases. To remove all gross tumor, concomitant resection of adjacent organs is required more than 75% of the time. Partial excision or debulking procedures do not improve survival over the results obtained with biopsy alone. Irradiation of macroscopic residual tumor in the retroperitoneum has been almost uniformly unsuccessful, emphasizing the importance of complete surgical resection. Because of the difficulty achieving wide resection margins, however, radiation therapy frequently is used as a postoperative adjuvant. The excellent local rates obtained with postoperative radiation therapy for lesions of the extremities have not been matched in the retroperitoneum. Several trials of postoperative adjuvant chemotherapy have not shown benefit for patients with retroperitoneal sarcoma.

ANSWER: d

REFERENCE: Chapter 106—Sarcomas of Bone and Soft Tissue: Management of Retroperitoneal Sarcomas

8. A 28-year-old woman has a painless mass in a cesarean section scar 18 months after delivery. Which of the following statements is/are true concerning diagnosis and management in this case?

a. The patient is likely to die of metastatic disease
b. Resection of the mass with a histologically negative margin usually is satisfactory treatment
c. Postoperative radiation therapy can be considered in the care of this patient if the resected specimen reveals close approximation between the tumor and the margin
d. Treatment with tamoxifen and sulindac is preferable to conventional chemotherapy in the care of patients with advanced forms of this tumor

COMMENT: Desmoid tumors are more common among women than among men and frequently manifest in the vicinity of a cesarean section scar within 1 to 2 years of delivery. These facts, combined with isolated reports of spontaneous regression of desmoid tumors at menopause and the finding of estrogen receptors on some tumors, suggest a hormonal component to their development. Because of these findings, hormonal therapy with a variety of agents, most notably tamoxifen, has been used with occasional success. Therapy with the nonsteroidal antiinflammatory drug sulindac alone or in combination with tamoxifen has led to objective regression in as many as 50% of cases of familial polyposis-associated desmoid tumors. Sporadic desmoid tumors not associated with familial polyposis also sometimes respond to this therapy. The surgical approach to resection of sporadic desmoid tumors is similar to that used for low-grade soft tissue sarcoma—resection with a histologically negative margin if possible but without sacrifice of major neurovascular structures or adjacent organs unless absolutely necessary. If pathologic analysis of the resected specimen shows close approximation between the tumor and the surgical margin, either reexcision or postoperative radiation therapy is used. Chemotherapy is a last resort when all other therapies have failed and the patient has severe symptoms or is in danger of dying because of compression of vital structures by the tumor. Unresectable or recurrent desmoid tumors, as well as those associated with familial polyposis, are managed first with a combination of tamoxifen and sulindac. Death due to desmoid tumors are infrequent but can occur owing to local recurrence in a critical area such as the neck. Desmoid tumors almost never metastasize, even after numerous local recurrences.

ANSWER: b, c, d

REFERENCE: Chapter 106—Sarcomas of Bone and Soft Tissue: Diagnosis and Management of Desmoid Tumors

9. A 14-year-old girl has a painful mass on her lower thigh just above the knee. Which of the following statements is/are true concerning diagnosis and management in this case?

a. A plain radiograph of the affected bone shows destruction of bone with new bone formation and periosteal reaction
b. Computed tomography is the most important modality in evaluation of the tumor
c. The preferable technique of biopsy is full-thickness biopsy of the bony tumor itself
d. Preoperative (neoadjuvant therapy) should be considered part of standard treatment
e. The use of preoperative neoadjuvant chemotherapy has replaced postoperative adjuvant chemotherapy in the care of most patients

COMMENT: Osteosarcoma is by far the most common primary malignant tumor of bone. Osteosarcoma occurs most commonly around the knee, in either the distal femur or the proximal tibia, but it can occur in any bone. Most cases of osteosarcoma occur among children and adolescents; approximately 80% of patients are younger than 20 years. A painful mass is the most common symptom of osteosarcoma of the extremities. Plain radiography of the affected bone is the first step in evaluating for suspected osteosarcoma. High-grade osteosarcoma leads to rapid destruction of bone with new bone formation and periosteal reaction. These changes manifest radiographically as an extensive, poorly defined destructive lesion, often with an extraosseous component. Computed tomography is the most important modality in the evaluation of sarcoma of the bone. It is excellent for assessing the degree of bony destruction, the extent of soft tissue involvement, and the relation of the tumor to adjacent neurovascular structures.

Radiologic evaluation should be completed before biopsy. The biopsy should be carefully planned not to jeopardize subsequent efforts at limb sparing. If an adequate amount of tissue can be obtained by means of sampling the extraosseous component, this is preferable to biopsy of the bone itself. If the cortex of bone is entered, a plug of methyl methacrylate can be used to seal the bone and prevent hemorrhage or tumor spillage.

Unlike therapy for soft tissue sarcoma, preoperative (neoadjuvant) chemotherapy is sufficiently well established to be considered standard management of osteosarcoma. Osteosarcomas of an extremity can be managed surgically by means of radical amputation or en bloc resection with limb sparing. Limb-sparing approaches can be considered for most patients with sarcoma of an extremity and no evidence of neurovascular involvement. Adjuvant chemotherapy has been proven to increase the survival rate after amputation or limb-sparing surgery among patients with osteosarcoma. Although most protocols incorporate preoperative chemotherapy, this does not replace postoperative treatment but can influence the duration and type of therapy given.

ANSWER: a, b, d

REFERENCE: *Chapter 106—Sarcomas of Bone and Soft Tissue: Diagnosis and Management of Primary Bone Sarcomas*

10. Which of the following statements is/are true concerning the management of recurrent and metastatic sarcoma?

    a. There is little role for postoperative follow-up care after management of the primary sarcoma

    b. Local and regional failure is most common with sarcoma of an extremity

    c. Aggressive resection of solitary or multiple metastatic lesions of the lung can be associated with cure in the care of as many as one third of patients

    d. All patients with local recurrence of sarcoma of an extremity need radical amputation

COMMENT: Many adult and pediatric patients with locally recurrent or even metastatic sarcoma can be cured with aggressive surgery, often combined with radiation therapy and chemotherapy. For this reason, all patients with sarcoma should be observed carefully for recurrence of the disease. Low-grade sarcoma can recur as long as 20 years after the original resection, so follow-up evaluation must be maintained long term. Despite aggressive multimodality therapy, local recurrence is a major cause of treatment failure among patients with sarcoma.

The risk of local recurrence after surgical treatment of soft tissue sarcoma varies according to a number of factors. The most important of these is site of origin of the tumor. Lesions of the head and neck, trunk, and retroperitoneum are associated with a higher risk of local recurrence than are lesions of the extremity. Local and regional sites have been found to be the first sites of recurrence after definitive resection in 50% of cases of sarcoma of the head, neck, and trunk and in 75% of cases of retroperitoneal tumor, compared with 15% of lesions of the extremities. Limb-sparing approaches can control and even cure local recurrence in the absence of distal metastasis. For patients treated with surgery alone who have local failures of therapy, multimodality therapy with repeat resection, radiation therapy, and sometimes chemotherapy is associated with survival rates close to those of previously untreated patients. Patients with recurrence after surgery and radiation are more likely to need radical amputation to control recurrence in an extremity but may still be candidates for salvage surgery.

The lungs are the most frequent site of distant spread of sarcoma and are often the only site of metastasis. Aggressive resection of solitary or multiple metastatic lesions of the lung is associated with cure in approximately 25% to 35% of cases of soft tissue and osteogenic sarcoma. Patients with unresectable pulmonary metastatic lesions or with extrapulmonary metastasis usually are treated with cytotoxic chemotherapy.

ANSWER: c

REFERENCE: *Chapter 106—Sarcomas of Bone and Soft Tissue: Management of Recurrent and Metastatic Sarcomas*

CHAPTER 107

PLASTIC AND RECONSTRUCTIVE SURGERY

1. The deleterious effects of aging are produced through numerous processes. Which of the following statements is/are true concerning skin changes with advancing age?
   a. Aging affects all cells equally
   b. Chronologic aging is the most important factor affecting these skin changes
   c. Ultraviolet radiation is the major offending agent in sunlight
   d. Sun exposure can cause vascular changes in the skin

COMMENT: The major events affecting the aging of skin occur in cells that are genetically directed to retard their own proliferation. Once proliferation has ceased, events within the cell induce accumulation of waste product pigments, an increase in the proportion of inactive enzymes, and the loss of important genes. The skin changes of advancing age result from the generalized aging process as well as the effect of sun exposure. Of the two, sun exposure appears more detrimental than chronologic aging alone. Ultraviolet radiation is the main offending agent in sunlight. It appears to be responsible for the observed skin changes of aging. In addition, sunlight can induce various benign, premalignant, and malignant neoplasms. Among its effects, sun exposure results in microvascular changes such as dilatation and tortuous arteries and veins.

ANSWER: c, d

REFERENCE: *Chapter 107—Plastic and Reconstructive Surgery: Biology of Aging Skin*

2. Blepharoplasty can remove excess skin and fat of the upper and lower eyelids and eliminate wrinkling. Which of the following statements is/are true concerning this procedure?
   a. The procedure can be performed with local or general anesthesia
   b. Lower lid ectropion is a complication of over-aggressive skin excision
   c. Lower lid ectropion necessitates reoperation
   d. Preliminary postoperative results can be apparent within a few weeks of the procedure

COMMENT: Patients seeking blepharoplasty are evaluated preoperatively for visual acuity, ptosis of the upper lids, and dry eye. Careful examination of the lower eyelids is performed to assess the extent of lower lid laxity. If considerable laxity exists and is unappreciated, ectropion of one or both lids can occur postoperatively. Overaggressive skin excision can result in lower lid ectropion. If lower eyelid ectropion does occur, it is managed by means of massage and taping. In rare instances, reoperation and placement of a skin graft are needed to correct the ectropion. Blepharoplasty can be performed with local or general anesthesia. Preliminary postoperative results are apparent approximately 3 weeks after the operation, when most of the swelling and discoloration have resolved.

ANSWER: a, b, d

REFERENCE: *Chapter 107—Plastic and Reconstructive Surgery: Regional Operative Procedures*

3. Which of the following statements is/are true concerning rhytidectomy, or face lift?

 a. A history of smoking or hypertension can adversely affect results
 b. The procedure must be performed with general anesthesia
 c. The postoperative results can be assessed within 1 month of the procedure
 d. Complications of the procedure include facial nerve injury

COMMENT: Age, gravity, and sun exposure combine to change facial appearance over time. Rhytidectomy can be sought by patients who seek a more youthful appearance to improve self image and compete successfully in business and social arenas. Preoperatively, the surgeon questions each patient regarding factors that may affect the outcome of surgery. Smokers are at increased risk of skin necrosis after rhytidectomy. A patient with hypertension is more likely to have postoperative hematoma. Rhytidectomy can be performed with local or general anesthesia. Bruising that occurs as a result of the surgical procedure usually resolves within 3 weeks. Much of the facial swelling is diminished by that time; however, gradual reduction in swelling and relaxation of the tightened skin occurs for several more months. In general, a stable postoperative result is achieved within 6 months of the procedure. Complications of rhytidectomy include bleeding and hematoma. Surgical wound infection is rare. Permanent injury to the facial nerve can occur, although the incidence appears to be less than 2% among patients undergoing their first operation.

ANSWER: a, d

REFERENCE: *Chapter 107—Plastic and Reconstructive Surgery: Regional Operative Procedures*

4. Which of the following statements is/are true concerning rhinoplasty?

 a. The procedure can be performed with local or general anesthesia
 b. Rhinoplasty is performed only for aesthetic purposes
 c. Either intranasal or external incisions can be used
 d. The final result usually is apparent with resolution of the swelling within 3 weeks of the operation

COMMENT: Rhinoplasty is a surgical procedure whereby the contour of the external nose is changed. The procedure can be performed with local or general anesthesia. Hemostasis is facilitated by the use of intranasal vasoconstrictors and epinephrine-containing anesthetic solutions injected into the nose. Access to the bones and cartilage composing the nasal dorsum can be obtained through an intranasal or an external incision.

Aesthetic rhinoplasty is directed at correction of deformities such as dorsal hump, refinement of the nasal tip, or correction of a drooping nasal tip. Among patients with obstructed breathing in association with an external deformity, a simultaneous procedure can be performed on the nasal septum to improve airflow. Much of the swelling resolves within 3 weeks of the operation. It takes several months, however, for the final result to declare itself. Because of persistent nasal swelling, the results of rhinoplasty may not be fully appreciated until 1 year after the procedure.

ANSWER: a, c

REFERENCE: *Chapter 107—Plastic and Reconstructive Surgery: Regional Operative Procedures*

5. The use of prostheses for breast augmentation has received tremendous discussion in both the medical literature and the general press. Which of the following statements is/are true concerning the risks of prosthetic breast implants?

   a. Strong evidence exists that the silicone implants can be carcinogenic
   b. The presence of an implant can complicate mammography and early detection of breast cancer
   c. Current U.S. Food and Drug Administration (FDA) recommendations have restricted the use of silicone gel implants because of the possible association with autoimmune disease
   d. Uncomfortable breast hardness can result from scar capsular contraction

COMMENT: Breast augmentation with a prosthesis can improve breast contour. The prosthesis is not totally inert, and each patient must be informed regarding the effects of its placement. Most implants placed since 1991 have been filled with saline solution. Before then, silicone gel-filled implants were in common use. Concerns were raised regarding the possible association between silicone gel and autoimmune disease, resulting in FDA recommendations for marked restriction in the use of this material in breast implants. The shell of most current implants is still composed of silicone rubber. However, evidence suggests that implants are neither carcinogenic nor likely to induce systemic illness. The implants do cause the body to form a scar capsule. In some patients, this capsule can contract and result in uncomfortable breast hardness or visual distortion of breast contour. The presence of an implant also can complicate mammography, and the patient should be aware of this fact.

ANSWER: b, c, d

REFERENCE: *Chapter 107—Plastic and Reconstructive Surgery: Regional Operative Procedures; Augmentation Mammoplasty*

6. Breast implants cause the body to form a scar capsule, which in some patients can contract. Which of the following statements can be associated with scar contracture?

   a. A smooth surface of the silicone shell is associated with a lower rate of capsular contraction
   b. Breast massage in the early postoperative period may reduce the incidence of capsular contracture
   c. Capsular contracture usually occurs after the first year after insertion of a breast implant
   d. If a breast implant is removed because of capsular contracture, reinsertion is contraindicated

COMMENT: The scar capsule that forms after insertion of a breast prosthesis can contract and cause uncomfortable breast hardness or a visual distortion. Implants vary in structure and content. The shell of most implants is composed of silicone rubber. This shell can be smooth or textured. The textured-surface implant seems to be associated with a lower rate of capsular contraction and breast firmness. Breast massage should be instituted during the first week postoperatively. Massage is believed to reduce the incidence of capsular contracture. If capsular contracture does occur, it usually is apparent within the first 6 months. Patients who request therapy for capsular contracture often undergo removal of the implant and repositioning of the existing implant or insertion of an implant with a different composition.

ANSWER: b

REFERENCE: *Chapter 107—Plastic and Reconstructive Surgery: Regional Operative Procedures; Augmentation Mammoplasty*

7. Which of the following statements is/are true concerning mastopexy and reduction mammoplasty?

   a. Mastopexy is used to manage isolated skin excess. It does reduce the overall size of the breast

   b. In mastopexy but not breast reduction, nipple viability can be expected

   c. Reduction mammoplasty is best performed with general anesthesia

   d. Breast-feeding usually is not possible after breast reduction

COMMENT: Obesity, pregnancy, and aging contribute to drooping of the breasts that is both functionally impairing and aesthetically displeasing. The deformity can be caused solely by an excess of skin. Isolated skin excess is managed by means of mastopexy. When other elements of breast enlargement are present, such as nipple enlargement, displacement of the nipple inferiorly on the breast, and an excess of breast tissue and fat, reduction mammoplasty is indicated. Mastopexy and breast reduction both decrease the size of the breast. Both operations also sustain nipple viability through maintenance of underlying or adjacent vascular tissue. The procedures usually are performed with general anesthesia. Complications include hematoma, infection, and wound breakdown. Breast-feeding may or may not be possible after breast reduction.

ANSWER: c

REFERENCE: *Chapter 107—Plastic and Reconstructive Surgery: Regional Operative Procedures; Mastopexy and Reduction Mammoplasty*

8. Which of the following statements is/are true concerning abdominoplasty?

   a. The procedure usually involves a diamond-shaped excision

   b. For most patients, a new umbilicus must be constructed

   c. Liposuction can be added to the procedure to further refine the abdominal contour

   d. The procedure can frequently be performed as an outpatient operation with the patient immediately returning to normal activity

COMMENT: Abdominoplasty involves a diamond-shaped excision. However, the umbilicus is circumscribed and left attached to the abdominal wall. The excess skin and fat are removed as a single unit with the remaining abdominal skin separate from the underlying abdominal wall cephalad to facilitate wound closure. The abdominal wall musculature can be tightened and further refined and the abdominal contour can be achieved by means of liposuction of the subcutaneous fatty layers at the margin of the flaps and along the midline. The patient is flexed at the waist, and wound closure is begun. An opening is made in the skin to allow insertion of the umbilicus. Postoperatively it is necessary for the patient to remain in a flexed position. Prophylaxis against venous thrombosis and pulmonary embolism is maintained in the postoperative period. Over a 1- to 2-week period, the skin stretches, and the patient can assume the erect position.

ANSWER: a, c

REFERENCE: *Chapter 107—Plastic and Reconstructive Surgery: Regional Operative Procedures; Abdominoplasty*

9. Suction-assisted lipectomy (liposuction) is the technique that allows removal of localized fat deposits from parts of the body. Which of the following statements is/are true concerning liposuction?

   a. Age is not a factor in predicting success after liposuction
   b. In large-volume procedures, blood transfusion may be necessary
   c. Several weeks or months may be required to assess the final appearance
   d. Rippling or irregularities of the overlying skin can result in a less than desirable appearance

COMMENT: The ideal patient for liposuction is a young person with good skin tone who has localized fat deposits. Skin tone is important because the skin must contract and assume an improved contour once the underlying fat is removed. Rippling and irregularities of the overlying skin can occur if skin laxity was present preoperatively or if adequate shrinkage of skin does not take place. Several weeks or months may be required to assess the final appearance of liposuction. After 1,500 to 1,800 mL of tissue, fluid, and blood are removed, blood transfusion usually is necessary.

ANSWER: b, c, d

REFERENCE: *Chapter 107—Plastic and Reconstructive Surgery: Regional Operative Procedures; Liposuction*

10. Tissue flaps can be classified according to vascular supply. Which of the following anatomic variations can serve as the vascular supply for a tissue flap?

    a. Direct cutaneous arteries
    b. Septal perforators
    c. Indirect vascularization through arterioles from subadjacent muscles
    d. None of the above

COMMENT: Skin territories can be fed by direct cutaneous arteries, by septal perforators, or indirectly through arterioles from subadjacent muscles. An example of a direct cutaneous system is the deltopectoral flap, fed by the second, third, or fourth intercostal perforator from the internal mammary artery. A musculocutaneous flap has skin perforators from the underlying muscle, which is supplied by a major vascular pedicle. An example of this is the latissimus dorsi flap, in which the skin is supplied by perforators from the latissimus dorsi muscle, which is supplied by the thoracodorsal artery and vena comitans. A fasciocutaneous flap has skin supplied by perforators that pass to the surface along fascial septa and between adjacent muscle bellies and arborize at the level of the deep fascia to form a plexus from which branches supply subcutaneous tissues and dermis.

ANSWER: a, b, c

REFERENCE: *Chapter 107—Plastic and Reconstructive Surgery: Principles of the Flap*

11. Which of the following statements is/are true concerning the excursion of tissue flaps?

  a. With a transposition flap, the resulting defect is covered with a skin graft or adjacent tissue rearrangement
  b. An advancement flap is lifted on its blood supply and advanced into an adjacent defect.
  c. Island pedicle flaps can be transferred over longer distances
  d. A free flap involves amputation of the flap from its origin and transplantation to another site

COMMENT: Flaps can be described not only on the basis of their blood supply but also on the basis of their excursion. A transposition flap is composed of tissue moved to an adjacent soft tissue defect, and the resulting defect is covered with either skin graft or rearrangement of adjacent tissue. An advancement flap is lifted on its blood supply and advanced into an adjacent defect. An example is the V/Y flap used for ischial pressure sores. Island pedicle flaps imply that a block of tissue is raised on an artery and vena comitans and transposed over longer distances. The radial forearm flap for hand coverage is an example of this flap. A free tissue transplant, or free flap, is a flap isolated on the arterial and vena comitans to that block of tissue. It is amputated from its blood supply and transplanted with microsurgical techniques from one site to another.

ANSWER: a, b, c, d

REFERENCE: *Chapter 107—Plastic and Reconstructive Surgery: Principles of the Flap*

12. Which of the following statements is/are true concerning the progression of wound closure techniques?

  a. Delayed primary closure occurs when a wound is closed 24 to 48 hours after the original incision
  b. Wound closure by secondary intention avoids trapping of bacteria by means of wound contraction
  c. No particular care is necessary in preparation of the bed before skin grafting
  d. Free flaps involve transfer of only muscle and skin

COMMENT: Most wounds can be closed by means of primary closure. In instances of infection or contamination, delayed primary closure can be considered. With this technique, the patient is returned to the operating room 24 to 48 hours after the original operation, and the wound is closed. Healing by secondary intention allows small open areas or wounds to heal spontaneously. This technique avoids trapping of bacteria as wound contraction and epithelialization take place. In instances of larger defects, skin grafting can be performed, provided the bed is appropriate to receive a graft. Clean granulation and good vascular inflow are necessary for inosculation of the graft. If skin grafting is not satisfactory or when a cavity defect exists, a local rotation flap, such as a muscle flap or fasciocutaneous flap, can be considered for closure. The highest rung on the reconstructive ladder, and one used quite frequently by reconstructive plastic surgeons, is free tissue transfer. Any tissue can be transplanted, including bowel, muscle, skin, bone, or fascia, or any combination of these. These composite flaps restore form and provide functional restoration.

ANSWER: a, b

REFERENCE: *Chapter 107—Plastic and Reconstructive Surgery: Reconstructive Ladder*

13. Which of the following statements is/are true concerning reconstruction after resection for malignant disease of the head and neck?

  a. Previous radiation has no effect on reconstruction after resection of a head and neck tumor.
  b. Frozen section diagnosis should be obtained to ensure negative margins before reconstruction
  c. Free jejunal flaps can serve as a conduit from the oropharynx to the esophagus
  d. Recipient vessels for head and neck reconstruction are the external carotid, facial, and thyroid arteries
  e. Tracheostomy is seldom necessary after intraoral or mandibular reconstruction

COMMENT: Microsurgical reconstruction has become the standard for extirpation of tumors of the head and neck. Patients with head and neck cancer often have a history of smoking and may have undergone radiation therapy. Resection of this area should be reconstructed with vascularized tissue imported from outside the region. The pectoralis major flap, the trapezius flap, and the latissimus dorsi island pedicle flap can be used for lower neck reconstruction. For all patients with a head and neck cancer, negative surgical margins should be obtained before reconstruction. This usually is done by means of frozen section, or the wound can be packed or dressed for 24 to 48 hours until the final pathology report becomes available. In instances of hypopharyngeal, pharyngeal, or laryngeal resection, free jejunum or radial forearm flaps can provide a conduit from the oropharynx to the esophagus. Recipient vessels for head and neck reconstruction include the external carotid, facial, and thyroid arteries. These should be preserved whenever possible during resection. Prophylactic tracheostomy should be considered, particularly in instances of mandibular and intraoral reconstruction, because of often massive swelling that occurs after these procedures.

ANSWER: b, c, d

REFERENCE: *Chapter 107—Plastic and Reconstructive Surgery: Head and Neck*

14. Congenital anomalies managed by pediatric plastic and reconstructive surgeons include:

  a. Cleft lip
  b. Craniofacial deformities of Apert's syndrome
  c. Syndactyly
  d. Radial club hand

COMMENT: Pediatric plastic surgery is a subspecialty of plastic surgery. Craniofacial and other congenital defects, such as cleft lip and palate, fall under the domain of the plastic surgeons working with specialists in otolaryngology, audiology, orthodontics, and speech pathology. In cases of cleft lip and cleft palate, failure of fusion of mesodermal segments during gestation result in a facial cleft involving the palate, the lip, or both. The lip usually is repaired first. Palate repair is next, and correction of velopharyngeal incompetence, alveolar bone grafting for dental arch formation, and among adolescents, nasal reconstruction of the cleft lip (rhinoplasty) are performed later. Craniofacial deformities, such as those of Crouzon's or Apert's syndrome, are best managed by a craniofacial surgeon. These children may or may not have normal intelligence and may have other congenital problems. Congenital anomalies of the hand include syndactyly, polydactyly, and radial club hand. The trend is to release syndactyly before the first year of age, if possible, to take advantage of the properties of fetal wound healing that allow wounds to heal with less scarring.

ANSWER: a, b, d

REFERENCE: *Chapter 107—Plastic and Reconstructive Surgery: Pediatric Plastic Surgery*

15. Which of the following statements is/are true concerning breast reconstruction?

    a. The conventional transverse rectus abdominis muscle (TRAM) flap is based on the superior epigastric artery

    b. A free TRAM flap is based on the superior epigastric artery

    c. A superior gluteal or lateral thigh flap can be used as an alternative to a TRAM flap

    d. Construction of a nipple-areolar complex should be deferred until several months after completion of the TRAM flap

COMMENT: The TRAM flap provides skin and subcutaneous tissue as well as muscle for postmastectomy reconstruction if expanders and saline-filled implants are not desired. Experience with free tissue transfer after mastectomy has been excellent. Free flaps such as the TRAM flap, superior gluteal flap, or lateral thigh flap can be used to provide tissue for breast construction when a conventional TRAM flap cannot be performed. The conventional TRAM flap is based on the superior epigastric artery. The free TRAM flap is based on the deep inferior epigastric artery, which usually is anastomosed to the axillary artery or a branch of the thoracodorsal artery. Breast reconstruction is completed with a tattoo or surgical construction of a nipple-areolar complex. This can be done at the same time as the TRAM flap. Contralateral breast augmentation or reduction may be needed depending on the nature of the breast cancer and the patient's desires.

ANSWER: a, c

REFERENCE: *Chapter 107—Plastic and Reconstructive Surgery: Trunk/Chest*

16. Reconstructive microsurgery has been used to treat patients with lymphedema of both the upper and the lower extremities. Which of following statements is/are true concerning management of this condition?

    a. Lymphangiography should be performed pre-operatively in all cases

    b. Microlymphaticovenous anastomosis results in improvement for most patients

    c. Substantial volume changes in the extremity occur among most patients

    d. Additional surgical procedures to reduce extremity volume can be used as an adjunct to microlymphaticovenous anastomosis

COMMENT: Selected patients with lymphedema can be treated with microscopic venolymphatic bypass. In a series of more than 100 patients with lymphedema treated with microlymphaticovenous anastomosis, objective assessment of volume and circumferential extremity measurement were performed. Lymphangiography was used initially but discontinued because it caused sclerosis of the lymphatic drainage system. Most patients (73%) had improvement after anastomosis. However, volume changes occurred among only 42% of patients. Reduction procedures can be performed as an adjunct for these patients. Patients who underwent earlier operations had better results than patients treated late in the disease.

ANSWER: b, d

REFERENCE: *Chapter 107—Plastic and Reconstructive Surgery: Venous Lymphatic Insufficiency*